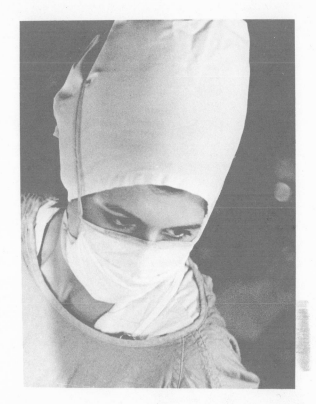

Mosby's Comprehensive Review of Nursing

EIGHTH EDITION

The C.V. Mosby Company

SAINT LOUIS 1973

EIGHTH EDITION

Previous editions copyrighted 1949, 1951, 1955,
1958, 1961, 1965, 1969

Distributed in Great Britain by Henry Kimpton,
London

Library of Congress Cataloging in Publication Data

Mosby (C. V.) Company.
  Mosby's comprehensive review of nursing.

  (Mosby's comprehensive review series)
  Includes bibliographies.
  1. Nurses and nursing—Examinations, questions,
etc. 2. Nurses and nursing—Outlines, syllabi, etc.
I. Title. [DNLM: 1. Nursing—Outlines. WY 100
M894c 1973]
RT55.M6   1973   610.73'076   73-1291
ISBN 0-8016-3528-4

CB/CB/B 9 8 7 6 5 4 3 2

EDITORIAL PANEL

PREFACE

TO EIGHTH EDITION

The preparation of the eighth edition of *Mosby's Comprehensive Review of Nursing* continues to reflect the most current information concerning nursing. Several changes have been made in organization and several chapters have been redone. Communicable diseases and orthopedics have been removed as separate discussions, and pertinent information from these content areas has been placed primarily with medical-surgical nursing and pediatric nursing. Principles of restorative care has been replaced with a new chapter on rehabilitation nursing. Fundamentals of nursing has been completely revised. All review questions in nutrition and almost all review questions in pharmacology have been integrated in the clinical nursing content areas. Material throughout the book has been brought up to date.

The International Business Machines Corporation has graciously given permission for the continued use of their answer sheet. Familiarity with this type of answer sheet, which is used extensively by many schools, colleges, and examining boards, should be valuable to all nurses.

The contributors hope that the changes made will increase the value of the book to the student or graduate nurse in reviewing subject matter and in preparing for examinations.

Editorial panel

PREFACE
TO FIRST EDITION

This book is intended to be a study outline for those nurses, student and graduate, who wish a clear, authoritative summary of the subjects taught in the basic course in nursing. Subject matter has been organized and references given so that students or graduates may be helped in reviewing any of these subjects. Material has been selected and presented so that students may get help in integrating basic science courses and nursing arts with clinical nursing subjects.

Graduate nurses may find this book helpful in preparing for special examinations.

It may also be valuable to graduates who wish to get a quick review of any subject, particularly if they are taking refresher, supplementary, or postgraduate courses in nursing.

Each member of the editorial panel was selected because of her experience as a teacher in her special fields as well as because of her knowledge in the subjects. No attempt has been made to have each subject fit into any set pattern. Each contributor has been given freedom to present the subject matter as, from her experience, she has found it to be most effective.

CONTENTS

GENERAL INTRODUCTION

The licensing examination

THE LICENSING EXAMINATION

Comprehensive guide for the understanding of examination procedures including maintenance of security and the administration of the State Board Test Pool Examinations, ANA publication (Code B-31), 1964.*

Gibbs, G. E.: Will continuing education be required for license renewal? American Journal of Nursing 71:2175, Nov., 1971.

Let's examine (a series of articles in Nursing Outlook):

Safety and effectiveness of practice, 10:679, Oct., 1962.

Preparing to take State Boards, 10:807, Dec., 1962.

Why one licensure examination? 11:749, Oct., 1963.

The State Board Test Pool, 11:811, Nov., 1963.

The origin of the State Board Test Pool Examination service, 12:55, July, 1964.

The history of plans for licensure tests in professional nursing, 12:55, Aug., 1964.

Policies of N.L.N. test services, 12:56, Sept., 1964.

Separate licensure examinations for diploma and degree program graduates, 13:7, July, 1965.

Who constructs those tests? 18:66, Feb., 1970.

Licensure tests—an N. L. N. service, Nursing Outlook 10:609, Sept., 1962.

Selden, W. K.: Licensing boards are archaic, American Journal of Nursing 70:124, Jan., 1970.

FUNCTION OF LICENSURE

Licensure in nursing, as in any of the other professions, is a state function under the police powers granted by the Constitution of the United States. Those police powers require the states to protect the health and the welfare of their citizens. As part of the fulfillment of this function, licensure is widely used as a means of guaranteeing a safe level of practice in many occupations, including the professions. A common portal of entry to a profession is the licensing examination.

In the United States, the law in all but 3 of the 54 states and territories which include the District of Columbia and the Virgin Islands, makes it mandatory for an individual engaged in the practice of registered nursing to be licensed; similar laws are being sought in the remaining states, in which a graduate nurse now can hold certain positions without registration.

Regardless of whether the licensing law is permissive or mandatory in the jurisdiction in which a graduate registered nurse wishes to practice, it is to her advantage to become registered as soon as possible after completing her basic program and to keep her license in effect throughout her life. This enables her to return to active nursing at any time, without undue difficulty, if she so desires. It also tends to minimize the potential difficulties in moving from one jurisdiction to another.

In meeting the licensing requirements, a nurse demonstrates to herself and to all the residents of the jurisdiction in which she wishes to practice that she can contribute significantly to the health and welfare of the community in which she is employed. In taking the licensing examination, she has an opportunity to provide evidence that she will be safe in the practice of nursing as measured by the criteria accepted by the profession. Her scores on this examination give her a basis for comparing her knowledge and understanding with that of other

---

*Currently under revision; to be issued as a manual when completed.

nurses seeking licensure. They provide a relative index of her competence to meet the nursing needs of patients.

DEVELOPMENT OF THE LICENSING EXAMINATION

The official title of the licensing examination under discussion is the State Board Test Pool Examination. It is so called because the state boards of nursing that use it participate in its preparation in cooperation with the American Nurses' Association and the National League for Nursing. New forms are introduced at frequent intervals, both to safeguard test security and to permit test questions to reflect the latest concepts concerning the care of the ill and the promotion of health.

This examination is used in all 54 jurisdictions except Puerto Rico, where (because of language difficulties) an examination of their own choice is used, to determine whether graduates of schools of nursing meet minimum requirements for licensure.

Many values accrue as a result of a large number of jurisdictions' using the same licensing examination. The test scores permit a direct comparison of the performance of each candidate with that of a large representative sample of all candidates seeking licensure. This information can be definitely useful to the individual candidate in making professional plans. It may be of some help to faculties of basic nursing programs. It aids each licensing authority in establishing the minimum standards that will best meet the nursing needs of its jurisdiction. It facilitates mobility of nurses, since the score a candidate earns in one jurisdiction can be utilized by every other jurisdiction using this examination in determining whether or not she meets its minimum test standards for licensure. It gives the profession pertinent information concerning the feasibility of establishing common minimum standards of eligibility for initial licensure and licensure by endorsement in all jurisdictions using the same licensing examination.

CONTENT AND ORGANIZATION OF THE LICENSING EXAMINATION

The State Board Test Pool Examination consists of five tests—one in each of the major clinical fields: medical, surgical, obstetric, pediatric, and psychiatric nursing. Most of the questions in each test are concerned with the nursing care of particular patients described therein, patients who are representative of common health problems on a national basis. The questions are designed to evaluate a candidate's skill in recognizing and utilizing pertinent principles of the physical, biologic, and social sciences, as well as her understanding of specific nursing skills and abilities involved in meeting the needs of a patient safely and effectively. For example, candidates may be asked to indicate the position that is most therapeutic for a certain patient to assume or indicate the reason why a patient needs to be kept in a certain position. To answer such questions appropriately, a candidate needs to understand and correlate certain aspects of anatomy and physiology, basic nursing, the effects of medication administered to the patient, his attitude toward his illness, and other pertinent factors. Most questions are based on nursing situations similar to those with which candidates have had experience. Some, however, require candidates to apply basic principles and techniques to clinical situations with which they have had little or no experience.

All the tests are objective in form; that is, several suggested answers, one of which nursing authorities agree is superior to the others, are given for each question. Candidates are asked to designate the reply that best answers each question. The number of questions in the five tests varies, but the total is such that they all can be administered within a 1½- or 2-day period and still give all candidates an opportunity to attempt each question.

PREPARATION FOR TAKING THE EXAMINATION

Because of the many ways in which her performance on the licensing examination can influence her professional career, it is important for each graduate nurse to see that her scores are as high as she is capable of earning. The entire basic program in nursing is designed to enable students to gain the information and skills necessary to practice nursing safely and effectively, and the student who applies herself efficiently throughout this program will be well prepared by the time of graduation to begin her nursing career and to take the licensing examination to demonstrate her competence. Nevertheless, many candidates believe they can do better on this examination if they undertake some special preparation for it. Such individuals are likely to find it most profitable to concentrate their efforts in two areas: (1) review of any part of the curriculum that they have found particularly difficult and (2) identification and thorough understanding of basic facts and principles involved in giving safe, efficient nursing care.

A few individuals can improve their scores significantly by a highly concentrated period of study immediately before taking an examination. The majority, however, profit more by spreading their review over a much longer period of time, and the best time to begin studying for state boards is the first class attended in the school. Many candidates profit from devoting the evening immediately preceding the examination to a pleasant diversion that is completed in time to permit a good night's rest.

TAKING THE LICENSING EXAMINATION

The most crucial requisite for doing well in this examination is to bring to it a sound understanding of the subject and a high level of reading comprehension. Determination to do well and confidence that she will do so further enhance the well-prepared individual's chances of earning high scores.

At least three other requirements must be met if an individual's performance is to reflect accurately her professional competence. First, she must follow explicitly all the directions given by the examiner and those printed at the beginning of each test, as well as any that refer to a specified group of questions. Second, she must read each question carefully to make certain that she understands it before deciding how to answer it. Third, she must record her answers in the space and manner specified. Some candidates find it helpful to glance over a test before starting to answer the questions. It enables them to answer the questions in the order most efficient and comfortable for them.

The score a candidate earns on each test is the number of questions to which she gives the best of the suggested answers minus a deduction for each other answer given. Therefore, a candidate reduces her score if she gives more than one reply to any question. Although there is a possibility

of her also lowering her score by answering any question about which she is uncertain of the best reply, it is generally to her advantage to answer such questions, since her knowledge and understanding of nursing increase her likelihood of giving the expected (best) answer more often than would be expected by chance alone. Accordingly, a candidate increases her chances of earning the highest score of which she is capable by omitting only those questions about which she has absolutely no information and making certain that she gives only one reply to each question she answers.

INTERPRETATION OF SCORES

The licensing authority in each jurisdiction decides the minimum score that a candidate must have, on each test, to qualify as a registered nurse. It also decides what information is to be given to each candidate about her performance on the licensing examination. In the most widely used reporting system, the average score on each test is assigned an equivalent standard score of 500 and the other scores are spread out in a systematic manner so that more than half are between 400 and 600 and practically all are between 200 and 800. (See diagram.)

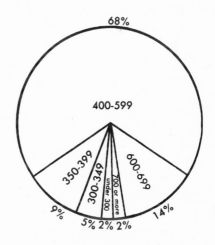

CONCLUSIONS

By meeting the standards required for licensure, a registered nurse demonstrates to herself, her colleagues, and the public that she is qualified to practice her profession in the community of her choice. Although she has already learned much that she needs to know to give safe and effective nursing care, she must continue to learn throughout her career if she is to make the greatest professional contribution of which she is capable. This is especially true as the explosion of knowledge continues at geometric rates and the life-span of the utility of learning decreases. These factors may account for the rising pressure to require evidence of continuing education for the renewal of registration of the license to practice nursing.

THE BIOLOGIC
AND
PHYSICAL SCIENCES

Anatomy and physiology

Microbiology

Chemistry

CHAPTER

1

ANATOMY

AND

PHYSIOLOGY

Anthony, C. P., and Kolthoff, N. J.: Textbook of anatomy and physiology, ed. 8, St. Louis, 1971, The C. V. Mosby Co.

Best, C. H., and Taylor, N. B., editors: Physiological basis of medical practice, ed. 8, Baltimore, 1966, The Williams & Wilkins Co.

Guyton, A. C.: Textbook of medical physiology, ed. 4, Philadelphia, 1971, W. B. Saunders Co.

Mountcastle, V. B., editor: Medical physiology, ed. 12, vols. 1 and 2, St. Louis, 1968, The C. V. Mosby Co.

Ruch, T. C., and Patton, H. D.: Physiology and biophysics, ed. 19, Philadelphia, 1965, W. B. Saunders Co.

Trumbore, R. H.: The cell, St. Louis, 1966, The C. V. Mosby Co.

MAJOR CONCEPTS ABOUT THE BODY

1. **Organization a prime characteristic of both structure and function of the body**
   Because of organization, the body is a structural and functional unit and not merely a chaotic collection of countless smaller units
2. **Four kinds of smaller units organized to form the body**
A. Cells—smallest units that can maintain life and reproduce
B. Tissues—organizations of many similar cells with nonliving intercellular substance between them
C. Organs—organizations of several different kinds of tissues so arranged that they can perform more complex functions than any individual tissue
D. Systems—organizations of different kinds of organs so arranged that they can perform more complex functions than any individual organ
3. **Structure the determinant of function**
4. **Body structure (and, therefore, function) changed gradually but in many ways throughout life**
5. **Survival—the body's prime function, survival of the individual and of the species**
6. **All body functions—cell functions**
   Each cell performs self-serving functions to maintain its own life and also specializes in some body-serving function to help maintain the body's life
7. **Body functions changed in response to changes in the environment**
   Usually the responses are adaptive; that is, they maintain or quickly restore homeostasis (relative constancy of the internal or cellular environment)

Cells

1. **Structure** (Fig. 1-1 and Table 1-1)
2. **Functions**
A. Movement of substances through cell membrane—accomplished by physical and physiologic processes: main physical processes—diffusion and osmosis; main physiologic processes—active transport

9

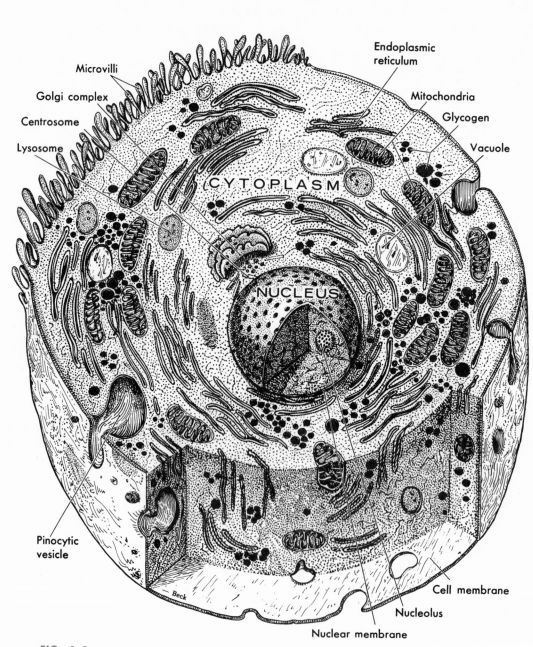

FIG. 1-1

Modern diagram of a typical cell, based on what is seen under an electron microscope. The mitochondria are the sites of the oxidative reactions that provide the cell with energy. The dots that line the endoplasmic reticulum are ribosomes, the sites of protein synthesis. (From Anthony, C. P., and Kolthoff, N. J.: Textbook of anatomy and physiology, ed. 8, St. Louis, 1971, The C. V. Mosby Co.)

TABLE 1-1

CELL STRUCTURES AND FUNCTIONS

Name of structure	Description	Function
1. Cell membrane	1. About 3/10,000,000 inch thick 2. Consists, according to triple-layer hypothesis, of inner and outer layers of protein molecules with double layer of lipid molecules between them 3. Few tiny pores or openings in membrane	1. Maintains cell's wholeness and organization 2. Determines what substances can enter and leave cell

2. Cytoplasm	1. Body of cell, exclusive of nucleus
	2. Contains thousands of organelles ("little organs")
	  a. Membranous organelles: endoplasmic reticulum, Golgi apparatus, mitochondria, lysosomes
	  b. Nonmembranous organelles: ribosomes, centrosome	

3. Cytoplasmic organelles a. Endoplasmic reticulum (ER)	Complicated network of canals, extending through cytoplasm and opening at cell's surface	Serves as cell's circulatory system, in that some substances are transported through ER
b. Golgi apparatus	Membranous vesicles near nucleus	Synthesizes large carbohydrate molecules, combines them with proteins, secretes products
c. Mitochondria	Sacs whose walls consist of outer and inner membranes separated by fluid; enzyme molecules attach to these membranes	Serve as cell's "powerhouses"; enzymes of mitochondria catalyze series of chemical reactions known as the citric acid cycle and these reactions provide about 95% of cell's energy supply
d. Lysosomes	Membranous sacs; contain enzymes	Enzymes in lysosomes digest substances that enter them; under some conditions, digest and thereby destroy cells
e. Ribosomes	Tiny granules, large numbers of which dot surfaces of endoplasmic reticulum; others scattered through cytoplasm	Cell's "protein factories"; ribosomes attached to ER synthesize proteins, which move through ER to Golgi apparatus and then are secreted by cell; ribosomes lying free in cytoplasm synthesize proteins for cell's own use (its enzymes and structural proteins)
f. Centrosome (centrosphere)	Spherical body near center of cell (i.e., the nucleus)	Plays part in formation of spindle fibers during cell reproduction (mitosis)
4. Nucleus	Spherical body in center of cell; enclosed by pore-containing membrane; contains *chromosomes* and *nucleoli;* segments of DNA molecule called *genes;* chromosomes composed mainly of DNA molecules; genes are segments of DNA molecules; nucleoli composed mainly of RNA	Genes determine heredity by complex mechanism that transcribes DNA into RNA and then translates RNA into proteins; each of thousands of kinds of proteins synthesized performs specific function

mechanisms, phagocytosis, pinocytosis; energy for physical processes comes from random, never-ceasing movements of atoms, ions, and molecules; energy for physiologic processes comes from chemical reactions of catabolism carried on by living cells

1. Diffusion—movement of solutes and water in all directions within a fluid and in both directions through membrane; net movement of each substance, however, occurs from area where that substance is more concentrated into one in which it is less concentrated; hence, net diffusion of solute across a membrane is from more to less concentrated solution, but net diffusion of water is from less to more concentrated solution (because water molecules are more concentrated in less concentrated solution); diffusion tends to equilibrate concentrations of two solutions separated by membrane (e.g., water and oxygen diffuse through cell membranes)

2. Osmosis—diffusion of water through a membrane that maintains at least one concentration gradient across the membrane; direction of net osmosis: down the water concentration gradient; i.e., more water osmoses out of the more dilute solution into the more concentrated one than osmoses in the opposite direction; pressure developed in a solution, as result of net osmosis into it, called *osmotic pressure;* net osmosis occurs into a hypertonic solution from a solution that is hypotonic to it; *hypertonic solution:* one that has greater potential osmotic pressure because it has higher concentration of solute particles than solution to which it is hypertonic; *hypotonic solution:* one that has lower potential osmotic pressure and lower solute concentration than solution to which it is hypotonic

3. Active transport mechanisms ("pumps") —devices that move ions or molecules through cell membranes against their concentration gradients (i.e., in direction opposite from net diffusion or net osmosis; energy supplied by catabolism of cell)

4. Phagocytosis—movement of relatively large particles (e.g., bacteria and fragments of disintegrating cells) into cell; a segment of cell membrane encircles particle, then pinches off from rest of membrane and migrates into cytoplasm of cell

5. Pinocytosis—physiologic process similar to phagocytosis, except that pinocytosis moves fluid into cell whereas phagocytosis moves particles

B. Cell metabolism—consists of two processes, catabolism and anabolism

1. Catabolism—complex process that releases energy stored in food molecules; part of this energy is released as heat but a little more than half of it is immediately put back in storage in unstable, high-energy bonds of ATP molecules; as cells need energy, ATP high-energy bonds break down rapidly, supplying the energy that does all kinds of cellular work

   a. Consists of two series of chemical reactions: glycolysis and the citric acid cycle; *glycolysis*—anaerobic (nonoxygen-utilizing) reactions that convert 1 glucose molecule to 2 pyruvic acid molecules and yield small amount of ATP and heat

   b. Citric acid cycle—series of aerobic reactions that use oxygen to oxidize 2 pyruvic acid molecules to 6 carbon dioxide molecules and 6 water molecules and yield about 95% of the ATP and heat formed during catabolism

2. Anabolism—series of chemical reactions by which cell synthesizes complex chemical compounds (e.g., enzymes, structural proteins, secretions); anabolism is one kind of cellular work for which catabolism supplies energy via ATP

C. Cell reproduction—accomplished by mitosis, process in which chromosomes (DNA molecules) duplicate themselves before cell divides to form two new cells, each of which receives a full set of chromosomes: 46 chromosomes in normal human cells other than mature ova and sperm, which contain 23 chromosomes

Tissues

See Table 1-2 for names of four main kinds of tissues, some subtypes of each, and examples of location and function.

TABLE 1-2

TISSUES

Tissues	Main locations	Functions
1. Epithelial		
a. Simple squamous (single layer flat cells)	1. Alveoli of lungs	1. Diffusion of gases between air and blood
b. Stratified squamous (several layers cells)	1. Outer layer of skin (epidermis)	1. Protection
c. Simple columnar	1. Secreting cells of glands	1. Secretion
2. Muscle		
a. Skeletal (voluntary or striated)	1. Attached to bones 2. Extrinsic eyeball muscles 3. Upper one third of esophagus	1. Movement of bones 2. Eye movements 3. First part of swallowing
b. Visceral (involuntary or smooth)	1. Upper walls of tubular viscera 2. In walls of blood vessels and large lymphatics 3. In ducts of glands 4. Intrinsic eye muscles (iris and ciliary body) 5. Arrector muscles of hairs	1. Movement of substances along tubes 2. Changes in size of blood vessels 3. Movement of substances along ducts 4. Changes in size of pupils and in shape of lens 5. Erection of hairs (gooseflesh)
c. Cardiac (branching)	1. Wall of heart	1. Contraction of heart
3. Connective Most widely distributed of all tissues		
a. Areolar (loose connective tissue)	1. Between other tissues 2. Between organs 3. Superficial fascia	1. Cement various parts of body together
b. Adipose (fat)	1. Subcutaneous 2. Padding at various points	1. Protection 2. Insulation 3. Support 4. Reserve food
c. Dense fibrous	1. Tendons 2. Ligaments 3. Aponeuroses 4. Deep fascia 5. Scars 6. Capsule of kidney, etc.	1. Furnish flexible but strong connection
d. Hemopoietic (1) Myeloid	1. Bone marrow	1. Forms red blood cells, most white blood cells (i.e., neutrophils, eosinophils, basophils), and platelets
(2) Lymphatic or lymphoid	1. Lymph nodes 2. Spleen 3. Thymus gland 4. Tonsils and adenoids	1. Form lymphocytes, monocytes, and plasma cells; filter lymph 2. Forms lymphocytes, monocytes, and plasma cells; filters blood 3. Forms lymphocytes 4. Form lymphocytes and plasma cells
e. Bone	1. Skeleton	1. Support 2. Protection
f. Cartilage (1) Hyaline	1. Part of nasal septum 2. Covering articular surfaces of bones 3. Larynx 4. Rings in trachea and bronchi	1. Furnish firm but flexible support

Continued.

TABLE 1-2

TISSUES—cont'd

Tissues	Main locations	Functions
3. Connective—cont'd f. Cartilage—cont'd (2) Fibrocartilage	1. Discs between vertebrae 2. Symphysis pubis	
(3) Elastic	1. External ear 2. Eustachian (auditory) tube	
4. Nervous	1. Brain 2. Spinal cord 3. Nerves	1. Receive and transmit stimuli

Skeletal system

1. Functions
A. Furnishes supporting framework
B. Affords protection for viscera, brain, etc.
C. Provides levers for muscles to pull on to produce movements
D. Hemopoiesis by red bone marrow—formation of all kinds of blood cells except lymphocytes and monocytes
2. Structure of long bones (Fig. 1-2)
3. Names and numbers of bones (Table 1-3)
4. Differences between male and female skeletons
A. Male skeleton larger and heavier than that of female
B. Male pelvis deep and funnel-shaped with narrow pubic arch; female pelvis shallow, broad, and flaring with wider pubic arch
5. Age changes in skeleton
A. From infancy to adulthood, not only do bones grow, but also their relative sizes change; head becomes proportionately smaller, pelvis relatively larger, legs proportionately longer, etc.
B. From young adulthood to old age, bone margins and projections change gradually; bone piles up along them (marginal lipping and spurs), thereby restricting movement
6. Joints
A. Types
  1. Diarthroses (freely movable joints) —most joints of body diarthroses; many subtypes (e.g., ball-and-socket, hinge, pivot)
  2. Synarthroses
    a. Cartilaginous type—slightly movable joints; e.g., intervertebral discs (between bodies of vertebrae)

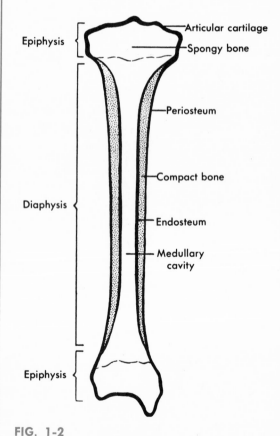

FIG. 1-2

Diagram to show structure of long bone as seen in longitudinal section.

TABLE 1-3
BONES OF THE BODY

Part of body	Name of bone	Number	Description
1. Axial skeleton a. Skull (1) Cranium	1. Frontal 2. Parietal 3. Temporal 4. Occipital 5. Sphenoid 6. Ethmoid	1 2 2 1 1 1	1. Forehead bone 2. Bulging bones that form top sides of cranium 3. Form lower sides of cranium and part of cranial floor 4. Forms posterior part of cranial floor and walls 5. Forms mid portion of cranial floor 6. Composes part of anterior portion of cranial floor; lies anterior to sphenoid, posterior to nasal bones
(2) Face	1. Nasal 2. Maxillary 3. Zygomatic (malar) 4. Mandible 5. Lacrimal 6. Palatine 7. Inferior conchae (turbinates) 8. Vomer	2 2 2 1 2 2 2 1	1. Form upper part of bridge of nose 2. Upper jaw bones 3. Cheek bones 4. Lower jaw bone 5. Fingernail-shaped bones posterior and lateral to nasal bones, in medial wall of orbit 6. Form posterior part of hard palate 7. Thin scroll of bone along inner surface of side wall of nasal cavity 8. Lower, posterior part of nasal septum
(3) Ear ossicles	1. Malleus (hammer) 2. Incus (anvil) 3. Stapes (stirrups)	2 2 2	Tiny bones in middle ear cavity in temporal bone; resemble, respectively, miniature hammer, anvil, and stirrups
b. Hyoid bone		1	U-shaped bone in neck between mandible and upper part of larynx; only bone in body that forms no joints with any other bones
c. Vertebral column	1. Cervical vertebrae 2. Thoracic vertebrae 3. Lumbar vertebrae 4. Sacrum 5. Coccyx	7 12 5 1 1	1. Upper 7 vertebrae 2. Next 12 vertebrae, ribs attached to these 3. Next 5 vertebrae, located in "small" of back 4. In embryo, 5 separate vertebrae, but fused in adult into 1 wedge-shaped bone 5. In embryo, 4 or 5 separate vertebrae, but fused in adult into 1 bone
d. Ribs and sternum	1. True ribs 2. False ribs 3. Sternum	7 pairs 5 pairs 1	1. Upper 7 pairs fastened to sternum by costal cartilages 2. Do not attach to sternum directly; upper 3 pairs of false ribs attached by means of costal cartilage of seventh ribs; last 2 pairs not attached at all and therefore called "floating" ribs 3. Breast bone
2. Appendicular skeleton a. Upper extremities	1. Clavicle 2. Scapula 3. Humerus 4. Radius 5. Ulna 6. Carpals	2 2 2 2 2 16	1. Collar bone; shoulder girdle fastened to axial skeleton by articulation of clavicle with sternum 2. Shoulder blade 3. Long bone of upper arm 4. Thumb side of forearm 5. Little finger side of forearm 6. Wrist bones; arranged in 2 rows at proximal end of hand

Continued.

TABLE 1-3

BONES OF THE BODY—cont'd

Part of body	Name of bone	Number	Description
2. Appendicular skeleton —cont'd			
a. Upper extremities —cont'd	7. Metacarpals	10	7. Long bones; form framework of palm of hand
	8. Phalanges	28	8. Miniature long bones of fingers; 3 in each finger, 2 in each thumb
b. Lower extremities	1. Os coxae, or pelvic bone	2	1. Large hip bones; lower extremities attached to axial skeleton by articulation of pelvic bones with sacrum
	2. Femur	2	2. Thigh bone
	3. Patella	2	3. Kneecap
	4. Tibia	2	4. Shin bone
	5. Fibula	2	5. Long, slender bone of lateral side of lower leg
	6. Tarsals	14	6. "Ankle" bones; form heel and proximal end of foot
	7. Metatarsals	10	7. Long bones of feet
	8. Phalanges	28	8. Miniature long bones of toes
	Total	206°	

°Sesamoid bones (rounded bones found in various tendons) have not been counted except for patellae, which are largest sesamoid bones; number of these bones varies greatly between individuals. Wormian bones (small islets of bones in some cranial sutures) have not been counted because of variability of occurrence.

b. Fibrous type—immovable joints; e.g., sutures between skull bones

B. Structure of 2 types of joints
1. Diarthroses—joint cavity or space between articular surfaces of 2 bones united by joint, thin layer of hyaline cartilage covering articular surfaces of joining bones; bones held together by fibrous capsule lined with synovial membrane and ligaments
2. Synarthroses—no joint cavity, no capsule; joining bones held together by fibrous tissue (e.g., sutures of skull) or cartilage (e.g., between bodies of vertebra)

C. Kinds of movement possible at diarthrotic joints
1. Flexion—bending one bone upon another; e.g., bending forearm on upper arm
2. Extension—stretching one bone away from another; e.g., straightening lower arm out from flexed position
3. Abduction—moving bone away from body's midline; e.g., moving arms straight out from sides
4. Adduction—moving bone back toward body's midline; e.g., bringing arms back to sides of body from outstretched or abducted position
5. Rotation—pivoting bone upon its axis; e.g., partial rotation—turning head from side to side
6. Circumduction—describing surface of cone with moving part; e.g., moving arm around so that hand describes circle
7. Special movements
   a. Supination—forearm movement turning palm forward
   b. Pronation—forearm movement turning back of hand forward
   c. Inversion—ankle movement turning sole of foot inward
   d. Eversion—ankle movement turning sole of foot outward
   e. Protraction—moving part, such as lower jaw, forward
   f. Retraction—pulling part back; opposite of protraction

7. **Ossification**
Process that changes cartilage or fibrous tissue to bone; skeleton originally formed of fibrous membranes and hyaline cartilage, most of which undergoes ossification before birth; ossification not com-

TABLE 1-4

TYPES OF MUSCLE TISSUE COMPARED

	Striated	Smooth	Branching
Microscopic structure	Long, multinuclear cells with cross-striae	Long, tapering cells, single nucleus, no cross-striae	With light microscope cells seem to branch into each other but electron microscope shows separate, individual cardiac cells; cross-striae
Macroscopic structure	Many small bundles of muscle fibers (cells) held together by fibrous covering (epimysium); extensions of epimysium in form of tendons and aponeuroses attach muscles to bones, cartilage, fascia, or skin Each skeletal muscle consists of three parts: origin, body, and insertion; contraction of muscle pulls insertion toward origin	Occurs as thin layers of tissue in walls of various hollow organs such as intestines and arteries	Composes heart, structure of which is discussed on p. 49
Nerve control	By voluntary nervous system via somatic motoneurons in spinal and some cranial nerves	By autonomic nervous system via autonomic motoneurons in autonomic, spinal, and some cranial nerves; not under voluntary control (with rare exceptions)	By autonomic nervous system via autonomic motoneurons in autonomic, spinal, and some cranial nerves; not under voluntary control (with rare exceptions)

pleted, however, until about age 25; two processes accomplish ossification: formation of bone matrix and then its calcification

A. Formation of bone matrix (the intercellular substance of bone, made up of collagen fibers and a cementlike substance)—osteoblasts (bone-forming cells) synthesize collagen and cement substance from proteins provided by the diet; vitamin C promotes formation of bone matrix; exercise and estrogens act in some way to stimulate osteoblasts to form bone matrix

B. Calcification of bone matrix—calcium salts deposited in the bone matrix; vitamin D promotes calcification

C. Growth

1. In length—by continual thickening of epiphyseal cartilage followed by ossification; as long as bone growth continues, epiphyseal cartilage grows faster than it can be replaced by bone; therefore, line of cartilage persists between diaphysis and epiphy-

ses and can be seen on x-ray film; sometime during adolescence cartilage is completely transformed into bone, at which time bone growth is complete

2. In diameter—osteoclasts destroy bone surrounding medullary cavity, thereby enlarging the cavity; at same time, osteoclasts add new bone around outer surface of the bone

Muscular system

1. Functions

A. Movement

B. Posture

C. Heat production—catabolism in muscle cells produces relatively large share of body heat

2. **Comparison of three types of muscle tissue** (Table 1-4)

3. **Basic principles about skeletal muscle actions**

A. Skeletal muscles contract only if stimulated; i.e., a skeletal muscle and its motor nerve function as a physiologic unit—either useless without the other's functioning

Corollary: Anything that prevents impulse conduction to a skeletal muscle paralyzes the muscle

B. Most skeletal muscles attach to at least two bones; as a muscle contracts and pulls on its bones, it moves the bone that moves most easily; the bone that moves is called the muscle's *insertion* bone, and the bone that holds stationary is its *origin* bone

C. Bones serve as levers, and joints as fulcrums of these levers (lever—any rigid bar free to turn about a fixed point, or fulcrum); a muscle's contraction exerts a pulling force on its insertion bone at the point where the muscle inserts, pulling that point nearer the muscle's origin bone

D. Skeletal muscles almost always act in groups rather than singly; members of groups are classified as follows:
1. Prime movers—the muscle or muscles whose contraction actually produces the movement
2. Synergists—muscles that contract at the same time as the prime mover, helping it produce the movement or stabilizing the part (i.e., holding it steady) so the prime mover can produce a more effective movement
3. Antagonists—muscles that relax while the prime mover is contracting (exception: antagonist contracts at the same time as the prime mover when a part needs to be held rigid, as the knee joint does in standing); antagonists have directly opposite actions and usually opposite locations with reference to bones they move; e.g., muscle that flexes lower arm lies on anterior surface of upper arm bone, whereas that which extends lower arm lies on posterior surface of upper arm

E. The body of a muscle usually does not lie over the part moved by the muscle; instead it lies above or below, or anterior or posterior to, the part; thus the body of a muscle that moves the lower arm will not be located in the lower arm but in the upper arm; e.g., biceps and triceps brachii muscles

F. Contraction of a skeletal muscle either shortens the muscle, producing movement, or increases the tension (tone) in the muscle; contractions are classified according to whether they produce movement or increase muscle tone as follows:
1. Tonic contractions—produce muscle tone; do not shorten the muscle so do not produce movements; only a few fibers contract at one time and this produces a moderate degree of muscle tone; in the healthy, awake body, all muscles exhibit tone
2. Isometric contractions—increase the degree of muscle tone; do not shorten the muscle so do not produce movements; daily repetition of isometric contractions gradually increases muscle strength—the purpose of isometric exercises
3. Isotonic contractions—muscle shortens, thereby producing movement; all movements are produced by isotonic contractions

4. **Origins, insertions, functions of main skeletal muscles**
Grouped according to functions (Table 1-5)

5. **Weak places in abdominal wall where hernia may occur**
A. Inguinal rings—right and left internal, right and left external
B. Femoral rings—right and left
C. Umbilicus

6. **Bursae**
A. Definition—small sacs lined with synovial membrane and containing synovial fluid
B. Locations—wherever pressure is exerted over moving parts
1. Between skin and bone
2. Between tendons and bone
3. Between muscles, or ligaments, and bone
C. Names of bursae that frequently become inflamed (bursitis)
1. Subacromial—between deltoid muscle and head of humerus and acromion process
2. Olecranon—between olecranon process and skin; inflammation called "student's elbow"
3. Prepatellar—between patella and skin; inflammation called "housemaid's knee"

TABLE 1-5

ORIGINS, INSERTIONS, AND FUNCTIONS OF MAIN SKELETAL MUSCLES

Part of body moved	Movement	Muscle	Origin	Insertion
Upper arm	Flexion	1. Pectoralis major	1. Clavicle (medial half) 2. Sternum 3. Costal cartilages of true ribs	1. Humerus (greater tubercle)
	Extension	1. Latissimus dorsi	1. Vertebrae (spines of lower thoracic, lumbar, and sacral) 2. Ilium (crest) 3. Lumbodorsal fascia	1. Humerus (inter-tubercular groove)
	Abduction	1. Deltoid	1. Clavicle 2. Scapula (spine and acromion)	1. Humerus (lateral side on deltoid tubercle)
	Adduction	1. Latissimus dorsi contracting with 2. Pectoralis major	See above See above	See above See above
Shoulder	Shrugging, elevating	1. Trapezius	1. Occipital bone 2. Vertebrae (cervical and thoracic)	1. Scapula (spine and acromion) 2. Clavicle
	Lowering	1. Pectoralis minor	1. Ribs (second to fifth)	1. Scapula (coracoid)
		2. Serratus anterior	1. Ribs (upper 8 or 9)	1. Scapula (anterior surface)
Lower arm	Flexion (With forearm supinated)	1. Biceps brachii	1. Scapula (supra-glenoid tuber-osity) 2. Scapula (coracoid)	1. Radius (tubercle at proximal end)
	(With forearm pronated)	2. Brachialis	1. Humerus (distal half, anterior surface)	1. Ulna (front of coronoid process)
	(With forearm semisupinated or semipronated)	3. Brachioradialis	1. Humerus (above lateral epicondyle)	1. Radius (styloid process)
	Extension	1. Triceps brachii	1. Scapula (infragle-noid tuberosity) 2. Humerus (posterior surface–lateral head above radial groove; medial head, below)	1. Ulna (olecranon process)
Thigh	Flexion	1. Iliopsoas (iliacus and psoas major)	1. Ilium (iliac fossa) 2. Vertebrae (bodies of twelfth thoracic to fifth lumbar)	1. Femur (small trochanter)
		2. Rectus femoris	1. Ilium and anterior, inferior iliac spine	1. Tibia (by way of patellar tendon)

Continued.

TABLE 1-5

ORIGINS, INSERTIONS, AND FUNCTIONS OF MAIN SKELETAL MUSCLES—cont'd

Part of body moved	Movement	Muscle	Origin	Insertion
Thigh— cont'd	Extension	1. Gluteus maximus	1. Ilium (crest and posterior surface) 2. Sacrum and coccyx (posterior surface) 3. Sacrotuberous ligament	1. Femur (gluteal tuberosity) 2. Iliotibial tract
		2. Hamstring group (see below)	1. Ischium (tuberosity) 2. Femur (linea aspera)	1. Fibula (head of) 2. Tibia (lateral condyle, medial condyle, and medial surface)
	Abduction	1. Gluteus medius and minimus	1. Ilium (lateral surface)	1. Femur (greater trochanter)
		2. Tensor fasciae latae	1. Ilium (anterior part of crest)	1. Iliotibial tract
	Adduction	1. Adductor group a. Brevis b. Longus c. Magnus	1. Pubic bone	1. Femur (linea aspera)
Lower leg	Flexion	1. Hamstring group a. Biceps femoris b. Semitendinosus c. Semimembranosus	1. Ischium (tuberosity) 2. Femur (linea aspera)	1. Fibula (head of) 2. Tibia (lateral condyle, medial condyle, and medial surface)
		2. Gastrocnemius	1. Femur (condyles)	1. Tarsal bone (calcaneus by way of tendo calcaneus)
	Extension	1. Quadriceps femoris group a. Rectus femoris b. Vastus lateralis c. Vastus medialis d. Vastus intermedius	1. Ilium (anterior, inferior spine) 2. Femur (linea aspera and anterior surface)	1. Tibia (by way of patellar tendon)
Foot	Flexion (dorsiflexion)	1. Tibialis anterior	1. Tibia (lateral condyle)	1. First cuneiform tarsal 2. Base of first metatarsal
	Extension (plantar flexion)	1. Gastrocnemius	1. Femur (condyles)	1. Calcaneus, by way of tendo calcaneus
		2. Soleus	1. Tibia	1. Same as gastrocnemius, but underneath
Head	Flexion	1. Sternocleidomastoid	1. Sternum 2. Clavicle	1. Temporal bone (mastoid process)
	Extension	1. Trapezius	1. Vertebrae (cervical) 2. Scapula (spine and acromion) 3. Clavicle	1. Occiput

TABLE 1-5

ORIGINS, INSERTIONS, AND FUNCTIONS OF MAIN SKELETAL MUSCLES—cont'd

Part of body moved	Movement	Muscle	Origin	Insertion
Abdominal wall	1. Compress abdominal cavity; therefore assists in straining, defecation, forced expiration, childbirth, posture, etc.	1. External oblique	1. Ribs (lower 8)	1. Innominate bone (iliac crest and pubis by way of inguinal ligament) 2. Linea alba
		2. Internal oblique	1. Innominate bone (iliac crest, inguinal ligament) 2. Lumbodorsal fascia	1. Ribs (lower 3) 2. Pubic bone 3. Linea alba
		3. Transversus	1. Ribs (lower 6) 2. Innominate bone (iliac crest, inguinal ligament) 3. Lumbodorsal fascia	1. Pubic bone 2. Linea alba
		4. Rectus abdominis	1. Innominate bone (pubic bone and symphysis pubis)	1. Ribs (costal cartilage of fifth, sixth, seventh)
Chest wall	1. Elevate ribs, thereby enlarging anteroposterior and anterolateral dimensions of chest and causing inspiration	1. External intercostals	1. Ribs (lower border of all but twelfth)	1. Ribs (upper border of rib below origin)
	2. Depress ribs	1. Internal intercostals	1. Ribs (inner surface, upper border of all except first)	1. Ribs (lower border of rib above origin)
	3. Pull floor of thorax downward, thereby enlarging vertical dimension of chest and causing inspiration	1. Diaphragm	1. Lower circumference of rib cage	1. Central tendon of diaphragm
Trunk	1. Flexion	1. Iliopsoas	1. Femur (small trochanter)	1. Ilium 2. Vertebrae (bodies of twelfth thoracic to fifth lumbar)
	2. Extension	1. Sacrospinalis a. Iliocostalis (lateral) b. Longissimus (medial)	1. Vertebrae (posterior surface of sacrum, spinous processes of lumbar and last 2 thoracic)	1. Ribs (lower 6)
				1. Vertebrae (transverse processes of thoracic) 2. Ribs (backs of)
			2. Ilium (posterior part of crest)	1. Vertebrae (spines of thoracic
		2. Quadratus lumborum	1. Ilium (posterior part of crest) 2. Vertebrae (lower 3 lumbar)	1. Ribs (twelfth) 2. Vertebrae (transverse processes of first 4 lumbar)

D. Function—act as cushions, relieving pressure between moving parts

7. **Tendon sheaths**
A. Definition and location—tube-shaped structures that enclose certain tendons, notably those of wrist and ankle; made of connective tissue lined with synovial membrane
B. Function—facilitate gliding movements of tendon

INTEGRATION AND CONTROL OF THE BODY
Nervous system

Because the body is made up of innumerable smaller units, mechanisms for controlling these so that they function as one large unit are essential. The nervous system provides one kind of control or integrating mechanism; and chemicals (mainly hormones but also carbon dioxide and various other substances) provide another kind.

1. **Cells**
A. Kinds—neurons and neuroglia the main kinds of cells composing nervous system organs
B. Neuroglia—connective tissue cells found only in nervous system; support neurons and connect them to blood vessels; *microglia* (one type of neuroglia) carry on phagocytosis in inflamed or degenerating brain tissue
C. Neurons (nerve cells)
   1. Kinds
      a. Sensory (afferent) neurons—transmit impulses to spinal cord or brain
      b. Motoneurons (motor or efferent neurons)—transmit impulses away from brain or spinal cord toward or to muscles or glands
         (1) Somatic motoneurons—transmit impulses from cord or brainstem to skeletal muscle
         (2) Visceral or autonomic motoneurons—transmit impulses from cord or brainstem to smooth muscle, cardiac muscle, or glands
      c. Interneurons (internuncial or intercalated neurons)—transmit impulses from sensory neurons to motoneurons
   2. Structure
      a. Main structural difference from other cells is that threadlike structures (called dendrites and axons,

or nerve fibers) extend out from opposite ends of neuron cell bodies; this unique structural feature makes neuron well-suited to its special function of transmitting impulses over distances
      b. Note following structures in Fig. 1-3:
         (1) Dendrites—fibers that conduct impulses to neuron cell body; most neurons have several dendrites
            (a) Receptors—the beginnings of dendrites of sensory neurons, the part that receives stimuli; impulse conduction normally begins in receptors
         (2) Axons—fibers that conduct impulses away from neuron cell bodies; each neuron has only one axon, but this may have one or more branches
         (3) Myelin sheath—segmented covering around nerve fiber
         (4) Neurilemma — continuous sheath around segmented myelin sheath; essential for nerve fiber regeneration; absent from brain and spinal cord fibers; these are not known to regenerate if destroyed by disease or injury
         (5) Synapse—contact points between endings of axon of one neuron and dendrites or cell body of another neuron
         (6) Effector—structure in which motoneuron axons terminate; specifically, either muscle or gland
   3. Function—impulse conduction

2. **Nerve impulse (action potential)**
A. Definitions
   1. Resting potential—the difference in electric charge that exists between the outer and inner surfaces of a neuron cell membrane when it is "resting"— in other words, when the neuron is not conducting impulses; resting potential normally equals about 70 to 90 millivolts, with the outside of the membrane positive to the inside (or, if you prefer, with the inside negative to the outside)
   2. Action potential—synonym for nerve impulse; a self-propagating wave of

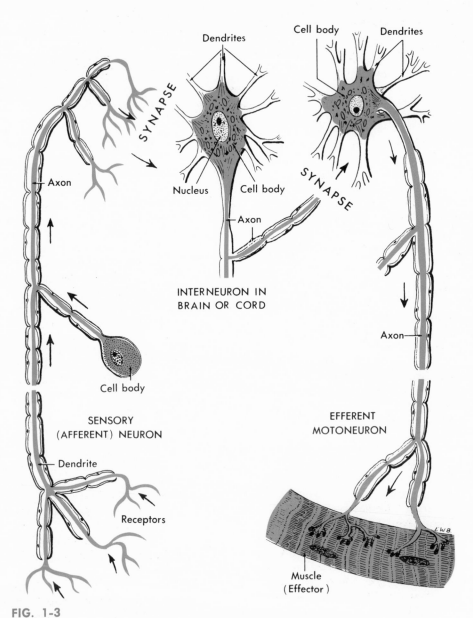

FIG. 1-3

Diagrammatic representation of a three-neuron reflex arc. Note that each neuron has three parts: a cell body and two extensions, dendrite(s) and an axon. (From Anthony, C. P., and Kolthoff, N. J.: Textbook of anatomy and physiology, ed. 8, St. Louis, 1971, The C. V. Mosby Co.)

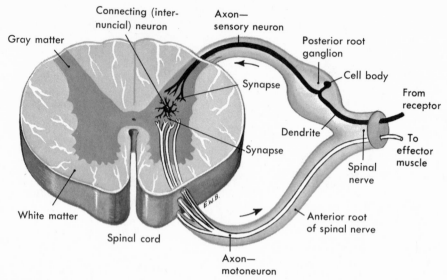

FIG. 1-4

Three-neuron reflex arc, consisting of a sensory neuron, a connecting (internuncial) neuron, and a motoneuron. Note the presence of two synapses in a three-neuron arc—(1) between sensory neuron axon terminals and internuncial neuron dendrites and (2) between internuncial axon terminals and motoneuron dendrites or cell bodies (located in anterior gray matter). Nerve impulses conducted over such arcs produce many spinal reflexes. Example: withdrawing the hand from a hot object. (From Anthony, C. P., and Kolthoff, N. J.: Textbook of anatomy and physiology, ed. 8, St. Louis, 1971, The C. V. Mosby Co.)

negativity that travels along the surface of a neuron's membrane
B. Basic route of impulse conduction—the reflex arc
1. Description—impulse conduction
   a. Starts in receptors
   b. Continues over reflex arc(s)
   c. Terminates in effectors (muscles and glands)
   d. Results in a reflex; i.e., a response by muscles or glands in which impulse terminates; a reflex, therefore, is either contraction of muscle or secretion by gland
   e. Not all impulses, of course, result in reflexes; many are inhibited at some point along the reflex arc
2. Types of reflex arcs
   a. Two-neuron (monosynaptic) reflex arc—simplest arc possible; consists of at least one sensory neuron, one synapse, and one motoneuron; synapse is region of contact between axon terminals of one neuron and dendrites or cell body of another neuron
   b. Three-neuron arc (Fig. 1-4)—con-

sists of at least one sensory neuron, synapse, interneuron, synapse, and motoneuron
   c. Complex, multisynaptic neural pathways also exist; many not yet clearly mapped
C. Conduction across synapses
1. When impulse reaches axon terminals, a chemical—e.g., acetylcholine or norepinephrine—is ejected from them into the microscopic synaptic space
2. Chemical released from many axon terminals has a stimulating effect on adjacent neurons (presumably this stimulating chemical is either acetylcholine or norepinephrine); chemical released from other axon terminals has an inhibitory effect on adjacent neurons; gamma-aminobutyric acid (GABA) is one inhibitory chemical
3. Axons that release acetylcholine called cholinergic fibers; those that release norepinephrine called adrenergic fibers
4. Termination of action of chemical transmitters

a. Acetylcholine inactivated in synapses by cholinesterase

b. Most norepinephrine leaves synapses to reenter axons, where some of it is again stored in small vesicles, and some is inactivated by monoamine oxidase in mitochondria; some norepinephrine inactivated in synapses by catechol-O-methyl transferase (COMT)

D. Speed of impulse conduction

  1. The larger the diameter of an axon the faster it conducts impulses; largest, fastest-conducting fibers—e.g., axons of somatic motoneurons—transmit impulses at speed of about 100 meters per second (more than 200 miles per hour)

  2. The smaller an axon's diameter, the slower it conducts impulses; smallest, slowest-conducting fibers transmit impulses at speed of about 1 mile per hour

3. Organs of nervous system

A. Spinal cord, brain, nerves, and ganglia

B. Spinal cord and brain constitute the central nervous system (CNS); nerves and ganglia constitute the peripheral nervous system (PNS)

C. Definitions

  1. White matter—bundles of myelinated nerve fibers

  2. Gray matter—clusters of neuron cell bodies mainly

  3. Nerves—bundles of myelinated nerve fibers located outside CNS

  4. Tracts—bundles of myelinated nerve fibers located within CNS

  5. Ganglia (singular ganglion)—macroscopic structures consisting of neuron cell bodies mainly; located outside CNS

D. Spinal cord

  1. Location—in spinal cavity, from foramen magnum to first lumbar vertebra

  2. Structure

    a. Deep groove (anterior median fissure) and more shallow groove (posterior median sulcus) incompletely divide cord into right and left symmetric halves

    b. Inner core of cord consists of gray matter shaped like a three-dimensional letter H

    c. Long columns of white matter surround the cord's inner core of gray matter; namely, right and left anterior, lateral, and posterior columns; composed of numerous sensory and motor tracts (Fig. 1-5)

  3. Functions

    a. Sensory tracts conduct impulses up cord to brain; motor tracts conduct impulses down cord from brain

    b. Gray matter of cord contains reflex centers for all spinal cord reflexes

E. Brain

  1. Divisions of brain (named in order—from below up—medulla, pons, midbrain, cerebellum, diencephalon, and cerebrum)

  2. Medulla

    a. Part of brain formed by enlargement of cord as it enters cranial cavity

    b. Consists mainly of white matter (sensory and motor tracts); also contains reticular formation (mixture of gray and white matter); some important reflex centers located in reticular formation: cardiac, vasomotor, respiratory, and swallowing centers

    c. Functions—contains centers for vital heart, blood vessel diameter (blood pressure), and respiratory reflexes; also centers for vomiting, coughing, swallowing, etc.; conducts impulses between cord and brain (both sensory and motor)

  3. Pons

    a. Part of brain located just above medulla; consists mainly of white matter (sensory and motor tracts) interspersed with gray matter (reflex centers)

    b. Conducts impulses between cord and various parts of brain and contains reflex centers for cranial nerves V, VI, VII, and VIII

  4. Midbrain

    a. Part of brain located between the pons, which lies below it, and the diencephalon and cerebrum, which lie above it; consists namely of white matter with scattered bits of gray matter

    b. Conducts impulses between cord and various parts of brain and contains reflex centers for cranial nerves III and IV (thus for pupillary reflexes and eye movements)

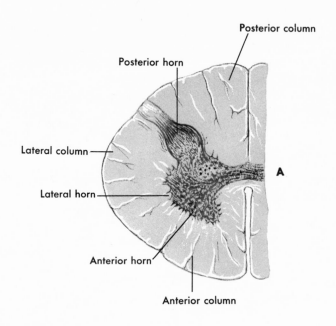

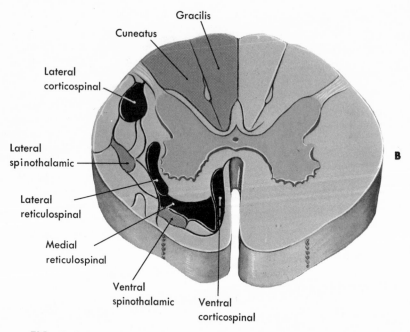

FIG. 1-5

A, Distribution of gray matter (horns) and white matter (columns) in a section of the spinal cord at the thoracic level. **B,** Location in the spinal cord of some major projection tracts. Black areas, descending motor tracts. Shaded areas, ascending sensory tracts. (From Anthony, C. P., and Kolthoff, N. J.: Textbook of anatomy and physiology, ed. 8, St. Louis, 1971, The C. V. Mosby Co.)

5. Diencephalon
   a. Thalamus and hypothalamus are major parts of the diencephalon
   b. Thalamus
      (1) Large rounded mass of gray matter in each cerebral hemisphere, lateral to third ventricle
      (2) Functions—conscious recognition of crude sensations of pain, temperature, and touch; relays almost all sensory impulses to cerebral cortex; responsible for emotional component of sensations (i.e., feelings of pleasantness or unpleasantness associated with them)
   c. Hypothalamus
      (1) Gray matter that forms floor of third ventricle and lower part of its lateral walls
      (2) Functions
         (a) Contains many higher autonomic reflex centers; these centers integrate autonomic functions—by sending impulses to each other and to lower autonomic centers—and they form a crucial part of the neural path by which emotions and other cerebral functions can alter vital, automatic functions such as the heartbeat, blood pressure, peristalsis, and secretion by glands and, thereby, produce psychosomatic diseases; neural path for psychosomatic disease—impulses from cerebral cortex to autonomic centers in hypothalamus, to lower autonomic centers in brainstem and cord, to visceral effectors (i.e., heart, smooth muscle, glands)
         (b) Helps control both the anterior pituitary gland and the posterior pituitary gland; certain neurons in hypothalamus release secretions into the pituitary portal veins, which transport them to the anterior pituitary gland where they influence its secretion of various important hormones; e.g., hypothalamic neurons secrete CRF (corticotropin-releasing factor) into pituitary portal veins, and CRF stimulates the anterior pituitary gland to secrete ACTH into the blood; neurons in the supraoptic nucleus of the hypothalamus synthesize ADH (antidiuretic hormone); from the cell bodies of these neurons, ADH migrates down their axons into the posterior pituitary gland, from which it is released into the blood; in short, hypothalamic neurons make ADH, but the posterior pituitary gland secretes it
         (c) Certain hypothalamic neurons serve as an "appetite center" and others function as a "satiety center"; together these centers regulate appetite and food intake
         (d) Certain hypothalamic neurons serve as heat-regulating centers by relaying impulses to lower autonomic centers for vasoconstriction, vasodilation, and sweating, and to somatic centers for shivering
         (e) Maintains waking state; constitutes part of the arousal or alerting neural pathway
6. Cerebrum
   a. Hemispheres, fissures, and lobes—longitudinal fissure divides cerebrum into 2 hemispheres connected only by corpus callosum; each cerebral hemisphere divided by fissures into 5 lobes: frontal, parietal, temporal, occipital, and island of Reil (insula)

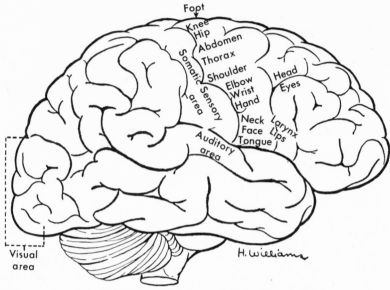

Foot
Knee
Hip
Abdomen
Thorax
Shoulder
Elbow
Wrist
Hand
Head
Eyes
Somatic Sensory area
Neck
Face
Tongue
Larynx
Lips
Auditory area
Visual area
H. Williams

FIG. 1-6

Localization of function in cerebral cortex. Conduction by precentral gyrus (frontal lobe) is necessary for voluntary or willed movements; by postcentral gyrus (parietal lobe) for general sensations such as pain, temperature, touch, kinesthesia; by transverse gyrus (temporal lobe) for hearing; by lingual gyrus and cuneus (occipital lobe) for vision. (From Francis, C. C: Introduction to human anatomy, ed. 6, St. Louis, 1973, The C. V. Mosby Co.)

b. Cerebral cortex—outer layer of gray matter arranged in ridges called convolutions or gyri
c. Cerebral tracts—bundles of axons compose white matter in interior of cerebrum; ascending projection tracts transmit impulses toward or to brain; descending projection tracts transmit impulses down from brain to cord; commissural tracts transmit from one hemisphere to other; association tracts transmit from one convolution to another in same hemisphere
d. Basal ganglia (or cerebral nuclei)—masses of gray matter embedded deep inside white matter in interior of cerebrum; caudate, putamen, and pallidum; putamen and pallidum constitute lenticular nucleus
e. Functions—in general, all conscious functions—e.g., analysis, integration, and interpretation of sensations, control of voluntary movements, use and understanding of language, and all other mental functions

7. Cerebellum
a. Structure—second-largest part of human brain; surface marked with sulci (grooves) and very slightly raised, slender convolutions; internal white matter forms pattern suggestive of veins of leaf
b. Functions
(1) The cerebellum exerts synergic control over skeletal muscles; this means that impulses conducted by cerebellar neurons coordinate skeletal muscle contractions to produce smooth, steady, and precise movements
(2) Because it coordinates skeletal muscle contractions, the cerebellum plays an essential part in
(a) Producing normal postures
(b) Maintaining equilibrium
8. Cord and brain coverings
a. Bony—vertebrae around cord; cranial bones around brain
b. Membranous—called meninges; consist of three layers

TABLE 1-6

DISTRIBUTION AND FUNCTION OF CRANIAL NERVE PAIRS

Name and number	Distribution	Function
Olfactory (I)	Nasal mucosa, high up along the septum especially	Sense of smell (sensory only)
Optic (II)	Retina of eyeball	Vision (sensory only)
Oculomotor (III)	Extrinsic muscles of eyeball, except superior oblique and external rectus; also intrinsic eye muscles (iris and ciliary)	Eye movements; constriction of pupil and bulging of lens, which together produce accommodation for near vision
Trochlear (IV) (smallest cranial nerve)	Superior oblique muscle of eye	Eye movements
Trifacial (V) (or trigeminal) largest cranial nerve	Sensory fibers to skin and mucosa of head and to teeth; muscles of mastication (sensory and motor fibers)	Sensations of head and face; chewing movements
Abducens (VI)	External rectus muscle of eye	Abduction of eye
Facial (VII)	Muscles of facial expression; taste buds of anterior two thirds of tongue; motor fibers to submaxillary and sublingual salivary glands	Facial expressions; taste; secretion of saliva
Auditory (VIII) (acoustic)	Inner ear	Hearing and equilibrium (sensory only)
Glossopharyngeal (IX)	Posterior one third of tongue; mucosa and muscles of pharynx; parotid gland; carotid sinus and body	Taste and other sensations of tongue; secretion of saliva; swallowing movements; functions in reflex arcs for control of blood pressure and respiration
Vagus (X) (or pneumogastric)	Mucosa and muscles of pharynx, larynx, trachea, bronchi, esophagus; thoracic and abdominal viscera	Sensations and movements of organs supplied; for example, slows heart, increases peristalsis and gastric and pancreatic secretion; voice production
Spinal accessory (XI)	Certain neck and shoulder muscles (muscles of larynx, sternocleidomastoid, trapezius)	Shoulder movements; turns head; voice production; muscle sense
Hypoglossal (XII)	Tongue muscles	Tongue movements, as in talking; muscle sense

Note: The first letters of the words in the following sentence are the first letters of the names of the cranial nerves, and many generations of anatomy students have used it as an aid to memorizing the names: "On Old Olympus Tiny Tops, A Finn and German Viewed Some Hops." (There are several slightly different versions of this sentence.)

(1) Dura mater—white fibrous tissue, outer layer

(2) Arachnoid membrane—cobwebby middle layer

(3) Pia mater—innermost layer of meninges; adheres to outer surface of cord and brain; contains blood vessels

9. Cord and brain fluid spaces

a. Subarachnoid space around cord

b. Subarachnoid space around brain

c. Central canal inside cord

d. Ventricles and cerebral aqueduct inside brain; 4 cavities within brain

(1) First and second (lateral ventricles)—large cavities, one in each cerebral hemisphere

(2) Third ventricle—vertical slit in cerebrum beneath corpus callosum and longitudinal fissure

(3) Fourth ventricle—diamond-shaped space between cere-

bellum and medulla and pons; is expansion of central canal of cord

10. Formation and circulation of cerebrospinal fluid
    a. Formed by plasma filtering from network of capillaries (choroid plexus) in each ventricle
    b. Circulates from lateral ventricles to third ventricle, cerebral aqueduct, fourth ventricle, central canal of cord, subarachnoid space of cord and brain; returns to blood via venous sinuses of brain

F. Cranial nerves—12 pairs (Table 1-6)
G. Spinal nerves—31 pairs
Each nerve attaches to cord by 2 short "roots," anterior and posterior; posterior roots marked by swelling, namely, spinal ganglion; branches of spinal nerves form plexuses (intricate networks of fibers, e.g., brachial plexus), from which nerves emerge to supply various parts of skin, mucosa, and skeletal muscles; since all spinal nerves are mixed nerves (i.e., composed of both sensory dendrites and motor axons), they function in both sensations and movements

4. **Sensory neural (conduction) pathways**
A. Sensory pathways to the cerebral cortex from the periphery consist of relays of at least 3 neurons, which we shall identify by Roman numerals
    1. Sensory neuron I—conducts from the periphery to the cord or to the brainstem
    2. Sensory neuron II—conducts from the cord or brainstem to the thalamus
    3. Sensory neuron III—conducts from the thalamus to the general sensory area of the cerebral cortex (areas 3, 1, 2 in the postcentral gyrus of the parietal lobe) (Figs. 1-6 and 1-7)
B. Crude awareness of sensations occurs when impulses reach the thalamus
C. Full consciousness of sensations with accurate localization and discrimination of fine details occurs when impulses reach the cerebral cortex
D. Most sensory neuron II axons decussate; so one side of the brain registers mainly sensations for the opposite side of the body
E. The principle of divergence applies to sensory neural pathways; each sensory

neuron synapses with many neurons and therefore impulses may diverge from any sensory neuron and be conducted to many effectors
F. Impulses that produce pain and temperature are conducted up the cord to the thalamus by the lateral spinothalamic tracts (Fig. 1-7)
G. Impulses that produce touch and pressure sensations are conducted up the cord to the thalamus by the following two pathways
    1. Impulses that result in the discriminating touch and pressure sensations (such as stereognosis, precise localization, and vibratory sense) are conducted by the medial lemniscal system, which consists of the fasciculi cuneatus and gracilis and the medial lemniscus; the fasciculi cuneatus and gracilis are the tracts of the posterior white columns of the cord; they conduct up the cord to the medulla; the medial lemniscus is a tract that conducts from the medulla to the thalamus
    2. Impulses that result in crude touch and pressure sensations are conducted up the cord to the thalamus by fibers of the ventral spinothalamic tracts
H. Sensory impulses that result in conscious proprioception or kinesthesia (sense of position or movement of body parts) are conducted over the same pathway as are impulses that result in discriminating touch and pressure sensations—by way of the fasciculi cuneatus and gracilis and the medial lemniscus
I. Sensory impulses, in addition to being conducted to the cerebral cortex by 3-neuron relays such as described above (in A, F, G, and H), are also conducted to it via complex multineuron pathways known as the reticular activating system; spinoreticular tracts relay sensory impulses up the cord to the brainstem reticular gray matter, and from here other neurons relay them to the hypothalamus, thalamus, and probably other parts of the brain, then finally to the cerebral cortex; conduction by the reticular activating system is essential for producing and maintaining consciousness; presumably, general anesthetics produce unconsciousness by inhibiting conduction by the reticular activating

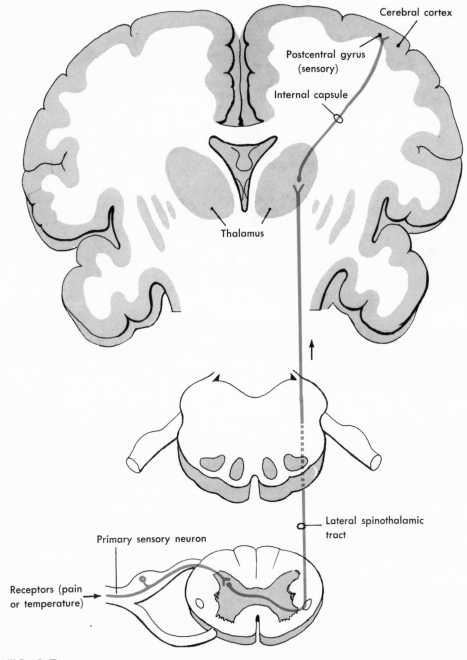

FIG. 1-7

The right and left lateral spinothalamic tracts (axons of sensory neurons II) relay sensory impulses from pain and temperature receptors. (From Anthony, C. P., and Kolthoff, N. J.: Textbook of anatomy and physiology, ed. 8, St. Louis, 1971, The C. V. Mosby Co.)

system; conversely, amphetamines and norepinephrine are thought to produce wakefulness by stimulating the reticular activating system

5. **Motor neural pathways to skeletal muscles**
A. Principle of the final common path—the final common path for impulse conduction to skeletal muscles consists of anterior horn neurons (i.e., motoneurons whose dendrites and cell bodies lie in the anterior gray columns of the cord and whose axons extend out through the anterior roots of spinal nerves and their branches to terminate in skeletal muscles); besides being referred to as the final common path and as anterior horn cells, these neurons are also called lower motoneurons and somatic motoneurons
B. Principle of convergence—axons of many neurons converge on (i.e., synapse with) each anterior horn motoneuron
C. Motor pathways from the cerebral cortex to anterior horn cells are classified according to the route by which the fibers enter the cord:
   1. Pyramidal tracts (or corticospinal tracts)—axons of neurons whose dendrites and cell bodies lie in the cerebral cortex; axons descend from cortex through internal capsule, pyramids of medulla, and spinal cord; a few of these axons synapse with anterior horn cells, but most of them synapse with internuncial neurons that synapse with anterior horn cells; conduction by pyramidal tracts must occur in order for willed movements to occur; hence one cause of paralysis is interruption of pyramidal tract conduction
   2. Extrapyramidal tracts—all tracts that conduct between the motor cortex and anterior horn cells, except the pyramidal tracts; upper extrapyramidal tracts relay impulses between the cortex, basal ganglia, thalamus, and brainstem; reticulospinal tracts (the main lower extrapyramidal tracts) relay impulses from the brainstem to the anterior horn cells in the cord; impulse conduction via extrapyramidal tracts is essential for producing normal large, automatic movements (e.g., walking, swimming) and for producing facial expressions and movements that characterize many emotions

D. The motor conduction pathway from the the cerebral cortex primary motor area to skeletal muscles via pyramidal tracts consists of a 2-neuron relay; an upper motoneuron conducts impulses from cerebrum to cord, and a lower motoneuron (anterior horn cell) conducts from cord to skeletal muscle (Fig. 1-8)
E. The motor conduction pathway from the cerebral cortex via extrapyramidal tracts consists of complex multineuron relays; several upper motoneurons relay impulses through basal ganglia, thalamus, and brainstem, and down the cord to the lower motoneuron
F. Motor pathways from the cerebral cortex to anterior horn cells are classified according to their influence on anterior horn cells as follows
   1. Facilitatory tracts—conduct impulses that have a facilitating or stimulating effect on anterior horn cells; main facilitatory tracts are the pyramidal tracts and the facilitatory reticulospinal tracts
   2. Inhibitory tracts—conduct impulses that have an inhibiting effect on anterior horn cells: main inhibitory tracts are the inhibitory reticulospinal tracts; interruption of inhibitory reticulospinal tracts results in spasticity (rigidity)
G. The ratio of facilitatory and inhibitory impulses impinging on anterior horn cells determines their activity (i.e., whether they are facilitated, stimulated, or inhibited)

6. **Autonomic nervous system**
A. Definition—the autonomic nervous system is the division of the nervous system that conducts impulses from the brainstem or cord out to visceral effectors. Visceral effectors are cardiac muscle, smooth muscle, and glandular tissue; briefly, then, the autonomic nervous system is the division of the nervous system that controls the body's automatic parts, those not controlled by the individual's will (with a few rare exceptions)
B. Divisions—autonomic nervous system consists of two divisions: the sympathetic (or thoracolumbar) system and the parasympathetic (or craniosacral) system
C. Organs
   1. Sympathetic system
      a. Sympathetic ganglia—two chains

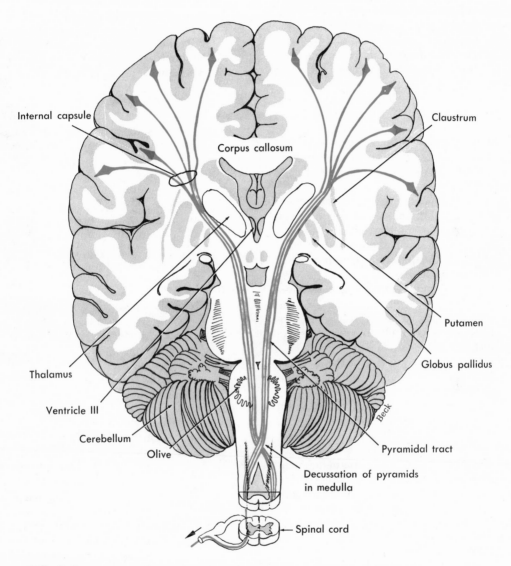

Internal capsule

Corpus callosum

Claustrum

Putamen

Globus pallidus

Thalamus

Ventricle III

Cerebellum

Olive

Pyramidal tract

Decussation of pyramids
in medulla

Spinal cord

Beck

FIG. 1-8

The crossed pyramidal tracts (lateral corticospinal), the main motor tracts of the body. Axons that compose pyramidal tracts come from neuron cell bodies in the cerebral cortex (mainly in motor area 4). After they descend through the internal capsule of the cerebrum and the white matter of the brainstem, about ¾ of the fibers decussate—cross over from one side to the other—in the medulla, as shown here. Then they continue downward in the lateral corticospinal tract on the opposite side of the cord. Each lateral corticospinal tract, therefore, conducts motor impulses from one side of the brain to skeletal muscles on the opposite side of the body. (From Anthony, C. P., and Kolthoff, N. J.: Textbook of anatomy and physiology, ed. 8, St. Louis, 1971, The C. V. Mosby Co.)

of 21 or 22 ganglia located immediately in front of the spinal column, one chain to the right, one to the left of it

  b. Collateral ganglia—located a short distance from the cord; e.g., celiac ganglia (solar plexus), superior and inferior mesenteric ganglia
  c. Sympathetic nerves—e.g., splanchnic nerves, cardiac nerves
 2. Parasympathetic system
  a. Parasympathetic ganglia—located at a distance from the spinal column, in or near visceral effectors; e.g., ciliary ganglion in posterior part of the orbit, near the iris and ciliary muscle (visceral effectors of the eye)
  b. Parasympathetic nerves—e.g., vagus nerve, called the "great parasympathetic nerve" of the body
D. Neurons
 1. Preganglionic sympathetic neurons— dendrites and cell bodies lie in lateral gray columns of thoracic and lumbar segments of cord; axons conduct from cord to sympathetic ganglia or to collateral ganglia
 2. Postganglionic sympathetic neurons— dendrites and cell bodies lie in sympathetic ganglia or in collateral ganglia; axons conduct to visceral effectors
 3. Preganglionic parasympathetic neurons—dendrites and cell bodies of some of these neurons lie in gray matter of brainstem and others lie in gray matter of sacral segments of cord; conduct impulses from brainstem or cord to parasympathetic ganglia
 4. Postganglionic parasympathetic neurons—dendrites and cell bodies lie in parasympathetic ganglia; axons conduct to visceral effectors
E. Some principles about the autonomic nervous system
 1. Dual autonomic innervation—both sympathetic and parasympathetic fibers supply most visceral effectors
 2. Single autonomic innervation—only sympathetic fibers supply sweat glands and probably the smooth muscles of hairs and of most blood vessels; preganglionic sympathetic fibers terminate in adrenal medulla (not postganglionic fibers as in other glands)

 3. Autonomic chemical transmitters—all preganglionic axons are cholinergic fibers, as are most (or perhaps all) parasympathetic postganglionic axons and a few sympathetic postganglionic axons (to sweat glands, external genitalia, and to smooth muscle in walls of blood vessels located in skeletal muscles); sympathetic postganglionic axons are the only adrenergic (i.e., release norepinephrine) fibers; but, as just mentioned, a few of them are cholinergic
 4. Autonomic antagonism and summation—sympathetic and parasympathetic impulses tend to produce opposite effects; algebraic sum of two opposing tendencies determines response made by doubly innervated visceral effector
 5. The principle of parasympathetic dominance of the digestive tract: normally, parasympathetic impulses to digestive tract glands and smooth muscle dominate over sympathetic impulses to them—dominance of parasympathetic impulses promotes digestive gland secretion, peristalsis, and defecation
 6. The principle of sympathetic dominance in stress: under the condition of stress, sympathetic impulses to visceral effectors generally increase greatly and dominate over parasympathetic impulses; notable exception —in some individuals under stress, parasympathetic impulses via the vagus nerve to glands and smooth muscle of the stomach greatly increase, causing increased hydrochloric acid secretion and increased gastric motility that eventually cause peptic ulcer, a condition that may aptly be called the great parasympathetic stress disease
 7. In general, when the sympathetic system dominates control of visceral effectors, it causes them to function in ways that enable the body to expend maximum energy as is necessary in strenuous exercise and other types of stress; see Table 1-7 for sympathetic effects on specific effectors
 8. Principle of nonautonomy—autonomic nervous system not autonomous; neither anatomically nor physiologically independent of rest of nervous sys-

TABLE 1-7

AUTONOMIC FUNCTIONS*

Visceral effectors	Parasympathetic (cholinergic) effects	Sympathetic (adrenergic or cholinergic) effects
Cardiac muscle	Slows heart rate; decreases strength of contraction	Accelerates rate; increases strength of contraction
Smooth muscle Of blood vessels in skin	No parasympathetic fibers	Adrenergic sympathetic fibers → stimulate → constrict skin vessels
Of blood vessels in skeletal muscles	No parasympathetic fibers	Adrenergic sympathetic fibers → stimulate → constrict skeletal muscle vessels Cholinergic sympathetic fibers → inhibit → dilate skeletal muscle vessels
Of blood vessels in brain, viscera, and genitalia	Parasympathetic fibers → inhibit → dilate vessels in brain, viscera, and genitalia	Adrenergic sympathetic fibers → stimulate → constrict vessels in brain and viscera Cholinergic sympathetic fibers → inhibit → dilate vessels in external genitalia
Of bronchi	Stimulates → bronchial constriction	Inhibits → bronchial dilatation
Of digestive tract	Stimulates → increased peristalsis	Inhibits → decreased peristalsis
Of anal sphincter	Inhibits → opens sphincter for defecation	Stimulates → closes sphincter
Of urinary bladder	Stimulates → contracts bladder	Inhibits → relaxes bladder
Of urinary sphincters	Inhibits → opens sphincter for urination	Stimulates → closes sphincter
Of eye (a) Iris	Stimulates circular fibers → constriction of pupil	Stimulates radial fibers → dilatation of pupil
(b) Ciliary	Stimulates → accommodation for near vision (bulging of lens)	Inhibits → accommodation for far vision (flattening of lens)
Of hairs (pilomotor muscles)	No parasympathetic fibers	Stimulates → "goose pimples"
Glands Sweat	No parasympathetic fibers	Cholinergic sympathetic fibers stimulate sweat glands
Digestive (salivary, gastric, etc.)	Stimulate secretion	Decrease secretion
Pancreas, including islets	Stimulates secretion	Decreases secretion
Liver	No parasympathetic fibers	Stimulates glycogenolysis which tends to increase blood sugar
Adrenal medulla	No parasympathetic fibers	Stimulates adrenaline secretion which tends to increase blood sugar, blood pressure, and heart rate and to produce many other sympathetic effects

*From Anthony, C. P., and Kolthoff, N. J.: Textbook of anatomy and physiology, ed. 8, St. Louis, 1971, The C. V. Mosby Co.

TABLE 1-8
RECEPTORS

Kinds	Locations	Stimulated by	Functions
Exteroceptors	Skin, mucosa, ear, eye	Changes in external environment (e.g., pressure, heat, cold, light waves, sound waves)	Initiate reflexes Initiate sensations of many kinds (e.g., pressure, heat, cold, pain, vision, hearing)
Visceroceptors (interoceptors)	Viscera	Changes in internal environment (e.g., pressure, chemical)	Initiate reflexes Initiate sensations of many kinds (e.g., hunger, sex, nausea, pressure)
Proprioceptors	Muscles, tendons, joints, semicircular canals of inner ear	Pressure changes	Initiate reflexes Initiate muscle sense, or sense of position and movement of parts; also called kinesthesia

tem; all parts of nervous system work together as single functional unit; e.g., dendrites and cells of all preganglionic neurons located in gray matter of brainstem or cord (lower autonomic centers) and influenced by impulses conducted to them from higher autonomic centers, notably in hypothalamus

9. Importance of autonomic nervous system to homeostasis—autonomic system plays major role in maintaining homeostasis; under usual conditions, autonomic impulses regulate activities of visceral effectors so that they maintain or quickly restore homeostasis; under highly stressful conditions, homeostasis may not be maintained

7. **Sense organs**
A. General remarks—millions of receptors distributed widely throughout skin, mucosa; muscles, tendons, joints, and viscera are "sense organs" of body (Table 1-8)
B. Sense organs of skin and mucosa—consist of receptors for spinal or cranial nerve branches; different types of receptors for different sensations such as heat, cold, pain, touch, and pressure; receptors unevenly distributed through skin and mucosa, joints, internal organs, etc.
C. Sense organs of muscles, tendons, and joints—(proprioceptors); several types, e.g., muscle and tendon "spindles," stimulated by so-called "stretch stimuli"; i.e.,

pressure on spindles due to stretching of muscles or tendons, during movements, initiates "stretch reflexes," e.g., knee jerk
D. Eye—highly specialized receptor
1. Anatomy
   a. Coats of eyeball (Table 1-9)
   b. Cavities and humors of eyeball (Table 1-10)
   c. Muscles of the eye (Table 1-11)
   d. Refractory media of eye
      (1) Cornea
      (2) Aqueous humor
      (3) Crystalline lens (has greatest refractive power)
      (4) Vitreous humor
   e. Accessory structures of eye
      (1) Eyebrows and lashes
      (2) Eyelids or palpebrae—lined with mucous membrane that continues over surface of eyeball, called conjunctiva; opening between lids—palpebral fissure; corners of eyes where upper and lower lids join, called inner and outer canthus, respectively
      (3) Lacrimal apparatus—lacrimal glands, ducts, sacs, and nasolacrimal ducts
2. Physiology of vision
   a. Formation of image on retina; accomplished by
      (1) Refraction (bending) of light rays as they pass through eye
      (2) Accommodation (i.e., bulging

TABLE 1-9

COATS OF THE EYEBALL

Location	Posterior portion	Anterior portion	Characteristics
Outer coat (sclera)	Sclera proper	Cornea	Protective fibrous coat; cornea, transparent; rest of coat, white and opaque
Middle coat (chorioid)	Chorioid proper	Ciliary body; suspensory ligament; iris (pupil, hole in iris); lens suspended in suspensory ligament	Vascular, pigmented coat
Inner coat (retina)	Retina	No anterior portion	Composed of three layers of neurons: visual receptors are called *rods* and *cones*; are beginnings of dendrites of photoreceptor neurons; cones most numerous in *fovea centralis,* a small depression in the *macula lutea* (yellowish area near center of retina); rods absent from fovea, numerous in peripheral areas of retina

TABLE 1-10

SUMMARY OF THE CAVITIES OF THE EYE

Cavity	Divisions	Location	Contents
Anterior	Anterior chamber Posterior chamber	Anterior to iris, posterior to cornea Posterior to iris, anterior to lens	Aqueous humor Aqueous humor
Posterior	None	Posterior to lens	Vitreous humor

TABLE 1-11

EYE MUSCLES

Location	Kind of muscle	Names	Functions
Extrinsic—attached to outside of eyeball and to bones of orbit	Skeletal (voluntary striated)	Superior rectus Inferior rectus Lateral rectus Mesial rectus Superior oblique Inferior oblique	Move eyeball in various directions
Intrinsic—within eyeball	Visceral (involuntary, smooth)	Iris Ciliary muscle	Regulates size of pupil Controls shape of lens, making possible accommodation for near and far objects

TABLE 1-12

DIVISIONS OF INTERNAL EAR (LABYRINTH)

Bony labyrinth (part of temporal bone)	Membranous labyrinth (inside bony labyrinth)
1. Vestibule Central section of bony labyrinth; oval and round windows are openings of middle ear into vestibule; bony semicircular canals also open into vestibule	1. Utricle—one of the parts of the membranous labyrinth contained in bony vestibule but separated from it by fluid called perilymph; utricle contains fluid called endolymph and structure called the macula, which is a sense organ (for the senses of equilibrium, head positions, and acceleration); vestibular nerve (branch of eighth cranial nerve) supplies macula 2. Saccule—another part of the membranous labyrinth within bony vestibule; separated from vestibule by perilymph; contains endolymph and macula
2. Cochlea A spiralling bony tube that resembles a snail shell in shape	3. Cochlear duct—membranous tube that forms shelf across interior of bony cochlea; contains endolymph and organ of Corti, the sense organ for hearing; cochlear nerve (branch of eighth cranial nerve) supplies organ of Corti; cochlear duct separated from bony cochlea by scala vestibuli and scala tympani, spaces that contain perilymph
3. Bony semicircular canals Three of these semicircular-shaped canals; each lies at approximately right angle to the others	4. Membranous semicircular canals—separated from bony semicircular canals by perilymph; contain endolymph and structure called the crista, a sense organ for the senses of equilibrium and head movements; vestibular nerve supplies crista

of lens for viewing near objects)

(3) Constriction of pupil; occurs simultaneously with accommodation, and in bright light

(4) Convergence of eyes for near objects in order that light rays from object may fall on corresponding points of two retinas; necessary for single binocular vision

b. Stimulation of retina; dim light causes breakdown of chemical rhodopsin present in rods, thereby initiating impulse conduction by rods, whereas bright light causes breakdown of chemicals in cones; hence, rods considered receptors for night vision and cones for daylight and color vision

c. Conduction to visual area in occipital lobe of cerebral cortex by fibers of optic nerves and optic tracts; vision occurs when impulses reach visual area

E. Ear

1. External ear—consists of auricle (or pinna) and external acoustic meatus (ear canal)

2. Middle ear—separated from external ear by tympanic membrane; middle ear contains auditory ossicles (malleus, incus, stapes) and openings from auditory (eustachian) tubes, mastoid cells, external ear, and internal ear (fenestra rotunda and ovalis); auditory tube, collapsible, lined with mucosa, extends from nasopharynx to middle ear; function—to equalize pressure on both sides of eardrum, as when tubes open during yawning or swallowing

3. Inner ear (or labyrinth)—composed of a bony labyrinth that has a membranous labyrinth inside it; parts of the inner ear (Table 1-12) are the following

a. Bony vestibule that contains the membranous utricle and saccule, each of which, in turn, contains a sense organ called the macula; vestibular nerve (branch of eighth cranial nerve) supplies the maculae; maculae are sense organs for three sensations: equilibrium, position of the head, and acceleration and deceleration

b. Bony semicircular canals that contain the membranous semicircular canals in which are located the *crista ampullaris,* the sense organ for sensations of equilibrium and head movements; vestibular nerve supplies the crista as well as the macula

   c. Bony *cochlea* that contains the membranous *cochlear duct* in which is located the *organ of Corti,* the hearing sense organ; cochlear nerve (branch of eighth cranial nerve) supplies the organ of Corti

4. Physiology of hearing

   a. Sound waves moving through air enter ear canal and move down it to strike against the tympanic membrane, causing it to vibrate

   b. Vibrations of tympanic membrane move the malleus, whose handle is attached to the membrane

   c. Movement of the malleus moves the incus, to which the head of the malleus attaches

   d. Incus attaches to the stapes; so as the incus moves, it moves the stapes against the oval window into which it fits; as the stapes presses inwardly on the perilymph around the cochlear duct, it starts a "ripple" in the perilymph

   e. Movement of the perilymph is transmitted to the endolymph inside the cochlear duct and stimulates the organ of Corti, which projects into the endolymph

   f. Cochlear nerve conducts impulses from the organ of Corti to the brain; hearing occurs when impulses reach the auditory area in the temporal lobe of the cerebral cortex

F. Olfactory sense organs—consist of receptors for first cranial nerves; located in nasal mucosa high along septum; highly sensitive to chemical stimuli, but easily fatigued

G. Gustatory sense organs—consist of receptors for cranial nerves VII and IX; called taste corpuscles, or taste buds; located in papillae of tongue, taste buds sensitive to sweet are most numerous at the tip of the tongue, those sensitive to sour and salt are most numerous at the tip and sides of the tongue, and those sensitive to bitter are most numerous at the back of the tongue; all tastes except sweet, sour, salt, and bitter result from fusion of two or more of these tastes plus olfactory stimulation

Endocrine system

1. **Organs—all ductless glands**
   Their secretions (hormones) enter blood, not ducts; see Table 1-13 for names of major endocrine glands and their hormones

2. **General functions**
   Same as general functions of nervous system: communication, control, integration

3. **Functions of anterior pituitary hormones**
   See Table 1-14

4. **Control of hormone secretion by anterior pituitary gland**

A. By the hypothalamus—certain neurons of hypothalamus synthesize and secrete chemicals into blood vessels (i.e., the hypothalamico-hypophyseal portal system), which transport them to the anterior pituitary, where they either stimulate or inhibit secretion of specific hormones; names of these chemicals and their effects are

   1. GH-RF (growth hormone–releasing factor) stimulates growth hormone secretion by anterior pituitary

   2. TRF (thyrotropin-releasing factor) stimulates thyrotropin secretion by anterior pituitary

   3. CRF (corticotropin, i.e., ACTH-releasing factor) stimulates ACTH secretion by anterior pituitary

   4. FSH-RF (follicle-stimulating hormone–releasing factor) stimulates FSH secretion by anterior pituitary

   5. LH-RF (luteinizing hormone–releasing factor) stimulates LH secretion by anterior pituitary

   6. PIF (prolactin-inhibiting factor) inhibits prolactin secretion by anterior pituitary; after childbirth, PIF secretion ceases, thereby allowing prolactin secretion and lactation

   7. MIF (melanocyte-stimulating hormone–inhibiting factor) inhibits MSH secretion by anterior pituitary

B. By negative feedback mechanisms as follows

   1. Between thyroid hormones and TSH; high blood levels of thyroid hormones inhibit TSH secretion by anterior

TABLE 1-13

ENDOCRINE GLANDS—LOCATIONS AND HORMONES

Endocrine glands	Location	Hormones
Anterior pituitary (adeno-hypophysis)	Cranial cavity, in sella turcica of sphenoid bone	1. Growth hormone (GH, somatotropin, somatropic hormone, STH) 2. Thyrotropin (thyroid-stimulating hormone or TSH) 3. Adrenocorticotropic hormone (ACTH, adrenocorticotropin) 4. Follicle-stimulating hormone (FSH) 5. Luteinizing hormone (LH) in female; interstitial cell–stimulating hormone (ICSH) in male 6. Prolactin (lactogenic hormone) 7. Melanocyte-stimulating hormone (MSH)
Posterior pituitary (neuro-hypophysis)		1. Antidiuretic hormone (ADH, vasopressin, Pitressin)° 2. Oxytocin
Thyroid	Neck	1. Thyroid hormones (thyroxine and triiodothyronine) 2. Thyrocalcitonin
Parathyroids		1. Parathyroid hormone (PTH, parathormone)
Adrenal cortex	Abdominal cavity	1. Glucocorticoids (mainly, cortisol and corticosterone) 2. Mineralocorticoids (mainly, aldosterone) 3. Sex hormones (small amounts of androgens and estrogens)
Adrenal medulla		1. Epinephrine (mainly) 2. Norepinephrine
Islands of Langerhans		1. Insulin (secreted by beta cells) 2. Glucagon (secreted by alpha cells)

Ovaries
  1. Graafian follicles
  2. Corpus luteum
	Pelvic cavity (female)	1. Estrogens
		2. Progesterone

Interstitial cells of testes	Scrotum (male)	1. Testosterone

°ADH and oxytocin are synthesized in the hypothalamus but are secreted by the posterior pituitary gland. Synthesis occurs in cell bodies of neurons of the supraoptic and paraventricular nuclei. From here they migrate down the neurons' axons into the posterior pituitary gland, which secretes them into the blood.

pituitary (either directly by inhibiting the anterior pituitary gland or indirectly by inhibiting the hypothalamus' secretion of TRF, or perhaps by both actions)

2. Between corticoids and ACTH; high blood levels of corticoids inhibit ACTH secretion by anterior pituitary either directly or indirectly by inhibiting CRF secretion by hypothalamus

3. Between progesterone and LH; high blood levels of LH directly or indirectly inhibit LH secretion by anterior pituitary

4. Between estrogens and FSH; high blood levels of estrogens directly or indirectly inhibit FSH secretion by anterior pituitary

C. By other mechanisms—for example, stress and low blood sugar are known to increase growth hormone secretion, and suckling increases prolactin secretion

5. **Functions of posterior pituitary hormones**
   See Table 1-15

6. **Control of hormone secretion by the posterior pituitary gland**

A. ADH secretion is controlled chiefly by the osmotic pressure and volume of the

TABLE 1-14
FUNCTIONS OF ANTERIOR PITUITARY HORMONES

Hormones	Functions	Hyposecretion effects	Hypersecretion effects
1. Growth hormone (GH)	a. Promotes protein anabolism (hence essential for normal growth) b. Promotes fat mobilization and catabolism; i.e., causes shift from carbohydrate catabolism to fat catabolism c. Slows carbohydrate metabolism; has anti-insulin, hyperglycemic, diabetogenic effect	Dwarfism (well-formed type)	Giantism (if occurs before skeleton full-grown) Acromegaly (if occurs in adult) Hyperglycemia; chronic excess GH may cause diabetes mellitus
2. TSH	a. Stimulates synthesis and secretion of thyroid hormones	Hypothyroidism; myxedema	Hyperthyroidism (exophthalmic goiter, various other names)
3. ACTH	a. Stimulates adrenal cortex growth and secretion of glucocorticoids	Atrophy of adrenal cortex and hyposecretion (e.g., Addison's disease) Increased skin pigmentation	Hypertrophy of adrenal cortex and hypersecretion (Cushing's syndrome)
4. FSH	a. Stimulates primary graafian follicle to start growing and to develop to maturity b. Stimulates follicle cells to secrete estrogens c. In male, FSH stimulates development of seminiferous tubules and spermatogenesis by them	Failure of follicle and ovum to grow and mature; sterility	
5. LH	a. Essential for bringing about complete maturation of follicle and ovum b. Causes ovulation; therefore, LH also known as the ovulating hormone c. Causes formation of corpus luteum in ruptured follicle following ovulation; hence the name, luteinizing hormone d. Stimulates corpus luteum to secrete progesterone e. In male, LH is called ICSH (interstitial cell–stimulating hormone) because it stimulates interstitial cells of testes to secrete testosterone		
6. Prolactin	a. Promotes breast development during pregnancy b. Initiates milk secretion after delivery of baby	Failure to lactate	
7. MSH (melanocyte-stimulating hormone)	a. Postulated to increase skin pigmentation by stimulating formation and dispersion of melanin granules in man, as it is known to do in lower animals		

TABLE 1-15
FUNCTIONS OF POSTERIOR PITUITARY HORMONES

Hormones	Functions	Hyposecretion effects	Hypersecretion effects
1. ADH (anti-diuretic hormone; vasopressin)	a. Increases water reabsorption by kidney's distal and collecting tubules, thereby producing anti-diuresis (less urine volume; name based on this effect)	Diuresis (polyuria); diabetes insipidus	Antidiuresis (oliguria)
2. Oxytocin (the "quick-birth hormone")	a. Stimulates powerful contractions by pregnant uterus; name oxytocin from Greek for "swift childbirth" b. Stimulates milk ejection from alveoli (milk-secreting cells) of lactating breasts into ducts; essential before milk can be removed by suckling		

TABLE 1-16
FUNCTIONS OF THYROID AND PARATHYROID HORMONES

Hormones	Functions	Hypofunction effects	Hyperfunction effects
1. Thyroid hormones (thyroxine and tri-iodothyronine)	a. Stimulate metabolic rate; therefore, essential for normal physical and mental development b. Inhibit anterior pituitary secretion of TSH	Cretinism, if occurs early in life; myxedema, if occurs in older children or adults	Hyperthyroidism
2. Thyrocalcitonin	a. Quickly decreases blood calcium concentration if it increases about 20% above normal level; presumably accelerates calcium movement from blood into bone		
Parathyroid hormones 1. Parathormone	a. Increases blood calcium concentration by accelerating following three processes:	Decreased blood calcium (hypocalcemia) which causes increased neural excitability and tetany	Increased blood calcium (hypercalcemia) which causes decreased neural excitability and muscle weakness
	(1) breakdown of bone with release of calcium into blood		Bone "softening"—decalcification
	(2) calcium absorption from intestine into blood		
	(3) kidney tubule reabsorption of calcium from tubular urine into blood, thereby decreasing calcium loss in urine		
	b. Decreases blood phosphate concentration by slowing its reabsorption by kidney tubules and thereby increasing phosphate loss in urine	Increased blood phosphorus (hyperphosphatemia)	Hypophosphatemia

TABLE 1-17

FUNCTIONS OF ADRENAL CORTEX HORMONES

Hormones	Functions	Hypofunction effects (e.g., in Addison's disease)	Hyperfunction effects (e.g., in Cushing's syndrome)
1. Glucocorticoids (GC's), mainly cortisol (hydrocortisone) and corticosterone	In general, a normal blood concentration of glucocorticoids promotes normal metabolism of all three kinds of foods and a high blood concentration produces various stress responses, e.g.:		
	a. Accelerates mobilization and catabolism of fats; i.e., causes shift from usual utilization of carbohydrates for energy to fat utilization		
	b. Accelerates tissue protein mobilization and catabolism; (tissue proteins hydrolyzed to amino acids which enter blood and are carried to liver for deamination and gluconeogenesis)		Muscle atrophy and weakness; osteoporosis
	c. Accelerates liver gluconeogenesis; i.e., formation of glucose from mobilized proteins (hyperglycemic effect)		Hyperglycemia
	d. Causes atrophy of lymphatic tissues, notably thymus and lymph nodes		Lymphocytopenia
	e. Decreases antibody formation (immunosuppressive, antiallergic effect)		Decreased immunity Decreased allergy
	f. Slows the proliferation of fibroblasts characteristic of inflammation (anti-inflammatory effect)		Spread of infections; slower wound healing
	g. Mild acceleration of sodium and water reabsorption and potassium excretion by kidney tubules		High blood sodium (hypernatremia; sodium retention); also water retention; low blood potassium (hypokalemia)
	h. Decreases ACTH secretion		
2. Mineralocorticoids (MC's), mainly aldosterone	a. Marked acceleration of sodium and water reabsorption by kidney tubules	Low blood sodium (hyponatremia); dehydration	High blood sodium (hypernatremia); water retention, edema
	b. Marked acceleration of potassium excretion by kidney tubules	High blood potassium (hyperkalemia)	Low blood potassium (hypokalemia)

extracellular fluid; a decrease in ECF volume and/or an increase in ECF osmotic pressure stimulates hypothalamic neurons (in supraoptic nuclei) to synthesize more ADH and, as a result, the posterior pituitary secretes more ADH

B. Oxytocin secretion is increased by stimulation of mother's nipples by baby's nursing

7. **Functions of thyroid and parathyroid hormones**
   See Table 1-16

8. **Control of thyroid secretion of hormones**

A. TRF (thyroid-releasing factor) from hypothalamus stimulates anterior pituitary secretion of TSH (thyroid-stimulating hormone), which stimulates thyroid secretion of thyroxine and triiodothyronine

B. Blood level of calcium ions controls thyroid secretion of thyrocalcitonin; high blood concentration of calcium stimulates thyroid secretion of thyrocalcitonin

9. **Control of hormone secretion by parathyroids**

A. Low blood calcium concentration stimulates parathyroids to secrete parathyroid hormone; high blood calcium concentration inhibits parathyroid hormone secretion

B. Parathyroids, unlike most other endocrines, are not controlled by an anterior pituitary hormone

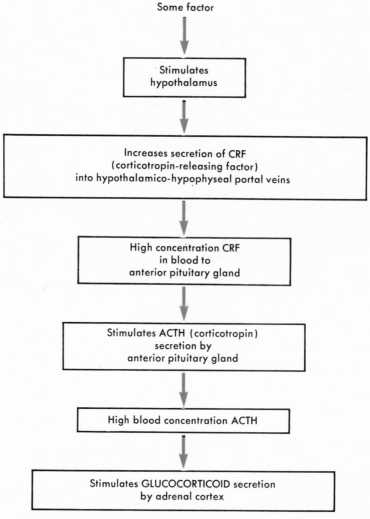

FIG. 1-9

Mechanism that controls glucocorticoid secretion.

10. **Functions of adrenal cortex hormones**
    See Table 1-17
11. **Control of hormone secretion by adrenal cortex**
A. Glucocorticoid secretion controlled by mechanism shown in Fig. 1-9
B. Aldosterone secretion controlled by mechanism shown in Fig. 1-10
12. **Functions of sex hormones**
    See Table 1-18
13. **Control of hormone secretion by ovaries**
A. Estrogens controlled by mechanism shown in Fig. 1-11
B. Progesterone—high blood concentration of LH (luteinizing hormone) stimulates progesterone secretion

14. **Control of testosterone secretion by interstitial cells of testes**
    High blood concentration of ICSH (interstitial cell–stimulating hormone, analogous to LH in female) stimulates testosterone secretion

MAINTAINING THE METABOLISM OF THE BODY
Circulatory system

1. **Functions**
A. Primary function—transportation of various substances to and from body cells
B. Secondary functions—contributes to all of body's functions: metabolism, water

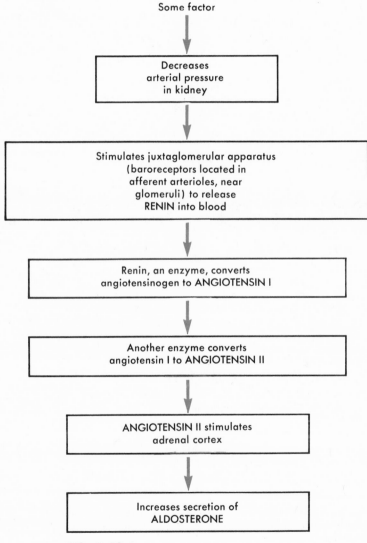

Some factor

Decreases
arterial pressure
in kidney

Stimulates juxtaglomerular apparatus
(baroreceptors located in
afferent arterioles, near
glomeruli) to release
RENIN into blood

Renin, an enzyme, converts
angiotensinogen to ANGIOTENSIN I

Another enzyme converts
angiotensin I to ANGIOTENSIN II

ANGIOTENSIN II stimulates
adrenal cortex

Increases secretion of
ALDOSTERONE

FIG. 1-10
Mechanism that controls aldosterone secretion.

TABLE 1-18

FUNCTIONS OF SEX HORMONES (OVARIAN AND TESTICULAR)

Hormones	Functions
1. Estrogens (secreted by graafian follicle and corpus luteum)	a. Stimulate proliferation of epithelial cells of female reproductive organs; e.g., thickening of endometrium, breast development b. Stimulate uterine contractions c. Accelerate protein anabolism (including bone matrix synthesis) so promote growth; but also promote epiphyseal closure so limit height d. Mildly accelerate sodium and water reabsorption by kidney tubules; increase water content of uterus e. High blood estrogen concentration inhibits anterior pituitary secretion of FSH and prolactin but stimulates its secretion of LH f. Low blood estrogen concentration after delivery of baby stimulates anterior pituitary secretion of prolactin
2. Progesterone (secreted by corpus luteum)	Name "progesterone" indicates hormone's general function, "favoring pregnancy," e.g.: a. Stimulates secretion by endometrial glands (thereby preparing endometrium for implantation of fertilized ovum) b. Inhibits uterine contractions (thereby favoring retention of implanted ovum) c. Promotes development of alveoli (secreting cells) of estrogen-primed breasts; necessary for lactation d. Protein-catabolic and salt and water-retaining effects similar to corticoids but milder; increases water content of endometrium
3. Testosterone (secreted by interstitial cells of testes)	a. Growth and development of male reproductive organs; promotes "maleness" b. Marked stimulating effect on protein anabolism, including synthesis of bone matrix; hence, promotes growth; however, it also tends to limit height by promoting epiphyseal closure c. Mild acceleration of kidney tubule reabsorption of sodium chloride and water d. Inhibits secretion of ICSH by anterior pituitary

balance, homeostasis of pH and temperature, defense against microorganisms, etc.
2. **Blood cells**
A. Kinds
  1. Red blood cells (erythrocytes)
  2. White blood cells (leukocytes)
    a. Neutrophils—constitute 65% to 75% of total white count
    b. Eosinophils—constitute 2% to 5% of total white count
    c. Basophils—constitute 0.5% to 1% of total white count
    d. Lymphocytes—constitute about 20% to 25% of total white count
    e. Monocytes—constitute 3% to 8% of total white count
B. Number (Table 1-19)
C. Function (Table 1-19)
D. Formation (hemopoiesis) (Table 1-19)
E. Destruction—see Table 1-19
3. **Blood types**
A. Names—indicate type antigens on or in red cell membrane; e.g., type A blood means that red cells have A antigens; type O means that red cells have no antigens

B. Every person's blood belongs to one of the four AB blood groups (type A, type B, type AB, or type O) and, in addition, is either Rh-positive or Rh-negative
C. Plasma—normally contains no antibodies against antigens present on its own red cells but does contain antibodies against other A or B antigens not present on its red cells; e.g., type A plasma does not contain antibodies against A antigen but does contain antibodies against B antigen
D. No blood ever normally contains anti-Rh antibodies, and Rh-positive blood never contains them; in short, only Rh-negative blood ever contains anti-Rh antibodies, and then only if previously the individual has either been transfused with Rh-positive blood or has carried an Rh-positive fetus
E. The potential danger in transfusing blood is that the donor's blood may be agglutinated (clumped) by the recipient's antibodies, and plug some vital small vessel
F. Universal donor—type O (because red

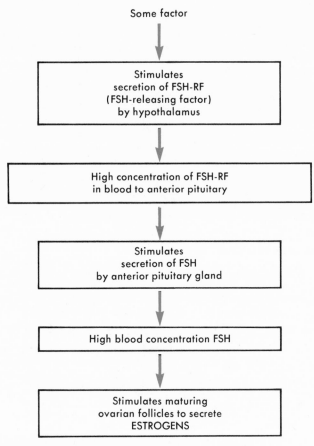

FIG. 1-11

Mechanism that controls estrogen secretion.

cells have neither A nor B antigens, they cannot be agglutinated if recipient's blood contains antibodies against them)

G. Universal recipient—type AB (red cells have both A and B antigens but agglutination of these not dangerous because too few recipient red cells can be clumped at one time by donor's antibodies to plug vessels)

4. **Blood plasma**

A. Definition—liquid part of blood or whole blood minus cells; constitutes more than half (normally, about 55%) of total blood volume; percentage of total blood volume composed of red cells (about 45%) referred to as hematocrit

B. Composition—about 90% water, 10% solutes (e.g., electrolytes, foods, gases, hormones, antibodies)

5. **Blood clotting**

A. Purpose—to plug up ruptured vessels and thus prevent fatal hemorrhage

B. Mechanism—swift, complex mechanism for changing soluble blood protein, fibrinogen, into insoluble protein, fibrin

C. Major events in blood clotting

1. The trigger that sets in operation the blood-clotting mechanism is the appearance of a "rough" spot in the lining of a blood vessel—e.g., patch-like deposits of a cholesterol-lipid substance as in atherosclerosis, or a cut edge of a vessel

2. Within a second or so, clumps of platelets adhere to the rough spot and their membranes rupture, releasing chemicals called "platelet factors," which act as the chemical trigger for starting a series of chemical reactions to follow in quick succession and bring about coagulation (Fig. 1-12)

D. Some facts about the blood proteins essential for clotting

1. Both prothrombin and fibrinogen are

TABLE 1-19

BLOOD CELLS*

Cells	Number	Function	Formation (hemopoiesis)	Destruction
Red blood cells (erythrocytes)	4½ to 5½ million per c.mm. (total of approximately 30 trillion in body)	Transport oxygen and carbon dioxide	Red marrow of bones (myeloid tissue)	By fragmentation in circulating blood and by macrophages of spleen, liver, and red bone marrow; thought to live about 120 days in bloodstream
White blood cells (leukocytes)	5 to 9 thousand per c.mm.	Play important part in producing immunity—e.g., phagocytosis mainly by neutrophils, lymphocytes, and monocytes; antibody formation by lymphocytes	Neutrophils, eosinophils, basophils formed in red marrow; original lymphocytes formed in thymus gland of fetus; postnatally, lymphocytes formed in lymph nodes and other lymphatic tissues	Not known definitely; probably some destroyed by phagocytosis and some by microorganisms
Platelets (thrombocytes)	250,000 to 450,000 per c.mm.; wide variation with different counting methods	Initiate blood clotting	Red marrow	Unknown

*Modified from Anthony, C. P., and Kolthoff, N. J.: Textbook of anatomy and physiology, ed. 8, St. Louis, 1971, The C. V. Mosby Co.

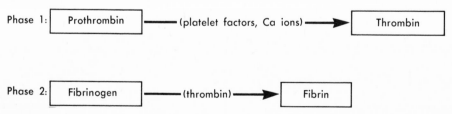

FIG. 1-12

Major chemical changes in blood clotting. Each equation summarizes a series of complex and still not completely understood chemical reactions.

soluble proteins normally present in blood in adequate amounts for clotting to occur at the normal rapid rate
2. Fibrin is an insoluble protein formed from the soluble protein fibrinogen, in the presence of the enzyme thrombin; fibrin appears as a tangled mass of threads having a jellylike texture; blood cells become enmeshed in these threads, and red cells give the clot its red color
3. Liver cells synthesize prothrombin and fibrinogen (as they do various other blood proteins); adequate amounts of vitamin K must be present in blood in order for the liver to make normal amounts of prothrombin
4. Normal blood prothrombin content: 10 to 15 mg. per 100 ml. plasma
5. Normal blood fibrinogen content: 350 mg. per 100 ml. plasma
E. Clinical applications
1. Hemophilia—hereditary disease characterized by defect in clotting ability of blood due to lack of a blood protein essential for clotting
2. Thrombosis—partial or complete occlusion of a blood vessel, due to presence of a stationary clot (thrombus)
3. Embolism—partial or complete occlusion of a blood vessel by a moving clot (embolus)
4. Atherosclerosis—plaques of lipoid material deposited in endothelium act as "rough" spots, causing platelet disintegration and thrombus formation; rough spots in blood vessel lining
5. Sluggish blood flow causes thrombus formation; frequent moving of a bed patient helps prevent sluggish blood flow, and thrombus formation
6. **Heart**
A. Location—in mediastinum with apex on diaphragm and pointing to left (apical beat may be counted by placing stethoscope in fifth intercostal space on line with left midclavicular point); two thirds of bulk of heart lies to left of midline of body, one third to right
B. Covering—pericardium
1. Structure
a. Fibrous pericardium—loose-fitting, inextensible sac around heart
b. Serous pericardium—consists of two layers
(1) Parietal layer—lines inner surface of fibrous pericardium

(2) Visceral layer (epicardium)—adheres to outer surface of the heart; pericardial space, lying between parietal and visceral layers, contains a few drops of lubricating pericardial fluid
2. Function—protects heart against friction by providing well-lubricated, smooth sac for heart to beat in
C. Structure of heart
1. Heart wall
a. Myocardium—composed of cardiac muscle cells
b. Endocardium—delicate endothelial lining of myocardium
2. Cavities
a. Upper 2 called atria (singular, atrium)
b. Lower 2 called ventricles
3. Valves and openings
a. Openings between atria and ventricles known as atrioventricular orifices
(1) Guarded by cuspid valves
(a) Tricuspid on right
(b) Mitral (bicuspid) on left
(2) Valves consist of 3 parts
(a) Flaps or cusps
(b) Chordae tendineae
(c) Papillary muscles
b. Opening from right ventricle into pulmonary artery guarded by pulmonary semilunar valves
c. Opening from left ventricle into great aorta guarded by aortic semilunar valves
4. Blood supply to myocardium (heart muscle)
a. By way of only 2 small vessels: the right and left coronary arteries, the first branches of the aorta
b. Both coronary arteries send branches to both sides of the heart
c. Right coronary branches supply right side of heart mainly, but also carry some blood to left ventricle (Table 1-20)
d. Left coronary branches supply left side of heart mainly but also, as Table 1-20 indicates, carry some blood to right ventricle
e. Most abundant blood supply of all goes to the myocardium of the left ventricle
f. Relatively few anastomoses (branches from one artery to another ar-

TABLE 1-20

CORONARY ARTERIES*

Right coronary artery	Left coronary artery
Divides into two main branches: 1. Posterior descending artery—sends branches to both ventricles 2. Marginal artery—sends branches to right ventricle and right atrium	Divides into two main branches: 1. Anterior descending artery—sends branches to both ventricles 2. Circumflex artery—sends branches to left ventricle and left atrium

*From Anthony, C. P., and Kolthoff, N. J.: Textbook of anatomy and physiology, ed. 8, St. Louis, 1971, The C. V. Mosby Co.

tery) exist between the larger branches of the coronary arteries; hence, if one of these vessels becomes occluded, little or no blood can reach the myocardial cells supplied by that vessel; deprived of an adequate blood supply, cells soon die (myocardial infarction)

5. Nerve supply to heart
   a. Sympathetic fibers (in cardiac nerves) and parasympathetic fibers (in vagus nerves) form cardiac plexuses
   b. Fibers from cardiac plexuses terminate mainly in SA node
   c. Sympathetic impulses tend to accelerate and strengthen heartbeat
   d. Parasympathetic (that is, vagal) impulses slow the heartbeat
6. Conduction system of heart
   Normally a nerve impulse begins its course through the heart in the heart's own pacemaker, i.e., in the SA (sinoatrial) node; it quickly spreads through both atria, via special conducting fibers, to the AV (atrioventricular) node; after a short delay in this node, the impulse is conducted by two branches of the AV bundle of His down both sides of the interventricular septum. From there, the impulse travels over Purkinje fibers to the lateral walls of the ventricles
   a. SA node—a cluster of cells located in the right atrial wall near the opening of the superior vena cava
   b. AV node—a small mass of special conducting cells located in the right atrium at the top of the interventricular septum
   c. AV bundle of His—special conducting fibers that originate in the AV node and extend by 2 branches down the 2 sides of the interventricular septum
   d. Purkinje fibers—special conducting fibers that extend from the AV bundle throughout the walls of the ventricles
   Impulse conduction through heart generates tiny electric currents that spread through surrounding tissues to the skin, from which visible records of conduction can be made with the electrocardiograph or oscillograph; conduction from the SA node through the atria causes atrial contraction and gives rise to the so-called P wave of the electrocardiogram; conduction from the AV node down the bundle of His and out the Purkinje fibers causes ventricular contraction and gives rise to the QRS wave

D. Physiology of heart
   1. Function—to pump varying amounts of blood through vessels as cells' needs change
   2. Cardiac cycle ("heartbeat")
      a. Nature—consists of systole (contraction) and diastole (relaxation) of atria and of ventricles; atria contract and as they relax ventricles contract
      b. Time required—about $\frac{4}{5}$ second for one cardiac cycle; so 70 to 80 cycles or heartbeats per minute

7. **Blood vessels**
A. Kinds
   1. Arteries—vessels that carry blood away from heart (all arteries except pulmonary artery carry oxygenated blood); arteries branch into smaller and smaller vessels called arterioles that branch into microscopic vessels, the capillaries
   2. Veins—vessels that carry blood toward heart (all veins except the pulmonary veins carry deoxygenated blood)
   3. Capillaries—microscopic vessels that carry blood from arterioles to venules; capillaries unite to form small veins or venules, which, in turn, unite to form veins; exchange of substances be-

TABLE 1-21
STRUCTURE OF THE BLOOD VESSELS

	Arteries	Veins	Capillaries
Coats	Lining (tunica intima) of endothelium Middle coat (tunica media) of smooth muscle, elastic, and fibrous tissues; this coat permits constriction and dilatation Outer coat (tunica adventitia or externa) of fibrous tissue; its firmness makes arteries stand open instead of collapsing when cut	Same 3 coats, but thinner and fewer elastic fibers; veins collapse when cut; semilunar valves present at intervals	Only lining coat present; therefore capillary wall only 1 cell thick
Blood supply	Endothelial lining cells supplied by blood flowing through vessels; cells of middle and outer coats supplied by tiny vessels known as the vasa vasorum or "vessels of the vessels"		
Nerve supply	Smooth muscle cells of middle coat innervated by autonomic fibers controlled by vasomotor center of medulla; able to cause either vasoconstriction or vasodilatation		
Abnormalities	Arteriosclerosis—hardening and thickening of walls of arteries Aneurysm—saclike dilatation of an artery wall Varicose veins—stretching of walls, particularly around semilunar valves Phlebitis—inflammation of vein; "milk leg," phlebitis of femoral vein of women after childbirth		

tween blood and interstitial fluid occurs in capillaries

B. Structure of blood vessels (Table 1-21)

C. Names of main blood vessels
1. Arteries (Fig. 1-13)
2. Veins—(Fig. 1-14) deep veins lie close to bones and many of them bear same name as corresponding artery; superficial veins lie near surface; veins in cranial cavity formed by dura mater, called sinuses

D. Fetal circulation—following structures essential for fetal circulation but normally cease to exist after birth
1. Umbilical arteries (2)—extensions of hypogastric arteries (internal iliacs) carry fetal blood to placenta
2. Placenta—attached to uterine wall
3. Umbilical vein—extends from placenta back to fetus' body; returns oxygenated blood from placenta to fetal circulation; 2 umbilical arteries and single umbilical vein constitute umbilical cord
4. Ductus venosus—small vessel that connects umbilical vein with inferior vena cava in fetus
5. Foramen ovale—opening in fetal heart septum between right and left atria
6. Ductus arteriosus—small vessel connecting pulmonary artery with descending thoracic aorta

Note: Only 2 fetal blood vessels carry pure, oxygenated blood—umbilical vein and ductus venosus; as soon as blood enters inferior vena cava from ductus venosus it becomes mixed with venous blood.

8. **Physiology of circulation**

A. Definitions
1. Circulation—blood flow through circuit of vessels
2. Systemic circulation—blood flow from left ventricle into aorta, other arteries, arterioles, capillaries, venules, and veins to right atrium of heart (Fig. 1-15)
3. Pulmonary circulation—blood flow from right ventricle to pulmonary artery to lung arterioles, capillaries, and venules, to pulmonary veins, to left atrium
4. Portal circulation—blood flow from capillaries, venules, and veins of stomach, intestines, and spleen into portal vein, liver arterioles, liver capillaries, to hepatic veins, to inferior vena cava

B. Principles of circulation
1. Blood circulates because a blood pressure gradient exists in its vessels; like all fluids, blood moves from region where its pressure is greater to region where pressure is less; because blood pressure highest in aorta and successively lower in arteries, arterioles, capillaries, venules, veins, and lowest in the central veins (venae

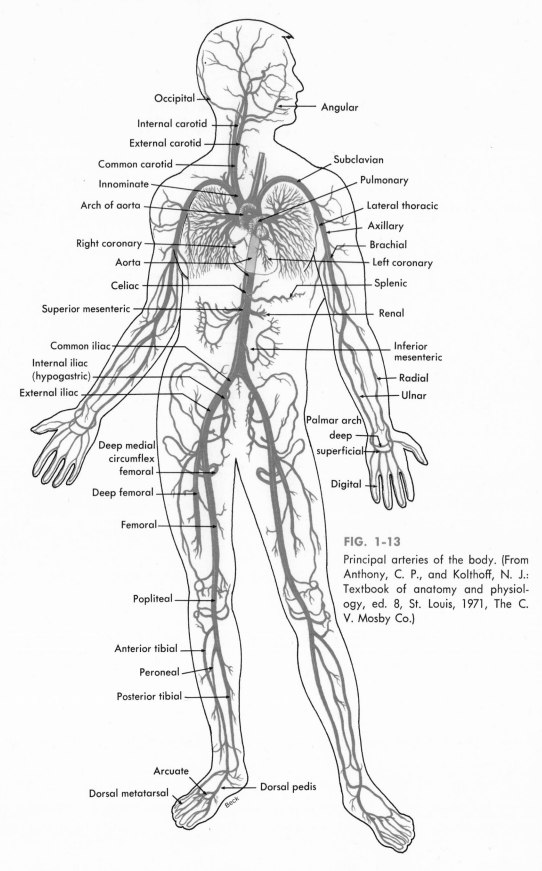

FIG. 1-13

Principal arteries of the body. (From Anthony, C. P., and Kolthoff, N. J.: Textbook of anatomy and physiology, ed. 8, St. Louis, 1971, The C. V. Mosby Co.)

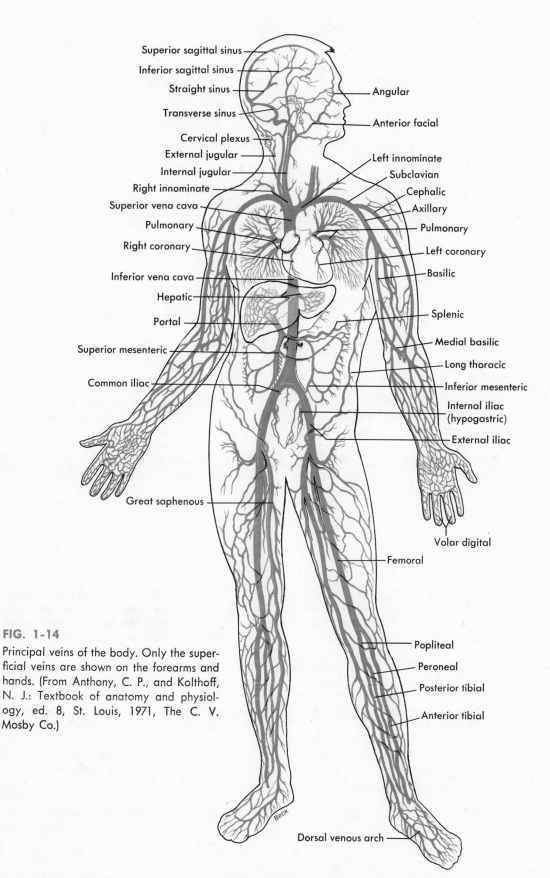

FIG. 1-14

Principal veins of the body. Only the superficial veins are shown on the forearms and hands. (From Anthony, C. P., and Kolthoff, N. J.: Textbook of anatomy and physiology, ed. 8, St. Louis, 1971, The C. V. Mosby Co.)

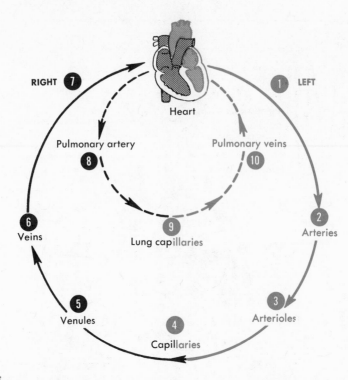

FIG. 1-15

Diagram showing the relation of systemic and pulmonary circulation. As indicated by the numbers, blood circulates from the left side of the heart to arteries, to arterioles, to capillaries, to venules, to veins, to the right side of the heart, to the lungs, and back to the left side of the heart, thereby completing a circuit. Refer to this diagram when tracing the circulation of blood to or from any part of the body. (From Anthony, C. P., and Kolthoff, N. J.: Textbook of anatomy and physiology, ed. 8, St. Louis, 1971, The C. V. Mosby Co.)

cavae), blood flows through vessels in this order (Figs. 1-15 and 1-16)
2. Normally systemic blood pressure gradient and mean arterial blood pressure about equal; reason—systemic blood pressure gradient equals mean arterial pressure minus central venous pressure (normally about zero)
3. Volume of blood circulating each minute varies directly with systemic blood pressure gradient and inversely with resistance opposing blood flow (peripheral resistance); principle is modification of Poiseuille's law; expressed as equation in simplest form and assuming central venous pressure of zero:

$$\text{Volume of blood circulating per minute} = \frac{\text{Arterial blood pressure}}{\text{Peripheral resistance}}$$

(Examine Fig. 1-17 to see what factors determine arterial pressure and peripheral resistance)
4. Arterial pressure determined directly, as Fig. 1-17 shows, by volume of blood in arteries; when arterial blood volume increases, arterial pressure tends to increase; when arterial blood volume decreases, arterial pressure tends to decrease
5. Arterial blood volume varies directly with cardiac minute output (rate × systolic discharge); anything that increases the heart rate or systolic discharge, therefore, tends to increase cardiac minute output, arterial volume, arterial pressure, systemic blood pressure gradient, and volume of blood circulating per minute
6. Heart rate is regulated mainly by pressoreflexes; briefly, increase in arterial pressure stimulates barorecep-

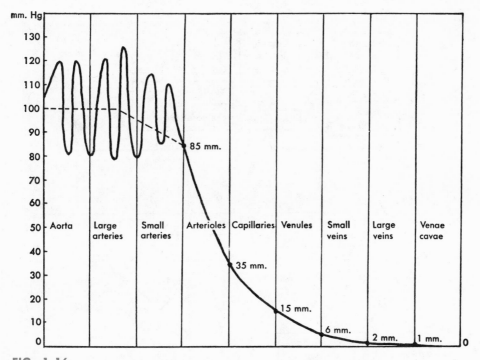

FIG. 1-16

Blood pressure gradient. Dotted line indicates average or mean systolic pressure in arteries.

tors in aorta and carotid sinus, which leads to increased parasympathetic impulses to heart (via vagus nerve), which slow the heart rate; a decrease in arterial pressure inhibits baroreceptors in aorta and carotid sinus and thereby leads to decreased parasympathetic impulses and increased sympathetic impulses to heart, which in turn causes a faster heart rate

7. Systolic discharge of heart is regulated mainly by ratio of sympathetic-parasympathetic impulses to it and by concentration of epinephrine in the blood; sympathetic dominance and a high blood epinephrine concentration increase systolic discharge; parasympathetic dominance decreases systolic discharge

8. Peripheral resistance varies directly with blood viscosity and inversely with diameter of arterioles; anything that increases blood viscosity tends to increase peripheral resistance, whereas anything that increases diameter of arterioles (dilates them) tends to decrease peripheral resistance; converse also true

9. Blood viscosity varies directly with blood protein concentration and number of blood cells; decrease in either tends to decrease blood viscosity; converse also true

10. Arteriole diameter is controlled mainly by vasomotor baroreflexes and chemoreflexes; in general, a decrease in arterial pressure initiates reflex vasoconstriction of small vessels in the so-called "blood reservoirs" (skin and abdominal viscera); conversely, an increase in arterial pressure initiates reflex vasodilatation in the skin and abdominal organs; hypoxia and hypercapnia cause vasoconstriction in the skin and abdominal organs but vasodilatation in skeletal muscles, heart, and brain

11. Increase in peripheral resistance, according to Poiseuille's law, tends to decrease circulation; at same time, however, an increase in peripheral resistance also tends to produce opposite effect; reason—increased peripheral resistance hinders blood flow out of arteries into arterioles, so more blood remains in arteries, and

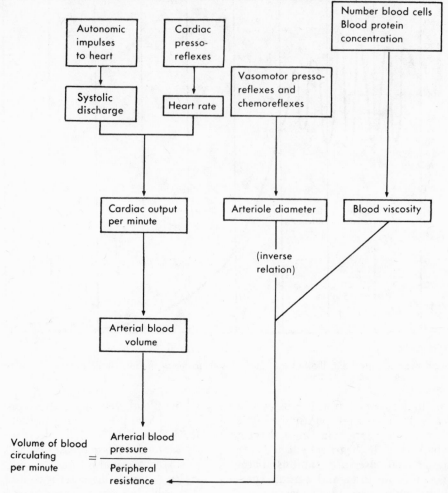

FIG. 1-17

Scheme to show some of the many parts of the complex circulation control mechanism. The volume of blood circulating through the body per minute is directly related to arterial blood pressure and inversely related to peripheral resistance. Note, however, that a great many factors act together to regulate these two factors.

this tends to increase arterial pressure and circulation; summarizing, an increase in peripheral resistance may decrease volume of blood circulating per minute, increase it, or not change it at all (Fig. 1-17)

C. Pulse
  1. Definition—alternate expansion and recoil of blood vessel
  2. Cause—variations in pressure within vessel due to intermittent injections of blood from heart into aorta with each ventricular contraction; pulse can be felt because of elasticity of arterial walls

  3. Where pulse can be felt—wherever artery lies near surface and over firm background, such as bone; some of those most easily palpated are listed below:
    a. Radial artery—at wrist
    b. Temporal artery—in front of ear, or above and to outer side of eye
    c. Common carotid artery—along anterior edge of sternocleidomastoid muscle, at level of lower margin of thyroid cartilage
    d. Facial artery—at lower margin of lower jaw bone, on line with corners of mouth, in groove in man-

dible about one third of way forward from angle of bone

   e. Brachial artery—at bend of elbow, along inner margin of biceps muscle

   f. Posterior tibial artery—behind medial malleolus (inner "ankle bone")

   g. Dorsalis pedis—on anterior surface of foot, just below the bend of the ankle

4. Venous pulse—in large veins only; produced by changes in venous pressure brought about by alternate contraction and relaxation of atria rather than of ventricles as in arterial pulse

9. **Lymphatic system**

Part of circulatory system; consists of lymphatic vessels, lymph nodes, lymph

A. Lymphatic vessels

   1. Structure—lymph capillaries similar to blood capillaries in structure; larger lymphatics similar to veins but are thinner walled, have more valves, and have lymph nodes in certain places along their course

   2. Names—largest lymphatic known as thoracic duct; drains lymph from entire body except upper right quadrant into left subclavian vein (where it joins the internal jugular); right lymphatic ducts drain lymph from upper right quadrant into right subclavian vein

   3. Functions

   Lymphatics return fluid and proteins to blood from interstitial fluid; about 60% of fluid filtered out of blood capillaries returns to circulation via lymphatics rather than by osmosis into venous ends of capillaries; about 50% of total blood proteins leak out of capillaries per day; since only way these large molecules can return to blood is via lymphatics, adequate lymph return is essential for maintaining homeostasis of blood proteins and, therefore, of blood volume

B. Lymph nodes

   1. Structure—lymphatic tissue, separated into compartments by fibrous partitions; afferent lymphatic vessels enter each node; one (usually) efferent vessel drains lymph out of node

   2. Location—usually in clusters; some of more important groups, from nursing viewpoint, listed below:

      a. Submental and submaxillary groups in floor of mouth; lymph from nose, lips, and teeth drains through these

      b. Superficial cervical nodes in neck, along sternocleidomastoid muscle; lymph from head and neck drains through these nodes

      c. Superficial cubital nodes at bend of elbow; lymph from hand and forearm drains through these nodes

      d. Axillary nodes in axilla; lymph from arm and upper part of chest wall, including breast, drains through these nodes (ones frequently removed during mastectomy for carcinoma)

      e. Inguinal nodes in groin; lymph from leg and external genitals drains through these nodes

   3. Functions

      a. Help defend body against injurious substances (notably, bacteria and tumor cells) by filtering them out of lymph and thereby preventing their entrance into bloodstream; also, phagocytes in lymph nodes destroy many of these substances by phagocytosis

      b. Lymphatic tissue of lymph nodes carries on process of hemopoiesis; specifically, it forms two types of white blood cells—lymphocytes and monocytes; some lymphocytes now thought to produce antibodies and some to become transformed into plasma cells which, in turn, produce antibodies; thus lymph nodes help defend the body in another way besides those mentioned under a, above—they also function as an important part of the immune response

C. Lymph

   1. Lymph—fluid in lymphatics

   2. Source of lymph is interstitial fluid; lymph is interstitial fluid that has entered the lymphatic capillaries

   3. Interstitial fluid is the fluid in the microscopic tissue spaces

   4. Source of interstitial fluid is blood plasma; interstitial fluid is formed by plasma filtering out of the blood capillaries into the tissue spaces (more about this on p. 83)

D. Spleen
   1. Location—left hypochondrium, above and behind cardiac portion of stomach
   2. Structure—lymphatic tissue, similar to lymph nodes; size varies; contains numerous spaces filled with venous blood
   3. Functions
      a. Defense—phagocytosis of particles such as microbes, red cell fragments, and platelets by reticuloendothelial cells* of spleen; antibody formation by plasma cells of spleen
      b. Hemopoiesis—lymphatic tissue of spleen, like that of the lymph nodes, forms lymphocytes and monocytes
      c. Spleen serves as blood reservoir; sympathetic stimulation causes constriction of its capsule, squeezing out an estimated 200 ml. of blood into general circulation within 1 minute's time

Respiratory system

1. **Function**
   To make possible exchange of gases between blood and air and thereby make possible cellular respiration
2. **Organs**
   Nose, pharynx, larynx, trachea, bronchi, lungs
A. Nose
   1. Structure
      a. Portions
         (1) Internal—in skull, above roof of mouth
         (2) External—protruding from face
      b. Cavities
         (1) Divisions—right and left
         (2) Meati—superior, middle, and lower; named for turbinates located above each meatus
         (3) Openings
            (a) To exterior—the anterior nares
            (b) To nasopharynx—the posterior nares
         (4) Conchae (turbinates)
            (a) Superior and middle processes of ethmoid bone;

inferior conchae, separate bones
            (b) Conchae partition each nasal cavity into 3 passageways or meati
         (5) Floor—formed by palatine bones and maxillae; these also act as roof of mouth
      c. Lining—ciliated mucosa
      d. Sinuses draining into nose (paranasal sinuses)
         (1) Frontal
         (2) Maxillary (antrum of Highmore)
         (3) Sphenoidal
         (4) Ethmoidal
   2. Functions
      a. Serves as passageway for incoming and outgoing air, filtering, warming, moistening, and chemically examining it
      b. Organ of smell (olfactory receptors located in nasal mucosa)
      c. Aids in phonation
B. Pharynx (throat)
   1. Structure—composed of muscle with mucous lining
      a. Divisions
         (1) Nasopharynx—behind nose
         (2) Oropharynx—behind mouth
         (3) Laryngopharynx—behind larynx
      b. Openings
         (1) In nasopharynx—4 openings— 2 auditory (eustachian) tubes and 2 posterior nares
         (2) In oropharynx—1 opening— fauces, archway into mouth
         (3) In laryngopharynx—2 openings —into esophagus and into larynx
      c. Organs in pharynx
         (1) In nasopharynx—pharyngeal tonsils (adenoids)
         (2) In oropharynx—palatine and lingual tonsils
   2. Functions of pharynx
      a. Serves as passageway for air, food, and liquid; i.e., serves as entrance to both respiratory and digestive tracts
      b. Aids in phonation
C. Larynx (voice box)
   1. Location—at upper end of trachea, just below pharynx

---

*Reticuloendothelial system—phagocytic cells, located mainly in liver, spleen, bone marrow, and lymph nodes; also, macrophages of connective tissue and microglia in brain and cord.

2. Structure
   a. Cartilages—9 pieces arranged in boxlike formation; thyroid largest of cartilages, "Adam's apple"; epiglottis, "lid" cartilage; cricoid, "signet ring" cartilage
   b. Vocal cords
      (1) False cords—folds of mucous lining
      (2) True cords—fibroelastic bands stretched across hollow interior of larynx; glottis is opening between true cords
   c. Lining—ciliated mucosa
3. Functions
   a. Voice production—during expiration, air passing through larynx causes vocal cords to vibrate; vibration of short, tense cords produces high pitch; long, relaxed cords, low pitch
   b. Serves as part of passageway for air; entrance to lower respiratory tract
D. Trachea (windpipe)
   1. Structure
      a. Walls—smooth muscle; contain C-shaped rings of cartilage at intervals; these keep tube open at all times
      b. Lining—ciliated mucosa
      c. Extent—from larynx to bronchi; about 4½ inches long
   2. Function—furnishes open passageway for air going to and from lungs
E. Lungs
   1. Structure
      a. Size—large enough to fill pleural divisions of thoracic cavity
      b. Shape—cone-shaped, with base downward
      c. Location—in pleural divisions of thorax; extend from slightly above clavicle to diaphragm; base of each lung rests on diaphragm
      d. Divisions
         (1) Lobes—3 in right lung, 2 in left
         (2) Root—consists of primary bronchus, pulmonary artery and veins bound together by connective tissue
         (3) Hilum—vertical slit on mesial surface of lung, through which root structures enter lung

         (4) Apex—pointed upper part of lung
         (5) Base—broad, inferior surface of lung
      e. "Bronchial tree"—consists of following:
         (1) Bronchi—right and left bronchi formed by branching of trachea; right bronchus slightly larger and more vertical than left; each primary bronchus branches, upon entering lung, into secondary bronchi
         (2) Bronchioles—small branches off secondary bronchi
         (3) Alveolar ducts—microscopic branches off bronchioles
         (4) Alveoli—microscopic sacs composed of single layer of simple squamous epithelial cells; each alveolar duct terminates in cluster of alveoli often likened to bunch of grapes; each alveolus enveloped by network of lung capillaries
      f. Covering of lung—visceral layer of pleura
   2. Function of lungs—furnish place where air and blood can come in close enough contact for rapid diffusion of gases to occur
      a. Bronchi, bronchioles, alveolar ducts—lower part of airway through which air moves into and out of alveoli
      b. Alveoli—microscopic sacs in which gases are exchanged very rapidly between air and blood; membranous walls of the millions of alveoli provide surface area large enough and thin enough to make possible rapid gas exchange
3. **Physiology of respiration**
A. Mechanism of inspiration (Fig. 1-18)
B. Mechanism of expiration (Fig. 1-19)
C. Amount of air exchanged in breathing
   1. Directly related to gas pressure gradient between atmosphere and alveoli and inversely related to resistance opposing air flow; the greater the difference between atmospheric pressure and alveolar pressure, the greater the amount of air exchanged in breathing; the greater the resistance opposing air flow to or from the lungs, the less air exchanged

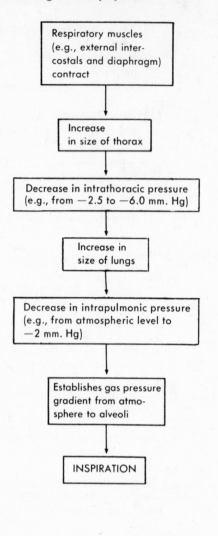

FIG. 1-18

Mechanism of inspiration.

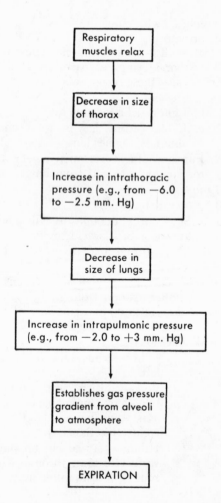

FIG. 1-19

Mechanism of expiration.

2. Measured by apparatus called spirometer
3. Tidal air—average amount expired after normal inspiration; approximately 500 ml.
4. Expiratory reserve volume—largest additional volume of air that can be forcibly expired after a normal inspiration and expiration; normal ERV, 1,000 to 1,200 ml.
5. Inspiratory reserve volume—largest additional volume of air that can be forcibly inspired after a normal inspiration; normal IRV, 3,000 to 3,300 ml.
6. Residual air—that which cannot be forcibly expired from lungs; about 1,200 ml.
7. Minimal air—that which can never be removed from alveoli if they have been inflated even once, even though lungs be subjected to atmospheric pressure that squeezes part of residual air out
8. Vital capacity—approximate capacity of lungs as measured by amount of air that can be forcibly expired after forcible inspiration; varies with size of thoracic cavity, which is determined by various factors (e.g., size of rib cage, posture, volume of blood and interstitial fluid in lungs, size of heart)

D. Diffusion of gases between air and blood
1. Where it occurs—across alveolar-capillary membranes, i.e., in lungs between air in alveoli and venous blood in lung capillaries
2. Direction of diffusion
   a. Oxygen—net diffusion down oxygen pressure gradient; i.e., from alveolar air to blood
   b. Carbon dioxide—net diffusion down carbon dioxide pressure gradient; i.e., from blood to alveolar air
3. Mechanism of oxygen diffusion (Fig. 1-20)
4. Mechanism of carbon dioxide diffusion (Fig. 1-21)

E. How blood transports oxygen
1. As solute—about 0.5 ml. of oxygen is dissolved in 100 ml. of blood; produces the blood P_{O_2}
2. As oxyhemoglobin—each gram of hemoglobin can combine with 1.34 ml. of oxygen; hence, with normal hemoglobin content (e.g., 15 grams per 100 ml. of blood) and 100% oxygen satu-

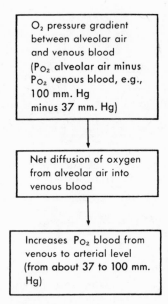

FIG. 1-20
Mechanism of oxygen diffusion.

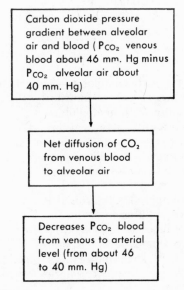

FIG. 1-21
Mechanism of carbon dioxide diffusion.

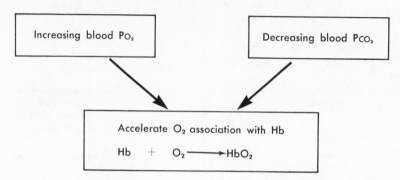

FIG. 1-22

Factors influencing rate of O_2 association with Hb.

ration, 15×1.34 (or about 20) ml. of oxygen is transported as oxyhemoglobin

$$Hb + O_2 \longrightarrow HbO_2$$
$$\text{Oxyhemoglobin}$$

3. Various factors influence rate at which oxygen associates with hemoglobin to form oxyhemoglobin (Figs. 1-22 and 1-24); also various factors influence oxygen dissociation from hemoglobin (Figs. 1-23 and 1-24)

F. How blood transports carbon dioxide
  1. As solute—small amount dissolves in plasma
  2. As bicarbonate ion—more than half of CO_2 in blood is present in the plasma as bicarbonate ion, formed by ionization of carbonic acid as follows:

$$CO_2 + H_2O \rightleftarrows H_2CO_3$$
$$\downarrow$$
$$H^+ + HCO_3^-$$

  3. As carbhemoglobin—less than one third of CO_2 is transported in combination with hemoglobin

G. Diffusion of gases between arterial blood and tissues (occurs in tissue capillaries)
  1. Oxygen—net diffusion of dissolved O_2 out of blood into tissues because of lower P_{O_2} there (perhaps 30 mm. Hg compared with arterial P_{O_2} of 100 mm. Hg); diffusion of dissolved oxygen out of blood lowers blood P_{O_2} from arterial to venous level (from 100 to 40 mm. Hg); decreasing P_{O_2} as blood moves through tissue capillaries causes oxygen to dissociate from hemoglobin, thereby releasing more oxygen for diffusion out of blood to tissue cells

  2. Carbon dioxide—net diffusion of CO_2 into blood because of lower P_{CO_2} there (40 mm. Hg compared with probably over 50 mm. Hg in tissues); diffusion of CO_2 into tissue capillaries increases blood P_{CO_2} from arterial to venous level (from 40 to 46 mm. Hg); increasing P_{CO_2}, like decreasing P_{O_2}, tends to accelerate oxygen dissociation from hemoglobin

H. Control of respirations
  1. Usual regulators of respirations are arterial blood P_{CO_2} and pH; increase in arterial P_{CO_2} or decrease in its pH has stimulating effect on respirations and is followed by hyperventilation (increased rate and depth of respirations), whereas decrease in arterial P_{CO_2} or increase in its pH leads to hypoventilation; presumably, increase in arterial P_{CO_2} or decrease in arterial blood pH stimulates neurons of respiratory center in two ways—directly and indirectly via stimulation of carotid and aortic chemoreceptors
  2. Emergency controller of respirations is arterial blood P_{O_2}; according to one authority,[*] the P_{O_2} of arterial blood has the following effects on neurons of the respiratory center and thereby on respirations: 100 to 80 mm. Hg, normal respirations; 79 to 30 mm. Hg, increasing stimulation; maximum stimulation of respirations (mild hypoxia) at 30 mm. Hg P_{O_2} arterial blood; below 30 mm. Hg (severe hypoxia), depression or cessation of respirations

---

[*]Selkurt, E. E., editor: Physiology, ed. 2, Boston, 1966, Little, Brown & Co.

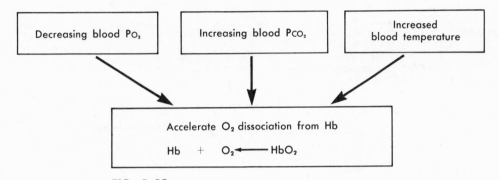

FIG. 1-23

Factors influencing rate of O_2 dissociation from Hb.

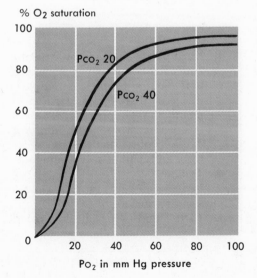

Po$_2$ in mm Hg pressure

FIG. 1-24

Oxygen association curves of human blood showing that the percentage of hemoglobin associated with oxygen depends upon both the oxygen and the carbon dioxide pressures of the blood. *Vertical coordinate,* %O_2 saturation (% of hemoglobin combined with oxygen). *Horizontal coordinate,* P_{O_2} in mm. Hg pressure. *Numbers on curves,* P_{CO_2} in mm. Hg pressure. *Interpretation:* When blood P_{O_2} is 40 and P_{CO_2} is also 40, about 75% of the hemoglobin is combined with O_2 (i.e., blood has about a 75% O_2 saturation). *Questions:* What is %O_2 saturation with blood P_{O_2} 40 and P_{CO_2} 20? Is it true that the lower the blood P_{CO_2}, the higher its O_2 saturation can be? (From Anthony, C. P., and Kolthoff, N. J.: Textbook of anatomy and physiology, ed. 8, St. Louis, 1971, The C. V. Mosby Co.)

TABLE 1-22

MODIFICATIONS OF COATS OF DIGESTIVE TRACT

Organ	Modifications		
	Mucous coat	*Muscle coat*	*Fibroserous coat*
Esophagus		Has 2 layers—inner one of circular fibers, outer one of longitudinal fibers; striated muscle in upper part, smooth in lower part of esophagus and in rest of tract	Outer coat, fibrous
Stomach	Arranged in temporary, longitudinal folds, called rugae; allow for distention Contains microscopic gastric and hydrochloric acid glands	Has 3 layers, instead of usual 2; circular, longitudinal, and oblique fibers; 2 sphincters—cardia at entrance of stomach, pylorus at its exit formed by circular fibers	Outer coat, visceral peritoneum; hangs in double fold from lower edge of stomach over intestines, forming apronlike structure, greater omentum, or "lace apron"
Small intestine	Contains permanent, circular folds, valvulae conniventes Microscopic, fingerlike projections, villi Microscopic intestinal glands (of Lieberkühn) Microscopic duodenal (or Brunner's) glands Clusters of lymph nodes, Peyer's patches Numerous single lymph nodes called solitary nodes	Has 2 layers—inner one of circular fibers, outer one of longitudinal fibers	Outer coat, visceral peritoneum
Large intestine	Solitary nodes Intestinal glands	Incomplete outer, longitudinall coat; present only in 3 tapelike strips that pull large intestine into small sacs (haustra); internal anal sphincter formed by circular smooth fibers; external anal sphincter, by striated fibers	Outer coat, visceral peritoneum

Digestive system

1. **Functions and importance**
A. Digestion of food, essential preparation for absorption and metabolism
B. Absorption of digested food
C. Elimination of wastes of digestion
2. **Coats composing wall of alimentary canal**
A. Mucous lining
B. Submucous coat of connective tissue—main blood vessels here
C. Muscle coat
D. Fibroserous coat
E. Modifications of coats (Table 1-22)
3. **Mouth (buccal cavity)**
A. Cheeks

B. Hard palate—formed by 2 palatine bones and palatine processes of maxillae
C. Soft palate—formed of muscle in shape of arch that forms partition between mouth and nasopharynx; fauces, archway, or opening, from mouth into oropharynx; uvula, conical shaped process suspended from midpoint of soft palate arch
4. **Tongue**
A. Papillae—many rough elevations on tongue's surface
B. Taste buds—specialized receptors of cranial nerves VII and IX; located in papillae
C. Frenum (or frenulum)—fold of mucous

TABLE 1-23
SALIVARY GLANDS

Name of gland	Location	Duct openings
Parotid	Below and in front of ear	On inside of cheek, opposite upper second molar tooth
Submandibular	Posterior part of floor of mouth	Floor of mouth, at sides of frenum
Sublingual	Anterior part of floor of mouth, under tongue	Several ducts open into floor of mouth

TABLE 1-24
DENTITION

Name of tooth	Number per jaw deciduous set	Number per jaw permanent set
Central incisors	2	2
Lateral incisors	2	2
Cuspids (canines)	2	2
Premolars (bicuspids)	0	4
Molars (tricuspids)	4	6
Total per jaw	10	16
Total per set	20	32

membrane that helps anchor tongue to mouth floor

5. **Salivary glands** (Table 1-23)
6. **Teeth**
A. Deciduous, or "baby teeth"—10 in each jaw, or 20 in set
B. Permanent—16 per jaw, or 32 in set (Table 1-24)
C. Eruption
  1. Deciduous—first one erupts usually at age 6 months, rest follow at intervals of one or more months; however, great individual variation in time of eruption of teeth; deciduous teeth shed between ages 6 and 13 years
  2. Permanent—usually between 6 years and about 17 years; third molars (wisdom teeth) last to erupt
D. Structure of tooth (Fig. 1-25)
7. **Pharynx (throat)**
8. **Esophagus**
A. Location and extent
  1. Posterior to trachea and heart
  2. Extends from pharynx through diaphragm to stomach—distance of approximately 10 inches

B. Structure—collapsible, muscle tube; (trachea noncollapsible tube due to presence of cartilaginous rings)
9. **Stomach**
A. Size, shape, position
  1. Size—varies in different persons and, also, according to whether distended or not
  2. Shape—elongated pouch, with greater curve forming lower, left border
  3. Position—in epigastric and left hypochondriac portions of abdominal cavity
B. Divisions
  1. Fundus—portion above esophageal opening
  2. Body—central portion
  3. Pylorus—constricted, lower portion
C. Curves
  1. Lesser—upper, right border
  2. Greater—lower, left border
D. Sphincters
  1. Cardiac—guarding opening of esophagus into stomach
  2. Pyloric—guarding opening of pylorus into duodenum
E. Coats of stomach—see Table 1-22
F. Glands of stomach—secrete gastric juice composed of mucus, hydrochloric acid, and enzymes; simple columnar epithelial cells form surface of gastric mucosa and secrete mucus; millions of microscopic gastric glands embedded in gastric mucosa composed of different types of cells, mainly chief cells (zymogen cells), that secrete gastric juice enzymes, and parietal cells that secrete hydrochloric acid
10. **Small intestine**
A. Size—approximately 1 inch in diameter, 20 feet in length when relaxed
B. Divisions
  1. Duodenum—joins pylorus of stomach; about 10 inches long; C-shaped

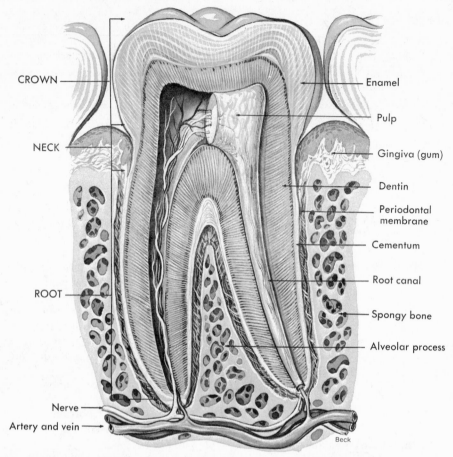

CROWN

NECK

ROOT

Nerve

Artery and vein

Enamel

Pulp

Gingiva (gum)

Dentin

Periodontal membrane

Cementum

Root canal

Spongy bone

Alveolar process

Beck

FIG. 1-25

A molar tooth, sectioned to show its bony socket and details of its three main parts: crown, neck, and root. The pulp contains nerves and blood vessels. (From Anthony, C. P., and Kolthoff, N. J.: Textbook of anatomy and physiology, ed. 8, St. Louis, 1971, The C. V. Mosby Co.)

2. Jejunum—middle section; about 8 feet long
3. Ileum—lower section; about 12 feet long; no clear boundary between jejunum and ileum

11. Large intestine

A. Size—approximately 2½ inches in diameter, but only 5 or 6 feet in length when relaxed

B. Divisions
1. Cecum—the first 2 or 3 inches of large intestine
2. Colon
   a. Ascending—extends vertically along right border of abdomen up to level of liver
   b. Transverse colon—extends horizontally across abdomen, below liver and stomach and above small intestine
   c. Descending colon—extends vertically down left side of abdomen to level of iliac crest
   d. Sigmoid colon—S-shaped part of large intestine curving downward below iliac crest to join rectum; lower part of sigmoid curve which joins rectum bends toward left (anatomic reason for placing patient on left side for giving enema—gravity thereby assists inflow of water)

3. Rectum—last 7 or 8 inches of intestinal tube

12. Liver

A. Location and size—occupies most of right hypochondrium and part of epigastrium; largest gland in body

B. Lobes—divided into lobules by blood vessels and fibrous "partitions"
   1. Right lobe—subdivided into 2 smaller lobes (caudate and quadrate) and right lobe, proper
   2. Left lobe—single lobe

C. Ducts
   1. Hepatic duct—from liver
   2. Cystic duct—from gallbladder
   3. Common bile duct—formed by union of hepatic and cystic ducts in Y formation; drains bile into duodenum at hepato-pancreatic papilla

D. Functions
   1. Liver is one of most vital organs because of its role in metabolism of proteins, carbohydrates, and fats
      a. Carbohydrate metabolism by liver cells
         (1) Glycogenesis—conversion of glucose to glycogen for storage; insulin tends to promote liver glycogenesis
         (2) Glycogenolysis—conversion of glycogen to glucose and release of glucose into blood; epinephrine and glucagon accelerate glycogenolysis
         (3) Gluconeogenesis—formation of glucose from proteins or fats; glucocorticoids (e.g., hydrocortisone, corticosterone) have accelerating effect on gluconeogenesis
      b. Fat metabolism by liver cells
         (1) Ketogenesis—first step in fat catabolism occurs mainly in liver cells; consists of series of reactions by which fatty acids are converted to ketone bodies (acetoacetic acid, acetone, beta-hydroxybutyric acid)
         (2) Fat storage
      c. Protein metabolism by liver cells
         (1) Anabolism—synthesis of various proteins, notably blood proteins (e.g., prothrombin, fibrinogen, albumins, most globulins)
         (2) Deamination—first step in protein catabolism; chemical reaction by which amino group is split off from amino acid to form ammonia and a keto acid
         (3) Urea formation—liver cells convert to urea most of the ammonia formed by deamination
   2. Secretes bile, substance important in digestion and absorption of fats, and as vehicle for excretion of cholesterol and bile pigments
   3. Detoxifies various harmful substances (e.g., drugs)

13. Gallbladder

A. Size, shape, location—approximately size and shape of small pear; lies on undersurface of liver

B. Structure—sac made of smooth muscle, lined with mucosa arranged in rugae (temporary, longitudinal folds)

C. Function—concentrates and stores bile

14. Pancreas

A. Size, shape, location—larger in men than in women, but considerable individual variation; fish-shaped, with body, head, and tail; located in C-shaped curve of duodenum

B. Structure—both duct and ductless gland
   1. Pancreatic cells—pour secretion, pancreatic juice, into duct that runs length of gland and empties into duodenum at hepato-pancreatic papilla
   2. Islands of Langerhans (or islet cells)—clusters of cells not connected with pancreatic ducts; 2 main types of cells compose islets, namely, alpha and beta cells; constitute endocrine glands

C. Functions
   1. Pancreatic cells connected with pancreatic ducts secrete pancreatic juice, enzymes of which help digest all 3 kinds of foods (Table 1-25)
   2. Islet cells constitute endocrine gland
      a. Alpha cells secrete hormone glucagon, which accelerates liver glycogenolysis; hence, tends to increase blood sugar
      b. Beta cells secrete insulin, one of most important metabolic hormones, which exerts profound influence over the metabolism of carbohydrates, proteins, and fats
         (1) Insulin accelerates active transport of glucose (along with potassium and phosphate ions)

TABLE 1-25

CHEMICAL DIGESTION

Digestive juices and enzymes	Food enzyme digests (or hydrolyzes)	Resulting product
1. Saliva a. Amylase (ptyalin)	Starch (polysaccharide, complex sugar)	Maltose (disaccharide, or double sugar)

2. Gastric juice
   a. Protease (rennin)
   b. Pepsin, plus hydrochloric acid
	Caseinogen (milk protein)
	Proteins, including casein
		Casein (curds)
		Proteoses and peptones (partially digested proteins)

c. Lipase (of little importance)	Emulsified fats (butter, cream, etc.)	Fatty acids and glycerol*
3. Bile (contains no enzymes)	Large fat droplets (unemulsified fats)	Small fat droplets, or emulsified fats
4. Pancreatic juice a. Protease (trypsin)	Proteins (either intact or partially digested)	Peptones, peptids, amino acids*
b. Lipase (steapsin) c. Amylase (amylopsin)	Bile-emulsified fats Starch	Fatty acids and glycerol* Maltose

5. Intestinal juice (succus entericus)
   a. Peptidases
   b. Sucrase
	Partially digested proteins
	Sucrose (cane sugar)
		Amino acids*
		Glucose and fructose* (monosaccharides, or simple sugars)

c. Lactase	Lactose (milk sugar)	Glucose and galactose* (monosaccharides)
d. Maltase	Maltose (malt sugar)	Glucose* (dextrose)

*"End products" of digestion or, in other words, completely digested foods ready for absorption.

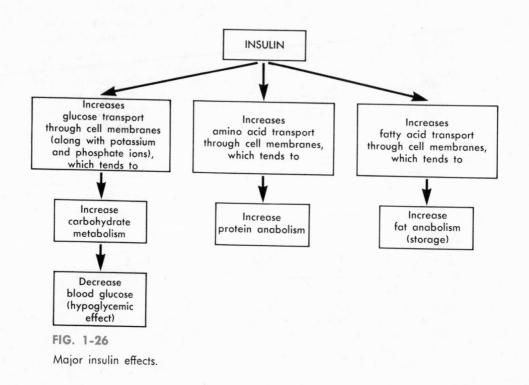

FIG. 1-26

Major insulin effects.

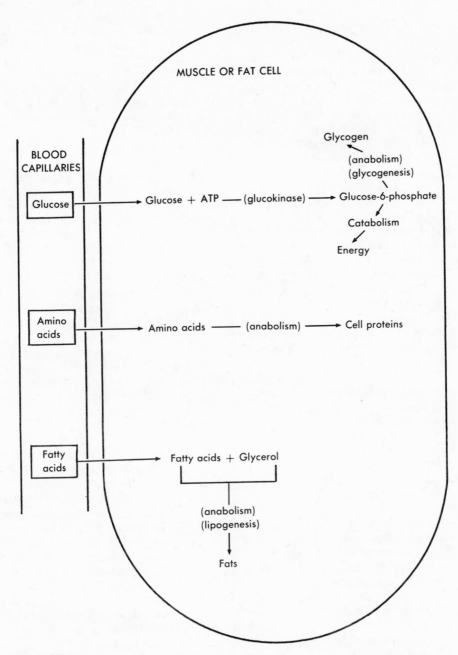

FIG. 1-27

Insulin effects. Insulin accelerates glucose, amino acid, and fatty acid transfer through cell membranes, therefore is essential for normal metabolism of all three kinds of food.

through cell membranes; therefore, it tends to decrease blood glucose (hypoglycemic effect) and to increase glucose utilization by cells either for catabolism or for anabolism (Fig. 1-26)

 (2) Insulin stimulates liver cell glucokinase; therefore, it promotes liver glycogenesis, another effect that tends to lower blood glucose (Fig. 1-27)

 (3) Insulin inhibits liver cell phosphatase and therefore inhibits liver glycogenolysis

 (4) Insulin accelerates rate of amino acid transfer into cells, so promotes protein anabolism within them (Fig. 1-27)

 (5) Insulin accelerates rate of fatty acid transfer into cells, promotes fat anabolism (also called fat deposition or lipogenesis), and inhibits fat catabolism (Fig. 1-27)

15. Vermiform appendix

A. Size, shape, location—about size and shape of large angleworm; blind-end tube off cecum just beyond ileocecal valve

B. Structure—wall, same coats as compose intestinal wall

16. Digestion

A. Definition—all changes that food undergoes in alimentary canal

B. Purpose—conversion of foods into chemical and physical forms that can be absorbed and metabolized

C. Kinds

 1. Mechanical digestion—all movements of alimentary tract that

  a. Change physical state of foods from comparatively large solid pieces into minute dissolved particles

  b. Propel food forward along alimentary tract, finally eliminating digestive wastes from body

   (1) Deglutition—swallowing

   (2) Peristalsis—wormlike movements that squeeze food downward in tract

   (3) Mass peristalsis—entire contents moved into sigmoid colon and rectum; usually occurs after meal

   (4) Defecation—emptying of rectum, so-called "bowel movement"

   c. Churn intestinal contents so all becomes well mixed with digestive juices and all parts of contents come in contact with surface of intestinal mucosa to facilitate absorption

 2. Chemical digestion—series of hydrolytic processes dependent upon specific enzymes; hydrolysis, decomposition of complex compound into 2 or more simple compounds by means of chemical reaction with water (Table 1-25)

D. Control of digestive gland secretion

 1. Saliva

  a. Secretion of saliva—neural control of this reflex results from parasympathetic impulses to glands, initiated by taste, smell, and sight of food

 2. Gastric juice

  a. Neural control similar to that of salivary glands

  b. Hormonal control—partially digested proteins cause gastric mucosa to release hormone, gastrin, into blood; gastrin stimulates gastric mucosa to secrete juice with high pepsin and hydrochloric acid content

 3. Pancreatic juice

  a. Hormonal control—hydrochloric acid (in chyme entering duodenum from stomach) causes intestinal mucosa to release hormone, secretin, into blood, secretin stimulates pancreatic cells to secrete juice high in sodium bicarbonate content (to neutralize hydrochloric acid) but low in enzymes; products of protein digestion (e.g., proteoses, peptones, and amino acids) cause intestinal mucosa to release another hormone, pancreozymin, which stimulates pancreatic cells to secrete enzymes

  b. Neural control—reflex secretion of pancreatic juice results from parasympathetic impulses via vagus nerve

 4. Bile—hormonal control of secretion

  a. Although bile is secreted continuously, secretin increases amount of bile secreted

TABLE 1-26
FOOD ABSORPTION

Form absorbed	Structures into which absorbed	Circulation
Protein—as amino acids	Into blood in intestinal capillaries	Portal vein, liver, hepatic vein, inferior vena cava to heart, etc.
Carbohydrate—as monosaccharides (glucose and fructose)	Same as amino acids	Same as amino acids
Fat—as glycerol and fatty acids Because fatty acids insoluble they first combine with bile salts to form water-soluble substance	Chiefly into lymph in intestinal lacteals; some into blood	During absorption, i.e., while in epithelial cells of intestinal mucosa, glycerol and fatty acids recombine to form microscopic particles of fats (chylomicrons); lymphatics carry them by way of thoracic duct to left subclavian vein, superior vena cava, heart, etc.

b. Presence of fats in intestine causes intestinal mucosa to release hormone, cholecystokinin, into blood; cholecystokinin stimulates smooth muscle of gallbladder to contract, ejecting bile into duodenum

5. Intestinal juice—control obscure but believed to be both reflex and hormonal; food in small intestine causes mucosa to release hormone, enterocrinin, into blood; enterocrinin stimulates intestinal glands to secrete

17. **Absorption**
A. Definition—passage of substances through intestinal mucosa into blood or lymph
B. How accomplished—probably mainly by active transport by intestinal cells; makes it possible for both water and solutes to move through intestinal mucosa in direction opposite that expected according to laws of osmosis and diffusion
C. Where absorption occurs—from small intestine, with exception of alcohol, certain drugs, and some water; alcohol, drugs, and some water absorbed from stomach; largest amount of water absorbed from large intestine
D. Absorption of each of three foods (Table 1-26)

18. **Metabolism**
A. Meaning—consists of two complex processes: catabolism and anabolism
B. Catabolism
1. Consists of complex series of chemical reactions that take place inside cells and yield energy, carbon dioxide, and water; about half of energy released

from food molecules by catabolism put back in storage in unstable, high-energy bonds of ATP molecules and the rest transformed to heat; energy in high-energy bonds of ATP can be released as rapidly as needed for doing cellular work

2. Two processes involved: glycolysis and Krebs' citric acid cycle (p. 72)
3. Purpose—to continually provide cells with utilizable energy (i.e., energy that can be supplied instantaneously to the energy-consuming mechanisms which do cellular work)
C. Anabolism—synthesis of various compounds from simpler compounds; an important kind of cellular work that uses some of energy made available by catabolism
D. Metabolism of carbohydrates
1. Consists of the following processes:
   a. Glucose transport through cell membranes and phosphorylation
      (1) Insulin promotes this transport through cell membranes
      (2) Glucose phosphorylation—conversion of glucose to glucose-6-phosphate, catalyzed by enzyme glucokinase (Fig. 1-27); insulin increases activity of glucokinase so promotes glucose phosphorylation; essential preliminary to both glycogenesis and glucose catabolism
   b. Glycogenesis—conversion of glucose to glycogen for storage; occurs mainly in liver and muscle cells

c. Glycogenolysis
  (1) In muscle cells—glycogen changed back to glucose-6-phosphate, which is then catabolized in the muscle cells (Fig. 1-27)
  (2) In liver cells—glycogen changed back to glucose; enzyme, glucose phosphatase, is present in liver cells and catalyzes final step of glycogenolysis, the changing of glucose-6-phosphate to glucose; this enzyme lacking in most other cells; glucagon and epinephrine accelerate liver glycogenolysis
d. Glucose catabolism
  (1) Glycolysis—series of anaerobic reactions that break 1 glucose molecule down into 2 pyruvic acid molecules with conversion of about 5% of energy stored in glucose to heat and ATP molecules
  (2) Krebs' citric acid cycle—series of aerobic chemical reactions by which 2 pyruvic acid molecules (from 1 glucose molecule) are broken down to 6 carbon dioxide and 6 water molecules with release of some energy as heat and some stored again in ATP; citric acid cycle releases about 95%, and glycolysis only about 5% of energy stored in glucose; citric acid cycle occurs in the mitochondria of cells
e. Gluconeogenesis—sequence of chemical reactions carried on in liver cells; process converts protein or fat compounds into glucose
f. Principles about normal carbohydrate metabolism
  (1) Principle of "preferred energy fuel"—cells first catabolize glucose, sparing fats and proteins; when their glucose supply becomes inadequate, they next catabolize fats, sparing proteins; and finally, when fats are used up, they catabolize their own cell proteins
  (2) Principle of glycogenesis—glucose in excess of about 120 to 140 mg. per 100 ml. blood brought to liver by portal veins enters liver cells where it undergoes glycogenesis and is stored as glycogen
  (3) Principle of glycogenolysis—when blood glucose decreases below midpoint of normal, liver glycogenolysis accelerates and tends to raise blood glucose concentration back toward midpoint of normal
  (4) Principle of gluconeogenesis—when blood glucose decreases below normal or when amount of glucose entering cells is inadequate, liver gluconeogenesis accelerates and tends to raise blood glucose concentration
  (5) Principle of glucose storage as fat—when blood insulin content adequate, glucose in excess of amount used for catabolism and glycogenesis is converted to fat, and stored in fat depots
E. Control of metabolism—primarily by hormones
  1. Pancreatic hormones
    a. Insulin—exerts predominant control over carbohydrate metabolism but also affects protein and fat metabolism; see pp. 68 and 69 and Figs. 1-26 and 1-27; in general, insulin accelerates carbohydrate metabolism by cells, thereby decreasing blood glucose
    b. Glucagon (secreted by alpha cells of islands of Langerhans)—accelerates liver glycogenolysis only
  2. Anterior pituitary hormones
    a. Growth hormone tends to
      (1) Accelerate protein anabolism; hence promotes growth of skeleton and soft tissues
      (2) Accelerate fat mobilization from adipose cells; this tends to bring about shift from use of glucose, the "preferred fuel" for catabolism, to catabolism of fats
      (3) Accelerate liver gluconeogenesis (from fats); this tends to increase blood glucose
      (4) Stimulate glucagon secretion, which in turn stimulates liver

glycogenolysis and glucose release into blood

b. ACTH (adrenocorticotropic hormone)—stimulates adrenal cortex secretion, especially of glucocorticoids

3. Adrenal cortex hormones—glucocorticoids (mainly cortisol and corticosterone) tend to

a. Accelerate fat mobilization and catabolism, thereby promoting shift to fat catabolism from glucose catabolism whenever latter is inadequate for energy needs

b. Accelerate tissue protein mobilization (catabolism)

c. Accelerate liver gluconeogenesis; presumably secondary effect, resulting from protein mobilization, tends to increase blood sugar

4. Adrenal medulla hormones—the catecholamines epinephrine and norepinephrine tend to accelerate both liver and muscle glycogenolysis with release of glucose from liver into circulation; therefore tend to increase blood sugar

5. Male sex gland hormone—testosterone; secreted by interstitial cells of testes; tends to accelerate protein anabolism

F. Metabolic rates

1. Meaning—calories of heat energy produced and expended per hour or per day

2. Ways of expressing

a. In kilocalories (1 kilocalorie = 1,000 calories = 1 Calorie)

b. As "normal" or as definite percentage above or below normal (e.g., plus 10% or minus 10%)

3. Basal metabolic rate—kilocalories heat produced when individual is awake but resting, 12 to 18 hours after last meal, in comfortably warm environment

a. Factors determining basal metabolic rates (Fig. 1-28)

(1) Size—BMR is directly related to square meters of surface area of body; the larger the surface area, the higher the BMR (surface area computed from height and weight)

(2) Sex—5% to 7% higher in male than in female of same size and age

(3) Age—BMR inversely related to age; as age increases BMR decreases

(4) Amount of thyroid hormones secreted; thyroid hormones accelerate BMR

(5) Body temperature—BMR directly related to body temperature; e.g., 1° centigrade increase in body temperature above normal is accompanied

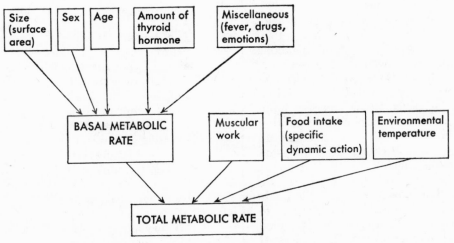

FIG. 1-28

Factors that determine basal and total metabolic rates.

by about 13% increase in BMR

(6) Miscellaneous factors such as sleep (decreases BMR), pregnancy, and emotions (increase BMR)

b. How basal metabolic rates are determined—by measuring the amount of oxygen inspired in a given time; for each liter of O_2 inspired, 4.825 kilocalories of heat is produced when diet is an ordinary mixed one

4. Total metabolic rate—kilocalories of heat energy expended per day; equal to basal metabolic rate plus number of kilocalories of energy used for muscular work, eating and digesting food, and adjusting to cool temperatures

5. Some principles about the metabolic rate and its relation to body weight

a. In order for body weight to remain constant (except for variations in water content), energy balance must be maintained; that is, the total kilocalories in the food ingested must equal the individual's total metabolic rate (expressed in kilocalories); in other words, body weight remains constant when energy input equals energy output

b. Whenever energy input (total kilocalories in food intake) is greater than the energy output (total metabolic rate), body weight increases
Corollary: Body weight does not increase (provided there is no water retention) unless energy input exceeds energy output.

c. Whenever energy input (total kilocalories in food intake) is less than the energy output (total metabolic rate), body weight decreases
Corollary: Body weight does not decrease (provided there is no water deficit) unless energy input is less than energy output; in other words, the only way anyone can lose weight (other than by dehydrating oneself) is to eat fewer kilocalories per day than one's own total metabolic rate (TMR); only then is stored fat catabolized to provide the energy not provided by catabolism of the food ingested
Example: If TMR for 1 day is 2,400 kilocalories and only 1,400 kilocal-

ories of food is ingested, then difference, 1,000 kilocalories, must be supplied by catabolism of stored fat, thereby producing weight loss; if you eat 500 kilocalories a day less than your TMR for 1 week, you will lose 1 pound of body fat

19. **Mechanisms for regulating food intake**

A. Thermostat theory holds that moderate decrease in blood temperature acts as stimulant to appetite center so increases appetite; and increase in blood temperature (fever) produces opposite effect

B. Glucostat theory postulates that low blood glucose concentration or low rate of glucose utilization (e.g., diabetes mellitus) acts as stimulant to appetite center so increases appetite; and high blood glucose level produces opposite effect

20. **Homeostasis of body temperature**

A. In order to maintain homeostasis of body temperature, heat production must equal heat loss

B. Heat is produced only by catabolism of foods—especially in skeletal muscles and liver

C. Heat is lost from the body

1. From the skin by the physical processes of evaporation, radiation, conduction, and convection; about 80% of the total heat lost from the body occurs through the skin

2. Through mucosa of respiratory, digestive, and urinary tracts, in warming cool inspired air, and cooling ingested foods and liquids

D. Thermostatic control of heat production and loss

1. The human "thermostat" consists of neurons located in the anterior part of the hypothalamus, which serve as thermal receptors; that is, they are stimulated by a slight increase in blood temperature (as little as 0.01° C.) and bring about two changes—sweating and dilatation of skin blood vessels—that increase the amount of heat lost from the body and thereby tend to decrease blood temperature back to normal

E. Heat-dissipating mechanism

1. Set in operation by an increase in blood temperature above the threshold of stimulation of thermal receptors in hypothalamus

2. Responses
   a. Increased sweating, which increases heat loss from skin by evaporation
   b. Dilatation of skin blood vessels, which increases heat loss from skin by radiation
F. Heat-gaining mechanism
   1. Details not established, but mechanism is activated by a decrease in blood temperature
   2. Responses
      a. Skin blood vessel constriction, which decreases heat loss from skin
      b. Shivering, which increases heat production
G. Skin thermal receptors—stimulation of these receptors gives rise to sensations of heat or cold and often initiates voluntary movements to reduce these sensations—e.g., fanning oneself to cool off or exercising to warm up

Urinary system

1. **Functions of urinary system**
A. Secrete urine
B. Eliminate urine from body (urination, micturition, or voiding)
2. **Kidneys**
A. Gross anatomy
   1. Size, shape, and location—about 4 × 2 × 1 inch; shaped like lima beans; lie against posterior abdominal wall, behind peritoneum at level of last thoracic and first 3 lumbar vertebrae; right kidney slightly lower than left
   2. External structure
      a. Hilum—concave notch on mesial surface; blood vessels and ureter enter kidney through this notch
      b. Renal capsule—protective capsule of fibrous tissue that envelops kidney
   3. Internal structure
      a. Cortex—outer layer of kidney substance; composed of renal corpuscles, convoluted tubules, and adjacent parts of loops of Henle
      b. Medulla—inner portion of kidney; composed of loops of Henle and collecting tubules
      c. Pyramids—triangular wedges of medullary substance; have striped appearance
      d. Papillae—apices of pyramids; collecting tubules open into renal pelvis here

      e. Columns—inward extensions of cortex between pyramids
B. Microscopic anatomy of kidney
   1. Glomerulus—cluster of capillaries, invaginated in Bowman's capsule
   2. Bowman's capsule—funnel-shaped upper end of urinary tubules
   3. Renal corpuscle—composed of Bowman's capsule and the glomerulus invaginated in it
   4. Nephron—physiologic unit of kidney, consists of renal corpuscle plus tubules
C. Physiology of kidney
   1. Function—excrete urine and thereby
      a. Excrete various normal and abnormal metabolic wastes
      b. Regulate composition and volume of blood and blood pressure; i.e., help maintain homeostasis, e.g., especially important in maintenance of fluid and electrolyte balance and acid-base balance
   2. Mechanism by which urine is formed (Fig. 1-29)
      a. In glomerulus—urine formation starts with process of filtration; water and solutes (except albumins, fibrinogen, and other blood proteins) filter out of blood into Bowman's capsule, passing through glomerular-capsular membrane
      b. In proximal tubule and loop of Henle
         (1) Reabsorption of glucose and other food molecules from tubule filtrate to blood in peritubular capillaries—probably mainly by active transport mechanisms
         (2) Reabsorption of electrolytes from tubule filtrate to blood in peritubular capillaries—cations (notably Na^+) are reabsorbed by active transport; anions (notably Cl^- and HCO_3^-) are reabsorbed by diffusion following cation transport
         (3) Reabsorption of water from tubule filtrate to blood in peritubular capillaries—by osmosis as result of electrolyte reabsorption
      c. In distal tubule
         (1) Reabsorption of electrolytes into blood as in proximal tubule

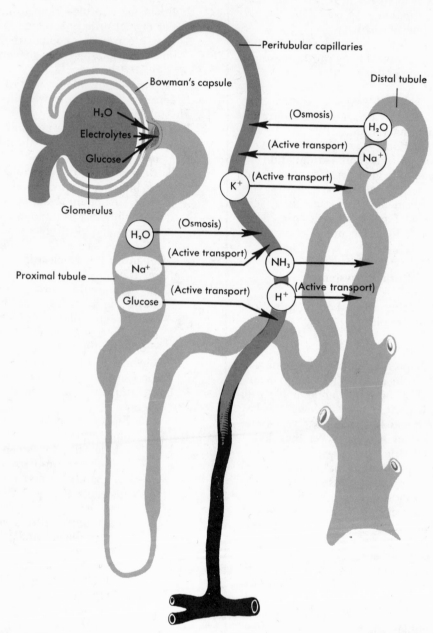

FIG. 1-29

Diagram showing glomerular filtration, tubular reabsorption, and tubular secretion—the three processes by which the kidneys secrete urine. In the proximal tubule, note that water is reabsorbed from the tubular filtrate into blood by osmosis, but sodium and glucose are reabsorbed mainly by active transport mechanisms. Note, too, that water and sodium are also reabsorbed from the distal tubule. Potassium and hydrogen ions and ammonia, in contrast, are secreted into the tubule from the blood. (From Anthony, C. P., and Kolthoff, N. J.: Textbook of anatomy and physiology, ed. 8, St. Louis, 1971, The C. V. Mosby Co.)

(2) Reabsorption of water into blood by osmosis; hormone, ADH, controls amount of water osmosing out of distal tubule (discussed under 3a below), whereas amount of electrolytes reabsorbed controls amount of osmosis out of proximal tubule

(3) Secretion of H^+, K^+, ammonia, and some other substances from blood in peritubular capillaries to tubule filtrate; secretion accomplished by active transport mechanism

3. Urine volume is controlled normally by mechanisms that regulate the amount of water reabsorbed by the kidney tubules; only under abnormal conditions does the glomerular filtration rate influence urine volume

a. The ADH mechanism—neurons in the hypothalamus (mainly in the supraoptic nucleus)—produces the antidiuretic hormone and the posterior pituitary gland secretes it into the blood; ADH secretion stimulated by two conditions, an increase in ECF osmotic pressure (for example, due to sodium retention) or a decrease in ECF volume; ADH acts on distal and collecting tubules, causing more water to osmose from the tubule filtrate back into the blood; this increased water reabsorption tends to increase the total volume of body fluid by decreasing the urine volume; in other words, ADH has both a water-retaining and an antidiuretic effect

Clinical applications: Anesthetics and some stress situations act in some way to stimulate ADH secretion and cause small urinary output. A decrease in ECF osmotic pressure, e.g., due to sodium loss, inhibits ADH secretion and results in diuresis (increased urine volume).

b. The aldosterone mechanism—an increase in aldosterone secretion (indirectly by a decrease in arterial blood pressure as shown in Fig. 1-10) tends to decrease urine volume by stimulating kidney tubules to reabsorb primarily more sodium and secondarily more water; thus aldosterone tends to produce sodium retention, water retention, and a low urine volume (antidiuresis)

c. Control by amount of solutes in tubule filtrate; in general, increase in tubule solutes causes decreased osmosis of water from proximal tubule back into blood and therefore increase in urine volume; e.g., in diabetes, excess glucose in tubule filtrate leads to increased urine volume (polyuria, diuresis)

d. Glomerular filtration rate normally is quite constant at about 125 ml. per minute, i.e., it does not vary enough to alter volume of urine produced, but in certain pathologic conditions glomerular filtration rate may change markedly and alter urine volume; e.g., in shock, glomerular filtration decreases or even ceases, causing decreased urine volume (oliguria) or urinary suppression (anuria)

3. **Ureters**
A. Location—lie behind parietal peritoneum; extend from kidneys to posterior part of bladder floor
B. Structure—ureter expands as it enters kidney to form renal pelvis; subdivided into calyces, each of which contains renal papilla; ureter walls composed of smooth muscle with mucosa lining and fibrous outer coat
C. Function—collect urine secreted by kidney cells and drain it into bladder

4. **Urinary bladder**
A. Location—behind symphysis pubis, below parietal peritoneum
B. Structure—collapsible bag of smooth muscle lined with mucosa arranged in rugae; 3 openings—1 into urethra and 2 from ureters
C. Functions
1. Reservoir for urine until sufficient amount accumulated for elimination
2. Expulsion of urine from body by way of urethra (urination, micturition, or voiding)

5. **Urethra**
A. Location
1. Female—behind symphysis pubis, in front of vagina

2. Male—extends through prostate gland, fibrous sheet, and penis

B. Structure—musculomembranous tube lined with mucosa; opening to exterior called urinary meatus

C. Functions
1. Female—passageway for expulsion of urine, only
2. Male—passageway for expulsion of both urine and male reproductive fluid

6. Urine

A. Physical characteristics

B. Chemical composition—urine consists of approximately 95% water which contains normally the following main substances:
1. Wastes
   a. From protein metabolism—urea, uric acid, creatinine, etc.
   b. Miscellaneous; e.g., hippuric acid formed in liver from detoxication of benzoates (in some foods)
2. Salts (electrolytes)
   a. Cations—Na^+ is most abundant; also K^+, NH_4^+, and others
   b. Anions—Cl^- most abundant; also bicarbonate, phosphate, and others
3. Pigments—urochrome is principal one
4. Hormones and products of their metabolism
   a. Pituitary gonadotropins
   b. Chorionic gonadotropins (in pregnancy, secreted by placenta; presence of chorionic gonadotropins in urine is basis for pregnancy tests)
   c. 17-ketosteroids from metabolism of corticoids and androgens
5. Abnormal constituents; e.g., glucose, albumin, red blood cells, casts, calculi

Reproductive system

1. Male reproductive organs

A. Glands
1. Main male sex glands (gonads) are the testes
2. Accessory glands
   a. Seminal vesicles (paired)
   b. Prostate gland
   c. Bulbourethral (Cowper's) glands (paired)

B. Ducts
1. Epididymis (paired)
2. Seminal ducts (vas deferens, ductus deferens) (paired)
3. Ejaculatory ducts (paired)
4. Urethra

C. Supporting structures
1. External
   a. Scrotum
   b. Penis
2. Internal—spermatic cords (paired)

D. Testes
1. Structure—fibrous capsule covers each testis and sends partitions into interior of gland, dividing it into lobules composed of tiny tubules called seminiferous tubules, embedded in connective tissue containing interstitial cells; few ducts emerge from top of gland to enter head of epididymis
2. Location—in scrotum, 1 testis in each of 2 compartments of scrotum
3. Functions
   a. Seminiferous tubules carry on spermatogenesis; that is, they form spermatozoa, the male sex cells or gametes
   b. Interstitial cells secrete testosterone, the main androgen or male hormone (see Table 1-17 for testosterone functions)
4. Structure of spermatozoon—consists of head, middle piece, and whiplike tail that propels sperm; microscopic in size

E. Epididymis
1. Location—lies along top and side of each testis
2. Structure—each epididymis consists of single, tightly coiled tube enclosed in fibrous casing
3. Function—conducts seminal fluid (semen) from testes to vas deferens; secretes small part of semen; stores semen prior to ejaculation, sperm becoming motile during this period

F. Vas deferens (seminal ducts)
1. Location—extend through inguinal canal into abdominal cavity, over top and down posterior surface of bladder to join ducts from seminal vesicles
2. Structure—pair of tubes or ducts
3. Function—conduct sperm and small amount of semen from each epididymis to an ejaculatory duct
4. Clinical application—vasectomy is the surgical procedure in which a short section of each vas is cut out and its separated ends tied off; as a result,

sperm cannot enter the ejaculatory ducts and be ejaculated; vasectomy produces only one important physiologic change—semen from a vasectomized male contains no sperm; hence vasectomy sterilizes a man, makes him infertile; it does not render him impotent; it does, however, slightly decrease the amount of semen ejaculated

G. Ejaculatory ducts—formed by union of each vas with duct from seminal vesicle; pass through prostate gland to terminate in urethra; function—ejaculate semen into urethra (urethra described under urinary system)

H. Seminal vesicles
  1. Location—on posterior surface of bladder
  2. Structure—convoluted pouches, mucous lining
  3. Function—secrete nutrient-rich fluid estimated to constitute about 30% of semen

I. Prostate gland
  1. Location—encircles urethra just below bladder
  2. Structure—doughnut-shaped gland with ducts opening into urethra
  3. Function—secretes estimated 60% of semen; prostatic secretion is alkaline in reaction, fact of functional importance, since acid lessens sperm motility; prostatic secretion contains abundance of enzyme, acid phosphatase; therefore, blood level of this enzyme increases in metastasizing cancer of prostate—fact of diagnostic importance

J. Bulbourethral glands (Cowper's)
  1. Location—just below prostate gland
  2. Structure—small, pea-shaped structures with duct leading into urethra
  3. Function—secrete alkaline fluid that forms part of semen

K. Scrotum—skin-covered pouch suspended from perineal region; divided into 2 compartments, each one containing testis, epididymis, and first part of seminal duct

L. Penis—made up of 3 cylindrical masses of erectile tissue that contain large vascular spaces; filling of these with blood causes erection of penis; 2 larger and upper cylinders named corpora cavernosa; smaller, lower one contains urethra, called corpus cavernosum; glans penis—a bulging structure at distal end of penis, over which double fold of skin, prepuce or foreskin, fits loosely

M. Spermatic cord—fibrous tube located in each inguinal canal; serves as casing around each vas deferens and its accompanying blood vessels, lymphatics, and nerves

2. **Female reproductive organs**
A. Names of main female reproductive organs—ovaries, uterus, uterine tubes, vagina, vulva, and breasts
B. Uterus
  1. Structure
    a. Shape and size—pear-shaped organ measuring $3 \times 2 \times 1$ inch in virginal state
    b. Divisions
      (1) Body—upper and main part of uterus; fundus bulging upper surface of body
      (2) Cervix—narrow, lower part of uterus; projects into vagina
    c. Walls—composed of smooth muscle (known as myometrium), lined with mucosa (known as endometrium); partial outer covering (i.e., over upper surface) of parietal peritoneum
    d. Cavities
      (1) Body cavity—small and triangular in shape with 3 openings into it; 2 from uterine tubes, 1 into cervical canal
      (2) Cervical cavity—canal with constricted opening, internal os, into body cavity, and another, external os, into vagina
  2. Location of uterus—in pelvic cavity between bladder and rectum
  3. Position of uterus—flexed between body and cervix, with body lying over bladder, pointing forward and slightly upward; cervix joins vagina at right angles; organ capable of considerable mobility; therefore, often gets in abnormal positions, such as retroverted (tilted backward)
  4. Ligaments of uterus—hold uterus in position; 8 ligaments; all but 2 are folds of parietal peritoneum
    a. Broad ligaments, 2—a double fold of parietal peritoneum that forms kind of partition across pelvic cavity, suspending uterus between its folds

b. Uterosacral ligaments, 2—foldlike extensions of peritoneum from posterior surface of uterus to sacrum, 1 on each side of rectum

c. Posterior ligament, 1—fold of peritoneum between posterior surface of uterus and rectum; forms deep pouch, cul-de-sac of Douglas (or rectouterine pouch); this pouch lowest point in pelvic cavity and, therefore, place where pus accumulates in pelvic inflammations; can be drained by posterior colpotomy (incision at top of posterior vaginal wall)

d. Anterior ligament, 1—fold of peritoneum between uterus and bladder; forms shallow cul-de-sac

e. Round ligaments, 2—fibromuscular cords from upper, outer angles of uterus, through inguinal canals, terminating in labia majora

5. Functions of uterus
  a. Menstruation
  b. Pregnancy
  c. Labor

C. Uterine tubes (fallopian tubes, oviducts)
1. Location—attached to upper, outer angles of uterus
2. Structure—same 3 coats as uterus; distal ends fimbriated and open into pelvic cavity; mucosal lining of tubes and peritoneal lining of pelvis in direct contact here, fact of importance in spread of infection from tubes to peritoneum
3. Function—serve as ducts through which ova travel from ovaries to uterus; fertilization normally occurs in tube

D. Ovaries—female gonads
1. Location—behind and below uterine tubes, anchored to uterus and broad ligaments
2. Size and shape of large almonds
3. Microscopic structure—each ovary of newborn female consists of several thousand graafian follicles embedded in connective tissue; follicles are epithelial sacs in which ova develop; usually, between years of menarche and menopause, 1 follicle matures each month, ruptures surface of ovary, and expels its ovum into pelvic cavity
4. Functions
  a. Oogenesis—formation of mature ovum in graafian follicle

b. Ovulation—expulsion of ovum from follicle into pelvic cavity

c. Secretion of female hormones; maturing follicle secretes estrogens; corpus luteum secretes progesterone and estrogens (see Table 1-18 for hormone functions)

E. Vagina
1. Location—between rectum and urethra
2. Structure—collapsible, musculomembranous tube, capable of great distention; outlet to exterior protected by fold of mucous membrane called hymen
3. Functions
  a. Receives semen from male
  b. Constitutes lower part of birth canal
  c. Acts as excretory duct for uterine secretions and menstrual blood

F. Vulva—consists of numerous structures that together constitute external genitals; main parts of vulva
1. Mons veneris—hairy, skin-covered pad of fat over symphysis pubis
2. Labia majora—hairy, skin-covered "lips"
3. Labia minora—small "lips" covered with modified skin
4. Clitoris—small mound of erectile tissue, below junction of 2 labia minora
5. Urinary meatus—just below clitoris; opening into urethra
6. Vaginal orifice—below urinary meatus; opening into vagina; hymen, fold of mucosa, partially closes orifice
7. Skene's glands—small mucous glands whose ducts open on either side of the urinary meatus
8. Bartholin's glands—two small, bean-shaped glands; duct from each gland opens on either side of the vaginal orifice; both Bartholin's glands and Skene's glands have clinical interest because they frequently become infected (especially by the gonococcus)

G. Breasts, or mammary glands
1. Location—just under skin, over pectoralis major muscles
2. Size—depends on deposits of adipose tissue rather than amount of glandular tissue
3. Structure—divided into lobes and lobules that, in turn, are composed of racemose glands; excretory duct leads from each lobe to open in nipple; cir-

cular, pigmented area, the areola, borders nipples

4. Function—secrete milk (lactation)
5. Control of lactation—briefly
    a. Shedding of placenta causes marked decrease in blood levels of estrogens and progesterone which, in turn, stimulates anterior pituitary to increase prolactin secretion; high blood level of prolactin stimulates alveoli of breast to secrete milk
    b. Suckling controls lactation in 2 ways: by acting in some way to stimulate anterior pituitary secretion of prolactin and to stimulate posterior pituitary secretion of oxytocin, which stimulates milk "letdown," i.e., release of milk out of alveoli into ducts from which infant can remove it by suckling

3. **Menstrual cycle**
A. Meaning—term menstrual cycle refers mainly to changes in the uterus and ovaries, which recur cyclically from the time of the menarche to the menopause; however, many related cyclic changes also occur, e.g., in breasts, vaginal epithelium, uterine contractions, body temperature, and emotional "tone"
B. Length of cycle—28 days, typical; considerable variation, however, between individuals and often in one individual from time to time
C. Hormonal control of menstrual cycle—not yet completely understood but following information is generally accepted as fact
    1. Menses—brought on by marked decrease in blood levels of progesterone and estrogens at about cycle day 25
    2. Growth of new follicle and ovum—the low blood concentration of estrogens present for a few days before and during the menses stimulates the anterior pituitary gland to secrete follicle-stimulating hormone (FSH); the resulting high blood concentration of FSH stimulates one or more primitive graafian follicles and their ova to start growing and also stimulates the follicle cells to secrete estrogens; this leads to a high blood concentration of estrogens which, in turn, has a negative feedback effect on FSH secretion by the anterior pituitary gland; i.e., a high blood concentration of estrogens inhibits anterior pituitary secretion of

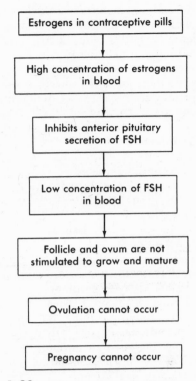

FIG. 1-30
One mechanism by which contraceptive pills may act to prevent pregnancy.

FSH whereas a high blood concentration of FSH stimulates follicular secretion of estrogens
    3. Endometrial thickening—in preovulatory phase is due to proliferation of endometrial cells stimulated by the increasing concentration of estrogens in blood; in premenstrual phase is due partly to endometrial cell proliferation and partly to fluid retention caused by increasing progesterone concentration
    4. Ovulation—brought on by high LH concentration
D. Clinical applications
    1. Contraceptive pills contain synthetic preparations of estrogen-like and/or progesterone-like compounds
    2. Most commonly used contraceptive pills prevent pregnancy by preventing ovulation (Fig. 1-30)
    3. Large doses of a synthetic estrogen-like compound (diethylstilbestrol or DES), given as an emergency measure after intercourse (e.g., after rape), prevent pregnancy by preventing implantation of a fertilized ovum

4. Recently, chemicals called prostaglandins (in the form of vaginal tablets) have been introduced; used the morning after intercourse, they prevent pregnancy by preventing implantation of a fertilized ovum; or prostaglandins may be used routinely on the 28th day of the menstrual cycle; the descriptive nicknames "morning-after pills," "once-a-month pills," and "menses-inducing pills" refer to prostaglandins

FLUID AND ELECTROLYTE BALANCE

1. **Introduction**
A. Meaning of fluid balance—same as homeostasis of fluids
   1. Total volume of fluid and total amount of electrolytes in body are normal and remain relatively constant
   2. Volume of blood plasma, interstitial fluid, and intracellular fluid and the concentration of electrolytes in each remain relatively constant, with homeostasis of distribution of fluid as well as of total volume
B. Fluid balance and electrolyte balance interdependent
2. **Some general principles about fluid balance**
A. Cardinal principle—intake must equal output
B. Fluid and electrolyte balance maintained primarily by mechanisms that adjust output to intake; secondarily by mechanisms that adjust intake to output
C. Fluid balance also maintained by mechanisms that control movement of water between fluid compartments
3. **Avenues by which water enters and leaves body**
A. Water enters body through digestive tract (both in liquids and in foods)
B. Water is formed in body by metabolism of foods
C. Water leaves body via kidneys, lungs, skin, and intestines
4. **Mechanisms that maintain homeostasis of total fluid volume**
A. The chief mechanisms for maintaining homeostasis of total fluid volume are those that regulate the amount of fluid lost by way of the urine, increasing or decreasing it to make the total fluid output volume equal the total fluid intake volume

B. Under abnormal conditions, various factors such as hyperventilation, hypoventilation, vomiting, diarrhea, and circulatory failure may alter the volume of fluid lost
C. Regulation of fluid intake
   1. Mechanism by which intake adjusted to output not completely known
   2. One controlling factor seems to be degree of moistness of mucosa of mouth—if output exceeds intake, mouth feels dry, sensation of thirst occurs, and individual ingests liquids
5. **Mechanisms that maintain homeostasis of fluid distribution**
A. Comparison of plasma, interstitial fluid, and intracellular fluid
   1. Plasma and interstitial fluid constitute extracellular fluid (ECF), internal environment of body or, in other words, environment of cells
   2. Intracellular fluid (ICF) volume largest, plasma volume smallest; ICF about 40% of body weight, IF about 16%, and plasma about 4%, or ICF volume about ten times that of plasma and IF volume about four times plasma volume
   3. Chemically, plasma and IF almost identical except that plasma contains slightly more electrolytes and considerably more proteins than IF; also blood contains somewhat more sodium and fewer chloride ions
   4. Chemically, ECF and ICF strikingly different; sodium main cation of ECF; potassium main cation of ICF; chloride main anion of ECF; phosphate main anion of ICF; protein concentration much higher in ICF than in IF
B. Control of water movement between plasma and interstitial fluid
   1. By four pressures—blood hydrostatic (BHP) and osmotic pressures (BOP) and interstitial fluid hydrostatic (IFHP) and osmotic pressures (IFOP); two of these pressures, namely BHP and IFOP, tend to move fluid out of the blood in the capillaries into the interstitial fluid; BOP and IFHP tend to move fluid back into the capillary blood from the interstitial fluid; therefore, as Starling's law of the capillaries states, equal amounts of water

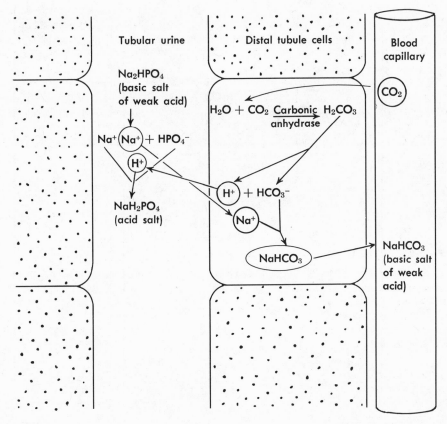

FIG. 1-31

Acidification of urine and conservation of base by distal renal tubule excretion of H ions into the urine and reabsorption of Na ions into the blood in exchange for the H ions excreted from it. (From Anthony, C. P., and Kolthoff, N. J.: Textbook of anatomy and physiology, ed. 8, St. Louis, 1971, The C. V. Mosby Co.)

move back and forth between blood and interstitial fluid only when BHP + IFOP equals BOP + IF; in other words, water balance exists between blood and IF only under these conditions; corollaries of Starling's law of the capillaries are that blood gains fluid from interstitial fluid whenever (BHP + IFOP) is less than (BOP + IFHP) and loses fluid to interstitial fluid whenever (BHP + IFOP) is greater than (BOP + IFHP)

2. Control of water movement through cell membranes, i.e., between extracellular and intracellular fluids: primarily by relative osmotic pressures of ECF and ICF, which depend mainly upon sodium concentration of ECF and potassium concentration of ICF; for example, if ECF sodium concentration increases, its volume also increases due to net osmosis into the ECF from the ICF; in contrast, if ICF potassium increases, its volume increases (while ECF volume decreases as it loses water to ICF due to net osmosis into ICF)

ACID-BASE BALANCE

1. **Some principles about acid-base balance**
A. Healthy survival depends upon the body's maintaining a state of acid-base balance; more specifically, healthy survival depends upon the maintenance of a relatively constant, slightly alkaline pH of blood and other body fluids
B. When the body is in a state of acid-base balance, it maintains homeostasis of the hydrogen ion concentration of body fluids; specifically, blood pH remains

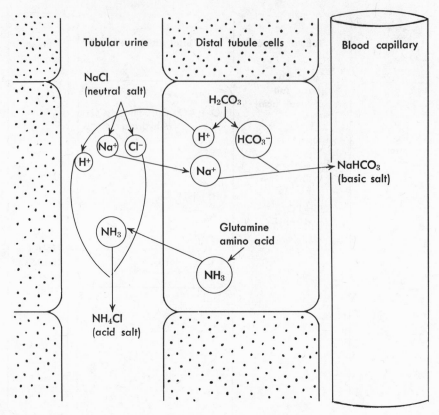

FIG. 1-32

Acidification of urine by tubule excretion of ammonia (NH₃). An acid (glutamine) leaves blood, enters a tubule cell, and is deaminized to form ammonia that is excreted into urine, where it combines with hydrogen to form NH₄ ion. In exchange for NH₄ ion, the tubule cell reabsorbs Na ion. (From Anthony, C. P., and Kolthoff, N. J.: Textbook of anatomy and physiology, ed. 8, St. Louis, 1971, The C. V. Mosby Co.)

relatively constant between 7.35 and 7.45
C. The body has three devices or mechanisms for maintaining acid-base balance; named in order of the speed with which they act they are the buffer mechanism, the respiratory mechanism, and the renal or urinary mechanism
D. A state of uncompensated acidosis exists if blood pH decreases below 7.35
E. A state of uncompensated alkalosis exists if blood pH increases above 7.45
2. **The buffer mechanism for maintaining acid-base balance**
A. The buffer mechanism consists of chemicals called buffers, which are present in the blood and other body fluids and which combine with relatively strong acids or bases to convert them to weaker acids or bases; hence, buffers function to prevent marked changes in blood

pH when either acids or bases enter the blood
B. A buffer is often referred to as a "buffer pair" because it consists of not one but two substances; the chief buffer pair in the blood consists of the weak acid, carbonic acid (H_2CO_3), and its basic salts, collectively called base bicarbonate ($B.HCO_3$); sodium bicarbonate ($NaHCO_3$) is by far the most abundant base bicarbonate present in blood plasma
C. When the body is in a state of acid-base balance, blood contains 27 mEq. base bicarbonate per liter and 1.35 mEq. carbonic acid per liter; usually this is written as a ratio, referred to as the base bicarbonate/carbonic acid ratio:

$$\frac{27 \text{ mEq. B.HCO}_3}{1.35 \text{ mEq. H}_2\text{CO}_3} = \frac{20}{1}$$

D. Whenever the base bicarbonate/carbonic acid ratio of blood equals 20/1, blood pH equals 7.4

E. Base bicarbonate buffers nonvolatile acids that are stronger than carbonic acid; it reacts with them to convert them to carbonic acid and a basic salt; for example, lactic acid (an acid produced during catabolism and added to blood as it flows through the tissue capillaries) is a stronger acid—i.e., adds more H^+ to blood—than carbonic acid; sodium bicarbonate buffers lactic acid as follows:

H. lactate + $NaHCO_3$ → H_2CO_3 + Sodium lactate
(lactic acid) (buffer)

Some facts to note about the changes in capillary blood produced by the buffering of blood by base bicarbonate:

1. Buffering does not prevent blood pH from decreasing, but it does prevent it from decreasing as markedly as it would without buffering; because carbonic acid is a weaker acid than lactic acid, it ionizes less, thereby adding fewer hydrogen ions to blood than lactic acid would have

2. Buffering removes some $NaHCO_3$ from blood and adds some H_2CO_3 to it; this necessarily decreases the base bicarbonate/carbonic acid ratio, which in turn necessarily decreases the pH of blood as it flows through capillaries (from its arterial level of about 7.4 to its venous level of about 7.38)

   Principle worth remembering: anything that decreases blood's base bicarbonate/carbonic acid ratio necessarily decreases blood pH, hence tends to produce acidosis; the *corollary* is also true: anything that increases the base bicarbonate/carbonic acid ratio necessarily increases blood pH, hence tends to produce alkalosis

3. **Respiratory mechanism for controlling acid-base balance**

A. Venous blood enters lung capillaries and as it flows through them, carbon dioxide moves out of the blood into the alveolar air and is blown out of the body in the expired air; this means that the arterial blood leaving the lung capillaries contains less carbon dioxide than does the venous blood entering them

B. Whenever blood's carbon dioxide content decreases, its hydrogen ion concentration also decreases, and therefore its pH increases because a decrease in the amount of carbon dioxide in blood causes the following reactions to reverse themselves (application of the law of mass action): i.e., to proceed toward the left, thereby decreasing the number of hydrogen ions remaining in the blood

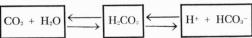

$$CO_2 + H_2O \rightleftharpoons H_2CO_3 \rightleftharpoons H^+ + HCO_3^-$$

Note: These equations show why the carbon dioxide content of blood and its hydrogen ion concentration are always directly related to each other; any increase in blood's carbon dioxide content drives the reactions to the right so increases blood's hydrogen ion concentration (i.e., decreases its pH); any decrease in blood's carbon dioxide decreases its hydrogen ion concentration (i.e., increases its pH)

4. **The renal or urinary mechanism for maintaining acid-base balance**

A. The renal mechanism is the most effective device the body has for maintaining acid-base balance; unless it operates adequately, acid-base balance cannot be maintained

B. The renal mechanism for maintaining acid-base balance makes the urine more acid and the blood more alkaline; the mechanism consists of two functions performed by the distal renal tubule cells, both of which remove hydrogen ions from blood to urine and in exchange reabsorb sodium ions from tubular urine to blood

1. Distal tubule cells secrete hydrogen ions and reabsorb sodium ions as shown in Fig. 1-31

2. Distal tubule cells form ammonia which combines with hydrogen ions they have secreted to form ammonium (NH_4) ions which are excreted in the urine in exchange for sodium ions which are reabsorbed into the blood as shown in Fig. 1-32

C. The preceding distal tubule functions produce the following results:

1. They increase blood's sodium bicarbonate content and decrease its carbonic acid content, thereby increasing the base bicarbonate/carbonic acid ratio and blood pH

2. They acidify urine, i.e., decrease urine pH

5. Clinical applications

The drug acetazolamide (Diamox) inhibits the enzyme carbonic anhydrase; as you can deduce from Fig. 1-31, inhibition of carbonic anhydrase will slow carbonic acid formation and hydrogen ion secretion into urine by the distal tubule cells; this, in turn, will slow sodium bicarbonate reabsorption and therefore water reabsorption from the urine into blood; results of carbonic anhydrase inhibition—urine becomes more alkaline, blood becomes less alkaline, urine volume increases (diuresis), and ECF volume decreases

REVIEW QUESTIONS FOR ANATOMY AND PHYSIOLOGY
Multiple choice

Read each question carefully and consider all possible answers. When you have decided which answer is best, blacken in the corresponding space on the answer sheet. There is only one best answer for each question (or implied question).

1. Which of the following is the smallest unit capable of maintaining life and reproducing itself?
   1. Cell
   2. Centrosome
   3. DNA
   4. RNA
2. What term refers to part of the chest cavity?
   1. Mediastinum
   2. Pelvis
   3. Pleural cavity
   4. Thoracic cavity
3. Which of the following organs does not lie in the mediastinum?
   1. Esophagus
   2. Pineal gland
   3. Thymus gland
   4. Trachea
4. To open the heart, a surgeon would have to cut through the
   1. Pericardium
   2. Peritoneum
   3. Pleura
   4. 1 and 3
5. Which word best describes the location of the stomach with reference to the pancreas?
   1. Anterior
   2. Distal
   3. Dorsal
   4. Superior
6. You would not look in the pelvic cavity to find the
   1. Ovaries
   2. Sigmoid colon
   3. Thymus gland
   4. Uterus
7. To find the spleen, you would look in which region of the abdominal cavity?
   1. Hypogastric
   2. Left hypochondriac
   3. Left lumbar
   4. Right hypochondriac
8. The title sagittal section of the brain means that the brain was cut
   1. Across horizontally
   2. Into anterior and posterior portions
   3. Into right and left portions
   4. Into sections suitable for microscopic examination

9. What term describes the location of the upper arm muscles with reference to the lower arm?
   1. Caudal
   2. Distal
   3. Dorsal
   4. Proximal
10. The term homeostasis means
    1. Cellular reproduction
    2. Constancy within a narrow range
    3. Energy release
    4. Unchanging
11. In order to survive in a healthy condition the body must maintain relative stability of its internal environment. This cardinal physiologic principle is known as
    1. Boyle's law or principle
    2. Starling's principle
    3. Principle of homeostasis
    4. Principle of integration
12. Delicate membranes compose the walls of most kinds of cytoplasmic organelles but not of the
    1. Golgi apparatus
    2. Lysosomes
    3. Mitochondria
    4. Ribosomes
13. "Protein factory" is a nickname for the
    1. Endoplasmic reticulum
    2. Golgi apparatus
    3. Lysosomes
    4. Ribosomes
14. "Cellular power plant" is a nickname for the
    1. Centrosome
    2. Golgi apparatus
    3. Lysosomes
    4. Mitochondria
15. Cellular digestive bag is a nickname for the
    1. Centrosome
    2. Golgi apparatus
    3. Lysosomes
    4. Mitochondria
16. What structure is now believed to synthesize carbohydrate, combine it with protein, and secrete the product in miniature, globular-shaped packages?
    1. Centrosome
    2. Endoplasmic reticulum
    3. Golgi apparatus
    4. Lysosomes
17. The small granules attached to the endoplasmic reticulum consist chiefly of
    1. ATP (adenosine triphosphate)
    2. DNA (deoxyribonucleic acid)
    3. Fat-splitting enzymes
    4. RNA (ribonucleic acid)
18. The small granules attached to the endoplasmic reticulum are
    1. Ribosomes
    2. Mitochondria
    3. Lysosomes
    4. Centrosomes
19. Which of the following does not require the presence of a living cell?
    1. Active transport
    2. Metabolism
    3. Mitosis
    4. Osmosis
20. Which molecules can duplicate or "reproduce" themselves?
    1. All molecules
    2. ATP
    3. DNA
    4. DNA and ATP
21. A cell can still live in a healthy condition without performing one of the following functions. Which one?
    1. Active transport
    2. Anabolism
    3. Catabolism
    4. Mitosis
22. Which part of the cell plays the most important part in heredity?
    1. Cytoplasm
    2. Golgi apparatus
    3. Lysosome
    4. Nucleus

23. Which tissue performs the functions of secretion and absorption?
    1. Columnar epithelial
    2. Simple squamous epithelial
    3. Lymphoid
    4. Reticular
24. Which sentence states a truth about osmosis?
    1. Both water and solute particles can osmose through some membranes
    2. If a membrane freely permeable to water and to all solutes present separates two solutions, water does not osmose through this membrane but, rather, diffuses through it
    3. If water osmoses through a membrane, it osmoses through it in only one direction
    4. Net osmosis occurs from a more concentrated solution into a more dilute one
25. Substances can enter or leave a living cell but not a dead one by
    1. Diffusion   3. Mitosis
    2. Osmosis   4. Phagocytosis
26. The accompanying diagram represents a cell immersed in a 10% sodium chloride solution. Assume that the cell membrane permits free movement of both water and NaCl through it. Water will move through the cell membrane by
    1. Dialysis   10% NaCl
    2. Diffusion   0.85% NaCl
    3. Osmosis
    4. Both 2 and 3
27. NaCl would move through the membrane of the cell shown in question 26 in which direction?
    1. Both into and out of the cell
    2. Into the cell
    3. Out of the cell
28. Under the conditions specified in question 26, net movement of NaCl would
    1. Occur in both directions through the membrane
    2. Occur into the cell
    3. Occur out of the cell
    4. Not occur
29. Under the conditions specified in question 26, net movement of water would
    1. Occur in both directions
    2. Occur into the cell
    3. Occur out of the cell
    4. Not occur
30. If the cell membrane shown in item 26 were impermeable to NaCl
    1. More water would move into the cell than out of it
    2. The net movement of water would occur down the water concentration gradient, which is up the solute concentration gradient
    3. Water would move through the membrane by osmosis
    4. Both 2 and 3
31. Which of the following is false?
    1. Net diffusion of water occurs only in one direction
    2. Net diffusion of water occurs down a water concentration gradient, which is up a solute concentration gradient
    3. Net diffusion continues even after two solutions separated by a membrane have equilibrated
    4. Net diffusion of water and net diffusion of solute through a membrane both tend to equilibrate the two solutions separated by the membrane
32. Which of the following is true?
    1. The direction of net osmosis through a suitable membrane is down the solute concentration gradient
    2. To say that water osmoses through a membrane that maintains a solute concentration gradient is preferable to saying that it diffuses through this membrane
    3. Both 1 and 2
    4. Neither 1 nor 2
33. Which of the following results from smooth muscle contraction?
    1. Vasoconstriction
    2. Gooseflesh
    3. Both of the preceding
    4. None of the preceding
34. Which of the following states a truth about red bone marrow?
    1. Also referred to as hemopoietic tissue and myeloid tissue
    2. Located in the medullary cavity of long bones
    3. Forms all red blood cells in infants but not in adults
    4. Serves as the main storage depot for iron
35. The scientific name for bone-forming cells is
    1. Haversian cells   3. Osteoclasts
    2. Osteoblasts   4. Osteocytes
36. In the adult, red bone marrow is present
    1. In the diaphyses and epiphyses of long bones
    2. Only in the diaphyses of long bones
    3. Only in the epiphyses of certain long bones
    4. None of the preceding
37. The layman's name for the clavicle is
    1. Collar bone   3. Shin bone
    2. Kneecap   4. Shoulder blade
38. The scientific name for the shin bone is
    1. Femur   3. Patella
    2. Fibula   4. Tibia
39. The scientific name for the socket for the humerus is
    1. Acetabulum   3. Glenoid cavity
    2. Crista galli   4. Sella turcica
40. What bat-shaped bone forms the midportion of the cranial floor?
    1. Atlas   3. Ethmoid
    2. Calcaneus   4. Sphenoid
41. What bone or bony projection lies behind the point where the wrist artery is palpated for counting the pulse?
    1. One of the carpal bones
    2. One of the tarsal bones
    3. Radius
    4. Ulna
42. The sella turcica
    1. Contains the pineal body
    2. Contains the pituitary body
    3. Is a depression in the ethmoid bone
    4. More than one of the preceding is true
43. Which of the following is true about diarthrotic joints?

1. All of them permit flexion, extension, abduction, and adduction
2. Ligaments hold the joining bones together
3. Synovial membrane lines the joint cavity
4. Both 2 and 3

44. One of the bones of the face is the
    1. Astragalus   3. Malar
    2. Calcaneus   4. Malleus
45. Which of the following is a bone in neither the upper nor the lower extremity?
    1. Calcaneus   3. Hyoid
    2. Fibula   4. Patella
46. Which movements can you perform at both your hip and knee joints?
    1. Abduction and adduction
    2. Abduction and extension
    3. Circumduction and rotation
    4. Flexion and extension
47. Which of the following is (are) not part of the ethmoid bone?
    1. Cribriform plate   3. Sinuses
    2. Crista galli   4. Sella turcica
48. Which muscle does not function as an extensor?
    1. Rectus abdominis   3. Sacrospinalis
    2. Rectus femoris   4. Trapezius

Situation: Mrs. Adams, a 70-year-old woman, fell and fractured the neck of her right femur. Questions 49 to 53 relate to this situation.

49. The neck of the femur
    1. Is also called the shaft or diaphysis of the femur
    2. Lies at the distal end of the femur, a short distance above the knee joint
    3. Lies between the greater and the lesser trochanter of the femur
    4. Lies between the head of the femur and the greater trochanter
50. The hip joint
    1. Is a ball-and-socket type amphiarthrosis
    2. Is a pivot type synarthrosis
    3. Like all diarthroses, is enclosed by a fibrous capsule lined with synovial membrane
    4. Joins the femur to the pelvic bone, with the head of the femur fitting into the glenoid cavity
51. Structure of the hip joint makes possible
    1. Abduction, adduction, flexion, and extension of the thigh
    2. Circumduction and rotation of the thigh
    3. Both of the preceding
    4. None of the preceding
52. Mrs. Adams' injured leg cannot support her weight so she cannot walk even though her leg muscles can still contract. When a person steps forward, contraction of the
    1. Biceps femoris and other hamstring muscles extend the thigh and lower leg
    2. Iliopsoas flexes the thigh, and the rectus femoris extends the lower leg
    3. Rectus femoris flexes the thigh and lower leg
    4. Sartorius muscle flexes the thigh and extends the lower leg
53. One of the muscles of the quadriceps femoris group
    1. Contracts to produce the knee-jerk reflex

2. Is located on the front of the thigh
3. Serves as the antagonist to the hamstring group of muscles
4. All of the preceding

54. The part of a neuron that conducts impulses away from its cell body is called
    1. An axon   3. An effector
    2. A dendrite   4. A neurilemma
55. The terminals of axons supplying skeletal muscle
    1. Release acetylcholine
    2. Release ATP
    3. Release cholinesterase
    4. Release epinephrine or closely related compound
56. In what ways does the interior surface of the membrane of a nonconducting neuron differ from the external surface?
    1. Negatively charged and contains less sodium
    2. Positively charged and contains less sodium
    3. Negatively charged and contains more sodium
    4. Positively charged and contains more sodium
57. What force(s) regulate the passage of sodium ions across a nerve cell membrane?
    1. Electric charge
    2. Sodium concentration gradient
    3. Sodium pump
    4. All of the above
58. What is an action potential?
    1. A series of events marked by change in polarization of cell membrane
    2. Transmission of a nerve impulse across a synapse
    3. Recovery of the nerve following passage of an impulse
    4. None of the above
59. The presence of myelin on a nerve fiber gives what characteristics?
    1. Gray color and regeneration of fibers
    2. White color and increased rate of impulse transmission
    3. White color and regeneration of fibers
    4. Gray color and increased rate of impulse transmission
60. A neuron cannot regenerate if
    1. Its cell body has been destroyed
    2. Its axon has no myelin sheath
    3. Its axon has no neurilemma
    4. Both 1 and 3
61. Which is not true about all reflex arcs?
    1. Include a sensory and a motor neuron
    2. Consist of at least 3 neurons
    3. Have their centers in gray matter of the brain or spinal cord
    4. Terminate in muscle or gland
62. The knee-jerk in response to a sharp tap over the patellar tendon
    1. Is an autonomic reflex
    2. Is a conditioned reflex
    3. Is mediated by a 3-neuron reflex arc
    4. Has its reflex center in the spinal cord
63. Which of the following is not necessary for any responses called reflexes?
    1. Autonomic nerves   3. Effectors
    2. Cerebral cortex   4. Synapses

64. If the anterior root of a spinal nerve were cut, what would be the result in the regions supplied by that spinal nerve?
    1. Complete loss of sensation
    2. Complete loss of movement
    3. Complete loss of sensation and movement
    4. Complete loss of sensation, movement, and autonomic control of blood vessels and sweat glands
65. The hypothalamus
    1. Receives impulses from the cerebral cortex
    2. Sends impulses to many autonomic centers
    3. Helps control body temperature and appetite
    4. All of the preceding
66. Almost all sensory impulses pass through what structure on their way to the cerebral cortex?
    1. Corpus striatum   3. Thalamus
    2. Hypothalamus   4. Pallidum
67. Feeling of pleasantness or unpleasantness (varying in degree from mild to intense) occurs when sensory impulses reach the
    1. Basal ganglia   3. Hypothalamus
    2. Cerebral cortex   4. Thalamus

Situation: Mrs. Burt was unconscious when admitted to the hospital. Questions 68 through 76 refer to this patient.

68. Unconsciousness indicates nonfunctioning of
    1. Cerebellum   3. Cerebral nuclei
    2. Cerebral cortex   4. Hypothalamus
69. Mrs. Burt's right eye stayed open and its pupil appeared dilated. Nonconduction by which cranial nerve would explain the fact that Mrs. Burt could not close her right eye?
    1. Second   3. Fourth
    2. Third   4. Seventh
70. Nonconduction by which cranial nerve would explain Mrs. Burt's dilated right pupil?
    1. Second   3. Fourth
    2. Third   4. Seventh
71. Mrs. Burt's mouth was drawn over to the left, a fact suggesting nonconduction by which cranial nerve?
    1. Left facial   3. Right abducens
    2. Right facial   4. Right trigeminal
72. Tendon reflexes—for example, the knee-jerk—on the right side of Mrs. Burt's body were found to be exaggerated. Therefore which of the following structures must still be conducting impulses?
    1. Anterior horn neurons
    2. Basal ganglia
    3. Pyramidal tracts
    4. Upper motoneurons
73. The knee-jerk is
    1. A contralateral reflex, not an ipsilateral one
    2. A flexor reflex
    3. Mediated by a 2-neuron reflex arc
    4. Mediated by a 3-neuron reflex arc
74. When Mrs. Burt regained consciousness, she had a spastic type paralysis of the right side of her body. Spasticity results from nonconduction by certain
    1. Extrapyramidal pathways
    2. Lower motoneurons
    3. Spinothalamic tract fibers
    4. Pyramidal tract fibers
75. Mrs. Burt's paralysis resulted from nonconduction by
    1. Left extrapyramidal tract fibers
    2. Left lower motoneurons
    3. Neurons in left postcentral gyrus
    4. Neurons with cell bodies in left precentral gyrus and axons in pyramidal tracts
76. Mrs. Burt's physician performed a lumbar puncture on her. To do this procedure, he inserted a needle into the
    1. Aqueduct of Sylvius
    2. Foramen ovale
    3. Subarachnoid space
    4. Pia mater
77. Cell bodies of sensory neurons are found in
    1. Anterior root spinal ganglia
    2. Cranial nerve ganglia
    3. Posterior root spinal ganglia
    4. 2 and 3
78. In order for a sensory impulse to travel from receptors in the hand to the cerebral cortex it must pass over
    1. At least 3 neurons
    2. At least 2 neurons
    3. More than 3 neurons
    4. Only 1 neuron
79. What part of the cerebral cortex registers general sensations such as heat, cold, pain, and touch?
    1. Frontal lobe   3. Parietal lobe
    2. Occipital lobe   4. Temporal lobe
80. Which of the following conducts impulses initiated by stimulation of pain receptors?
    1. Lateral spinothalamic tracts
    2. Posterior white columns
    3. Reticulospinal tracts
    4. Ventral spinothalamic tracts

Situation: Mr. Brown suffered severe head injuries in an automobile accident. Questions 81 through 85 relate to Mr. Brown.

81. Because Mr. Brown was still unconscious when he was placed on a cart to move him from the emergency room to the division, the nurse made sure his arms would not hang down over the edge of the cart. By taking this precaution she prevented injury to which plexus?
    1. Basilic   3. Celiac
    2. Brachial   4. Solar
82. Because the part named contains the vital respiratory, cardiac, and vasomotor centers, injury to this part of the brain is particularly likely to cause death. Which part?
    1. Medulla   3. Pons
    2. Midbrain   4. Thalamus
83. Mr. Brown's temperature, soon after admission to the hospital, registered 39° C., a fact suggesting injury of the
    1. Hypothalamus   3. Temporal lobe
    2. Pallidum   4. Thalamus
84. After Mr. Brown recovered consciousness, he complained of hearing ringing noises, a fact suggesting injury of
    1. Cranial nerve VI   3. Frontal lobe
    2. Cranial nerve VIII   4. Occipital lobe
85. Mr. Brown had no paralysis after his accident, a fact suggesting no injury to the
    1. Basal ganglia

2. Parietal lobe
3. Precentral gyrus
4. Postcentral gyrus

86. Pyramidal tract fibers
   1. Are axons of neurons whose cell bodies lie in the cerebral cortex
   2. Are long fibers that extend all the way from the cerebral cortex down through the internal capsule and brainstem and terminate in the spinal cord
   3. Conduct impulses that make willed movements possible
   4. All of the preceding

87. The ability to sense vibrations depends upon conduction by
   1. Association tracts
   2. Posterior gray columns of the cord
   3. Posterior white columns of the cord
   4. Ventral spinothalamic tracts

88. For a motor impulse to travel from the primary motor area of the cerebral cortex to skeletal muscle cells, it must pass over
   1. At least 4 neurons
   2. At least 3 neurons
   3. At least 2 neurons
   4. Only 1 neuron

Situation: Mrs. Johns tells the nurse preparing her for surgery that she is "terribly scared." Questions 89 through 93 relate to Mrs. Johns.

89. The nurse knows that one of the following statements does not accurately describe the autonomic nervous system. Which one?
   1. Both sympathetic and parasympathetic impulses continually play on most visceral effectors
   2. Sympathetic impulses tend to stimulate and parasympathetic impulses tend to inhibit the functioning of any visceral effector
   3. The autonomic nervous system does not function autonomously but is regulated by impulses from the hypothalamus and other parts of the brain
   4. Visceral effectors (namely, cardiac muscle, smooth muscle, and glandular epithelial tissue) receive impulses only via autonomic neurons

90. Which of the following is not a visceral effector?
   1. Blood vessels
   2. Heart
   3. Pancreas
   4. Soleus

91. The nurse knows that various changes in nervous system functioning occur during stress. For example
   1. A change occurs in the ratio of parasympathetic to sympathetic impulses conducted to most viscera
   2. Conduction by the autonomic nervous system is initiated by stress
   3. Conduction by parasympathetic neurons ceases
   4. Conduction by sympathetic neurons begins

92. In caring for Mrs. Johns, the nurse observed the following indication of sympathetic control
   1. Mrs. Johns' pupils appeared no bigger than the head of a common pin
   2. Her skin appeared very pale

3. Her skin felt very dry
4. She had a pulse rate of 60

93. Which of the following indicate parasympathetic dominance?
   1. Excess epinephrine secretion, causing vasoconstriction and leading to hypertension
   2. Excess hydrochloric acid secretion, leading to stomach ulcer
   3. Constipation
   4. Goose pimples

94. A nurse is caring for a patient with a tumor of the cerebellum. In view of the functions of this organ, what symptom(s) should she expect to observe?
   1. Absence of the knee-jerk and other reflexes
   2. Inability to execute smooth, precise movements
   3. Inability to execute voluntary movements
   4. Unconsciousness

95. A patient, asked to stand still with eyes closed, starts to sway and almost falls. One of the following spinal cord structures is diseased in this patient. Which one?
   1. Anterior gray columns
   2. Anterior white columns
   3. Posterior gray columns
   4. Posterior white columns

96. Which of the following must function for hearing to take place?
   1. Cochlear nerve
   2. Organ of Corti
   3. Both of the preceding
   4. Vestibular and organ of Corti nerve

97. Which part of the ear contains the receptors for hearing?
   1. Cochlea
   2. Middle ear
   3. Tympanic cavity
   4. Utricle

98. Cones are
   1. Absent from the fovea centralis of the retina
   2. Most numerous in the optic disc area of the retina
   3. Not stimulated by dim light
   4. Specialized structures in the organ of Corti

99. The cornea is
   1. The colored part of the eye
   2. The white part of the eye
   3. Transparent and lies over the colored part of the eye
   4. Transparent and lies under the colored part of the eye

100. When the ciliary muscles of the eye contract
   1. The lens bulges
   2. The lens flattens
   3. The pupils constrict
   4. The pupils dilate

101. When the ciliary muscles contract
   1. They bring about convergence of the two eyes
   2. They close the eyelids
   3. They focus the lens on distant objects
   4. They focus the lens on near objects

102. Failure to feel pain from an abscessed tooth might be due to disease of which cranial nerve?

1. Facial   3. Third
2. Second   4. Fifth

103. The anterior pituitary gland does not secrete
    1. Antidiuretic hormone
    2. Follicle-stimulating hormone, luteinizing hormone, and lactogenic hormone
    3. Growth hormone
    4. Thyroid-stimulating hormone

Situation: Mr. Pierce, a patient who has acromegaly and diabetes mellitus, has had a hypophysectomy by means of yttrium 90 rods implanted in his pituitary gland. Questions 104 through 110 relate to Mr. Pierce.

104. Presumably an oversecretion of which hormone produces acromegaly?
    1. Growth hormone
    2. Thyroid hormone
    3. Thyroid-stimulating hormone
    4. Testosterone

105. Which of the following hormones is not secreted by the anterior pituitary gland?
    1. ACTH
    2. Aldosterone
    3. Growth hormone
    4. Interstitial cell–stimulating hormone

106. Hormones secreted by the anterior pituitary gland are essential for stimulating growth and hormone secretion by certain other endocrine glands—for example, by which of the following?
    1. Adrenal medulla
    2. Islands of Langerhans
    3. Parathyroids
    4. Thyroid, gonads, and adrenal cortex

107. Which of the following will not be true of Mr. Pierce following his hypophysectomy? He will
    1. Be sterile for the rest of his life
    2. Have to take cortisone (or similar preparation) for the rest of his life
    3. Have to take thyroxin (or similar preparation) for the rest of his life
    4. Require larger doses of insulin than he did preoperatively

108. Mr. Pierce might develop any of the following conditions except one as the result of his hypophysectomy. Which one could not result from the hypophysectomy?
    1. Adrenal crisis (marked hypocorticoidism)
    2. Diabetes insipidus
    3. Diabetes mellitus
    4. Hypothyroidism

109. Increased blood concentration of cortisol (hydrocortisone)
    1. Decreases anterior pituitary secretion of ACTH
    2. Makes the body less able to resist stress successfully
    3. Tends to accelerate wound healing
    4. Tends to decrease liver gluconeogenesis

110. Corticoids do not produce
    1. Anabolic effect
    2. Anti-immunity effect
    3. Hyperglycemic effect
    4. Potassium-losing effect

111. ICHS (interstitial cell–stimulating hormone) is the male counterpart of which of the following in the female?
    1. FSH
    2. Lactogenic hormone
    3. Luteinizing hormone
    4. Progesterone

112. Which of the following secretes an antidiuretic substance important for maintaining fluid balance?
    1. Anterior pituitary
    2. Adrenal cortex
    3. Adrenal medulla
    4. Posterior pituitary

113. Parathyroid hormone is the hormone that tends to
    1. Accelerate bone breakdown with release of calcium into the blood
    2. Decrease blood calcium concentration
    3. Decrease blood phosphate concentration
    4. Increase calcium absorption into bone

114. The hormone that tends to decrease blood calcium concentration is
    1. Aldosterone
    2. Thyrocalcitonin
    3. Parathyroid hormone
    4. Thyroid hormone

115. High concentration of estrogens in the blood
    1. Causes ovulation
    2. Inhibits anterior pituitary secretion of FSH
    3. Is one of the causes of osteoporosis
    4. Stimulates lactation

116. Blood sugar tends to decrease following increased secretion of
    1. ACTH
    2. Adrenaline
    3. Glucagon
    4. None of the preceding

117. If a young man weighs 70 kg., which of the following would be considered a normal total blood volume for his body?
    1. 1,000 ml.   3. 5 L.
    2. 5 gal.   4. 10 L.

118. Myeloid tissue is another name for
    1. Connective tissue
    2. Lymphatic tissue
    3. Red bone marrow
    4. Red or yellow bone marrow

119. If 75% of your white blood cells were which of the following, it would be considered normal
    1. Erythrocytes   3. Monocytes
    2. Lymphocytes   4. Neutrophils

120. Reticulocyte is a synonym for
    1. Platelet
    2. One type of immature monocyte
    3. One type of immature red blood cell
    4. None of the preceding

121. Whole-body irradiation injures or destroys bone marrow, making it unable to function normally. As a result, which of the following would you expect to develop?
    1. Anemia
    2. Decreased susceptibility to infections
    3. Increased tendency for bones to break
    4. Increased blood viscosity

122. The more blood cells per cubic millimeter of blood
    1. The greater the blood viscosity

2. The higher the hematocrit
3. Both of the preceding
4. None of the preceding

123. Which function(s) do red blood cells perform?
1. Hemopoiesis
2. Synthesis of antibodies
3. Transport of carbon dioxide and oxygen
4. Transport of oxygen but not of carbon dioxide

124. Which of the following is thought to stimulate red blood cell formation?
1. Corticoid deficiency
2. Hypercapnia
3. Hypoxia
4. Irradiation

125. Type AB blood
1. Contains A and B antibodies
2. Contains A and B antigens
3. Is universal donor type blood
4. More than one of the preceding

126. When blood clots, what soluble substance becomes an insoluble gel?
1. Fibrin   3. Prothrombin
2. Fibrinogen   4. Thrombin

127. Vitamin K is essential for normal blood clotting because it promotes
1. Ionization of blood calcium
2. Platelet disintegration
3. Fibrinogen formation by liver
4. Prothrombin formation by liver

128. What substance formed in blood acts as a catalyst for the final blood-clotting reaction?
1. Fibrinogen   3. Prothrombin
2. Prothrombinase   4. Thrombin

129. Jaundiced patients are susceptible to postoperative hemorrhage because their blood does not clot normally. Why?
1. Excess bile salts in blood inactivate prothrombinase
2. Excess bile salts in blood inhibit liver synthesis of prothrombin
3. Excess bile salts in blood inhibit liver synthesis of vitamin K
4. Lack of bile in intestines causes inadequate vitamin K absorption, which causes inadequate prothrombin synthesis by liver

Situation: Mr. James lost a large volume of blood as a result of injuries sustained in an automobile accident. Assume that normally Mr. James had the pressures shown below in the two columns at the left and that immediately following his blood loss they changed as shown in the two columns on the right. (Figures indicate mm. Hg pressure.) Questions 130 through 135 relate to Mr. James.

	HP	OP	HP	OP
Capillary blood	24	25	18	25
Interstitial fluid	4	5	4	5

130. According to Starling's law of the capillaries
1. Blood hydrostatic pressure (BHP) tends to move fluid out of blood into interstitial fluid, and interstitial fluid hydrostatic pressure (IFHP) tends to move fluid in the opposite direction
2. Blood osmotic pressure (BOP) tends to draw fluid into capillary blood from interstitial fluid, and interstitial fluid osmotic pressure (IFOP) tends to draw fluid out of capillary blood into interstitial fluid
3. The total force tending to move fluid out of blood into interstitial fluid is the sum of BHP + IFOP
4. All of the preceding are true

131. In order for blood and interstitial fluid to exchange even amounts of fluid
1. (BHP + IFOP) minus (IFHP + BOP) must equal zero
2. (BHP + IFOP) must equal (IFHP + BOP)
3. Both of the preceding
4. None of the preceding

132. Before Mr. James' accident
1. The sum of the pressures that tended to move fluid out of his blood into his interstitial fluid was 28 mm. Hg
2. The sum of the pressures that tended to move fluid into his capillary blood from his interstitial fluid was 30 mm. Hg
3. Both of the preceding
4. The sum of the pressures that tended to move fluid into blood was 29 mm. Hg

133. Immediately after Mr. James had lost a large volume of blood
1. A net force of 6 mm. Hg pressure caused his blood to gain fluid from his interstitial fluid
2. His blood volume decreased even further due to operation of Starling's law of the capillaries
3. The sum of the two pressures that tended to cause blood to lose fluid to interstitial fluid equalled 14 mm. Hg pressure
4. The sum of the two pressures that tended to cause blood to gain fluid from interstitial fluid equalled 20 mm. Hg

134. Within a few hours enough fluid had shifted into Mr. James' blood from his interstitial fluid to raise capillary hydrostatic pressure to 24 mm. Hg. At that point, which of the following was not true?
1. No more water moved between Mr. James' blood and his interstitial fluid
2. The sum of the pressures tending to move fluid out of Mr. James' blood into his interstitial fluid equalled 29 mm. Hg
3. The sum of the pressures tending to move fluid into Mr. James' blood from his interstitial fluid equalled 29 mm. Hg
4. The amount of fluid exchanged between Mr. James' blood and his interstitial fluid became equal

135. According to Starling's law of the capillaries
1. Any factor that decreases capillary osmotic pressure tends to cause edema by decreasing the amount of fluid moving into blood from interstitial fluid
2. Any factor that increases capillary hydrostatic pressure tends to cause edema by increasing the amount of fluid moving out of blood into interstitial fluid

3. Both of the preceding
4. Neither of the preceding

136. An artificial pacemaker is used in some patients to perform the function normally performed by the
    1. Accelerator nerves to the heart
    2. Atrioventricular node
    3. Bundle of His
    4. Sinoatrial node

137. Intravenous infusions in the adult are usually given into the
    1. Brachial artery
    2. Brachial vein
    3. Median basilic vein
    4. Radial vein

138. Which chamber of the heart ejects oxygenated blood into the general systemic circulation?
    1. Left atrium   3. Right atrium
    2. Left ventricle   4. Right ventricle

139. What part of the heart does blood enter when returning from the lungs?
    1. Left atrium   3. Right atrium
    2. Left ventricle   4. Right ventricle

140. Which chamber of the heart receives most of the returning venous blood?
    1. Left atrium   3. Right atrium
    2. Left ventricle   4. Right ventricle

141. Which of the following statements is not true about blood pressure?
    1. Is highest in the arteries, lowest in the capillaries
    2. Is due largely to the pumping action of the heart
    3. Varies with the amount of blood in the arteries; the fuller the arteries, the higher the arterial blood pressure
    4. Decreases as a result of generalized vasodilatation

142. In certain kinds of kidney diseases blood albumin is lost in the urine. Which of the following conditions does this lead to?
    1. Decreased blood osmotic pressure
    2. Decreased blood volume
    3. Edema
    4. All of the preceding

143. Which of the following homeostatic mechanisms are initiated by a decrease in arterial blood pressure (e.g., after hemorrhage)?
    1. Reflex acceleration of the heart
    2. Reflex vasoconstriction in skin and other blood reservoirs
    3. Both of the preceding
    4. Reflex slowing of the heart and vasodilatation in skin and other blood reservoirs

144. Which of the following is a false statement about blood proteins?
    1. Contribute to blood viscosity
    2. Do not function to help the body resist infectious diseases
    3. Help maintain normal blood volume
    4. Play a major part in blood clotting

145. In general, the higher the red blood cell count
    1. The greater the blood viscosity
    2. The higher the blood pH
    3. The less it contributes to immunity
    4. The lower the hematocrit

146. Lymph nodes do not
    1. Carry on phagocytosis
    2. Filter particles out of lymph
    3. Form lymphocytes that may become plasma cells and produce antibodies
    4. Form neutrophils

147. In the adult, the spleen normally does not
    1. Destroy platelets and worn-out red blood cells by phagocytosis
    2. Form monocytes, lymphocytes, and plasma cells
    3. Form red blood cells
    4. Serve as a storage depot for blood

148. What structure(s) is (are) located on the posterior wall of the nasopharynx?
    1. Adenohypophysis
    2. Adenoids
    3. Pineal gland
    4. Tonsils

149. The amount of oxygen dissolved in plasma
    1. And that combined with hemoglobin are about equal
    2. Is only a small fraction of the amount combined with hemoglobin
    3. Is much greater than the amount combined with hemoglobin
    4. Is slightly less than the amount combined with hemoglobin

150. Blood samples from the right atrium, right ventricle, and pulmonary artery are analyzed for their oxygen content during cardiac catheterizations. Normally
    1. All contain about the same amount of oxygen
    2. All contain about 20 vol.% oxygen
    3. Pulmonary artery blood contains the most oxygen of these samples
    4. All contain more oxygen than pulmonary vein blood

151. Which of the following contains the most carbon dioxide?
    1. Alveolar air
    2. Interstitial fluid
    3. Intracellular fluid
    4. Pulmonary vein blood

152. Oxygen and carbon dioxide are exchanged in the lungs by
    1. Active transport mechanism
    2. Diffusion
    3. Filtration
    4. Osmosis

153. Oxygen and carbon dioxide pass through normal living cell membranes by
    1. Active transport mechanisms
    2. Diffusion
    3. Filtration
    4. Both 1 and 2

154. Cutting the left phrenic nerve
    1. Is done to relieve pain in the left side of the chest
    2. Paralyzes left diaphragm, so collapses left lung
    3. Collapses right lung
    4. Paralyzes the diaphragm on the opposite side

155. The physical examination reveals that a patient's tidal air is normal. What is "tidal air"?
    1. Amount of air exhaled normally after a normal inspiration

2. Amount of air that can be exhaled forcibly after a normal inspiration
3. Amount of air that can be forcibly inspired over and above a normal inspiration
4. Amount of air trapped in the alveoli, which cannot be expired

156. Which of the following indicates a normal adult vital capacity?
    1. 500 ml.   3. 3,500 ml.
    2. 1,500 ml.   4. 10,000 ml.
157. Which of the following is not true? Contraction
    1. Of the diaphragm is caused by impulses over the vagus nerves
    2. Of the diaphragm enlarges the thoracic cavity
    3. Of the diaphragm causes inspiration
    4. Of the entire diaphragm is possible only if the phrenic nerves are intact
158. What is the usual stimulant for the respiratory center?
    1. Calcium ions   3. Lactic acid
    2. Carbon dioxide   4. Oxygen

Data: Typical normal oxygen pressures in air and blood are 40, 95, 100, and 158 mm. Hg. Questions 159 through 162 relate to this fact.

159. 40 mm. Hg is a normal oxygen pressure in
    1. Alveolar air   3. Atmosphere
    2. Arterial blood   4. Venous blood
160. 100 mm. Hg is a normal oxygen pressure in
    1. Alveolar air
    2. Arterial blood
    3. Both of the preceding
    4. None of the preceding
161. 158 mm. Hg is a normal oxygen pressure in
    1. Alveolar air   3. Atmosphere
    2. Arterial blood   4. Venous blood
162. 95 mm. Hg is a normal oxygen pressure in
    1. Alveolar air   3. Atmosphere
    2. Arterial blood   4. Venous blood

Typical normal carbon dioxide pressures in air and blood are 40 and 46 mm. Hg. Questions 163 and 164 relate to this fact.

163. 40 mm. Hg is a normal carbon dioxide pressure in
    1. Alveolar air
    2. Arterial blood
    3. Both of the preceding
    4. Venous blood
164. 46 mm. Hg is a normal carbon dioxide pressure in
    1. Alveolar air   3. Atmosphere
    2. Arterial blood   4. Venous blood
165. What outcome of cellular respiration is most useful to the body?
    1. Carbon dioxide discharge
    2. Energy release from foods
    3. Food intake
    4. Oxygen intake
166. Which is the greatest amount of pressure?
    1. Alveolar pressure during expiration
    2. Intrathoracic (intrapleural) pressure during expiration
    3. Intrathoracic pressure during inspiration
    4. Atmospheric pressure

167. Oxygen dissociation from hemoglobin and therefore oxygen delivery to the tissues are accelerated by
    1. A decreasing oxygen pressure in the blood
    2. A decreasing oxygen pressure and/or an increasing carbon dioxide pressure in the blood
    3. An increasing oxygen pressure and/or a decreasing carbon dioxide pressure in the blood
    4. An increasing carbon dioxide pressure in the blood
168. Which of the following contain(s) lipase?
    1. Bile
    2. Bile and gastric juice
    3. Bile and pancreatic juice
    4. Gastric juice and pancreatic juice
169. Normal fat catabolism produces
    1. Energy, carbon dioxide, and water
    2. Ketones
    3. Both of the preceding
    4. Fatty acids and glyceryl
170. Obstruction of which of the following would cause jaundice?
    1. Common bile duct   3. Hepatic duct
    2. Cystic bile duct   4. 1 or 3
171. To what part of the alimentary tract is the appendix attached?
    1. Cecum   3. Ileum
    2. Colon   4. Jejunum
172. A tumor in the region of the hepato-pancreatic papilla (of Vater) would probably interfere with the flow of
    1. Bile into the intestine
    2. Bile and pancreatic juice into the intestine
    3. Intestinal juice into the intestine
    4. 2 and 3
173. What function(s) does the liver perform?
    1. Produces urea
    2. Produces fibrinogen and prothrombin
    3. Helps maintain normal blood sugar level; also plays important part in protein and fat metabolism
    4. All of the preceding
174. Which of the following is not a normal function of the adult liver?
    1. Forms ammonia in first step of protein catabolism
    2. Glycogenesis, glycogenolysis, gluconeogenesis, ketogenesis
    3. Produces red blood cells
    4. Synthesizes bile
175. Which of the following does not help digest carbohydrates?
    1. Gastric juice   3. Pancreatic juice
    2. Intestinal juice   4. Saliva
176. Why are jaundiced patients given low-fat diets? Because
    1. Fats irritate inflamed bile ducts
    2. They cannot metabolize fats
    3. They can neither digest nor absorb fats normally
    4. All of the preceding
177. Which of the following is a partially digested form of food?
    1. Amino acids   3. Glucose
    2. Fatty acids   4. Lactose
178. Which digestive juice contains no digestive enzymes?

1. Bile
2. Gastric juice
3. Intestinal juice
4. Saliva

179. By what mechanism(s) are water and digested foods absorbed?
　　1. Active transport only
　　2. Diffusion and active transport
　　3. Diffusion only
　　4. Osmosis and diffusion

180. An increase in blood temperature above normal
　　1. Decreases the rate of catabolism
　　2. Slows enzyme activity
　　3. Stimulates thermal receptors located in the thalamus
　　4. Stimulates thermal receptors located in the hypothalamus

181. If an individual has a consistently higher than normal blood sugar, he
　　1. Has diabetes insipidus
　　2. May have an epinephrine deficiency
　　3. Has hyperinsulinism
　　4. May have an oversecretion of ACTH, cortisol, or growth hormone

182. Only one digestive juice contains protein-, carbohydrate-, and fat-digesting enzymes—which one?
　　1. Gastric juice
　　2. Intestinal juice
　　3. Pancreatic juice
　　4. Saliva

183. Which of the following is false?
　　1. Under basal conditions a large person produces more calories of heat per hour than a small one, other things being equal
　　2. Per kilogram of body weight, a large person produces more calories than a small one, other things being equal
　　3. The BMR of a woman is lower than that of a man, other things being equal
　　4. Fever increases the BMR

184. Which of the following occurs in insulin deficiency?
　　1. Decreased anabolism of carbohydrates, proteins, and fats
　　2. Decreased catabolism of carbohydrates
　　3. Increased catabolism of fats with increased ketone body formation
　　4. All of the preceding

Data: Assume that your energy output per day—i.e., your total metabolic rate—is 2,000 kilocalories. The diet you have been eating has supplied a total of 2,000 kilocalories per day. Protein foods have contributed 200 kilocalories of this total. Now you decide to change to a "high-protein diet." You will still eat a total of 2,000 kilocalories per day. But in your new diet, proteins will contribute 300 kilocalories.

185. Which statement is false?
　　1. Your weight will stay constant on your new high-protein diet if it did on your former diet, since both diets supply the same number of kilocalories
　　2. Whenever energy output equals energy input, body weight necessarily remains constant (assuming no change in its fluid content)
　　3. Energy output equals energy input when the total metabolic rate equals the total caloric intake per day
　　4. Body weight always decreases if the total metabolic rate exceeds the total caloric intake per day (assuming no change in fluid content)

186. Which statement is true?
　　1. It is impossible to lose weight unless you "eat less"—unless you decrease your total caloric intake
　　2. Exercise increases the total metabolic rate
　　3. You can lose weight by either decreasing your total caloric intake or increasing your total metabolic rate
　　4. Both 2 and 3

187. As the amount of antidiuretic hormone in blood increases
　　1. Glomerular filtration tends to decrease
　　2. Tubular reabsorption of potassium and water increases
　　3. Tubular reabsorption of sodium and water increases
　　4. Urine concentration tends to decrease

188. Which of the following statements is not true about urine formation?
　　1. Slightly less than half of the water filtered from the blood in urine formation is reabsorbed into the blood
　　2. The first step in urine formation is filtration of blood plasma from the glomeruli into the Bowman's capsules
　　3. The second step in urine formation is the reabsorption of water and some of the solutes by the tubule cells
　　4. The tubule cells also help form urine by secreting varying substances; e.g., hydrogen ions

189. Which of the following statements is not true about urine formation?
　　1. The amount of water reabsorbed by distal renal tubules is controlled by a hormone secreted by the neurohypophysis
　　2. The amount of sodium ions reabsorbed by the tubules is controlled largely by aldosterone
　　3. The most important determinant of the amount of urine excreted is the rate of glomerular filtration
　　4. When the osmotic pressure of the blood decreases, less antidiuretic hormone (ADH) is secreted, so more urine is excreted

190. Which statement is true?
　　1. Bowman's capsule is the fibrous capsule around the kidney
　　2. A glomerulus, Bowman's capsule, and renal tubules together constitute a nephron
　　3. Nephrons are about the only structures, if not the only ones, in which active transport of substances through cell membranes does not occur
　　4. The renal cortex secretes hormones called corticoids

191. Which statement is false?
　　1. When renal blood pressure increases above normal, the kidneys release a substance called renin into the blood
　　2. The substance renin from the kidneys changes a normal blood protein to a substance that tends to constrict blood vessels
　　3. Glucose is reabsorbed into the blood only in the proximal tubules

4. Urine always has an acid reaction

192. Which statement is true?
    1. Glomeruli are small arteries present in the kidney
    2. The volume of urine secreted is regulated mainly by mechanisms that control the glomerular filtration rate
    3. An increase in the hydrostatic pressure in Bowman's capsule tends to increase the glomerular filtration rate
    4. A decrease in blood protein concentration tends to increase the glomerular filtration rate

Data: Mrs. A is to be treated with an artificial kidney. Her blood will flow through cellophane tubing immersed in a dialyzing fluid. The amounts of a few of the substances in her blood are listed below in the column on the left. The amounts of these substances in the dialyzing fluid are listed in the column on the right. The cellophane used for the tubing is permeable to all the substances listed but is not permeable to blood proteins or to red blood cells.

Mrs. A's plasma	Dialyzing fluid
mEq./L.	*mEq./L.*
130------------------Na$^+$------------------140	
6.5--------------- K$^+$---------------- 3	
mg./100 ml.	*mg./100 ml.*
90---------------Glucose----------------1,750	
40--------------- Urea ---------------- 0	

Questions 193 through 197 apply to the given data:

193. Ions will pass through the cellophane tubing
    1. In both directions   3. By osmosis
    2. By diffusion   4. Both 1 and 2
194. Glucose will pass through the cellophane tubing
    1. By active transport
    2. By osmosis
    3. In both directions, but more into than out of blood
    4. None of the preceding
195. Which process or processes can occur through the cellophane tubing?
    1. Diffusion and osmosis
    2. Sodium and potassium transport
    3. Neither of the preceding
    4. Both 1 and 2
196. More of which substance(s) will leave than enter Mrs. A's blood?
    1. Glucose
    2. Potassium and urea
    3. Sodium
    4. Both glucose and sodium
197. More of which substance(s) will move into than out of Mrs. A's blood?
    1. Glucose
    2. Potassium and urea
    3. Sodium
    4. Both glucose and sodium
198. Which of the following produces sperm?
    1. Epididymis
    2. Interstitial cells of testis

3. Seminal vesicle
4. Seminiferous tubules

199. Human sperm and ova are similar, in that
    1. About the same number of each is produced
    2. They are cells of about the same size
    3. They have about the same ability for locomotion
    4. They have the same number of chromosomes
200. What structure encircles the male urethra?
    1. Bulbourethral gland
    2. Epididymis
    3. Prostate gland
    4. Seminal vesicle
201. Which is a temporary endocrine gland?
    1. Neurohypophysis   3. Epididymis
    2. Corpus luteum   4. Seminal vesicle
202. Menstruation usually occurs two or three days after a marked
    1. Decrease in the blood concentration of estrogens and progesterone
    2. Decrease in the blood concentration of follicle-stimulating hormone
    3. Decrease in the blood concentration of luteinizing hormone
    4. Increase in the blood concentration of estrogens and progesterone
203. A normal mature sperm is now believed to contain
    1. 23 chromosomes
    2. 24 chromosomes
    3. 23 pairs of chromosomes
    4. 24 pairs of chromosomes
204. Testosterone is secreted by
    1. Adrenal medulla
    2. Interstitial cells of testes
    3. Seminiferous tubules of testes
    4. More than one of the preceding
205. In what structure(s) does fertilization normally occur?
    1. Cervix   3. Uterine tubes
    2. Ovaries   4. Vagina
206. Progesterone is secreted by the
    1. Adenohypophysis and corpus luteum
    2. Corpus luteum and graafian follicle
    3. Corpus luteum
    4. Graafian follicle
207. After which of the following would menstruation still occur?
    1. Bilateral salpingectomy
    2. Bilateral oophorectomy
    3. Cervical hysterectomy (uterine body but not cervix removed) and bilateral oophorectomy
    4. Unilateral oophorectomy and hysterectomy (entire uterus removed)
208. If a woman has had both her ovaries removed, which of the following is false?
    1. The concentration of estrogens, progesterone, and FSH in her blood will remain low
    2. She will no longer menstruate
    3. She will not be able to become pregnant
    4. Both 2 and 3
209. Mrs. A menstruates regularly every 30 days. Her last menses started on January 1. When will she most probably ovulate next?
    1. January 5 or 6   3. January 17
    2. January 15   4. January 28

Situation: Mrs. Parks has been brought into the hospital in a state of diabetic acidosis. Questions 210 through 217 relate to Mrs. Parks.

210. Which of the following represents a typical normal pH for arterial blood?
   1. 7.0
   2. 7.35
   3. 7.42
   4. 7.45

211. In her state of uncompensated acidosis, which of the following might represent the arterial blood pH of Mrs. Parks?
   1. 6.45
   2. 7.2
   3. 7.48
   4. None of the preceding

212. Larger than normal amounts of acetoacetic acid have been entering Mrs. Parks' blood as one of the indirect results of her insulin deficiency. Like lactic acid and other nonvolatile acids, acetoacetic acid is buffered in the blood chiefly by
   1. Carbon dioxide
   2. Potassium salt of hemoglobin
   3. Sodium bicarbonate
   4. Sodium chloride

213. As a result of the buffering of acetoacetic acid
   1. Mrs. Parks' blood pH remains unchanged
   2. Mrs. Parks' blood pH increases slightly
   3. The carbonic acid content of her blood remains unchanged
   4. The sodium bicarbonate content of Mrs. Parks' blood necessarily decreases and its carbonic acid content increases

214. An increase in blood's carbonic acid content
   1. Automatically increases its carbon dioxide content which, in turn, stimulates respirations
   2. Tends to increase the ratio of base bicarbonate/carbonic acid present in blood
   3. Tends to increase blood pH
   4. All of the preceding

215. Which of the following is not true about hyperventilation?
   1. May produce acidosis, if it continues too long
   2. Hyperventilation results from acidosis and tends to compensate for it

   3. Tends to decrease blood's carbon dioxide and carbonic acid content
   4. Tends to increase blood pH

216. The most effective device the body has for preventing blood pH from decreasing below normal is
   1. Almost instantaneous buffering of acids as they enter blood
   2. Hyperventilation
   3. Hypoventilation
   4. Secretion of hydrogen ions and ammonium ions by distal renal tubules in exchange for sodium ions

217. Acetazolamide (Diamox) inhibits the enzyme carbonic anhydrase. Which of the following changes does not result directly or indirectly from this action?
   1. Carbonic acid content of blood decreases
   2. Distal renal tubules form less carbonic acid from carbon dioxide and water, excrete fewer hydrogen ions, and reabsorb fewer sodium ions
   3. Urine becomes alkaline; blood becomes less alkaline
   4. Patient may develop acidosis

218. Which of the following correctly compares blood plasma and interstitial fluid?
   1. Both contain the same kinds of ions
   2. Plasma contains slightly more of each kind of ion than interstitial fluid
   3. Plasma exerts lower osmotic pressure than interstitial fluid
   4. The main cation in plasma is sodium, whereas the main cation in interstitial fluid is potassium

219. Which play(s) the major role in maintaining fluid balance?
   1. Heart
   2. Kidneys
   3. Liver
   4. Lungs

220. If a patient hyperventilates for an extended period of time, he will
   1. Probably develop acidosis and become dehydrated
   2. Probably develop alkalosis and become dehydrated
   3. Probably maintain acid-base balance but become dehydrated
   4. Probably develop alkalosis only

NAME _____ DATE _____

LAST FIRST MIDDLE

SCHOOL _____ CITY _____

AGE _____ SEX _____ M or F

DATE OF BIRTH _____

GRADE OR CLASS _____ INSTRUCTOR _____

NAME OF TEST _____ PART _____

SAMPLE:

1—1 a country
1—2 a mountain
1—3 an island
1—4 a city
1—5 a state

1. Chicago is

DIRECTIONS: Read each question and its numbered answers. When you have decided which answer is correct, blacken the corresponding space on this sheet with the special pencil. Make your mark as long as the pair of lines, and move the pencil point up and down firmly to make a heavy black line. If you change your mind, erase your first mark completely. Make no stray marks; they may count against you.

BE SURE YOUR MARKS ARE HEAVY AND BLACK.
ERASE COMPLETELY ANY ANSWER YOU WISH TO CHANGE.

	1 2 3 4 5		1 2 3 4 5		1 2 3 4 5		1 2 3 4 5		1 2 3 4 5
151		181		211		241		271	
152		182		212		242		272	
153		183		213		243		273	
154		184		214		244		274	
155		185		215		245		275	
156		186		216		246		276	
157		187		217		247		277	
158		188		218		248		278	
159		189		219		249		279	
160		190		220		250		280	
161		191		221		251		281	
162		192		222		252		282	
163		193		223		253		283	
164		194		224		254		284	
165		195		225		255		285	

BE SURE YOUR MARKS ARE HEAVY AND BLACK.
ERASE COMPLETELY ANY ANSWER YOU WISH TO CHANGE.

	1 2 3 4 5		1 2 3 4 5		1 2 3 4 5		1 2 3 4 5		1 2 3 4 5
166		196		226		256		286	
167		197		227		257		287	
168		198		228		258		288	
169		199		229		259		289	
170		200		230		260		290	
171		201		231		261		291	
172		202		232		262		292	
173		203		233		263		293	
174		204		234		264		294	
175		205		235		265		295	
176		206		236		266		296	
177		207		237		267		297	
178		208		238		268		298	
179		209		239		269		299	
180		210		240		270		300	

2

MICROBIOLOGY

Gebhardt, L. P.: Microbiology, ed. 4, St. Louis, 1970, The C. V. Mosby Co.
Lyles, S. T.: Biology of microorganisms, St. Louis, 1969, The C. V. Mosby Co.
Smith, A. L.: Microbiology and pathology, ed. 10, St. Louis, 1972, The C. V. Mosby Co.

SOME GENERAL FACTS AND PRINCIPLES ABOUT MICROORGANISMS

1. **Definitions**
A. Microbe, or microorganism—animal or plant so small that it can be seen only by aid of microscope
B. Microbiology—science or study of microbes; branch of larger science, biology, because it studies living things
C. Pathogens—microbes capable of producing disease
D. Nonpathogens—microbes not capable of producing disease
2. **Distribution of microbes**
A. Microbes present nearly every place where life is possible
B. The following parts of the body, however, normally sterile; that is, contain no microbes: blood, cerebrospinal fluid, gastric juice, pleural fluid, pericardial fluid, peritoneal fluid, urine, mucous membrane of the urinary tract, and serous and synovial membranes
3. **Classification of microbes**
A. Most human pathogens belong to the plant kingdom, but a few very important ones belong to the animal kingdom
B. Both plant and animal kingdoms consist of various subdivisions as follows
   1. Phyla—names of plant phyla end in *phyta;* e.g., human pathogens belong to either the plant phyla named protophyta and thallophyta or to the animal phylum protozoa
   2. Classes—subdivisions of a phylum; e.g., schizomycetes constitute a major class of protophyta
   3. Orders—subdivisions of classes; eubacteriales and actinomycetales are orders of the schizomycetes class
   4. Families—subdivisions of orders; names end in *aceae;* e.g., micrococcaceae is one of several families of eubacteriales
   5. Genera—subdivisions of families; the first name of a specific microorganism names its genus and is always capitalized; e.g., Staphylococcus
   6. Species—subdivision of genera; the last name of a specific microorganism names its species and is not capitalized; e.g., the word aureus names the species of the microbe, *Staphylococcus aureus*
C. Microbes are classified according to their food supply as
   1. Saprophytes—those that live on nonliving organic matter, such as bread, milk, dead animals; true saprophytes nonpathogenic
   2. Parasites—those that live on living organisms; pathogens primarily parasites although many can live and multiply on nonliving culture media
D. Microbes are classified according to their oxygen requirements as
   1. Aerobes—organisms that require free oxygen for survival
   2. Anaerobes—organisms that grow only when no free oxygen present

3. Microaerophils—require free oxygen for growth but in an amount less than present in air
E. Microbes classified according to their ability to form spores: either *spore-formers* or *nonsporeformers*
F. Microbes classified according to their reaction to acid-fast staining: either *acid-fast* or *nonacid-fast* organisms
G. Microbes classified according to their reaction to Gram's stain: either *gram-positive* or *gram-negative* organisms
H. Most species of microbes are not pathogenic to man but are either harmless or actually useful to him; for example, microbes produce penicillin, streptomycin, and various other antibiotics; microbes perform essential parts of the processes used to make bread, beer, wine, cheese, and leather

4. **Methods of studying and identifying microbes**
A. Kinds of methods used
  1. Microscopic examination
  2. Cultures
  3. Biochemical reactions
  4. Animal inoculations
B. Microscopic examinations
  1. Kinds of microscopes
    a. Compound—usual laboratory microscope; magnification seldom over ×1,000
    b. Electron microscope
      (1) Cost prohibitive for most laboratories
      (2) Great magnification (up to ×2 million) possible with best techniques
      (3) Reveals objects that are too small to be measured in microns (μ) and are measured instead in Angstroms (1/10,000μ, or 1/10,000,000 mm., or about 1/254,000,000 inch)
  2. Preparation of slides for microscopic examination
    a. Without stains
      (1) Hanging-drop preparations—useful to observe motility of living organisms
      (2) Dark-field illumination—microscopic background appears dark and microbes appear bright silvery color due to angle at which rays of light strike them through substage condenser; useful in examining *Treponema pallidum* especially
    b. With stains—before staining, film or smear of material to be stained must be fixed (usually by flaming, i.e., passing slide through flame slowly 2 or 3 times) in order to kill microbes and stick them to slide
      (1) General stains—such as methylene blue, gentian violet, carbolfuchsin, and safranine; these stain most bacteria, but not capsules, spores, or flagella
      (2) Differential stains—more complicated to do, but valuable because help in identifying bacteria by dividing them into different groups according to reaction to differential stains
        (a) Gram's staining method —consists of staining microbes first with purplish stain (such as methyl violet or gentian violet), setting stain with Gram's iodine solution, decolorizing with alcohol or acetone, and then counterstaining with red stain (usually carbolfuchsin or safranine); some organisms positively stained with first stain when iodine applied; therefore do not decolorize with alcohol or acetone and so cannot take counterstain; such organisms appear purplish from original stain; said to be gram-positive; other bacteria do not take fixed color with first stain and Gram's iodine but, instead, become decolorized by alcohol or acetone and take counterstain; therefore appear reddish; said to be gram-negative; Gram's staining method particularly valuable clinically in helping to identify gonococci and men-

ingococci, both gram-negative diplococci

(b) Acid-fast staining—consists of staining smear with carbolfuchsin (red), decolorizing with acid-alcohol, then counterstaining with methylene blue; "acid-fast" organisms retain original red dye, remaining fast even in presence of acid that decolorizes other organisms that then counterstain blue; method particularly valuable for identifying tuberculosis bacilli (*Myobacterium tuberculosis*) in sputum, the only acid-fast rods commonly found in sputum; *Bacillus leprae* also acid-fast

(3) Negative staining—consists in mixing drop containing bacteria with black dye, nigrosin, or India ink, then smearing mixture on slide; bacteria appear colorless against black background; particularly useful in examining *Treponema pallidum* and other spirochetes

C. Studying microbes by cultures
  1. Definitions
    a. Cultures—growths of large numbers of microbes on suitable food media: broth, agar, milk, etc.
    b. Culture media—food substances in or on which cultures grown
    c. Colony—cluster of millions of microbes, presumably all descendants from single bacterium; visible to naked eye
  2. Types of culture media commonly used
    a. Liquid—beef broth in tubes or flasks, litmus milk, peptone water
    b. Solid—beef broth with agar added to cause it to solidify; various other substances such as blood, gelatin, and sugars (dextrose, lactose, maltose, etc.) often added to either liquid or solid culture media
      (1) Agar broth poured into test tube and allowed to solidify on slant, called agar slant

      (2) When poured into Petri dish, called agar plate
      (3) Beef agar inoculated with bacteria before it solidifies, spoken of as pour plate
      (4) When inoculated by streaking after hardened, known as streak plate
    c. Living tissue cultures—used to grow rickettsiae and viruses
  3. Special kinds of culture media
    a. Selective media—promote growth of 1 kind of microbe, inhibit growth of others in same culture; e.g., bismuth sulfite agar promotes growth of typhoid bacilli while inhibiting growth of other organisms present in feces
    b. Differential media—differentiate certain organisms from others growing in same culture; e.g., EMB (eosin–methylene blue) agar differentiates gram-negative bacteria of intestinal tract; differential media especially valuable for helping diagnose respiratory and intestinal infections
  4. Types of cultures
    a. Classified according to number of kinds of bacteria
      (1) Pure cultures—contain only 1 kind of bacteria, e.g., *Staphylococcus epidermidis*
      (2) Mixed cultures—contain 2 or more kinds of bacteria
    b. Classified according to species of bacteria: e.g., *Staphylococcus epidermidis* culture, *Bacillus subtilis* culture
  5. Ways in which cultures studied
    a. Smears made and microbes studied microscopically either with or without staining
    b. Cultural characteristics observed
      (1) Media most favorable to growth
      (2) Appearance of colonies—whether large or small, smooth or rough, moist or dry
      (3) Oxygen requirements (anaerobic or aerobic)
D. Studying microbes by biochemical reactions such as
  1. Fermentation reactions (anaerobic oxidation reactions by which some organisms use carbohydrates to gen-

erate energy-rich ATP molecules); various kinds of fermentation reactions are useful for identifying different groups of microorganisms, as
a. Nonfermenters
b. Fermenters that produce acid only
c. Fermenters that produce acid and gas—e.g., *Escherichia coli,* a normal inhabitant of intestinal tract
d. Lactose fermenters—e.g., *E. coli* and other nonpathogens in intestinal tract
e. Nonlactose fermenters—e.g., *Shigella* and *Salmonella,* pathogens in intestinal tract
2. Urea-splitting reaction—identifies organisms as
a. Urease-positive organisms (contain enzyme urease, which catalyzes conversion of urea of ammonia); e.g., *Proteus* bacilli (gram-negative, normal inhabitants of intestinal tract)
b. Urease-negative organisms—do not contain urease so cannot convert urea to ammonia; e.g., *Salmonella* and *Shigella,* pathogens in intestinal tract
E. Studying microbes by inoculating animals
1. Material suspected of containing microbes is injected into a laboratory animal; animal is then kept under observation for effects: its blood or other body fluids may be examined, smears may be examined microscopically, cultures may be made, etc.
2. Animal inoculation is best method yet devised for detecting presence of certain microbes in certain organs—for example, for detecting presence of *Mycobacterium tuberculosis* in the kidney
3. Animal inoculation is easiest way of obtaining pure culture of certain organisms—for example, pure cultures of *Diplococcus pneumoniae*
5. **Structure of microbes**
A. Microbes are unicellular organisms except for molds and 2 families of bacteria—namely, the Actinomycetaceae and Streptomycetaceae families (of the Actinomycetales order)
B. Microbes vary in size but are so small they are measured in microns and millimicrons (1 micron = 1/1,000 milli-

meter, or about 1/25,000 inch; 1 millimicron = 1/1,000 micron, or about 1/25,000,000 inch); some viruses have diameters of only a few millimicrons and are only slightly larger than largest protein molecules
C. Microbes contain nuclear material (deoxyribonucleic or ribonucleic acids—DNA, RNA), but nucleus usually not visible except in molds, yeasts, and protozoa
D. Special structures characterize certain kinds of microorganisms; examples
1. Molds
a. Mycelium
(1) Fluffy-looking growth formed by branching and interlacing threads of mold
(2) Mycelium gives mold characteristic appearance
(3) Often highly colored; e.g., green, orange, black, or white
b. Hyphae
(1) Single threads form mycelium
(2) Hyphae unicellular and multinucleated, or multicellular
(3) Usually grow mainly on surface of organic matter but may penetrate material
2. Bacteria
a. Spores
(1) Small, glistening, round or ovoid bodies within bacteria
(2) Sporeforming human pathogens cause only 4 important diseases—tetanus, gas gangrene, botulism, and anthrax
(3) Spores can resist highly unfavorable conditions such as prolonged boiling, drying, and action of some chemicals
(4) Spores are dormant—do not grow and reproduce; but if favorable environment is restored, they return to vegetative form of the bacterium and start to reproduce again; spores, like seeds, can lie dormant almost indefinitely and again "sprout" or come to life when growth conditions become favorable
(5) Molds also form spores; however, these are not dormant, resistant bodies but reproduc-

tive bodies that form new molds

b. Capsule—starchy or gelatinous casing that forms around certain species of bacteria; encapsulated bacteria not so readily ingested by phagocytes as nonencapsulated ones; capsules, therefore, considered "earmark of virulence"; most prominent in organisms that have just recently left body

c. Flagella—fine, hairlike extensions of cytoplasm from bacterial cell; not all bacteria show flagella, but some have several; by lashing movements flagella propel organism in various directions

3. Protozoa

a. Cilia—fine, hairlike processes that propel organism

b. Flagella—long, hairlike extensions of protoplasm of cell; may be several on single protozoon; propel organism by whiplash movement

c. Pseudopods—literally, false feet; irregular, changing projections of organism's protoplasm

d. Cyst—protective covering that forms around organism; enables it to resist unfavorable conditions better than can active, vegetative form of organism

6. **Physiology of microorganisms**

A. Compared with physiology of higher forms of life

1. Like all living things, microorganisms carry on functions, such as

a. Digestion, absorption, and metabolism of food and excretion of wastes

b. Respiration

c. Reproduction

2. As in all forms of life, enzymes play vital role in physiology of microorganisms; they catalyze chemical reactions necessary for life, e.g., the chemical reactions of digestion and metabolism

3. Like all living things, microorganisms can survive in healthy condition only when environment remains relatively stable as to various factors

a. Temperature

b. pH (H ion concentration)

c. Oxygen content

d. Food content

e. Water content

4. Many microorganisms use simple inorganic compounds for metabolism, whereas higher forms of life can use only complex organic compounds

a. Nitrogen-fixing bacteria can synthesize protoplasm (anabolism) out of simple inorganic substances

(1) Nitrogen

(2) Carbon dioxide

(3) Water

b. Higher forms of life can use for anabolism only the more complex organic compounds

(1) Proteins

(2) Carbohydrates

(3) Fats

5. Mechanisms by which microorganisms carry on various functions differ from those of more complex forms of life; for example

a. Microorganisms secrete digestive enzymes into medium surrounding them, where the enzymes digest foods before foods enter the microorganism

b. More complex forms of life take undigested foods into bodies, then digest them

B. Metabolism of microorganisms—produces various kinds of substances, notably

1. Exotoxins—powerful poisons excreted into surrounding medium by the following pathogens

a. *Corynebacterium diphtheriae*

b. *Clostridium tetani*

c. *Clostridium botulinum*

d. Clostridia of gas gangrene (*Clostridium perfringens,* and a few others)

2. Endotoxins—poisons probably contained in most pathogenic bacteria but do not leave the bacterial cell until it disintegrates

3. Antibiotics—substances that inhibit multiplication of other microbes; produced by certain bacteria and molds; e.g., *Streptomyces griseus* produces streptomycin; the mold *Penicillium notatum* produces penicillin

4. Pigments—colored substances produced by some bacteria; e.g., *Staphylococcus aureus* produces golden pigment

C. Respiration of microorganisms

1. Aerobes—require free oxygen from environment for catabolism
2. Anaerobes—use oxygen from chemical compounds; obligate anaerobes cannot multiply in presence of free oxygen; facultative anaerobes can live in absence of free oxygen but ordinarily do not

D. Reproduction of microorganisms
   1. Molds—special reproductive cells (spores) form on ends of hyphae; appear as familiar colored or black dots seen on molds
   2. Yeasts—usually reproduce by budding, kind of fission in which small "daughter cell," or "bud," forms and then pinches off from parent yeast cell; under unfavorable conditions yeasts may reproduce by spore formation
   3. Bacteria—asexual, by direct fission—simple division of 1 organism into 2
      a. Rate of multiplication very rapid
      b. Each generation produces new generation in about 20 to 30 minutes
      c. Natural checks on breathtaking rate of multiplication: depletion of foods and increase of injurious wastes
   4. Rickettsiae
      a. Reproduce inside living cells, with rare exceptions
      b. Unlike most bacteria, cannot grow in artificial media
      c. Grow only in living tissues such as chick embryo tissue
   5. Viruses—method not fully understood; probably not simple fission
      a. Viruses reproduce only inside living cells
      b. Like rickettsiae, viruses cannot be grown in artificial media
      c. Grow only in living tissues or tissue cultures; e.g., poliomyelitis viruses used to prepare Salk vaccine grown in monkey kidney tissue cultures

MICROORGANISMS AND DISEASE

1. **Definitions**
A. Infection or infectious disease—a condition resulting when microorganisms enter the body, multiply in the body, and produce a reaction by the body
B. Communicable disease—an infectious disease caused by an organism that has been transmitted to the individual directly or indirectly from another host, usually of the same species, but not always
C. Contagious disease—a term usually used to indicate an infectious disease that is spread easily and directly from one person to another

2. **Sources or reservoirs of infectious organisms**
A. The ultimate sources of almost all infectious organisms are human beings or animals who either have the disease (sometimes unrecognized) or are carriers of the disease organism
B. Plants may be a reservoir of some fungus infectious organisms

3. **Ways in which microorganisms are transmitted to the body**
A. Microbes are often transmitted directly from one body to another by actual contact, or droplets (Fig. 2-1)
B. Microbes are often transmitted indirectly from one body to another, by means of some other agent (Fig. 2-2); some important middlemen in microbe transfer are
   1. Fingers—touch wastes from infected bodies, or articles contaminated with excretions; later touch other persons or objects used by them
   2. Fomites—articles contaminated with excretions from infected person
   3. Foods, especially milk
   4. Water
   5. Soil
   6. Insects

4. **Microbe transfer by foods**
A. Sources of microbes transferred to foods are numerous; especially important are the fingers of food workers and transfers from flies, rats, mice, roaches, dishes, cow udders, dust, etc. (Fig. 2-2)
B. Microbes transferred by foods cause various diseases—notably
   1. Certain infections of the digestive tract—examples: typhoid, undulant fever (usually transmitted through milk), dysentery (usually through milk), cholera, paratyphoid
   2. Certain infections of the respiratory tract—examples: septic sore throat, diphtheria, scarlet fever
   3. Certain intoxications (poisonings)
      a. Most commonly, food intoxications

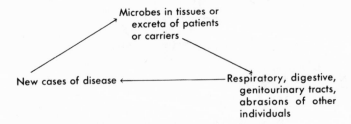

FIG. 2-1

Direct transfer of pathogens.

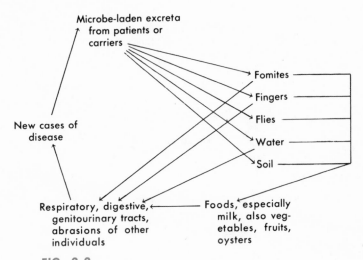

FIG. 2-2

Indirect transfer of pathogens.

probably result from contamination of foods by certain strains of staphylococci, which multiply in foods and release exotoxins into them; after ingestion, these potent poisons act as enterotoxins—that is, they produce diarrhea and vomiting; symptoms may be severe but usually last only a few hours and rarely result in death

b. Less common, but much more serious form of food intoxication—botulism; microbe named *Clostridium botulinum*, when it contaminates food, releases into it exotoxins that are said to be the most deadly poisons known; they are neurotoxins that act on the central nervous system

C. Disease transfer by foods can be prevented by the following

1. Cleanliness in preparation and serving of foods—especial attention to hands, habits, and health of food workers; cleanliness of dishes, utensils; protection of food from flies, rats, roaches

2. Prompt and continued refrigeration of foods until ready to be prepared for consumption

3. Thorough cooking

4. Special precautions for milk necessary because it is excellent culture medium for microbes and is often consumed raw; inspection of farms and dairies, bacteria counts, pasteurization

5. **Microbe transfer by water**

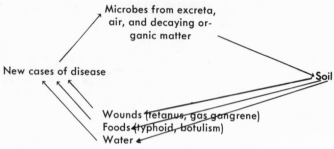

FIG. 2-3

Transfer of pathogens by soil.

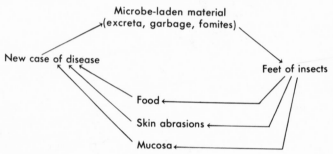

FIG. 2-4

Mechanical transfer of pathogens by insects.

A. Microbes are transferred to water from human or animal excreta; microbes may enter water directly in sewage disposal or indirectly by drainage through soil from outhouses or manure piles into wells, springs, or other sources of water supply

B. Diseases commonly transmitted through water are those whose causative organisms leave body in feces—notably
   1. Typhoid fever
   2. Paratyphoid fever
   3. Dysentery—amebic and bacillary
   4. Cholera

C. Microbe transfer by water can be prevented by using various water purification methods; approved methods for
   1. Community use—filtration, sedimentation, chemicals
   2. Home use—boiling

6. **Microbe transfer by the soil**

A. Microbes are transferred to the soil from human and animal excreta, decaying plants and animals, and from the air (Fig. 2-3)

B. Certain diseases are commonly transmitted through microbes in the soil—notably
   1. Diseases caused by sporeformers—tetanus, anthrax, gas gangrene, and botulism
   2. Diseases caused by nonsporeformers—typhoid fever and histoplasmosis

7. **Microbe transfer by insects (arthropods)**

A. Insects can transfer microbes by mechanical and by biologic methods
   1. Mechanical transfer—insects' feet act as mechanical conveyors for microbes of any kind (Fig. 2-4)
   2. Biologic transfer—insect bites patient, thereby getting microbes into insect's body where they undergo separate cycle of development for definite length of time; after that time, when insect bites another individual, microbes are injected and produce new case of disease (Fig. 2-5 and Table 2-1)

B. Theoretically, any kind of insect can mechanically transfer any kind of mi-

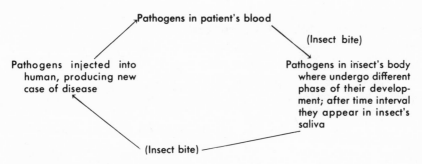

FIG. 2-5

Biologic transfer of pathogens by insects.

TABLE 2-1

DISEASES TRANSMITTED BY BIOLOGIC TRANSFER BY INSECTS

Disease	Pathogen	Insect that biologically transfers pathogen
Malaria	Protozoa (*Plasmodium malariae* and *vivax* mainly)	Female *Anopheles* mosquito (12-day cycle for microbe's development in mosquito's body)
Yellow fever	Virus	*Aedes aegypti* mosquito (12-day cycle in insect's body); some other mosquitoes
Typhus fever	Rickettsia (*Rickettsia prowazekii*)	Body louse, or head louse, occasionally; also rat flea
African sleeping sickness (trypanosomiasis)	Protozoa (*Trypanosoma gambiense* and *rhodesiense*)	Tsetse fly
Plague (bubonic)	Bacillus (*Pasteurella pestis*)	Rat flea, from rats and other rodents to man or from man to man by rat flea

crobe; practically, flies and roaches are the insects that most often mechanically transfer microbes

C. Relatively few kinds of insects can biologically transfer relatively few kinds of microbes (Table 2-1)

8. **Microbe transfer by air**

A. Air transfer of microbes seldom results in disease, since most human pathogens survive only a short time in the air (drying and ultraviolet rays kill them)

B. Exception: air transfer of the *Mycobacterium tuberculosis* often spreads the disease

9. **Microbe transfer by carriers**

A. Carriers—persons who harbor in their bodies certain pathogens but who do not have the related disease

   1. Contact (or "healthy") carriers—persons who have never had disease but have acquired organisms merely by contacting patients with disease

   2. Incubatory carriers—those in the incubation stage of a disease before symptoms have developed

   3. Chronic carriers—those who have recovered from a disease but continue to harbor its causative organisms for indefinite time

B. Diseases most frequently spread by carriers

   1. Typhoid fever

   2. Diphtheria

   3. Meningitis

   4. Pneumonia

   5. Dysentery

C. Importance of carriers in transmission of disease—highly important because they contact other persons freely, since unsuspected of spreading pathogens; often difficult to identify and isolate

TABLE 2-2

PATHOGEN TRANSFER IN SEVERAL TYPES OF DISEASES

Type disease	Route by which pathogens leave body	Usual method of transfer	Preferred portal of entry
Respiratory infections, including common communicable diseases	Discharges from nose and mouth	Droplets, kissing, fingers, fomites, foods	Respiratory mucosa, by way of nose or mouth
Gastrointestinal infections	Feces and urine	Fomites, foods, water, kissing	Mouth, swallowing
Genitourinary tract infections	Discharges from lesions or genitourinary mucosa	Direct contact (e.g., sexual relations, kissing); also, probably by fomites	Directly into blood or tissues through abrasions or through genitourinary mucosa

10. **Microbe entry into and exit from the body** (Table 2-2)

A. Microbes enter the body by way of several "portals of entry," the chief ones of which are the mucous membrane linings of the respiratory, digestive, and genitourinary tracts

B. Each human pathogen has a preferred portal of entry into the body and usually does not cause disease unless it enters through its preferred portal
   1. Preferred portal of entry for microbes that cause respiratory infections is the mucous lining of the respiratory tract
   2. Preferred portal of entry for microbes that cause gastrointestinal infections is the mucous lining of the digestive tract
   3. Preferred portal of entry for microbes that cause genitourinary infections is the mucous lining of the genitourinary tract

C. Some pathogens invade through more than one portal of entry and cause different infections for different portals; e.g., streptococci enter via skin abrasions or mucosa of respiratory tract; if skin portal of entry, streptococci may cause either local inflammation or general one, septicemia; in contrast, they may produce pneumonia if respiratory tract portal of entry

D. Any microbe may enter the body by way of cuts or abrasions in the skin but almost none can penetrate the intact skin; tularemia organisms and hookworm larvae, however, are notable exceptions to this rule; they can enter the body through the intact skin

E. Most pathogens cannot go through placenta into fetal body; 3 pathogens, however, constitute notable exceptions to this principle—those causing syphilis, smallpox, and rubella

F. Most microbes leave the body in its excreta although some make their exit by way of blood
   1. Nose and mouth discharges—portals of exit for organisms that cause respiratory infections and communicable diseases
   2. Feces—portal of exit for organisms that cause gastrointestinal infections, poliomyelitis, tetanus and sometimes for tuberculosis organisms and hepatitis virus A
   3. Urine—portal of exit for organisms that cause gastrointestinal and urinary tract infections, undulant fever and sometimes for tuberculosis organisms
   4. Vaginal discharges—portal of exit for organisms that infect female reproductive tract
   5. Pus and exudates—portals of exit for miscellaneous pathogens
   6. Vomitus—portal of exit for organisms that cause digestive tract infections
   7. Blood—portal of exit for pathogens transferred by insects (e.g., malaria organism) and for various others such as pathogens of syphilis and rickettsial infections

11. **Relation between microbe invasion of the body and disease**

A. Entry of microbes into the body does not always result in disease

B. Whether or not microbes produce an infection when they enter the body and also the severity of the infection depend upon the following 4 factors

1. Portal of entry—microbes must enter body via suitable portal to survive, multiply, and cause infection; e.g., typhoid pathogens entering via digestive tract often produce typhoid fever, whereas those entering via skin abrasion do not
2. Number of microbes entering—the larger the number, the greater the probability that they will cause disease
3. Virulence (or pathogenicity) of pathogens—their ability to overcome body defenses and invade tissues, multiply in them, and cause disease; the greater the virulence of the invading pathogens, the greater the probability that they will cause disease when they enter the body
   a. A pathogen's degree of virulence seems to be determined largely by the kind of chemicals it produces; pathogens that tend to be highly virulent are those which produce the following: kinases, hyaluronidase, leukocidins, capsules, and exotoxins; pathogens that produce endotoxins but not exotoxins tend to be less virulent than the exotoxin producers
      (1) Kinases (also called fibrinolysins)—chemicals that dissolve blood or fibrin clots; hence, increase virulence by making it easier for organisms to spread through tissues; the virulence of streptococci, staphylococci, and some other bacteria stems in part from the kinases they produce
      (2) Hyaluronidase — ("spreading factor")—a chemical that decreases the viscosity of intercellular substance, thereby making it easier for pathogens to invade and spread through tissues; the virulence of pneumococci and streptococci stems partly from the hyaluronidase they produce
      (3) Leukocidins—chemicals that kill many of the white blood cells, thereby leaving fewer of them to destroy the pathogens by phagocytosis; the virulence of pneumococci, streptococci, and staphylococci stems partly from the leukocidins they produce
      (4) Capsules—formations that increase the virulence of pathogens possessing them, apparently making the organisms less vulnerable to destruction by phagocytosis; more of the organisms, therefore, survive to cause disease; pneumococci and some other bacteria produce enveloping capsules
      (5) Exotoxins—extremely powerful poisons (protein compounds) that quickly destroy large numbers of body cells; only living microbes and only a few species liberate exotoxins
      (6) Endotoxins — poisons (lipopolysaccharides) released from dead, disintegrating microbe cells; not so lethal to body cells as exotoxins
   b. The virulence of different members of the same species of pathogens varies according to several factors—for example
      (1) Pathogens tend to be most virulent when freshly discharged from the body of a person sick with an infectious disease
      (2) Pathogens have low virulence if they have come from a carrier's body
      (3) Pathogens tend to be more virulent, the more rapidly and the more repeatedly they have been transferred from one individual to another; for example, the pathogens transmitted later in an epidemic are usually more virulent than those transmitted earlier
      (4) Pathogens are less virulent if they have been exposed to unfavorable conditions such as drying, cold temperature, sunlight, and certain chemicals
4. Resistance of the body—the body has several defense mechanisms that tend

to prevent microbe invasion and multiplication and, therefore, tend to prevent or lessen the severity of infectious disease

Note: These are included in the discussion on resistance and immunity.

C. Koch's postulates—4 requirements that, if fulfilled, are accepted as proof that given organism produces given disease

1. Particular microbe must be found in every case of the particular disease investigated
2. Particular microbe must be isolated and grown in pure culture
3. Particular microbe must cause particular disease after it is inoculated into susceptible animal
4. Particular microbe must be recovered from inoculated animal and its identity established

12. **How microbes cause disease**
Microbes cause disease by means of the above discussed chemicals

RESISTANCE AND IMMUNITY

1. **Defense mechanisms by which the body resists microbes and develops immunity**
A. Defense mechanisms against microbes operate in two general ways

1. External defenses—function as barriers that tend to prevent microbes from invading body tissues; external defenses are nonspecific; that is, they operate to prevent entry of all kinds of microbes; the following are highly effective external defenses
   a. Intact skin and mucosa
   b. Various secretions — examples: tears, gastric juice, vaginal secretions
   c. Cilia of the respiratory mucosa
2. Internal defenses—act against microbes after they have invaded body tissues; they make them unable to cause disease; internal defenses consist of many parts

B. The body's external defenses and most of its internal defenses against microbes are nonspecific; in other words, they operate either to keep out or to destroy all kinds of microbes

C. One kind of internal defense, the immune response, is a specific defense; that is, a specific pathogen stimulates formation of a specific kind of chemical (called an antibody or immune body),

which destroys that pathogen or neutralizes its toxins

D. Immunity means a high degree of resistance to a particular species of pathogens; synonym for immunity is nonsusceptibility

E. Immunity results from operation of the body's various defenses against microbes, mainly from phagocytosis and the immune response, but also from other factors (described in the next few paragraphs)

2. **Internal defenses against microbes**
A. Phagocytosis—ingestion of microbes and destruction of them by certain cells called phagocytes (mainly the white blood cells called neutrophils, lymphocytes, and monocytes and various reticuloendothelial cells, notably the macrophages and microglia)

B. Leukocytosis—increase in number of white blood cells in circulating blood, thereby making more of them available to carry on phagocytosis

C. Properdin—a globulin normally present in blood; it functions in some way to kill gram-negative organisms such as *Escherichia coli* and also to inactivate viruses; it is known that properdin must associate with complement and magnesium ions (the so-called "properdin system") to become active and that irradiation decreases the properdin content of blood

D. Interferon—virus invasion stimulates production of this protein (perhaps by macrophages); interferon inhibits virus multiplication inside cells

E. The immune response—a complex, still incompletely understood series of events; important among these are the formation of immune bodies (antibodies) and the various antigen-antibody reactions that follow

1. An antigen is any substance that stimulates the formation of antibodies against it
2. Antigens are usually foreign proteins, e.g., cell proteins of microbes, and some toxins
3. Antibodies are proteins of the globulin type; therefore, also called immunoglobulins (or Ig); most antibodies are gamma globulins
4. Antigens are recognized as foreign to the body, by certain lymphocytes, and

this acts in some way to trigger formation of antibodies capable of reacting with the specific antigens
5. The tailor-made antibodies then react with the antigen to destroy it or make it harmless to the body
6. Antibodies are classified as follows according to the kind of antigen-antibody reaction they produce
   a. Antitoxins—antibodies that react with antigens called toxins to neutralize them; that is, to make them harmless to body tissues
   b. Agglutinins—antibodies that cause agglutination of microbes or other insoluble antigens when they react with them (agglutination means a sticking together of particles to form clumps of them; facilitates phagocytosis)
   c. Precipitins—antibodies that react with soluble antigens in a filtrate of bacterial growth, precipitating them out of solution
   d. Lysins (or cytolysins)—antibodies that lyse (dissolve) bacteria or other cells, when free complement is present
   e. Opsonins—antibodies that react with antigens to make them more easily destroyed by phagocytosis; the presence of complement increases opsonin activity
   f. Virus-neutralizing antibodies—antibodies that react with viruses in some way to make them unable to cause disease
6. Complement, a protein present in fresh blood serum; complement is necessary for the so-called complement-fixing antibodies (specifically, lysins and opsonins) to complete their reaction with their antigens, as shown by the following equation

Antigen + Antibodies + Complement

$$\downarrow$$

Antigen-antibody-complement combination (i.e., complement fixation or inactivation)

7. Antibodies differ as to length of time they remain in body
   a. Some antibodies remain in body very short time (e.g., those formed against influenza, pneumonia, venereal disease organisms)
   b. Some antibodies usually remain in body throughout life (antibodies against organisms of typhoid fever, smallpox, and many others)
   c. Small quantity of antibodies formed after first injection of vaccine consisting of killed microorganisms disappears from blood in few weeks; after second or third injections, large quantities of antibodies formed and may continue in blood for year or many years; practical application—vaccines of killed organisms (e.g., typhoid vaccine, Salk vaccine for poliomyelitis) are usually given in 3 doses, spaced from 1 week (typhoid vaccine) to 1 month (Salk vaccine) apart, and followed several months later by another "booster dose"
   d. After injection of weakened (attenuated) live organisms, body usually continues to form antibodies throughout life
8. Thymus gland—plays a crucial part in producing immunity; it produces lymphocytes (called T cell lymphocytes to indicate that they came from the thymus); T cell lymphocytes leave the thymus to migrate by way of the blood and lymph to the lymphatic tissues of the body—chiefly lymph nodes and spleen; those T cells that contact an appropriate antigen in the lymphatic tissues multiply; some of their descendants, according to one postulate, become plasma cells that secrete antibodies against the antigen that initiated the multiplication of the T cell lymphocytes; some evidence suggests that the thymus gland may also function another way to produce immunity—that is, it produces a chemical (hormone) that stimulates lymphocyte multiplication in lymphatic tissues; this increases the supply of lymphocytes available for taking part in antibody production; some T cell lymphocytes leave the thymus to recirculate over and over again; they also function to bring about transplant rejections and delayed hypersensitivity, but exactly how they do this is still uncertain
9. Antigen-antibody reactions form the

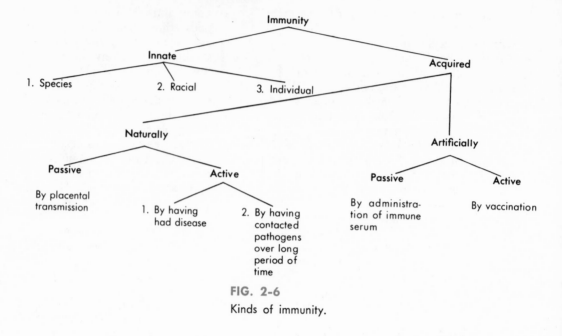

FIG. 2-6

Kinds of immunity.

basis for various tests used to diagnose disease or susceptibility to disease

  a. Agglutination tests—known antigens are mixed with patient's serum; if serum contains related agglutinin type antibodies, they agglutinate the molecules of the known antigen—cause them to stick together to form visible clumps; example: Widal test for typhoid fever—typhoid bacilli are mixed with patient's serum; if patient has or has had typhoid fever, his serum will contain agglutinins and will cause agglutination of the typhoid bacilli mixed with his serum

  b. Precipitation tests—based on precipitation of soluble antigens mixed with patient's serum; examples: Kahn and VDRL tests for syphilis

  c. Lysis or complement-fixation tests—based on lysis of known antigens mixed with patient's serum; example: Kolmer test for syphilis

3. Immunity

A. Immunity is classified according to whether it is natural or acquired, and according to whether it is active or passive

  1. Natural immunity is due to inherited characteristics so is innate or inborn; that is, present at birth

  2. Acquired immunity—due to acquired antibodies, not to inherited characteristics; may be acquired by

    a. Recovery from disease

    b. Harboring or contacting particular pathogen in numbers sufficient to stimulate antibody formation but not to cause illness; e.g., most urban adults relatively immune to tuberculosis because of this mechanism

    c. Transfer of antibodies from mother to fetus by way of placenta

    d. Vaccination

    e. Administration of immune serum

  3. Active immunity—any immunity in which person's body manufactures own antibodies; thus, the immunities due to recovery from disease, to contacting pathogens over long period of time, and to vaccination are all active immunities

  4. Passive immunity—any immunity produced by "ready-made" antibodies (from human being or animal) having been injected into body; passive immunity lasts shorter time than active; passive immunity is always acquired immunity—acquired in 2 ways

    a. By transfer of antibodies from mother to fetus by way of placenta; e.g., passive immunity of young in-

fants to measles, smallpox, etc. acquired in this way
b. By injection of serum from actively immunized animal or human being; e.g., injection of diphtheria antitoxin provides temporary passive immunity to diphtheria
B. Vaccines—antigens that are purposefully introduced into the body to stimulate it to form antibodies against the antigens introduced and thus to develop active immunity against diseases caused by those antigens; the antigens contained in vaccines consists of any one of the following
1. Weakened live organisms—various methods used to weaken organisms; for rabies vaccine, e.g., organisms are weakened by drying so that unable to cause rabies but still able to stimulate body to form antibodies against rabies organisms; smallpox viruses are weakened by growth in cow before use as vaccines; Sabin and Cox poliomyelitis vaccines contain weakened live virus
2. Dead microorganisms—killed by heat or chemicals; incapable of causing disease but still capable of stimulating body to form antibodies against them—examples: Salk poliomyelitis, typhoid, and pertussis vaccines
3. Toxins or modified toxins—toxoids (or anatoxins)—toxin plus chemical such as formaldehyde or alum that weakens toxin enough so it cannot produce disease but is still able to stimulate antibody production against it, e.g., diphtheria and tetanus toxoids (For more specific information about vaccines, see p. 115.)
C. Immune serum
1. An immune serum is either animal or human blood serum that is known to contain antibodies against specific antigens because the serum has come from an animal or human who has been actively immunized by vaccination or by having had the disease
2. Immune serum preparations are used mainly to treat disease and sometimes to prevent its development after exposure
3. Some of the main kinds of immune serum preparations are the following
a. Antitoxins—most widely used are diphtheria and tetanus antitoxins
b. Antirabies hyperimmune serum—contains antibodies against the rabies virus
c. Hyperimmune human antipertussis serum—contains antibodies against bacteria that cause whooping cough
d. Immune serum globulin (human)—the gamma globulin fraction of blood with which antibodies are associated; used to prevent or decrease the severity of a few diseases—examples: measles, infectious hepatitis, poliomyelitis
4. Allergy or hypersensitivity
A. Definition—allergy, or hypersensitivity, is an increased susceptibility to an antigen (in this case called an allergen); in other words, hypersensitivity is the condition opposite to immunity, which is an increased resistance to an antigen
B. Hypersensitivity, like immunity, is produced by antigen-antibody reactions
C. Two main kinds of allergy are the
1. Immediate type allergy—allergen-antibody reaction that occurs shortly after the allergen has entered the bloodstream; the antibody is of the type known as circulating or humoral antibody
2. Delayed type—reaction occurring several hours after entrance of the allergen; the antibodies that react with the allergen are carried by lymphatic cells and cannot be demonstrated as present in the body fluids
D. When an antigen-antibody reaction results in hypersensitivity, tissue cells have been injured by the reaction; in contrast, when an antigen-antibody reaction produces immunity, tissue cells have been protected from injury
E. Hypersensitivity manifests itself in various forms, some of the commonest ones being hay fever, asthma, hives (urticaria), and serum sickness
F. Allergy or hypersensitivity tests—based on antigen-antibody reactions producing allergic responses (that injure tissue cells) rather than immune responses (that protect tissue cells from injury)
Examples: tests done to detect hypersensitivity to wide variety of allergens; also, tuberculin test used to detect past or present tuberculosis depends upon allergic response to antigen-antibody re-

action between tuberculin and tuberculosis antibodies

DESTRUCTION AND INHIBITION OF MICROBES

1. Definitions

A. Contamination—presence of living microbes
B. Sterile—free from presence of all living microbes
C. Sterilize—to carry out process that leaves article treated free from presence of all living microbes, including spore forms
D. Disinfect—to carry out process that leaves article free from presence of all living pathogens
E. Aseptic—free from presence of all living pathogens; anything sterile, of course, aseptic
F. Antiseptic—able to prevent multiplication of pathogens
G. Bacteriostasis—condition in which bacteria remain static, i.e., do not grow or multiply
H. Bactericide (also bacteriocide)—agent able to kill all bacteria

2. Different situations require different types of control of microorganisms

A. Sterilization necessary in
1. Surgical procedures
2. Microbiologic laboratory procedures
3. Canning nonacid foods such as peas, beans, meats
B. Disinfection necessary in
1. Care of communicable diseases
2. Personal and public sanitation
C. Antisepsis and bacteriostasis necessary in
1. Controlling microorganisms in or on body (sterilizing or disinfecting likely to injure tissues)
2. Preserving foods and textiles

3. Kinds of agents used to destroy or inhibit microbes

A. Physical agents—heat, cold, ultraviolet light, drying, ionizing radiations, ultrasonic waves and agitation
B. Chemical agents—salts of heavy metals, oxidizing agents, carbon compounds, dyes, antibiotics, etc.

4. Heat as a sterilizing agent

A. Heat may be applied in the form of moist heat or dry heat
B. Moist heat is applied in the form of hot water or steam (either under pressure or free-flowing)

C. Dry heat may be applied by baking or burning
D. Moist heat and baking kill microbes by coagulating their cell proteins; burning destroys them by oxidation
E. The effectiveness of heat in destroying microbes is directly related to temperature, time, and moisture
1. At a given temperature, moist heat kills faster than dry heat
2. The higher the temperature, the shorter the time it must be applied to kill microbes—examples, moist heat
a. 62° C. (143° F.) applied for 30 minutes kills vegetative forms of most pathogens
b. 72° C. (161° F.) applied for 15 seconds kills vegetative forms of most pathogens
c. 100° C. (212° F.) applied for a few minutes kills vegetative forms of pathogenic bacteria, fungi, and most viruses; hepatitis viruses killed in about 30 minutes; boiling for many hours, however, may not destroy all spore forms present, so cannot be depended upon to sterilize
d. 121° C. (249.8° F.)—the temperature of steam under 15 pounds pressure—applied for about 45 minutes sterilizes; that is, kills all microbes, including spores
e. 135° C. (275° F.)—the temperature of steam under pressure of 28 to 30 pounds—applied for about 3 minutes sterilizes
F. Precautionary principle of great practical importance—for heat to sterilize, necessary temperature must contact all parts of material being sterilized for necessary length of time; therefore, in autoclaving
1. Large packages require more time to kill microbes
a. Sufficient degree of heat must penetrate interior
b. Heat must be applied about 45 minutes to an hour for packages more than 6 inches in diameter
2. Space must be left between small packages
3. Flat packages should be stacked on edge
a. Heat currents flow vertically
b. Helps penetration of desired degree of heat

G. Special points about each method of applying heat
1. Burning—or flaming
   a. Most effective possible method of sterilization
   b. Not practical for most objects
   c. Useful for sputum cups, gauze, garbage, paper articles and, in laboratory, for flaming needles and loops
2. Baking
   a. Useful mainly in home nursing and in sterilizing glassware for laboratory use
   b. Temperature of 350° F. (about 175° C.) for 2½ hours needed to sterilize (kill all spores and vegetative forms); higher temperature for longer time necessary because of lack of hydration
   c. If no oven thermometer available, slight charring of cotton or paper can be taken as indication of sufficient exposure at high enough temperature for sterilization
3. Boiling (100° C. or 212° F.)
   a. Most common method of applying moist heat
   b. Great practical value because easy, cheap, rapid, and effective against all vegetative forms
4. Steam under pressure—when applied correctly, most effective form of moist heat for sterilizing
5. Fractional sterilization (or intermittent or discontinuous sterilization)
   a. Limited usefulness because of time consumed
   b. Consists of boiling or steaming (100° C. or 212° F.) for 30-minute periods on 3 successive days
   c. Intervals (24-hour) allow spores to vegetate, and successive heating periods destroy newly formed vegetative forms
6. Pasteurization
   a. Kills nonspore forms of all pathogenic bacteria
   b. Useful mainly for making milk safe for human consumption
   c. Two methods
      (1) Flash method—heat cooled milk to at least 72° C. (161° F.), hold at least 15 seconds, cool rapidly
      (2) Holding method—heat cooled milk to at least 62° C. (143° F.), hold at least 30 minutes, cool rapidly
5. Cold
A. Mainly a bacteriostatic agent; does not sterilize
B. Prevents growth and multiplication of microbes by slowing down metabolism
C. Temperatures of freezing and below slowly kill many microbes
D. Tests show many organisms survive after 2 years' freezing
E. Cold used mainly for preventing bacterial spoilage of organic material such as foods and sera
6. Ultraviolet rays
A. Useful mainly in meat storage, treatment of certain skin infections, and in purifying water for pools
B. When not cut off by glass, dust, smoke particles, etc., ultraviolet rays kill organisms on surfaces of objects exposed
7. Drying
A. Useful mainly for food preservation
B. Bacteriostatic action because metabolism of organisms cannot continue without water
C. Some vegetative forms (gonococci, e.g.) killed in a few hours, or less, by drying
D. Spores known to survive complete drying for many years
8. Ionizing radiations
A. Methods that ensure safety still in experimental stages
B. Kill all microorganisms exposed
9. Ultrasonic waves and agitation
A. Methods used primarily in research
B. Injure microorganisms or kill them by rupturing cell membrane
10. Chemical agents used to destroy or inhibit microorganisms outside body
A. How chemicals inhibit or destroy microorganisms
   1. Most chemicals used as disinfectants or antiseptics, not as sterilizing agents, because most not reliable for killing spores
   2. Some chemicals thought to combine with proteins or lipids of cell membrane, thereby altering permeability
   3. Some combine with enzymes or genes or other proteins within organisms, making them unable to carry on vital functions, resulting either in death of organism or inability to multiply
B. Effectiveness of chemicals in destroying microorganisms depends upon various factors

1. Certain characteristics of the microorganisms present
   a. Species
      (1) Some species hard to kill with chemicals (e.g., virus of hepatitis)
      (2) Some moderately hard to kill with chemicals (e.g., *Staphylococcus aureus* and *Escherichia coli*)
      (3) Some easy to kill (e.g., pneumococci and gonococci)
   b. Number of organisms present—in general, more organisms present, longer the time necessary for chemical to kill all
   c. Whether or not organisms have capsules or spores—in general, these structures make it harder to kill organisms with chemicals
   d. Gram stain reaction of organisms present—in general, gram-positive organisms more easily killed by chemicals than gram-negative organisms
2. Concentration of chemical used—optimal concentration different for different chemicals; determined experimentally; e.g., alcohol most effective in concentrations of 70% and higher; cresol in 2% to 5%
3. Time and "contact"
   a. No chemical can kill any organism unless in contact with it; liquids with low surface tension spread better than those with high surface tension; therefore, low surface tension liquids more sure of making the close contact with microbes necessary to kill them
      (1) Wetting agents—liquids with low surface tension; e.g., soap
      (2) Detergents—wetting agents used mainly for cleaning but many are also antiseptics
   b. No chemical can kill instantaneously
   c. Important that chemical contact organisms long enough time to act
   d. Minimum effective time differs for different chemicals; determined experimentally
   e. In general the longer the time of contact, the more organisms killed
4. Temperature
   a. Warmer temperatures accelerate chemical reactions

   b. Temperatures of less than room temperature (68° F. or 20° C.) slow reactions sufficiently to decrease effectiveness of chemical disinfectants
5. Nature of material being disinfected —if organic material present, chemical may coagulate it, thereby forming protective coating around microorganisms, which prevents chemical from contacting them; skin almost impossible to disinfect because of resident bacteria within glandular structures
C. Factors governing selection of suitable chemical for various purposes (Table 2-3)
   1. Material to be treated—consider such factors as whether
      a. Heat possible
      b. Liquid or some other type chemical desirable
      c. Much organic matter present
   2. Relative advantages and disadvantages of chemical
      a. Cost
      b. Bleaching effects
      c. Irritating effects
      d. Corrosive effects on metals
      e. Staining
      f. Instability
      g. Difficulty or ease of preparing
      h. Odor
      i. Deodorizing qualities
D. Phenol coefficient—number that expresses power of chemical to prevent growth of microorganisms as compared with power of phenol to do this; e.g., if chemical kills in dilution of 1 to 300 whereas phenol tested under same experimental circumstances kills in dilution of 1 to 50, chemical said to have phenol coefficient of 6.0

11. Chemotherapy
Treatment or prevention of infections— by chemicals that inhibit or destroy pathogens in body (Table 2-4)

IMPORTANT FACTS ABOUT
DISEASE-PRODUCING MICROBES
SUMMARIZED

1. Infectious diseases produced by various pathogens (Table 2-5)
2. Anaerobic, disease-producing microbes
A. *Clostridium tetani*
B. *Clostridium perfringens* and other gas gangrene-producing organisms

TABLE 2-3
CHEMICALS WIDELY USED FOR DESTROYING MICROORGANISMS OUTSIDE THE BODY

Name of chemical	Uses	Characteristics
Hexachlorophene (G-11) pHisoHex (proprietary name for mixture pHisoDerm and 3% hexachlorophene)	Surgical scrubbing, pre-operative preparation of skin	Advantages—antibacterial action on skin persists for some time; decreases time necessary for surgical scrubbing; less time required with pHisoHex than with soap Disadvantage—some recent findings indicate continued use may have injurious effects
Soaps	Cleaning, scrubbing	Advantage—helps washing, scrubbing actions mechanically remove microbes; main reason for using soap Disadvantages—may not kill all pathogens; soap not properly dispensed may itself be source of infection; continued use removes natural secretions and may "dry out" skin
Coal tar derivatives Phenol (carbolic acid)	Excreta, utensils, fabrics, instruments	Advantages—can be used on wide variety of objects; cheap Disadvantages—even dilute solutions injurious to tissues if in contact more than about ½ hour; strong odor
Cresols (Lysol, trade name of cresol, soap, and alcohol preparation)	Excreta, utensils, instruments, fabrics	Advantages—less toxic to tissues than phenol; many uses, cheap Disadvantage—odor
Cationic detergents (Quaternary ammonium compounds or "quats") e.g., Zephiran, Phemerol, Roccal	Skin, variety of objects	Effective against gram-positive and gram-negative bacteria Less effective against acid-fast bacteria Ineffective against bacterial spores and viruses
Halogens Chlorinated lime (bleaching powder)	Excreta	Advantages—cheap, fast-acting Disadvantages—bleaches and rots fabrics; corrosive to tissues and metals; unstable in solution
Chloramines	Wounds, instruments, utensils	Less irritating to tissues and more stable than chlorinated lime solutions
Tincture of iodine	Skin	One of best skin disinfectants but may "burn" skin, especially if area tightly covered after application; stains
Salts of heavy metals Bichloride of mercury (mercuric chloride, corrosive sublimate)	Skin, glassware, thermometers	Advantages—cheap, odorless Disadvantages—corrodes metals, irritating to skin, highly poisonous; unreliable for excreta and other organic wastes because coagulates protein, forming protective coating around microorganisms
Merthiolate, Metaphen, Mercurochrome	Skin	Less toxic and corrosive than bichloride of mercury but effectiveness commonly overrated

Continued.

TABLE 2-3

CHEMICALS WIDELY USED FOR DESTROYING MICROORGANISMS OUTSIDE THE BODY—cont'd

Name of chemical	Uses	Characteristics
Salts of heavy metals—cont'd Silver nitrate	Eyes of newborn Gonorrheal infections	Advantage—particularly effective against gonococcus Disadvantages—decomposes in light; stains skin and fabrics
Miscellaneous Aerosols and chemical mists; e.g., propylene glycol, triethylene glycol	Air disinfection in isolation wards, barracks, etc.	Advantages—odorless, cheap, rapid-acting, low toxicity
Alcohol	Skin, thermometers	Disadvantages—expensive, slow-acting, evaporates; unreliable for organic wastes because coagulates protein, forming protective coating around microorganisms
Ethylene oxide	Surgical instruments and dressings Plastic and rubber goods	Gas, mixed with carbon dioxide to decrease flammability, used in new "cold sterilizers" for articles such as rubber and plastic goods that would be damaged by heat sterilization

TABLE 2-4

CHEMOTHERAPY

Chemicals	Source	Used mainly against
Antibiotics (Chemicals produced by living organisms) 1. Penicillin	*Penicillium notatum* (a mold)	Gram-positive bacteria—e.g., pneumococci, *Bacillus diphtheriae*, staphylococci Also, effective against gram-negative meningococci and gonococci and against *Treponema pallidum*
2. Streptomycin	*Streptomyces griseus* (an actinomycete)	*Haemophilus influenzae* *Mycobacterium tuberculosis* *Pasteurella pestis*
3. Tetracyclines Chlortetracycline (Aureomycin)	*Streptomyces aureofaciens* (an actinomycete)	Broad-spectrum antibiotics, effective against gram-negative bacteria; also, rickettsiae and some large viruses
Oxytetracycline (Terramycin)	*Streptomyces rimosus* (an actinomycete)	
4. Chloromycetin	Now produced synthetically *Streptomyces venezuelae*	Broad-spectrum antibiotics effective against most bacteria (except acid-fast), rickettsiae, and some large viruses
5. Bacitracin	*Bacillus licheniformis*	Inhibits many gram-positive organisms and certain gram-negative cocci (notably gonococci and meningococci) but not other gram-negative organisms

TABLE 2-4

CHEMOTHERAPY—cont'd

Chemicals	Source	Used mainly against
Chemicals not produced by living organisms		
1. Sulfa drugs (sulfonamides); e.g., sulfadiazine, sulfones		Meningococci, shigellae (dysentery bacilli)
2. Isoniazid (isonicotinyl-hydrazine)		Most effective agent against *Mycobacterium tuberculosis*
3. PAS (para-amino-salicylic acid)		*Mycobacterium tuberculosis;* often used with isoniazid
4. Arsenic compounds (e.g., Neosalvarsan)		*Treponema pallidum*
5. Atabrine, chloroquine, pyrimethamine, etc.		*Plasmodium malariae*
6. Ipecac (emetine hydrochloride)		*Entamoeba histolytica* (organism of amebic dysentery)

TABLE 2-5

SPECIFIC PATHOGENS AND INFECTIOUS DISEASES PRODUCED

Pathogens	Diseases produced
Molds	
1. Several species of genus *Microsporum*	1. Ringworm of skin and hair
2. Several species of genus *Epidermophyton*	2. Ringworm of skin and nails
3. Several species of genus *Trichophyton*	3. Ringworm of skin, hair, and nails
4. *Histoplasma capsulatum*	4. Histoplasmosis
Yeasts	
1. *Monilia albicans* (or *Candida albicans*)	1. Thrush and sprue
Bacteria	
1. Acid-fast	
a. *Mycobacterium tuberculosis* var. *hominis, bovis, avium*	a. Tuberculosis
b. *Mycobacterium leprae* (or *Bacillus leprae*)	b. Leprosy
2. Spirochetes	
a. *Treponema pallidum*	a. Syphilis
b. *Treponema pertenue*	b. Yaws
c. Several species of genus *Leptospira*	c. Hemorrhagic jaundice (Weil's disease or Fort Bragg fever)
3. Gram-negative, nonsporeforming bacilli	
a. *Salmonella typhosa*	a. Typhoid fever
b. *Salmonella paratyphi* and *schottmuelleri*	b. Paratyphoid fever
c. Several species of genus *Salmonella*	c. Salmonellosis (*Salmonella* food infection)
d. Several species of genus *Salmonella*	d. *Salmonella* enteritis (diarrhea)
e. Several species of genus *Shigella*	e. Shigellosis (bacillary dysentery)
f. *Haemophilus pertussis* and *parapertussis*	f. Pertussis (whooping cough)
g. *Brucella melitensis, abortus, suis*	g. Brucellosis (undulant fever or Malta fever)
h. *Pasteurella tularensis*	h. Tularemia (rabbit fever or deer fly fever)
i. *Pasteurella pestis*	i. Plague (bubonic plague or black death)
j. *Vibrio comma*	j. Cholera

Continued.

TABLE 2-5

SPECIFIC PATHOGENS AND INFECTIOUS DISEASES PRODUCED—cont'd

Microorganisms	Diseases produced
Bacteria—cont'd	
4. Gram-positive, sporeforming bacilli	
a. *Bacillus anthracis*	a. Anthrax
b. *Clostridium botulinum* (anaerobic)	b. Botulism (a food poisoning, not an infection)
c. *Clostridium tetani* (anaerobic)	c. Tetanus (lockjaw)
d. *Clostridium perfringens, septicum,* and others	d. Gas gangrene
5. Gram-positive, nonsporeforming bacilli	
a. *Corynebacterium diphtheriae*	a. Diphtheria
6. Gram-positive cocci	
a. *Micrococcus epidermidis* and *aureus* (or *Staphylococcus epidermidis* and *aureus*)	a. Many infections of skin (wounds, boils, acne, etc.), of blood (septicemia), of bone (osteomyelitis), of mucosa (otitis media, tonsillitis, sinusitis, conjunctivitis), and many others
b. *Streptococcus hemolyticus* (beta type) or *Streptococcus pyogenes*	b. Many infections such as scarlet fever, streptococcal sore throat, wound infections
c. Pneumococcus	c. Pneumonia and various other infections of respiratory tract
7. Gram-negative cocci	
a. Gonococcus (or *Neisseria gonorrhoeae*)	a. Gonorrhea
b. Meningococcus (or *Neisseria meningitidis*)	b. Epidemic meningitis
Viruses	
1. Herpesvirus varicellae (varicella-zoster or VZ virus)	1. Chickenpox and herpes zoster (shingles)
2. Poxvirus variolae	2. Smallpox (variola)
3. Measles virus	3. Measles (rubeola)
4. Rubella virus	4. German measles (rubella)
5. Adenoviruses (APC viruses—from adenoids, pharynx, conjunctiva)	5. Severe upper respiratory infections
6. Myxovirus influenzae	6. Influenza
7. Psittacosis virus	7. Psittacosis (parrot fever)
8. Poliomyelitis viruses	8. Poliomyelitis
9. Encephalitis viruses	9. Viral encephalitis
10. Rabies virus	10. Rabies
11. Yellow fever virus	11. Yellow fever
12. Myxovirus parotiditis	12. Mumps (infectious parotitis)
13. Infectious hepatitis viruses	13. Infectious hepatitis (catarrhal jaundice)
14. Coxsackie viruses	14. Herpangina, pleurodynia (devil's grippe)
Protozoa	
1. *Entamoeba histolytica*	1. Amebiasis (amebic dysentery)
2. *Plasmodium vivax, malariae, falciparum,* and *ovale*	2. Malaria
3. *Trypanosoma gambiense* and *rhodesiense*	3. African sleeping sickness
4. *Trichomonas vaginalis*	4. Vaginitis

C. *Clostridium botulinum*
3. **Spore-forming, disease-producing microbes**
A. *Clostridium tetani*
B. *Clostridium perfringens* and other pathogens of gas gangrene
C. *Clostridium botulinum*
D. *Bacillus anthracis*
4. **Acid-fast pathogens**
   Retain original red dye even though treated with acid-alcohol and counterstained
A. *Mycobacterium tuberculosis*
B. *Mycobacterium leprae*
C. *Treponema pallidum* and several other spirochetes
5. **Gram-positive, disease-producing microbes**
   Retain original purplish stain even though treated with alcohol or acetone and counterstained
A. *Mycobacterium tuberculosis*
B. *Corynebacterium diphtheriae*
C. All spore-forming, disease-producing microbes (item 3)
D. All cocci except gonococci and meningococci

6. **Gram-negative, disease-producing microbes**
   Take counterstain, usually red, after decolorizing with alcohol or acetone
A. All bacilli except *Mycobacterium tuberculosis*, *Corynebacterium diphtheriae*, and sporeformers
B. Gonococci
C. Meningococci
D. *Vibrio cholerae*
E. Spirochetes
7. **Pathogens that are frequently encapsulated**
A. Pneumococci
B. *Bacillus anthracis*
8. **Exotoxin, disease-producing microbes**
   Exotoxins are poisonous chemicals released by a few species of living microbes into surrounding fluid; exotoxins are specific; for example, this means that the exotoxin from diphtheria organisms produces diphtheria and no other disease and that it stimulates formation of diphtheria antitoxin and no other; major exotoxin producers are listed below; see Table 2-6 on vaccines and antisera
A. *Corynebacterium diphtheriae*

TABLE 2-6
SOME IMPORTANT VACCINES AND ANTISERA

Vaccines		Antisera	
Disease vaccine protects against	Antigen in vaccine	Disease antiserum protects against	Type antiserum
Bacterial diseases			
Cholera	Killed bacteria	Botulism	Antitoxin
Diphtheria	Toxoid	Diphtheria	Antitoxin
Paratyphoid	Killed bacteria	Gas gangrene	Antitoxin
Pertussis	Killed bacteria	Tetanus	Antitoxin
Plague	Killed bacteria	Pertussis	Antibacterial
Tetanus	Toxoid		
Tuberculosis (BCG)	Weakened bacteria		
Typhoid	Killed bacteria		
Rickettsial diseases			
Typhus	Killed rickettsiae		
Viral diseases			
Measles	Weakened virus		
Mumps	Weakened virus	Rabies	Antiviral
Poliomyelitis		Infectious hepatitis	Concentrated gamma globulin
(Salk)	Killed virus		
(Sabin and Cox)	Weakened virus		
Rabies		Measles	Concentrated gamma globulin
(Pasteur treatment)	Killed virus		
Smallpox	Weakened virus		
Viral influenza	Weakened virus		
Yellow fever	Weakened virus		

TABLE 2-7
SUMMARY HISTORY OF MICROBIOLOGY

Date	Person	Event
1590	Jansen—Dutch optician	Used first compound microscope
1665	Hooke	Wrote *Micrographia,* book on microscope
1673	van Leeuwenhoek	Called "father of bacteriology" because was first to describe shapes of bacteria accurately; made simple microscope of greater magnification (about ×160) than any preceding ones; made first drawing of bacteria in 1683
1796	Edward Jenner	Made successful vaccination against smallpox by using pus from cowpox pustule
1855	Louis Pasteur (French chemist)	Disproved spontaneous generation theory as cause of disease through his work on fermentation
1867	Louis Pasteur	Devised "pasteurization" as means of preventing "diseases of wine"
1867	Lord Lister (English surgeon)	Called "father of antiseptic surgery"; used carbolic acid spray during operations and immersed hands and instruments in it before
1877	Louis Pasteur	Discovered bacillus of malignant edema
1879	Louis Pasteur	Discovered streptococci as causative agents of puerperal fever
1879	Neisser	Discovered gonococci
1880	Eberth	Discovered typhoid bacilli
1882	Koch (German scientist)	Formulated his postulates for proving given microbe cause of given disease; discovered tuberculosis bacillus, *Vibrio cholerae,* and bacillus of conjunctivitis
1883	Klebs	Discovered diphtheria bacteria
1884	Löffler	Cultivated diphtheria bacteria
1885	Louis Pasteur	Developed "Pasteur treatment" for rabies

B. *Clostridium tetani*

C. *Clostridium perfringens* and other gas gangrene organisms

D. *Clostridium botulinum* (not actually pathogen, since disease it produces is a food poisoning not an infection; pathogens produce infections)

E. Virulent strains of *Staphylococcus aureus* and *Streptococcus*

9. **Endotoxins**

   Poisonous substances released from all microorganisms upon disintegration; do not effectively stimulate formation of antitoxins

SOME IMPORTANT EVENTS IN THE HISTORY OF MICROBIOLOGY

Microbiology is a comparatively new science—not much over 100 years old; all the fundamental discoveries that gave birth to this science were made after 1860, although many discoveries that laid foundation upon which science of microbiology could be built were made during 17th and 18th centuries; Table 2-7 summarizes some outstanding events in the history of this young but important science.

REVIEW QUESTIONS FOR MICROBIOLOGY
Multiple choice

Read each item carefully and consider all possible answers. When you have decided which answer is best, blacken in the corresponding space on the answer sheet. There is only one best answer for each item.

1. Which microbes have a spiral shape?
   1. Bacilli and diplococci
   2. Spirochetes and vibrios
   3. Both 2 and 3
   4. Neither 2 nor 3
2. The body cannot readily destroy pneumococci by phagocytosis because they have which of the following structures?
   1. Capsules and spores
   2. Capsules only
   3. Spores only
   4. Flagella
3. Under normal, natural conditions, microbes are present
   1. In all parts of the body
   2. In air, soil, and water
   3. In all raw foods
   4. Both 2 and 3
4. What structures enable microbes to survive under such unfavorable conditions as drying and boiling temperatures?
   1. Capsules and spores

2. Capsules only
3. Spores only
4. Flagella
5. Which kind of microbe is classified as animal?
   1. Mold   3. Spirochete
   2. Protozoon   4. Virus
6. Which kind of microbe is multicellular?
   1. Mold
   2. Protozoon
   3. Spirochete
   4. None of the preceding
7. *Staphylococcus aureus* is the name of a well-known kind of microbe.
   1. A microbe's first name tells what genus the microbe belongs to
   2. A microbe's last name tells what species of microbe it is
   3. Both 1 and 2
   4. Neither 1 nor 2
8. Which of the following are normally sterile; i.e., contain no living organisms?
   1. Blood and pleural fluid
   2. Gastric juices
   3. Both 1 and 2
   4. Neither 1 nor 2
9. Microorganisms are so small that their size is usually measured in
   1. Angstroms   3. Microns
   2. Millimicrons   4. 2 and 3
10. Which of the following is true about the size of viruses?
    1. Even smaller than protein molecules
    2. Too small to be seen even with electron microscope
    3. Both of the preceding
    4. Slightly larger than largest protein molecule
11. The pathogens classified as sporeformers cause the following diseases:
    1. Anthrax, botulism, gas gangrene, and tetanus
    2. Tuberculosis and leprosy
    3. Both 1 and 2
    4. None of the preceding
12. Yeasts reproduce sexually by
    1. Budding   3. Hyphae
    2. Fission   4. Spores
13. Bacteria reproduce by
    1. Budding   3. Spore formation
    2. Capsule formation   4. Transverse fission
14. Any disease caused by microbes may properly be called
    1. A communicable disease
    2. A contagious disease
    3. An infection
    4. Any of the preceding
15. What diseases are caused by pathogens that produce powerful exotoxins?
    1. Botulism and gas gangrene
    2. Diphtheria and tetanus
    3. Both 1 and 2
    4. None of the preceding
16. A gram-negative microbe is one that
    1. Cannot be stained by Gram's method
    2. Retains the original stain when stained by Gram's method
    3. Takes the counterstain when stained by Gram's method
    4. Weighs less than a gram

17. An acid-fast microbe is one that
    1. Cannot be destroyed by acids
    2. Retains the original stain even though treated with acid-alcohol and counterstained
    3. Is destroyed quickly by acids
    4. Takes a counterstain after treatment with acid-alcohol
18. Which organisms reproduce only inside living cells?
    1. Fungi
    2. Vibrios
    3. Plasmodia
    4. All of the preceding
19. Pathogens form various substances that increase their virulence—their ability to produce disease; which of the following is not one of these substances?
    1. Hyaline   3. Kinase
    2. Hyaluronidase   4. Leukocidin
20. Tetanus is usually transmitted by way of
    1. Insects   3. The soil
    2. Milk   4. Water
21. Biologic transfer of malaria is carried on by what insect?
    1. *Anopheles* mosquito
    2. *Aedes aegypti* mosquito
    3. Rat flea
    4. Tsetse fly
22. Gram-negative diplococci found in a vaginal smear are presumed to be
    1. Gonococci
    2. Meningococci
    3. Pneumococci
    4. *Treponema pallidum*
23. Acid-fast rods found in sputum are presumed to be
    1. Influenza virus
    2. *Bordetella pertussis*
    3. Diphtheria bacillus
    4. *Mycobacterium tuberculosis*
24. What kind of organism causes measles?
    1. Bacteria   3. Rickettsiae
    2. Protozoa   4. Viruses
25. What kind of organism causes infectious hepatitis?
    1. Bacteria   3. Rickettsiae
    2. Molds   4. Viruses
26. What kind of organism causes mumps?
    1. Bacteria   3. Rickettsiae
    2. Molds   4. Viruses
27. Under certain circumstances the virus that causes chickenpox can cause
    1. Cold sores   3. Shingles
    2. Infectious hepatitis 4. German measles
28. Through which portal of entry do most microbes probably enter the body?
    1. Mucosa of digestive and respiratory tracts
    2. Reproductive tract
    3. Skin
    4. Urinary tract
29. Which of the following is true about exotoxins?
    1. Act as antigens
    2. Destroy white blood cells
    3. Dissolve blood clots
    4. Are produced by all microorganisms
30. Which of the following statements is true about microorganisms as agents that cause disease?

1. Microorganisms are able to invade the body via the skin or mucosa only through an abrasion
2. The portal by which microorganisms enter the body bears no relationship to their ability to produce disease
3. The number of microorganisms invading the body is directly related to their ability to produce disease
4. Microorganisms that have "rested" outside the body for awhile before entering another host have a greater ability to produce disease than those rapidly transmitted from one host to another

31. Typhoid fever spreads via
    1. Carriers   3. Insects
    2. Water and foods   4. All of the preceding
32. Human carriers are not known to transmit
    1. Diphtheria   3. Meningitis
    2. Dysentery   4. Typhus fever
33. Yellow fever is transmitted via
    1. *Anopheles* mosquito
    2. *Aedes aegypti* mosquito
    3. Louse
    4. Tsetse fly
34. Antigen-antibody reactions can
    1. Facilitate the phagocytosis of antigens
    2. Neutralize antigens
    3. Make antigens harmless to the body
    4. All of the preceding
35. If you have had an injection of a modified antigen, you might have been given
    1. Diphtheria toxoid 3. Both 1 and 2
    2. Smallpox vaccine   4. Tetanus antitoxin
36. African sleeping sickness is transmitted via
    1. *Anopheles* mosquito
    2. *Aedes aegypti* mosquito
    3. Tsetse fly
    4. Rat fleas
37. An example of a disease caused by protozoa is
    1. African sleeping sickness
    2. Plague
    3. Syphilis
    4. Yellow fever
38. The commonest portals of entry for organisms that cause most communicable diseases are
    1. Mouth and nose
    2. Mouth and eyes
    3. Mouth and genitourinary tract
    4. Mouth and skin
39. A substance classed as an antigen must
    1. Act as an irritant, stimulating formation of antibodies against itself
    2. Be a protein
    3. Be a natural constituent of the body
    4. All of the preceding
40. Antibodies are now thought to be produced by
    1. Plasma cells only
    2. Plasma cells and some lymphocytes
    3. Lymphocytes, neutrophils, and also plasma cells
    4. Erythrocytes in the spleen and lymph nodes
41. The substance that would be given to a young woman who is entering nursing and who is found to be susceptible to typhoid fever
    1. Contains antigens
    2. Is a vaccine
    3. Produces artificial, active immunity
    4. All of the preceding

42. Which of the following statements is not true about vaccines?
    1. Are used to treat some acute infectious diseases
    2. Are used most often prophylactically before exposure to a disease
    3. Are sometimes used prophylactically after exposure if the incubation period is long
    4. Contain antigens
43. Vaccines differ from antisera in that
    1. Antigens constitute the active ingredient of vaccines; antibodies, of antisera
    2. Vaccines are used only to prevent disease, whereas antisera are used mainly to treat disease
    3. Vaccines always confer active immunity, whereas antisera never do
    4. All of the preceding
44. The substance used most often in the Pasteur treatment against rabies
    1. Contains antibodies 3. Both of preceding
    2. Is an antiserum   4. Is a vaccine
45. What substance is used in a Dick test?
    1. Diphtheria antitoxin
    2. Diphtheria toxoid
    3. Scarlet fever antitoxin
    4. Scarlet fever toxin
46. Which of the following is true about the tuberculin test?
    1. Indicates susceptibility of children to tuberculosis
    2. Is valuable for diagnosing tuberculosis in adults only
    3. Is most valuable for diagnosing tuberculosis in children
    4. Indicates susceptibility of adults to tuberculosis
47. Allergy and immunity are alike in that both
    1. Are always induced by introduction of a given antigen into the body at least twice
    2. Result from antibodies combining with their specific antigen
    3. Usually require about 2 days to develop
    4. All of the preceding
48. An example of an allergic response to an antigen is
    1. The reaction of a tubercular person to the tuberculin test
    2. The reaction of a person susceptible to scarlet fever to the Dick test
    3. The reaction of a person who has typhoid fever to the Widal test
    4. All of the preceding
49. The pathogen responsible for this disease is a rickettsia transferred usually by lice
    1. Bubonic plague   3. Typhoid fever
    2. Malaria   4. Typhus fever
50. Procedures that sterilize
    1. Always disinfect also
    2. Are aseptic also
    3. May employ either chemicals or heat
    4. All of the preceding
51. Which of the following can be relied upon to sterilize?
    1. Autoclaving (assuming that it is done properly)
    2. Boiling 30 minutes
    3. Complete drying
    4. All of the preceding

52. Which of the following is true?
    1. Baking articles 10 minutes at 350° F. is a reliable method of sterilizing them
    2. Steam under pressure always has a temperature higher than free-flowing steam or boiling water
    3. The rapid microbe-killing power of steam under pressure is directly due to its higher-than-atmospheric pressure and not to its higher-than-boiling temperature
    4. All of the preceding
53. Baking
    1. Sterilizes if done at temperature of 212° F. (100° C.) for 2 hours
    2. Sterilizes if done at 350° F. (about 175° C.) for 30 minutes
    3. Neither 1 nor 2 if spores are present
    4. Sterilizes under conditions listed in either 1 or 2
54. Which of the following is true about the effectiveness of chemicals in inhibiting or destroying microorganisms?
    1. In general, there is a direct relation between the concentration of a chemical and its antiseptic or germicidal powers
    2. There is no relation between the deodorizing powers of a chemical and its antiseptic or germicidal powers
    3. Both of the preceding
    4. There is no relation between the length of time a chemical contacts microorganisms and its antiseptic or germicidal powers
55. Which chemical should not be used on metals because it corrodes them?
    1. Alcohol
    2. Bichloride of mercury
    3. Cresol
    4. Hydrogen peroxide
56. Which chemical is best suited to disinfecting feces and other organic wastes?
    1. Alcohol
    2. Bichloride of mercury
    3. Chlorinated lime
    4. Compound cresol solution
57. Which chemical is particularly effective against the gonococcus?
    1. Alcohol
    2. Bichloride of mercury
    3. Potassium permanganate
    4. Silver nitrate
58. A chemical with a phenol coefficient of 10
    1. Will theoretically prevent growth of microorganisms in one tenth as concentrated solution as phenol will
    2. Must theoretically be ten times as concentrated as phenol in order to prevent growth of microorganisms
    3. Takes one tenth the time to kill microorganisms as phenol does
    4. Takes ten times as long to kill microorganisms as phenol does
59. Which of the following is used externally to inhibit the growth and multiplication of microbes rather than to kill them?
    1. Boiling 10 minutes
    2. Chemotherapy
    3. Freezing
    4. All of the preceding
60. Why is autoclaving used for sterilizing surgical supplies more often than boiling? Because
    1. More articles can be sterilized at one time
    2. Pressurized steam is surer to penetrate all parts of the material
    3. Steam is less injurious to materials
    4. A higher temperature can be attained, assuring the destruction of spores
61. Why is there more danger of botulism from home-canned green beans than from commercially canned beans? Because
    1. The *Clostridium botulinum* is a spore-former and true anaerobe
    2. The *Clostridium botulinum* forms exotoxins
    3. Usual home-canning methods do not apply a high enough temperature to kill spores in the given time
    4. All of the preceding
62. Why could the *Clostridium botulinum* grow in canned beans and not in fresh green beans cooked one day and then refrigerated? Because
    1. The *Clostridium botulinum* is a spore-former
    2. It is a true anaerobe
    3. It forms exotoxins
    4. The low temperature inhibits the growth of the organism
63. Why is boiling used for sterilizing many articles instead of autoclaving?
    1. Boiling kills all vegetative forms of microbes
    2. Usually there are no pathogenic spore-formers present
    3. Boiling is cheaper and easier than autoclaving
    4. All of the preceding
64. Milk that has just been pasteurized
    1. Contains no living microorganisms
    2. Contains no living pathogens
    3. Contains no living nonsporeforming pathogens
    4. All of the preceding
65. What is the effect of freezing, at below 0° F., on microorganisms?
    1. Inhibits their growth and multiplication
    2. Kills all microorganisms
    3. Kills all pathogens
    4. Kills all but sporeformers
66. Scrubbing the hands with soap under running water for several minutes
    1. Sterilizes them
    2. Mechanically removes all microorganisms
    3. Inhibits microorganism growth and multiplication for a short time
    4. Mechanically removes most microorganisms
67. Which statement about viruses is true?
    1. They can be seen with a light microscope only under high power
    2. They multiply only inside living cells
    3. They cause disease by means of the powerful exotoxins they produce
    4. None of the preceding

SCORES

1	5
2	6
3	7
4	8

NAME _____ DATE _____
     LAST   FIRST   MIDDLE

SCHOOL _____ CITY _____

DATE OF BIRTH _____

GRADE OR CLASS _____ INSTRUCTOR _____

AGE _____ SEX _____ M OR F

PART _____

NAME OF TEST _____

SAMPLE:
1—1 a country
1—2 a mountain
1—3 an island
1—4 a city
1—5 a state

1. Chicago is   1 :::: 2 :::: 3 ■ 4 :::: 5 ::::

DIRECTIONS: Read each question and its numbered answers. When you have decided which answer is correct, blacken the corresponding space on this sheet with the special pencil. Make your mark as long as the pair of lines, and move the pencil point up and down firmly to make a heavy black line. If you change your mind, erase your first mark completely. Make no stray marks; they may count against you.

BE SURE YOUR MARKS ARE HEAVY AND BLACK.
ERASE COMPLETELY ANY ANSWER YOU WISH TO CHANGE.

3

CHEMISTRY

Arnow, L. E.: Introduction to physiological and pathological chemistry, ed. 8, St. Louis, 1972, The C. V. Mosby Co.

Brewster, R. Q., and McEwen, W. E.: Organic chemistry, ed. 3, Englewood Cliffs, N. J., 1961, Prentice-Hall, Inc.

Cantarow, A., and Schepartz, B.: Textbook of biochemistry, ed. 4, Philadelphia, 1967, W. B. Saunders Co.

Cantarow, A., and Trumper, M.: Clinical biochemistry, ed. 6, Philadelphia, 1962, W. B. Saunders Co.

Drobner, R. H., and Mock, G. V.: Roe's principles of chemistry, ed. 11, St. Louis, 1972, The C. V. Mosby Co.

Goostray, S., and Schwenck, J. R.: Textbook of chemistry, ed. 9, New York, 1966, The Macmillan Co.

Linstromberg, W. W.: Organic chemistry: a brief course, ed. 2, Lexington, Mass., 1970, D. C. Heath Co.

Mahler, H. R., and Cordes, E. H.: Biological chemistry, New York, 1966, Harper & Row, Publishers.

Nevill, W.: General chemistry, New York, 1967, McGraw-Hill Book Co.

Orten, J. M., and Neuhaus, O. W.: Biochemistry, ed. 8, St. Louis, 1970, The C. V. Mosby Co.

Routh, J. I.: Fundamentals of inorganic, organic and biological chemistry, ed. 5, Philadelphia, 1965, W. B. Saunders Co.

Taber, C. W.: Cyclopedic medical dictionary, Philadelphia, 1969, F. A. Davis Co.

GENERAL CONCEPTS IN CHEMISTRY

1. Definitions

A. Science—a field of activity dealing with the observation and interpretation of facts, and the formation of theories concerning these facts

B. Chemistry—one area of science
  1. Composition and properties of matter
  2. Changes that matter undergoes
  3. Energy changes involved
  4. Laws governing these changes
  5. Divisions of chemistry
    a. Inorganic—concerned with a study of elements and compounds other than carbon
    b. Organic—concerned with a study of carbon compounds

C. Energy—capacity to do work
  1. Kinds of energy
    a. Kinetic energy—the energy a body possesses by virtue of its motion, as that in a running motor
    b. Potential energy—the energy a body possesses because of its existence in a high-energy state, as the force present in water behind a dam
  2. Forms of energy
    a. Heat
    b. Radiant
    c. Electric
    d. Chemical
    e. Atomic
  3. Measurement of energy
    a. Small calorie (cal.)—the amount of heat necessary to raise 1 gm. of water 1° C. in temperature
    b. Large calorie (Cal. or kcal.)—a kilocalorie; equal to 1,000 small calories
    c. Average daily requirement for humans—2,500 cal.
    d. Protein—4 kcal./gm., carbohydrate —4 kcal./gm., fat—9 kcal./gm.

D. Matter—that which occupies space, has mass, and possesses inertia
  1. Properties of matter

a. Physical—color, odor, taste, melting point, density, etc.
b. Chemical—the tendencies of a substance to undergo chemical change

2. Changes in matter
   a. Chemical change—one in which the chemical and physical properties are changed and a new substance is formed; example:

   Iron + Oxygen $\longrightarrow$ Iron oxide
   (a new substance)

   b. Physical change—one in which the physical properties are changed but the chemical nature remains unchanged; examples:

   Liquid water turning into solid, ice, or into gas, steam

3. States of matter
   a. Solid—definite size and shape, particles tightly compact
      (1) Crystalline
      (2) Amorphous
   b. Liquid—mobility of particles, assumes shape of container while maintaining definite volume
   c. Gas—no fixed shape, particles move independently of each other
      (1) Compressible
      (2) Expandable
      (3) Fills container into which it is placed

4. Classes of matter
   a. Elements—substances that cannot be decomposed by chemical means into more simple substances, each element having a specific place in the periodic table of elements
   b. Compounds—2 or more elements chemically combined in definite proportion by weight into a new substance having chemical properties different from those of the elements uniting to form it
   c. Mixtures—physical combinations of 2 or more substances not chemically united

5. Structure of matter
   a. Atom—the smallest fundamental unit of an element and the particle of an element that takes part in chemical change
   b. Atomic weight unit of mass (a.w.u.) —approximately the weight of 1 hydrogen atom (lightest known element)

c. Subatomic particles
   (1) Electron—negligible weight, 1 negative electron charge
   (2) Proton—1 atomic weight unit of mass, 1 positive electric charge
   (3) Neutron—1 atomic weight unit of mass, no electric charge
d. Nucleus of the atom
   (1) Bulk of weight of atom here, composed of protons and neutrons in approximately equal numbers
   (2) Number of protons in the nucleus of atom same as the atomic number; example: carbon—6 protons and atomic number, 6
   (3) Enough neutrons in nucleus to make up the difference between the atomic number and the atomic weight; example: carbon, having an atomic weight of 12 a.w.u., an atomic number of 6, and 6 neutrons (Fig. 3-1)
   (4) Isotope—an atom of an element, having the same number of protons and electrons as

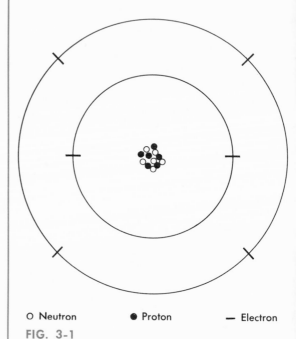

O Neutron   ● Proton   — Electron

FIG. 3-1

A carbon atom: atomic weight 12 a.w.u., atomic number 6.

other atoms of that element but possessing a different number of neutrons and a different atomic weight; some isotopes are radioactive

e. Outer energy orbitals of the atom
  (1) Electrons here
  (2) Chemical properties determined by number and arrangement of electrons in outer orbital
  (3) Arrangement of electrons: maximum of 2 in first orbital, maximum of 8 in second orbital, maximum of 18 in third orbital, maximum of 32 in fourth orbital, etc.
  (4) Element having 8 electrons in the outer orbital of its atom— a chemically inert element; exception is helium, which is inert and has 2 electrons in its first and only orbital

f. Number of protons always equal to number of electrons, so an atom is always electrically neutral

g. Recent discoveries show electrons in atom assume more complex spacing
  (1) Electrons occupy certain fixed areas away from nucleus
  (2) Energy required to move to other fixed areas farther from nucleus
    (a) Energy absorbed in packets called "quanta"
    (b) Absorbing quanta results in electrons' moving farther from nucleus
    (c) Electrons returning to original areas release energy
  (3) Closest position to nucleus that an electron can occupy called its "ground" or "stable" state

h. *Main quantum number* (n) represents lowest possible energy state of electron—ground state
  (1) n can be any *whole* number (1, 2, 3, etc.)
    (a) Number must be positive
    (b) Number cannot be zero
  (2) Other quantum numbers exist
    (a) $l = n - 1$ (0, 1, 2, etc.)
    (b) $m = +1, 0, -1$
    (c) $s = +\frac{1}{2}, -\frac{1}{2}$

  (3) For any value of main quantum number n, there exists a number representing how many electrons are needed to fill orbital in ground state
  (4) When $l = 0$, the energy level is called s; $l = 1$, the level is called p; $l = 2$, the level is called d; and for $l = 3$, the level is called f
  (5) Combining n and l values gives values for electron energy levels of atom

n	l	Energy levels possible	Number of electrons in energy levels
1	0	1s	2
2	1	2s, 2p	8
3	2	3s, 3p, 3d	18
4	3	4s, 4p, 4d, 4f	32

  (6) The s orbitals (1, 2, 3, etc.) are spherical in shape and hold a maximum of 2 electrons each (Fig. 3-2)
  (7) The p and d orbitals assume shapes as seen in Fig. 3-2, each shaded area holding a maximum of 1 electron

i. Difference between an atom of one element and an atom of another element is a result of the difference in number and arrangement of the subatomic particles in the respective atoms

j. Weight of an atom (mass number of atom) is the sum of all of the subatomic particles in that atom

k. By convention, the weight of an atom of the most plentiful carbon isotope is taken as 12 atomic weight units and all other atomic weights are based on this standard

l. Molecule—the smallest unit of a compound is formed by union of 2 or more atoms of different elements; a molecule of an element may be formed from 2 or more atoms of that element
  (1) Molecular weight—sum of all of the atomic weights of the atoms making up the molecule
  (2) Ion—an atom or molecule that has lost or gained an electron

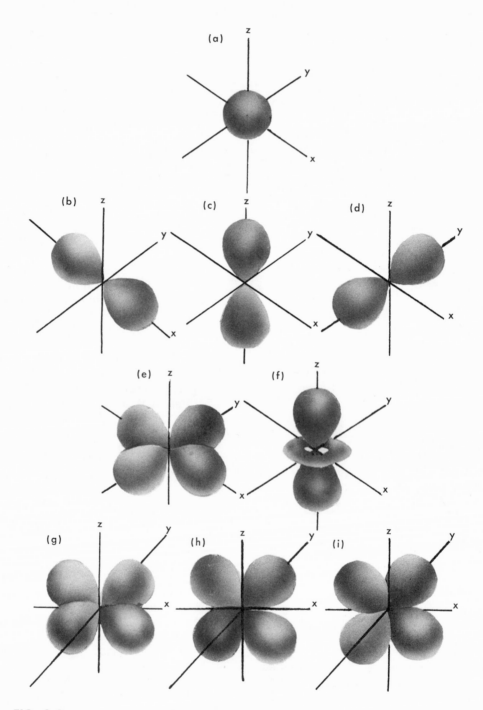

FIG. 3-2
Atomic electron orbitals: s orbital (a); p orbitals (b),(c),(d); and d orbitals (e),(f),(g),(h),(i).

TABLE 3-1
VALENCES SHOWN BY COMMON ELEMENTS AND RADICALS

1+	2+	3+
Ammonium, NH_4^+ Copper (I), Cu^+ Mercury (I), Hg^+ Potassium, K^+ Silver, Ag^+ Sodium, Na^+ Hydronium, H_3O^+	Barium, Ba^{++} Calcium, Ca^{++} Copper (II), Cu^{++} Iron (II), Fe^{++} Lead (II), Pb^{++} Magnesium, Mg^{++} Mercury (II), Hg^{++} Nickel (II), Ni^{++} Zinc, Zn^{++}	Aluminum, Al^{+++} Chromium (III), Cr^{+++} Iron (III), Fe^{+++}

1-	2-	3-
Acetate, $C_2H_3O_2^-$ Bicarbonate, HCO_3^- Bisulfate, HSO_4^- Bromide, Br^- Chlorate, ClO_3^- Chloride, Cl^- Fluoride, F^- Hydroxide, OH^- Iodide, I^- Nitrite, NO_2^- Nitrate, NO_3^-	Carbonate, $CO_3^=$ Chromate, $CrO_4^=$ Oxide, $O^=$ Peroxide, $O_2^=$ Sulfide, $S^=$ Sulfite, $SO_3^=$ Sulfate, $SO_4^=$	Phosphate, $PO_4^{\equiv}$

(or electrons) and thus has gained an electric charge (positive or negative)

m. Valence—the electric charge on an ion is called its *valence* (Table 3-1); term is also used to indicate the combining power of atoms that do not ionize

n. Radical—a group of 2 or more atoms or ions, chemically united and acting as a unit; has its own valence, which is the sum of the valences of the atoms or ions making up the radical

6. Chemical symbol—abbreviation for name of element, first letter always capitalized; example: Ca (calcium) stands for 1 atom of calcium

7. Formula—abbreviation of name of a compound, made up of chemical symbols for the atoms making up the molecule of the compound, with subscripts to show proportion of each element; example: $CaCl_2$ (calcium chloride) stands for 1 atom of calcium and 2 atoms of chlorine for each molecule of calcium chloride

8. Catalyst—substance entering into a reaction, speeding up or slowing down the reaction; catalyst is unchanged by the reaction; needed in small amounts

9. Enzyme—organic catalyst found in all living things

2. **Chemical bonding**

A. Electrovalent—type of bonding characterized by exchange of electrons between atoms of different elements

1. The atoms losing electrons become positively charged ions; atoms of metals form positive ions

2. The atoms gaining electrons become negatively charged ions; atoms of non-metals form negative ions

3. Molecules of compounds are then formed due to attractions between oppositely charged ions

4. Elements whose atoms can form either positive or negative ions are called amphoteric

B. Covalent—type of bonding common in atoms that do not lose or gain electrons readily; such atoms form molecules of compounds by sharing electrons, the shared electrons forming bonds between the atoms (Fig. 3-3)

3. **Chemical change**

A. Rules regulating chemical change

1. Law of conservation of energy—in any chemical reaction energy is neither created nor destroyed but only changed from one form of energy to another

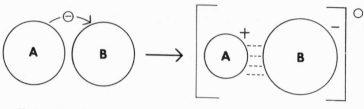

Electron(s) exchanged

Ions formed, are bound together by opposite charges, total molecule neutral in charge

ELECTROVALENT BONDING

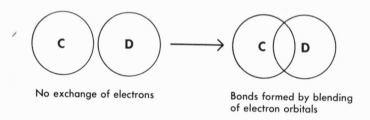

No exchange of electrons

Bonds formed by blending of electron orbitals

COVALENT BONDING

FIG. 3-3

Types of chemical bonding.

2. Law of conservation of matter—in a chemical reaction matter is neither created nor destroyed but only changed in form; the weight of the products equals the weight of the reactants

3. Law of definite composition—any given compound always contains same elements in same proportions by weight and united in the same manner

4. Law of multiple proportion—when 2 elements form more than 1 compound with each other, simple whole-number relationships exist in proportions of the elements whose amounts vary

5. Avogadro's hypothesis—equal volumes of gases under similar conditions of temperature and pressure contain the same number of molecules

6. Avogadro's number—at standard temperature (0° C.) and pressure (1 atmosphere) 22.4 liters of any gas contains 6.02×10^{23} molecules

B. Chemical equation
1. Function—symbolic expression of a chemical reaction
   a. Tells what elements or compounds react
   b. Tells what elements or compounds are formed
   c. Tells the amounts of reactants and products

2. Writing an equation
   a. On the left side are written symbols representing the reactants
   b. On the right side are written symbols representing the products
   c. For each element the number of atoms on left must equal the number of atoms on right
   d. In the formula of a compound, the positive valences must equal the negative valences
   e. An arrow shows direction of the reaction
   f. If more than 1 atom of an element is needed to balance valences in a molecule of a compound, small subscripts are used to indicate the number of atoms in the molecule; example: $CaCl_2$
   g. When a radical is used in a compound, the elements composing the radical are enclosed in parentheses if more than 1 particle of the radical

is needed to balance valences; example: ammonium carbonate—$(NH_4)_2CO_3$

C. Kinds of chemical reactions

1. Combination or synthesis

$$C \quad + \quad O_2 \quad \longrightarrow \quad CO_2$$

Carbon   Oxygen   Carbon dioxide

2. Decomposition or analysis

$$2HgO \quad \longrightarrow \quad 2Hg \quad + \quad O_2$$

Mercuric oxide   Mercury   Oxygen gas

3. Replacement or substitution

$$Zn \quad + \quad H_2SO_4 \quad \longrightarrow \quad ZnSO_4 \quad + \quad H_2$$

Zinc   Sulfuric acid   Zinc sulfate   Hydrogen gas

4. Double replacement

$$AgNO_3 \quad + \quad HCl \quad \longrightarrow \quad AgCl \quad + \quad HNO_3$$

Silver nitrate   Hydro-chloric acid   Silver chloride   Nitric acid

5. Irreversible reactions—if one of the products of a chemical reaction is a gas that can escape, a substance that is insoluble, or a substance that ionizes poorly, the reaction is irreversible; all other reactions are to some extent reversible

6. When the products of a reversible reaction are being formed at the same rate as the reactants are being re-formed, the reaction is said to be in *equilibrium;* example:

$$2NaNO_3 + K_2SO_4 \rightleftharpoons Na_2SO_4 + 2KNO_3$$

PERIODIC TABLE

1. **Chemical nature of elements depends on the number and position of electrons in orbitals outside nucleus**

A. Reactivity of elements depends especially on the number and position of electrons in the outermost electron orbital

B. Relationship exists between elements having same number of electrons in the outermost electron orbital

1. Sodium has 11 electrons with 1 electron in the outermost orbital

2. Potassium has 19 electrons with 1 electron in the outermost orbital

3. Chemically sodium and potassium react similarly, since each has 1 electron in the outermost orbital

2. **Chemical relationship is the basis of the periodic table**

A. Periodic table is a result of the work of many early scientists—the most lasting work being that of Mendeleev

B. Elements in vertical columns of table are similar to one another and are called families of elements

C. Knowing the chemical nature of one member of a family, you can predict the chemical nature of the rest of the family

IMPORTANT ELEMENTS IN PERIODIC TABLE

1. **Oxygen**

A. Physical properties

1. Colorless, odorless, and tasteless gas

2. Heavier than air

3. Slightly soluble in water

4. Liquefies and solidifies only at very low temperatures and high pressures

B. Chemical properties

1. Member of Group VI in periodic table

2. Has 8 electrons, 6 in the outermost orbital

3. Tends, in chemical reaction, to gain 2 electrons to complete outer orbital

   a. Becomes a negatively charged particle

   b. Reacts as a nonmetal

4. Can also form covalent bonds

5. Will not burn

6. Supports combustion

7. Unites with many elements to form oxides

   a. Oxides of metals are basic anhydrides; if put into water, they form bases

   b. Oxides of nonmetals are acid anhydrides; if put into water they form acids

   c. Many elements form more than 1 oxide; example: H_2O—water and H_2O_2—hydrogen peroxide

   d. The uniting of a substance with oxygen is called "oxidation"

C. Importance of oxygen

1. Forms about 21% of air

2. Forms about 50% of earth's crust

3. Is present in water—89% by weight, 33% by volume

4. Is present in foods, plant tissue, and animal tissue

5. Oxidation of organic compounds results in production of carbon dioxide, water, and energy

   a. Oxidation of food takes place in the

cells of living things and supplies the energy for life
  b. Oxidation of wood, coal, and other fuels supplies the energy for heat, functioning of machinery, movement of cars and buses, etc.
  c. Some oxidation is harmful
    (1) The rusting of iron can be prevented by coating the iron with material that reacts poorly with oxygen
    (2) Certain drugs are useless when oxidized; prevention lies in keeping bottles tightly closed to shut out air
D. Medical uses of oxygen
  1. Oxygen therapy used in many instances
    a. Lung congestion
    b. Cardiac failure
    c. Carbon monoxide poisoning
    d. In combination with anesthetics
    e. Newborn infants' breathing problems
    f. During and following operations, as a supportive measure
    g. To test for rate of cellular oxidation in basal metabolism test
E. Other uses of oxygen
  1. High-altitude aircraft
  2. Space capsules
  3. Oxyacetylene torches for welding
  4. Bleaching
  5. Antiseptic action
F. Preparation of oxygen
  1. Natural—green plants form oxygen as a product of photosynthesis
  2. Commercial
    a. Fractional distillation of liquid air
    b. Electrolysis of water
  3. Laboratory—heating an oxide to decompose it; example: potassium chlorate ($KClO_3$) with manganese dioxide as a catalyst decomposes to potassium chloride (KCl) and oxygen
G. Forms of oxygen
  1. Free
    a. Usually oxygen is found as a diatomic molecule (O_2), as is common to most gases
    b. Occasionally a triatomic molecule of oxygen (O_3) occurs; this is called *ozone* and represents an especially active form of oxygen
  2. Combined—oxygen forms many compounds called oxides

2. **Hydrogen**
A. Physical properties
  1. Odorless, tasteless, colorless gas
  2. Slightly soluble in water
  3. Lightest element
B. Chemical properties
  1. Is a member of Group IA or VIIA elements
  2. Has only 1 electron in its outer orbital—its only electron
  3. Usually loses this lone electron to become a positively charged ion (a metal) in chemical reaction
  4. Occasionally can gain an electron and become a negatively charged ion (a nonmetal) in chemical reaction
  5. By sharing its electron, can form covalent bond
  6. Burns with explosive force
  7. Does not support combustion
C. Importance of hydrogen
  1. Forms about 11% of water by weight, 66% by volume
  2. Is present in acids and in bases
  3. Is present in organic substances such as fuels and oils and other hydrocarbons
  4. Is present in foods and in cells of plants and animal tissues
  5. Uniting with nitrogen, hydrogen forms ammonia and amino acids (proteins)
  6. Acting as a reducing agent (opposite of oxidation), hydrogen removes oxygen from many oxides; example:

$$FeO \quad + \quad H_2 \quad \longrightarrow \quad Fe \quad + \quad H_2O$$

Iron oxide   Hydrogen   Iron   Water

  7. Added to liquid fat, hydrogen forms solid fat by process of hydrogenation
D. Preparation of hydrogen
  1. Naturally—in volcanic eruptions
  2. Commercially—electrolysis of water
  3. Laboratory
    a. Reaction of active metal with water

$$2Na \quad + \quad 2H_2O \quad \longrightarrow \quad H_2 \quad + \quad 2NaOH$$

Sodium   Water   Hydrogen   Sodium hydroxide

    b. Reaction of acids with metals

$$2HCl \quad + \quad Zn \quad \longrightarrow \quad H_2 \quad + \quad ZnCl_2$$

Hydrochloric acid   Zinc   Hydrogen   Zinc chloride

3. **Group IA—the alkali metals**

A. Sodium
  1. Important metal ion in plasma and intercellular fluids
  2. Basic forming element; forms antacid compounds
  3. With chlorine forms NaCl (table salt)
B. Potassium
  1. Important metal in body; found in intracellular areas
  2. Acts as a muscle relaxant
4. **Group IIA—the alkali earth metals**
A. Magnesium
  1. Forms part of the chlorophyll molecule
  2. Activator for many enzymes
  3. Present in bones
B. Calcium
  1. Needed for proper bone formation
  2. Activator for many enzymes
  3. Needed for lactation
  4. Essential for blood clotting
C. Strontium
  1. May substitute for calcium in body
  2. Radioactive isotope (strontium 90) can be a health hazard, forming pockets of radiation in tissues
D. Barium—used for outlining intestinal tract for x-ray studies
E. Radium—radiotherapy
5. **Group IIIA**
A. Boron—antiseptic, dentifrice, washing powders
B. Aluminum—alum, antacids, metal containers
6. **Group IVA**
A. Carbon—fuel (coal, coke), hydrocarbons, carbohydrates
B. Silicon—sandstone, sand, glass
C. Tin—tinfoil, dishes
D. Lead—piping, paint; some lead compounds poisonous
7. **Group V**
A. Nitrogen—forms 4/5 of air; found in amino acids and proteins
B. Phosphorus—bones and teeth
C. Arsenic—poison
  1. Used externally in medication
  2. Used to kill pests and vermin
8. **Group VI**
A. Oxygen—essential to life
B. Sulfur—vulcanizing rubber; local medication in skin diseases
9. **Group VIIA—the halogens**
A. Fluorine—to etch glass, to prevent tooth decay when added to water supply, etc.
B. Chlorine—bleach, poison gas, disinfectant, water purifier

C. Bromine—nerve medicine, photography
D. Iodine—local antiseptic, part of the thyroid hormone (thyroxine)
10. **Group IB**
A. Copper—wire, electric fixtures
B. Silver—filling for teeth, surgical mending of bone, photography
C. Gold—filling for teeth
11. **Inert gases**
A. Helium
  1. Lighter-than-air craft (will not burn)
  2. Used with oxygen in therapy for breathing difficulties
B. Neon—electric signs

OXIDATION-REDUCTION

1. **Uniting of oxygen with a substance results in oxidation**
2. **Uniting of hydrogen with a substance results in reduction**
3. **Basis of oxidation and reduction is transfer of electrons**
A. Removal of an electron from an atom of an element results in oxidation of that atom; example:

$$Na \quad - \quad 1e- \quad \longrightarrow \quad Na+$$

Sodium   Electron   Sodium
atom   ion

B. Addition of an electron to an atom of an element results in reduction of that element; example:

$$Cl_2 \quad + \quad 2e- \quad \longrightarrow \quad 2Cl-$$

Chlorine   Electrons   Chlorine ions

C. Substance that causes removal of an electron from an atom is called an *oxidizing agent*
D. Substance that adds an electron to an atom is called a *reducing agent*
E. Substances other than oxygen can act as oxidizing agents; example: chlorine—more effective than oxygen in removing electrons in many reactions
F. Substances other than hydrogen can act as reducing agents; examples: carbon and carbon monoxide
G. In an oxidation-reduction reaction, the oxidizing agent is itself reduced and the reducing agent is itself oxidized; example:

$$O_2 \quad + \quad 2H_2 \quad \longrightarrow \quad 2H_2O$$

Oxidizing   Reducing
agent   agent

The hydrogen becomes oxidized and the oxygen becomes reduced

4. **Oxidation-reduction reactions are important in body chemistry as a source of energy in the body through cellular oxidation of foods**
A. Oxygen is the usual oxidizing agent in cells
B. Some forms of life (anaerobes) can use substances other than oxygen for cellular oxidation

WATER

1. **A compound formed by chemical combination of oxygen and hydrogen**
A. Essential to life
B. Useful in many phases of living
C. Most abundant compound
2. **Physical properties**
A. Colorless, tasteless, odorless liquid
B. Exists chiefly as ice at low temperatures, liquid at moderate temperatures, and gas at elevated temperatures
   1. Water changes from liquid to solid at the *freezing point* (0° C. or 32° F.)
   2. Water changes from liquid to gas at the *boiling point* (100° C. or 212° F.)
   3. These transition points in the physical states of water are the basis of the centigrade and Fahrenheit temperature scales
   4. Conversion from one temperature scale to the other is accomplished by using formula:

$$1.8° \ C. = °F. - 32$$

3. **Chemical properties**
A. Water molecule is a *polar molecule*
   1. The water molecule has a special shape with a concentration of electrons in one area
   2. This gives the water molecule positive and negative poles; example:

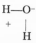

   3. Because of this molecular shape, water is an excellent solvent for ionic or slightly ionic substances
B. Water is a very stable compound; dissociates very slightly to H^+ and OH^- ions under normal conditions
C. Electrolysis can dissociate water into its components: hydrogen and oxygen
   1. Electrolysis gives 2 volumes of hydrogen for each volume of oxygen
   2. Electrolysis gives hydrogen and oxygen released from water in the ratio of 1 to 8 by weight
D. Many chemical reactions need water as a solvent before reaction will occur
E. Process of splitting a substance with the addition of water is called *hydrolysis*
F. Crystals formed including water in the molecule are called *hydrates*
   1. Water held in hydrates is called *the water of crystallization*
   2. When a hydrate loses the water of crystallization, it is called an *anhydride*
4. **Occurrence**
A. $5/7$ of earth is covered with water
B. Present in atmosphere, in crust of earth, in all plant and animal life
C. 68% of human body is water
D. All food and most materials used in everyday living contain some water
5. **Importance of water**
A. Necessary for life
B. Essential for many chemical reactions
C. Needed for digestion (hydrolysis) of food
D. Forms large percentage of plant and animal tissue
E. Necessary for circulation of blood; plasma a water solution
F. Necessary for elimination; urine, sweat, feces contain water
G. Lubricating fluid at joints (synovial fluid) contains water
6. **Evaporation—change of liquid water to water vapor**
Occurs at all temperatures but is rapid and complete at boiling point
7. **Solidification—change of liquid water to solid ice at freezing point**
A. Causes expansion; ice occupies larger volume than water that forms it
B. Freezing water can break pipes and vessels in which it is contained
C. Because of expansion, ice is lighter than water and floats on top of unfrozen water
8. **Amount of water vapor in the air is called the *humidity***
9. **Heat absorption**
A. Water has a great capacity for absorbing heat or giving off absorbed heat
B. Makes water (and ice) useful in ice packs, hydrotherapy, and hot compresses
10. **Water used as a standard**
A. Thermometer scales—the freezing and boiling points of water are used to standardize centigrade and Fahrenheit scales
B. Specific gravity—compares the density of

a volume of water to the density of the same volume of another substance
C. Weight—1 gm. the weight of 1 ml. of water at 4° C.
D. Calorie—(small calorie; cal.) the heat needed to raise 1 gm. of water 1° C.
E. pH—water acts as neutrality point on acid-base scale
11. Purifying water
A. Source of pure water necessary for health
B. Methods of purifying
  1. Filtration
  2. Chemical precipitation (aluminum sulfate)
  3. Chemical disinfection (chlorination)
  4. Boiling
  5. Distillation
  6. Ion exchange; resin filtration
12. Hard vs. soft water
A. Dissolved calcium or magnesium bicarbonates form "temporary" hard water; boiling or use of chemicals (washing soda) precipitates salts, leaving water "soft"
B. Dissolved calcium or magnesium sulfates form "permanently" hard water; chemical agents needed, to precipitate the salts
C. If unprecipitated, the dissolved salts react with soaps (but usually not with the newer detergents) and little lather can be obtained

IONIZATION

1. Ion
A. When an atom loses or gains an electron (electrons), it is no longer a neutral atom but a charged particle—an ion
B. The charge on this particle depends upon whether electrons are lost (+) or gained (−) and the number of electrons lost or gained
C. An electron is a negative particle; the loss of 1 electron makes ion positive (less negative) by 1; with loss of 2 electrons, ion is 2+, etc.
D. The gain of 1 electron makes ion negative by 1; with 2 electrons gained, the ion is 2−, etc.
2. Overall reaction
  In any chemical reaction the number of electrons lost by 1 atom is equal to gain by another atom; overall reaction neutral
3. Ionization and water
A. When certain compounds are placed in water, the polar water molecules dis-

sociate the molecules of the compound into ions—process is called ionization
B. A substance that will ionize when placed in water is called an electrolyte
C. A substance that will ionize in water (an electrolyte) will allow the passage of an electric current through its solution
D. Certain other compounds will dissolve in water but will not form ions
  1. These substances are called nonelectrolytes
  2. Their solutions will not allow the passage of an electric current
4. Acids, bases, and salts are electrolytes
A. They will ionize in water
B. Their water solutions will conduct an electric current
5. Electrolytes in water solutions are characterized by very rapid reactions—ions are free in solution to react
6. Factors that affect strength or weakness of an electrolyte
A. Amount of electrolyte present in solution
B. How well the electrolyte dissociates in solution—degree of ionization
  1. So-called "weak" electrolytes are substances that dissociate into ions to only a slight degree
  2. So-called "strong" electrolytes are substances that dissociate into ions to a larger degree

SOLUTIONS

1. Substances that dissolve in other substances form solutions
A. A solution can be classified as a homogeneous mixture
B. Solids, liquids, and gases can be dissolved in other solids, liquids, and gases
  1. Substance dissolved is called the *solute*
  2. Substance in which the solute is dissolved is called the *solvent*
  3. Common solution is one where a solid, liquid, or gas is dissolved in a liquid
2. Solubility is affected by various factors
A. Chemical and physical nature of the solvent
B. Chemical and physical nature of the solute
C. Amount of solvent vs. amount of solute
D. Temperature; warming aids some solutes (solids) to dissolve, cooling aids others (gases) to dissolve
E. Presence or absence of mixing; mixing usually speeds solution reaction

F. Pressure—especially when one of the components is a gas
3. **Water, having a polar molecule, acts as a solvent with many substances—especially with ionic compounds**
4. **Types of solutions**
A. Dilute—a small amount of solute in a relatively large amount of solvent
B. Concentrated—a large amount of solute in a relatively small amount of solvent
C. Unsaturated—a solution holding less solute than is possible for it to dissolve at a certain temperature and pressure
D. Saturated—a solution holding all the solute that it can dissolve at a certain temperature and pressure
E. Supersaturated solution—unique case of a solution holding more solute than it normally should for a particular temperature and pressure
 1. Very unstable condition
 2. Excess solute easily precipitates from solution
F. Percent solution—grams of solute per gram of solution; example: 10% sugar in water solution is 10 gm. of sugar in 100 gm. of sugar and water solution (10 gm. of sugar plus 90 gm. of water)
G. Molar solution—the number of gram-molecular weights of solute per liter of solution; symbol, M; example: 1M solution of NaCl is 58.5 (mol. wt.) gm. of NaCl in 1 liter of NaCl and water solution
H. Normal solution—the number of gram-equivalent weights of a solute per liter of solution; symbol, N
 1. An equivalent weight is that amount of a substance that is equivalent in chemical reactivity to 1 gram-atomic weight of hydrogen (a gram-atomic weight of hydrogen is 1.008 gm.)
 2. A gram-molecular weight of sulfuric acid (H_2SO_4) is 98.1 gm. and is equivalent to 2.016 gm. of hydrogen (2 atoms of hydrogen per molecule of H_2SO_4)
 3. An equivalent weight of sulfuric acid is

$$98.1 \times \frac{1.008}{2.016} \text{ or } 49.05 \text{ gm.}$$

 4. 49.05 gm. of sulfuric acid in 1 liter of sulfuric acid and water solution is a 1N solution of sulfuric acid
I. Molal solution—a gram-molecular weight of solute in 1,000 gm. of solvent
5. **Nonvolatile substances put into solution** These tend to raise the boiling point and lower the freezing point of the solvent in which they are dissolved; example: water and ethylene glycol (commercial antifreeze) freezes at a lower temperature and boils at a higher temperature than pure water
6. **Osmosis—process of selective diffusion**
A. More concentrated solution is separated from a less concentrated solution by a membrane that is permeable only to the solvent—*a semipermeable membrane*
B. Solvent moves more rapidly from the dilute solution into the concentrated solution than in the reverse direction
C. Pressure forcing the solvent across the membrane is called *osmotic pressure*

Cells stay normal size and shape

Cells shrivel and shrink

Cells swell and burst

Isotonic solution

Hypertonic solution

Hypotonic solution

FIG. 3-4

Effect of osmotic pressure of solutions upon cells placed in those solutions.

D. Isotonic solutions—when the osmotic pressures of 2 liquids are equal, the flow of solvent is equalized and the 2 solutions are said to be *isotonic* to each other
   1. Physiologic saline—0.89% NaCl in distilled water—is isotonic to blood and body tissues
   2. 5% dextrose in water is isotonic to blood and body tissues
   3. When isotonic solutions are administered intravenously, the blood cells remain intact

E. Hypertonic solutions—when 1 solution has less osmotic pressure (is more concentrated) than another, it draws fluid from the other and is said to be *hypertonic* to it

F. Hypotonic solutions—when 1 solution has more osmotic pressure (is more dilute) than another, it forces fluid into the other and is said to be *hypotonic* to it

G. Both hypertonic and hypotonic types of solution are destructive to body cells; they should not be used in intravenous injections (Fig. 3-4)

7. **Size of the particle of solute determines what type of solution exists**

A. Atomic, ionic, and most molecular-sized particles are extremely small particles—submicroscopic
   1. Particles are freely dispersed by solvent
   2. Particles are kept in solution by movement and attraction of solvent molecules
   3. Substances of this class are called *crystalloids*
   4. Crystalloids form true solutions
      a. Clear in appearance—particles cannot be seen
      b. Solute stays in solution as long as the solvent is not removed by evaporation or other means
      c. Solute accompanies solvent as it passes through filters and most membranes

B. Large particles of matter do not form solutions in the real sense of the term
   1. Solute particles easily settle out of solvent
   2. Solute particles can be seen by naked eye or with microscope, when suspended in solvent
   3. Solute can be removed by ordinary filtration
   4. Substances of this class are called coarse suspensions

C. The colloid particle
   1. Intermediate in size between the crystalloid and the coarse suspensoid
   2. Particle size much larger than that of crystalloid although smaller than particle of coarse suspensoid; diameter size of colloid around 0.0000001 to 0.00001 mm.
   3. Solutions of colloids
      a. Solute particles dispersed by solvent
      b. Solution—clear, cloudy, or opalescent
      c. Show bright path of reflected light when a beam of light is passed through solution—the Tyndall effect
      d. More stable than coarse suspensoids, less stable than true solutions
      e. With time, the colloid particles will settle out
      f. Affect osmotic pressure less than crystalloids
   4. Colloid particles will pass through ordinary filters, will be held back by most membranes
   5. Colloid particles carry electric charges on their surfaces—not to be confused with ionic charges
      a. Charges sometimes help keep particles in solution
      b. Colloid particles having charges that attract the solvent are called *lyophilic* (solvent-loving) colloids
      c. Colloid particles having charges that repel the solvent are called *lyophobic* (solvent-hating) colloids
      d. Lyophilic colloids form more stable solutions than do lyophobic colloids
      e. Lyophobic colloids easily separate out of solution
      f. Lyophobic colloid can be made to stay in solution by coating its particles with a layer of lyophilic colloid
      g. The stabilizing lyophilic colloid is called an *emulsifying agent*; the stabilized lyophobic colloid is said to have been *emulsified*; example:

      Oil and water make lyophobic colloid solution (separate easily)
      Oil, water, and soap—an emulsified solution, with the soap (lyophilic colloid) coating the oil (lyophobic colloid) and holding it in solution

6. Importance of colloid suspensions
   a. Proteins, fats, and many carbohydrates form molecules in the colloid range in size
   b. These form colloid solutions in the cells and body fluids
   c. Protoplasm of cell itself is a colloid
   d. Colloid chemistry is the chemistry of life
7. Sol-gel equilibrium
   a. Most colloids can exist in 2 forms, a sol and a gel
   b. Sol—a solution where the solid particles are suspended in a liquid
   c. Gel—a solution where the liquid particles are suspended in the solid medium
   d. Most of the physical and chemical characteristics of protoplasm can be explained by the equilibrium that exists between the sol and gel states

BASES, ACIDS, AND SALTS

1. Elements of the periodic table

A. Roughly divided into metals and non-metals
B. When a metal reacts with oxygen, it forms a metal oxide (basic anhydride); example:

$$2Ca + O_2 \longrightarrow 2CaO$$

1. A metal oxide placed in water forms a base; example:

$$CaO + H_2O \longrightarrow Ca(OH)_2$$

2. A base is a substance that usually adds an OH^- (hydroxyl) ion to any solution in which it is placed; example:

$$Ca(OH)_2 + Water \longrightarrow Ca^{++} + 2OH^-$$
$$(\text{in water solution})$$

C. Properties of a base
1. Bitter taste
2. Slippery feeling to touch
3. Electrolyte in water
4. Reacts with indicators, giving basic color
   a. Methyl orange—yellow
   b. Litmus—blue
   c. Phenolphthalein—red
5. Reacts with acids to form water and a salt (neutralization)
6. Reacts with certain metals to release hydrogen gas

7. Combines with organic acids (fatty acids) to form soaps
8. In high concentration destroys organic material; corrosive

D. Names and formulas of common bases —name usually formed by adding the word hydroxide to the name of the positive ion (metal or ammonium ion) forming the base
1. Calcium hydroxide ($Ca(OH)_2$)—water solution—called *lime water*
2. Sodium hydroxide ($NaOH$)—caustic soda
3. Potassium hydroxide (KOH)—soap making
4. Ammonium hydroxide (NH_4OH)—household cleaner
5. Magnesium hydroxide ($Mg(OH)_2$)—water solution marketed under trade name Milk of Magnesia—antacid, mild laxative
6. Aluminum hydroxide ($Al(OH)_3$)—component of antacid pills

2. When a nonmetal reacts with oxygen, it forms a nonmetal oxide (acid anhydride)
Example:

$$C + O_2 \longrightarrow CO_2$$

A. A nonmetal oxide placed in water forms an acid; example:

$$CO_2 + H_2O \longrightarrow H_2CO_3$$

B. An acid is ordinarily thought of as a substance that liberates an H^+ (hydrogen ion) to a solution in which it is placed; example:

$$H_2CO_3 + Water \longrightarrow H^+ + HCO_3^-$$
$$(\text{in water solution})$$

C. The hydrogen ion thus released does not remain alone but associates itself with some other particle, usually a water molecule; example:

$$H^+ + H_2O \longrightarrow H_3O^+ \ (\textit{hydronium} \text{ ion})$$

D. Properties of an acid
1. Sour taste
2. Reacts with indicators, giving an acid color
   a. Methyl orange—red
   b. Litmus—red
   c. Phenolphthalein—colorless
3. Combines with certain metals, releasing hydrogen gas
4. Reacts with bases to form water and a salt (neutralization)

5. Reacts with carbonates to give carbon dioxide gas
6. Acts as an electrolyte in water
7. In high concentration destroys organic materials—corrosive

E. Naming acids (Table 3-2)
1. An acid formed from hydrogen and a nonmetal is called a *binary* acid; name begins with "hydro" and ends in "ic"; example:

$$HCl—hydrochloric\ acid$$

2. Acids containing oxygen as well as hydrogen and the nonmetal are called *ternary* or *oxy* acids, are named for the nonmetal, and have the ending "ous" or "ic," showing less or greater concentration of oxygen; examples:

$$HClO_2—chlorous\ acid$$
$$HClO_3—chloric\ acid$$

3. An even smaller concentration of oxygen is indicated by the suffix "hypo," while an even greater concentration of oxygen is indicated by the suffix "per"; examples:

$$HClO—hypochlorous\ acid$$
$$HClO_4—perchloric\ acid$$

F. Names and formulas of common acids
1. Hydrochloric acid (HCl)—found in stomach, aids in digestion
2. Nitric acid (HNO_3)—used in test for proteins
3. Sulfuric acid (H_2SO_4)—in storage batteries
4. Carbonic acid (H_2CO_3)—one form in which carbon dioxide is transported in the blood
5. Boric acid (H_3BO_3)—mild antiseptic
6. Acetic acid ($C_2H_3O_2H$)—vinegar
7. Lactic acid ($C_3H_5O_3H$)—cause of muscle fatigue

3. **Strength or weakness of acids and bases depends on amount of ionization of the acid or base**
A. Poorly ionized acid is weak acid—less H^+
B. Poorly ionized base is weak base—less OH^-
C. Highly ionized acid is strong acid—more H^+
D. Highly ionized base is strong base—more OH^-

4. **For acid and base burns, flood with water and add the opposite weak chemical in diluted form**

A. Diluted weak acid on base burns
B. Diluted weak base on acid burns
5. **The compound (besides water) formed when an acid is neutralized by a base is a salt:**

$$HCl + KOH \longrightarrow H_2O + KCl$$

Acid   Base   Water   Salt

A. Properties of a salt
1. Crystalline in nature
2. Ionic even in the dry crystal
3. Electrolyte in solution
4. "Salty" taste
B. Reactions of salts
1. In water solution, salts may be acid, basic, or neutral
   a. The salt formed by the reaction between an acid and a base of equal degrees of ionization is usually neutral in solution; example:

$$HCl + NaOH \longrightarrow H_2O + NaCl$$

Highly   Highly   Water   Neutral salt
ionized   ionized   (sodium
acid   base   chloride)

   b. The salt formed by the reaction between a highly ionized acid and a poorly ionized base is an acid salt in solution; example:

$$HCl + NH_4OH \longrightarrow H_2O + NH_4Cl$$

Highly   Poorly   Water   Acid salt
ionized   ionized   (ammonium
acid   base   chloride)

   c. The salt formed by the reaction between a poorly ionized acid and a highly ionized base is a basic salt in solution; example:

$$H_2CO_3 + NaOH \longrightarrow H_2O + NaHCO_3$$

Poorly   Highly   Water   Basic salt
ionized   ionized   (sodium
acid   base   bicarbonate)

2. Salts can react chemically with acids, bases, and other salts to form new compounds
C. Naming salts (Table 3-2)
1. Binary salts—salts that contain 2 elements derive their names from the metal or ammonium ion of the base and the nonmetal of the acid that reacted to form them, with the ending of "ide"; example:

$$NaOH + HCl \longrightarrow H_2O + NaCl$$

Sodium   Hydro-   Water   Sodium
hydroxide   chloric   chlor*ide*
            acid

TABLE 3-2
NAMING OF ACIDS AND SALTS

	Formula of acid	Name of acid		Formula of corresponding salt	Name of salt
Binary acids	H_2S	Hydrosulfuric	Binary salts	Na_2S	Sodium sulfide
	HBr	Hydrobromic		NaBr	Sodium bromide
	HCl	Hydrochloric		NaCl	Sodium chloride
Ternary acids	HClO	Hypochlorous	Ternary salts	NaClO	Sodium hypochloride
	$HClO_2$	Chlorous		$NaClO_2$	Sodium chlorite
	$HClO_3$	Chloric		$NaClO_3$	Sodium chlorate
	$HClO_4$	Perchloric		$NaClO_4$	Sodium perchlorate
	$H_2N_2O_2$	Hyponitrous		$Na_2N_2O_2$	Sodium hyponitrite
	HNO_2	Nitrous		$NaNO_2$	Sodium nitrite
	HNO_3	Nitric (common)		$NaNO_3$	Sodium nitrate
	H_2SO_3	Sulfurous		Na_2SO_3	Sodium sulfite
	H_2SO_4	Sulfuric (common)		Na_2SO_4	Sodium sulfate
	$H_2S_2O_8$	Persulfuric		$Na_2S_2O_8$	Sodium persulfate

2. If the metal ion has more than 1 valence, the valence is indicated by a Roman numeral inserted in the name of the salt; example: iron has 2 valences—Fe^{++} and Fe^{+++}—and forms 2 salts with chlorine:

$FeCl_2$—iron (II) chloride (older name, ferrous chloride)
$FeCl_3$—iron (III) chloride (older name, ferric chloride)

3. An acid with 2 or more replaceable hydrogens forms a series of salts; incomplete replacement for the hydrogen leads to a "bi," "acid," or "hydrogen" salt; example:

H_2CO_3 +   NaOH $\longrightarrow$ H_2O + $NaHCO_3$

Carbonic   Sodium   Water   Sodium
acid   hydroxide   bicar-
                                    bonate
                                    Sodium
                                    acid car-
                                    bonate
                                    Sodium
                                    hydrogen
                                    carbonate

4. The oxygen-containing acids form a series of salts; the name of the salt with the lower oxygen content ends in "ite" while the name of the salt with the higher oxygen content ends in "ate"; example:

$AlPO_3$—aluminum phosphite
$AlPO_4$—aluminum phosphate

D. Important salts (Table 3-2)
 1. Sodium chloride (NaCl)—salt of intercellular and extracellular spaces

 2. Calcium phosphate ($CaPO_4$)—bone and tooth formation
 3. Potassium chloride (KCl)—salt of intracellular spaces
 4. Calcium carbonate ($CaCO_3$)—limestone
 5. Barium sulfate ($BaSO_4$)—when taken internally, outlines internal structures for x-ray studies
 6. Silver nitrate ($AgNO_3$)—antiseptic, photographic work
 7. Iron (II) sulfate ($FeSO_4$)—treatment of anemia
 8. Sodium bicarbonate ($NaHCO_3$)—antacid
 9. Calcium sulfate ($CaSO_4$)—hydrated form is plaster of Paris (casts for broken bones)
 10. Magnesium sulfate ($MgSO_4$)—Epsom salt

6. pH—Symbol of hydrogen ion concentration
A. A neutral solution has the same amount of acid reacting ions (H_3O^+) as basic reacting ions (OH^-)
B. An acid reacting solution has more H_3O^+ than OH^-
C. A basic reacting solution has more OH^- than H_3O^+
D. pH is used to represent these conditions
 1. The pH of a solution is defined as the logarithm of 1 divided by the concentration of H_3O^+:

$$\log \frac{1}{[H_3O^+]}$$

 2. A neutral solution has a pH of 7.00

3. An acid solution would have a pH in the range from 0 to 7.00; the lower the pH, the more acid the solution
4. A basic solution would have a pH in the range from 7.00 to 14.00; the higher the pH, the more basic the solution
5. Normal blood has a pH of 7.35 to 7.45
6. Many body fluids have varying pH ranges—gastric juice is acid, bile is basic, etc.

7. **Buffers**
A. A poorly ionized acid or base, plus a salt formed from that acid or base, acts as a buffer in solution
B. A buffer allows the addition of acid ions (H_3O^+) and basic ions (OH^-) without a change occurring in the pH of the solution to which the addition is made
C. A typical buffer of the blood is carbonic acid (H_2CO_3) plus its salt, sodium bicarbonate ($NaHCO_3$)
D. Many medications are buffered before administration; example: protamine zinc insulin

RADIOACTIVITY

1. **Certain elements (such as radium) have atoms whose nuclei are naturally unstable**
A. The nuclei of these atoms are constantly breaking down at a set rate
B. In the breakdown process these elements emit high-energy particles and rays that can penetrate other materials—radioactive rays
1. Alpha particle—fast-moving helium nucleus
a. Weight, 4 a.w.u. (atomic weight unit)
b. Charge, 2^+
c. Penetration, slight
2. Beta particle—fast-moving electron
a. Weight, practically 0 a.w.u.
b. Charge, 1^-
c. Penetration, moderate
3. Gamma ray—pentrating ray, similar to light ray
a. Weight, none
b. Charge, none
c. Highly penetrating
C. We have recently learned to use these radioactive elements; examples: radium treatment of cancer; radioactive bomb for defense

D. Measurement of radioactivity
1. The roentgen—1.6×10^{12} ion pairs/gm. of air (radioactive rays ionize gases)
2. The curie—37,000,000,000 nuclear disintegrations/sec.
3. The millicurie—0.001 of a curie
4. The microcurie—0.000001 of a curie
E. Certain radioactive materials take a long time to disintegrate; others take less than a second
1. The time during which one half of a certain radioactive material disintegrates is called its *half-life*
2. Determining the half-life of a radioactive element is used in dating fossils and telling the age of antiques
3. Short half-life elements are used on humans in medicine to cut down on the amount of exposure to radiation

2. **Radioactive isotopes**
A. In a certain element, 1 isotope may be nonradioactive and others be radioactive; example: the cobalt isotope Co^{59}, atomic weight 59 a.w.u., is nonradioactive but the cobalt isotope Co^{60}, atomic weight 60 a.w.u., is radioactive
B. Stable nuclei of nonradioactive elements can be made radioactive through bombardment by subatomic particles

3. **Uses of radioactivity in medicine**
A. Radium treatments for malignancy
B. Co^{60}—total body radiation for malignancy
C. Studies on body fluids, using radioactive isotope of sodium (Na^{24})
D. Leukemia, polycythemia, and bone cancer treatments with radioactive phosphorus (P^{32})
E. Tracing metabolic pathways of food and drugs by means of radioactive carbon (C^{14})
F. Studies on red cells (erythrocytes) and hemoglobin formation with radioactive iron (Fe^{59}) and radioactive chromium (Cr^{51})

4. **Protection from radiation**
A. Radiation danger decreases as distance from radioactive material increases
B. Heavy materials, can shield from radioactive rays; examples: lead, concrete
C. Radiation hazard increases with increase in time of exposure

5. **Nuclear fusion—lighter atoms can be made to combine to form heavier atoms under extreme physical conditions**

A. This releases great energy

B. It is thought that the sun's heat and light are caused by fusion of hydrogen atoms forming helium atoms; example:

$$4H_2 \longrightarrow 2He + 2 \text{ positrons}$$

C. Explosive power of the hydrogen bomb is related to this theory

ORGANIC CHEMISTRY

1. **Study of the carbon compounds**

A. Compounds thought at one time to be formed only by living organisms—thus "organic"

B. Carbon combines covalently with many other elements and with itself

C. Carbon forms a vast array of compounds

   1. Open straight chains; example:

Hexane

   2. Open branched chains; example:

Isopentane

   3. Ring or cyclic structures; example:

Cyclohexane

D. Carbon compounds exist as isomers—compounds containing the same number and kinds of atoms but differing in structure and in physical and chemical properties

Butane (normal butane)   Isobutane

2. **Hydrocarbons — compounds containing chiefly carbon and hydrogen**

A. Organic compounds form families of compounds, the larger differing from the next smaller by the addition of a definite number of carbon and hydrogen atoms

   1. These families of compounds are called "homologous" series

   2. They are classically named for the smallest member of the group

B. Saturated hydrocarbons

   1. If all of the bonds of carbon (4) are attached to other carbons, hydrogen, or other elements, we call this compound *saturated;* example:

   2. Saturated hydrocarbons are relatively unreactive and chemically stable

   3. Homologous series of saturated hydrocarbons—called the *paraffin, alkane* or *methane* series

      a. First member of the family is methane, CH_4

      b. Second member is ethane, C_2H_6

      c. Third member is propane, C_3H_8

      d. The difference between members is CH_2

      e. Higher members of the series can be formed by inserting a carbon and 2 hydrogen atoms into the chain of the next lowest paraffin

      f. The general formula for a paraffin is C_nH_{2n+2} where n is any positive number but zero

      g. Paraffins having chain lengths of C_1 to C_5 are gases at room temperature

      h. Paraffins having chain lengths of C_5 to C_{20} are liquids at room temperature

      i. Paraffins of longer chain length are solids at room temperature

   4. There are saturated hydrocarbons that do not fall into the general formula for a paraffin; these are cyclic hydrocarbons and form a series called *cycloparaffins;* example:

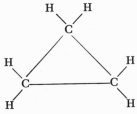

Cyclopropane (C_3H_6)
(an anesthetic)

C. Unsaturated hydrocarbons
1. When a hydrocarbon exists that does not have all of its carbon bonds attached to another carbon, a hydrogen, or another atom, the compound is called *unsaturated;* example:

$$H-\overset{|}{\underset{H}{C}}-\overset{|}{\underset{H}{C}}-H \quad or \quad H-\overset{|}{\underset{|}{C}}-\overset{|}{\underset{|}{C}}-H$$

2. Bonds that are unattached tend to combine with each other and form double or triple bonds; example:

$$H-\overset{|}{\underset{H}{C}}=\overset{|}{\underset{H}{C}}-H$$

Ethylene (C_2H_4)

$$H-C\equiv C-H$$

Acetylene (C_2H_2)

3. This forms 2 more homologous series:
   a. Double-bonded compounds form the *alkane, olefin,* or *ethylene* series; the general formula for olefins is C_nH_{2n}
   b. Triple-bonded compounds form the *alkyne* or *acetylene* series; the general formula for acetylenes is C_nH_{2n-2}
4. Unsaturated hydrocarbons are less stable and more chemically reactive than the saturated hydrocarbons; double and triple bonds tend to break and add in other atoms, becoming saturated
5. Unsaturated cyclic hydrocarbons
   a. Compound in which 6 carbons form a ring or cyclic shape and are surrounded by 6 hydrogen atoms is called benzene, C_6H_6
   b. Although highly unsaturated, benzene is not as reactive as would be expected
   c. The bonding in benzene gives stability to the double bonds
   d. Benzene is toxic, taken internally; prolonged breathing of fumes results in depression of blood-forming organs
   e. Benzene is useful as a fat solvent —used in the manufacturing of resins, paints, rubber
   f. Benzene is the first member of the *aromatic* series; other members are listed below
      (1) Naphthalene — moth-repellent and useful in the manufacture of resins, dyes, and plastics
      (2) Anthracene—used in the manufacture of dyes
      (3) Phenanthrene—basis for the biologic synthesis of sterols, steroid hormones, vitamins

3. **Functional groups**
A. If a hydrocarbon is treated with a halogen, 1 or more of the hydrogen atoms may be replaced—called *substitution;* example:

$$CH_4 \quad + \quad Cl_2 \quad \longrightarrow \quad CH_3Cl_4 \quad + \quad HCl$$
Methane   Chlorine   Chloroform   Hydro-
chloric
acid

B. Halogenated hydrocarbon is called an *alkyl halide*
C. Substituting halogen is called a *functional group*
D. Symbol "R" stands for a hydrocarbon residue
E. An R group can be any number of carbons in a straight chain, a branched chain, a ring form, or any combination of chain and ring groups
   1. Methyl group ($-CH_3$)
   2. Ethyl group ($-C_2H_5$)
   3. Propyl group ($-C_3H_7$)
   4. Phenyl group ($-C_6H_5$)—Ar used for R in this case
   5. Benzyl group ($-C_7H_7$)
F. Addition of a functional group to an R or Ar residue can make a vast number of important compounds (Table 3-3)
4. **Alkyl halides (R—X) have many uses**
A. Methyl chloride (CH_3Cl)—local anesthetic
B. Chloroform ($CHCl_3$)—general anesthetic
C. Carbon tetrachloride (CCl_4)—fat solvent
D. Ethyl chloride (C_2H_5Cl)—local anesthetic
E. Iodoform (CHI_3)—antiseptic
F. Ethylene dibromide ($C_2H_4Br_2$)—addition to gasoline

TABLE 3-3
ORGANIC DERIVATIVES AND GENERAL FORMULAS*

Functional group	Type of compound	General formula
—X (where X is F, Cl, Br, or I)	Alkyl halide	R—X
—OH	Alcohol	R—OH
$\overset{\displaystyle O}{\underset{\displaystyle }{—C—H}}$	Aldehyde	$\overset{\displaystyle O}{\underset{\displaystyle }{R—C—H}}$
$\overset{\displaystyle O}{\underset{\displaystyle }{—C—}}$	Ketone	$\overset{\displaystyle O}{\underset{\displaystyle }{R—C—R}}$
$\overset{\displaystyle O}{\underset{\displaystyle }{—C—OH}}$	Acid	$\overset{\displaystyle O}{\underset{\displaystyle }{R—C—OH}}$
$\overset{\displaystyle O}{\underset{\displaystyle }{—C—O—Y}}$ (where Y is a metal or ammonium ion)	Organic salt	$\overset{\displaystyle O}{\underset{\displaystyle }{R—C—O—Y}}$
$\overset{\displaystyle O}{\underset{\displaystyle }{—C—O—}}$	Ester	$\overset{\displaystyle O}{\underset{\displaystyle }{R—C—O—R'}}$
—O—	Ether	R—O—R'
—NH₂	Amine	R—NH₂
—SH	Thiol(mercaptan)	R—SH
—SO₃H	Sulfonic acid	R—SO₃H
—CN	Nitrile	R—CN
—NO₂	Nitro compound	R—NO₂

*R stands for a hydrocarbon residue; R' stands for a hydrocarbon residue, which may or may not be the same as R. (Ar is used in place of R when C_6H_5—needs to be indicated.)

G. Chlorobenzene (C_6H_5Cl)—preparation of phenol
5. **Alcohols (R—OH)**
A. Classification
  1. Primary alcohol—the functional group (—OH) on the end of a carbon chain; example:

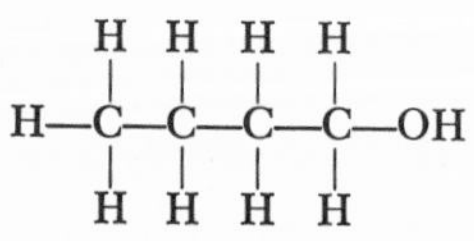

  H—C—C—C—C—OH (with H's)

  Primary butyl alcohol

  2. Secondary alcohol—the functional group (—OH) somewhere along the carbon chain, not at end; example:

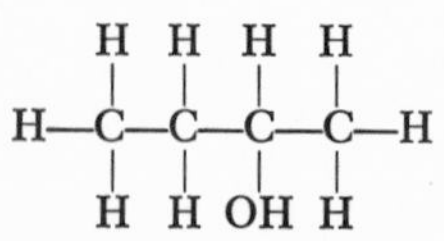

  Secondary butyl alcohol

  3. Tertiary alcohol—the functional group (—OH) on a carbon that also holds a branch chain; example·

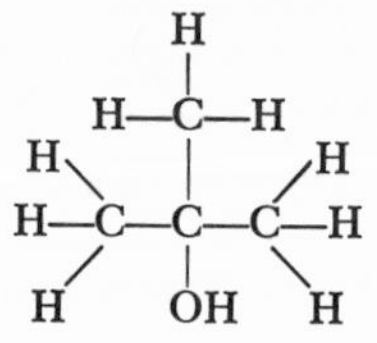

  Tertiary butyl alcohol

B. Reactions of alcohols
  1. Neutral in solution—neither acid nor base
  2. Intense oxidation causes alcohol to burn, as in alcohol lamps; example:

  $C_2H_5OH + 3O_2 \longrightarrow 2CO_2 + 3H_2O + Heat + Light$
  Ethyl alcohol

  3. Careful oxidation of primary alcohols

forms first aldehydes and then organic acids; example:

$$2CH_3CH_2OH + O_2 \longrightarrow$$

Ethyl alcohol   Oxygen

$$2CH_3\overset{\displaystyle O}{\overset{\|}{C}}—H + O_2 \longrightarrow$$

Acetaldehyde   Oxygen
and
H_2O

$$CH_3\overset{\displaystyle O}{\overset{\|}{C}}—OH$$

Acetic acid

4. Careful oxidation of secondary alcohols forms ketones; example:

$$2H—\overset{\displaystyle H}{\underset{\displaystyle H}{C}}—\overset{\displaystyle OH}{\underset{\displaystyle H}{C}}—\overset{\displaystyle H}{\underset{\displaystyle H}{C}}—H + O_2 \longrightarrow$$

Secondary
propyl
alcohol

$$2H—\overset{\displaystyle H}{\underset{\displaystyle H}{C}}—\overset{\displaystyle O}{\overset{\|}{C}}—\overset{\displaystyle H}{\underset{\displaystyle H}{C}}—H + 2H_2O$$

Acetone
(a ketone)

5. Alcohols react with inorganic acids to form alkyl halides or inorganic esters; example:

$$CH_3CH_2OH + HCl \longrightarrow CH_3CH_2Cl + H_2O$$

Ethyl alcohol   Ethyl
chloride

$$CH_3CH_2OH + HNO_2 \longrightarrow CH_3CH_2NO_2 + H_2O$$

Ethyl alcohol   Ethyl nitrite
(sweet spirits
of niter)

6. Alcohols react with organic acids to form esters; example:

$$CH_3CH_2OH + CH_3\overset{\displaystyle O}{\overset{\|}{C}}—OH \longrightarrow$$

Ethyl alcohol   Acetic acid

$$CH_3\overset{\displaystyle O}{\overset{\|}{C}}—O—CH_2CH_3 + H_2O$$

Ethyl acetate
(an ester)

C. Important alcohols
  1. Methyl alcohol—wood alcohol (CH_3 OH)—used as a solvent; poison if taken internally
  2. Ethyl alcohol—grain alcohol (CH_3CH_2OH)—used as a solvent for medications, as an antiseptic and rubbing compound; not poisonous; used as a beverage in social situations; large quantities taken internally cause the depression and confusion classified as "drunkenness"
  3. Propyl alcohol (C_3H_7OH)—used as a rubbing compound, industrial solvent, antiseptic
  4. Benzyl alcohol—local anesthetic; basis for the synthesis of ephedrine and the hormone epinephrine
  5. Glycerol—trihydric alcohol used in skin creams and as a solvent; nitrated form used in explosives; basis for synthesis of fats

$$\begin{array}{c} H \\ | \\ H—C—OH \\ | \\ H—C—OH \\ | \\ H—C—OH \\ | \\ H \end{array}$$

D. When an —OH (hydroxyl) group is attached directly to a benzene ring, a *phenol* is formed; example:

$$\begin{array}{c} H \\ | \\ C \\ \diagup \diagdown \\ H—C \quad C—OH \\ | \quad\quad | \\ H—C \quad C—H \\ \diagdown \diagup \\ C \\ | \\ H \end{array}$$

1. A phenol does not react as an alcohol, nor as a base, but as an acid; the H of the OH group ionizes and forms the hydronium ion in solution
2. As an acid, a phenol will react with bases to form an organic salt
3. Like any organic acid, phenols will undergo oxidation, reduction, substitutions; can react with other compounds to form esters and ethers
4. Important phenols
  a. Phenol (carbolic acid)—used as disinfectant, antiseptic, poison
  b. Cresol (Lysol)—disinfectant
  c. Resorcinol—antiseptic

6. **Aldehydes** $(R-\overset{\overset{\displaystyle O}{\|}}{C}-H)$—**formed by mild oxidation of primary alcohols**
A. Reactions of aldehydes
   1. Mild oxidation of aldehyde forms organic acid; example:

$$2R-\overset{\overset{\displaystyle O}{\|}}{C}-H + O_2 \longrightarrow 2R-\overset{\overset{\displaystyle O}{\|}}{C}-OH + 2H_2O$$

   2. Alkaline copper reagents cause this oxidation to occur—the basis of Benedict's (Fehling's, Clinitest) tests for aldehyde sugars; example:

$$2Cu(OH)_2 \quad + \quad R-\overset{\overset{\displaystyle O}{\|}}{C}-H \longrightarrow$$

   Copper (II)   Aldehyde
   hydroxide
   (blue)

$$Cu_2O \quad + \quad R-\overset{\overset{\displaystyle O}{\|}}{C}-OH \quad + \quad 2H_2O$$

   Copper (I)   Acid
   oxide
   (orange)

   3. Condensation (polymerization)—aldehydes will join with themselves and other aldehydes to form large aggregates
   4. Reduction forms a primary alcohol; example:

$$R-\overset{\overset{\displaystyle O}{\|}}{C}-H + H_2 \longrightarrow R-CH_2OH$$

   Aldehyde   Primary alcohol

B. Important aldehydes
   1. Formaldehyde $(H-\overset{\overset{\displaystyle O}{\|}}{C}-H)$—acrid-smelling gas; water solution of formaldehyde is called *formalin;* useful as an insecticide, fumigating agent, antiseptic, and disinfectant; also for fixing tissues for histologic examination
   2. Acetaldehyde $(CH-\overset{\overset{\displaystyle O}{\|}}{C}-H)$ — liquid with a sharp odor; polymerizes to paraldehyde; fumigation; forms chloral hydrate, a sedative and hypnotic; is used in manufacture of DDT, an insecticide
   3. Benzaldehyde—used for manufacture of drugs, dyes, perfumes
   4. Cinnamic aldehyde—active ingredient of oil of cinnamon
   5. Vanillin—active ingredient in vanilla extract

7. **Ketones** $(R-\overset{\overset{\displaystyle O}{\|}}{C}-R')$
A. Reactions of ketones
   1. Ketones are formed by the mild oxidation of secondary alcohols

   2. Reduction of ketones forms secondary alcohols

   3. Ketones are relatively unreactive
B. Some important ketones
   1. Acetone—solvent for paints and varnish; one end product of fat metabolism

   2. Dihydroxyacetone—intermediate product of carbohydrate metabolism

   3. Methyl ethyl ketone—solvent
   4. Benzophenone—perfumes, soaps, cosmetics
   5. Acetophenone—perfumes, soaps, cosmetics

8. **Organic (carboxylic)** $(R-\overset{O}{\underset{\|}{C}}-O-H)$

A. Reactions of organic acids

1. Organic acids are formed by mild oxidation of primary alcohols and aldehydes
2. Reduction of organic acids forms first aldehydes and then primary alcohols
3. The functional group is the carboxyl group

$$-\overset{O}{\underset{\|}{C}}-O-H$$

4. All organic acids ionize slightly (weak acids) to form hydronium ions (H_3O^+) in water solution
5. Formation of acyl halides by reacting with thionyl halides; example:

$$R-\overset{O}{\underset{\|}{C}}-O-H + SOX_2 \longrightarrow$$

Organic acid | Thionyl halide

$$R-\overset{O}{\underset{\|}{C}}-X \quad + \quad HX \quad + \quad SO_2$$

Acyl halide | Halide acid | Sulfur dioxide

$$CH_3-\overset{O}{\underset{\|}{C}}-O-H + SOCl_2 \longrightarrow$$

Acetic acid | Thionyl chloride

$$CH_3-\overset{O}{\underset{\|}{C}}-Cl \quad + \quad HCl \quad + \quad SO_2$$

Acetyl chloride | Hydrochloric acid | Sulfur dioxide

6. Formation of organic salts by reacting with a base

$$R-\overset{O}{\underset{\|}{C}}-O-H + NaOH \longrightarrow$$

Organic acid | Base

$$R-\overset{O}{\underset{\|}{C}}-O-Na + H_2O$$

Organic salt

$$CH_3-\overset{O}{\underset{\|}{C}}-O-H + NaOH \longrightarrow$$

Acetic acid | Sodium hydroxide

$$CH_3-\overset{O}{\underset{\|}{C}}-O-Na + H_2O$$

Sodium acetate

7. Important organic salts
   a. Lead acetate—making lead pigments, treating poison ivy dermatitis
   b. Sodium acetate—component of a well-known buffer
   c. Copper acetate—insecticide (Paris green)
   d. Aluminum acetate—dye making
   e. Calcium propionate—mold inhibitor in baked goods
   f. Calcium lactate—calcium therapy
   g. Ferric ammonium citrate—iron therapy
   h. Sodium citrate—anticoagulant in blood for transfusions
   i. Sodium oxalate—anticoagulant in blood for laboratory examinations
   j. Sodium benzoate—mold inhibitor for food
   k. Sodium salicylate—antipyretic, analgesic agent
8. Organic acids will react with alcohols to form *esters* and water

$$R'-\overset{O}{\underset{\|}{C}}-O-H + ROH \longrightarrow R'-\overset{O}{\underset{\|}{C}}-O-R + H_2O$$

$$CH_3-\overset{O}{\underset{\|}{C}}-O-H + CH_3OH \longrightarrow$$

Acetic acid | Methyl alcohol

$$CH_3-\overset{O}{\underset{\|}{C}}-O-CH_3 + H_2O$$

Methyl acetate (an ester)

B. Important organic acids

1. Formic acid $(H-\overset{O}{\underset{\|}{C}}-O-H)$—found in insect sting venom
2. Acetic acid $(CH_3-\overset{O}{\underset{\|}{C}}-O-H)$—acid of vinegar, used in manufacture of cellulose acetate
3. Lactic acid $(CH_3CH-\overset{O}{\underset{\|}{C}}-O-H)-$
   $\underset{H}{\overset{|}{O}}$
   acid of sour milk, intermediate in metabolism of carbohydrates

4. Oxalic acid ($H—O—\overset{\overset{\displaystyle O}{\|}}{C}—\overset{\overset{\displaystyle O}{\|}}{C}—O—H$)
—bleach
5. Citric acid

$(H—O—\overset{\overset{\displaystyle O}{\|}}{C}—CH_2—\overset{\overset{\displaystyle \overset{\displaystyle H}{|} \; O}{\|}}{C}—CH_2—\overset{\overset{\displaystyle O}{\|}}{C}—O—H)$

$\underset{\overset{\displaystyle \|}{O \quad OH}}{C}$

—acid in citrus fruits, intermediate in metabolism of carbohydrates, fats, and proteins (citric acid cycle)

6. Pyruvic acid ($CH_3—\overset{\overset{\displaystyle O}{\|}}{C}—\overset{\overset{\displaystyle O}{\|}}{C}—O—H$)
—intermediate in carbohydrate metabolism
7. Benzoic acid—synthesis of other products like the benzoate salts
8. Chaulmoogric acid—treatment of leprosy
9. Salicylic acid—synthesis of aspirin and sodium salicylate
10. Picric acid (2,4,6-trinitrophenol)—treatment of burns, precipitant of proteins in clinical test

C. Certain organic acids are produced from hydrolysis of fats and are called *fatty acids*
1. Butyric acid—C_3H_7COOH
2. Stearic acid—$C_{17}H_{35}COOH$
3. Palmitic acid—$C_{15}H_{32}COOH$
4. Oleic acid—$C_{17}H_{33}COOH$

9. **Esters** ($R—\overset{\overset{\displaystyle O}{\|}}{C}—O—R'$)

A. Reactions of esters
1. Esters formed in reaction between an acid and an alcohol
2. Esters easily hydrolyzed
   a. By acid (acid hydrolysis)

$CH_3—\overset{\overset{\displaystyle O}{\|}}{C}—O—CH_3 + HCl \longrightarrow$
Methyl acetate   Hydrochloric acid

$CH_3—\overset{\overset{\displaystyle O}{\|}}{C}—O—Na + CH_3OH$
Sodium acetate   Methyl alcohol

   b. By base (saponification)

$CH_3—\overset{\overset{\displaystyle O}{\|}}{C}—O—CH_3 + NaOH \longrightarrow$
Methyl acetate   Sodium hydroxide

$CH_3—\overset{\overset{\displaystyle O}{\|}}{C}—O—H + CH_3Cl$
Sodium acetate   Methyl chloride

c. When the ester contains the acid residue of a fatty acid, the hydrolysis of the ester by a base results in the formation of a *soap*—the basic salt of a fatty acid
3. When fatty acids react with the trihydroxy alcohol, glycerol, they form esters that are called *fats* or oils

$$H—\overset{\overset{\displaystyle H}{|}}{C}—OH$$
$$H—\overset{\overset{\displaystyle }{|}}{C}—OH + 3C_{17}H_{35}\overset{\overset{\displaystyle O}{\|}}{C}—OH \longrightarrow$$
$$H—\overset{\overset{\displaystyle }{|}}{\underset{\underset{\displaystyle H}{|}}{C}}—OH$$

Glycerol   Stearic acid (fatty acid)

$$H—\overset{\overset{\displaystyle H}{|}}{C}—O—\overset{\overset{\displaystyle O}{\|}}{C}—C_{17}H_{35}$$
$$H—\overset{\overset{\displaystyle }{|}}{C}—O—\overset{\overset{\displaystyle O}{\|}}{C}—C_{17}H_{35} + 3H_2O$$
$$H—\overset{\overset{\displaystyle }{|}}{\underset{\underset{\displaystyle H}{|}}{C}}—O—\overset{\overset{\displaystyle O}{\|}}{C}—C_{17}H_{35}$$

Glycerol tristearate   Water
(a fat)

B. Important esters

1. Ethyl acetate ($CH_3\overset{\overset{\displaystyle O}{\|}}{C}—O—CH_2CH_3$)
—solvent, stimulant, and antispasmodic

2. Butyl acetate ($CH_3\overset{\overset{\displaystyle O}{\|}}{C}—O—CH_2CH_2$)
—solvent
3. Ethyl nitrite ($CH_3CH_2NO_2$)—diuretic and antispasmodic
4. Amyl nitrite ($CH_3CH_2CH_2CH_2CH_2NO_2$)—lowers blood pressure, aids in asthma and angina pectoris
5. Glycerol trinitrate (nitroglycerin)—vasodilator, explosive

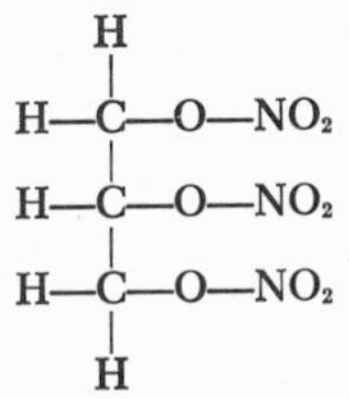

$$
\begin{array}{c}
H \\
| \\
H-C-O-NO_2 \\
| \\
H-C-O-NO_2 \\
| \\
H-C-O-NO_2 \\
| \\
H
\end{array}
$$

6. Methyl benzoate—perfumes and flavoring agents
7. Methyl salicylate—flavoring (oil of wintergreen)
8. Acetylsalicylic acid—aspirin

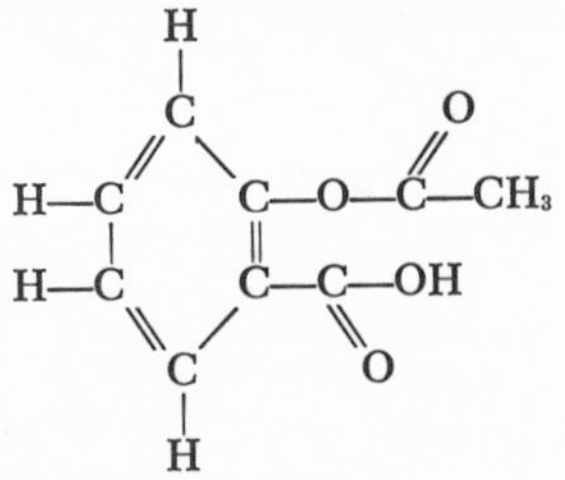

9. Phenolsulfonphthalein—an indicator for acid-base reactions
10. Many flavors and odors in foods, fruits, flowers, and perfumes are the result of volatile esters (amyl acetate, banana, ethyl butyrate, pineapple, etc.)

10. Ethers (R—O—R′)
A. Reactions of ethers
1. Ethers are formed from condensation of alcohol molecules with H_2SO_4 (sulfuric acid) acting as a catalyst; example:

$$R-OH + R'-OH \xrightarrow{H_2SO_4} R-O-R' + H_2O$$
Alcohols   Ether   Water

$$CH_3CH_2OH + CH_3CH_2OH \xrightarrow{H_2SO_4}$$
Ethyl   Ethyl
alcohol   alcohol

$$CH_3CH_2-O-CH_2CH_3 + H_2O$$
Diethyl ether   Water

2. Use of ether and oxygen in operating rooms makes for explosive conditions; care must be exercised preventing sparks
3. Ethers can cause nausea and irritation of tissues; cause much postoperative discomfort
B. Important ethers
1. Diethyl ether $(CH_3CH_2-O-CH_2CH_3)$—general anesthetic, solvent for fats
2. Dimethyl ether (CH_3-O-CH_3)—solvent
3. Divinyl ether $(CH_2=CH-O-CH=CH_2)$—anesthetic
4. Methyl propyl ether $(CH_3CH_2CH_2-O-CH_3)$—anesthetic

11. Amines (R—NH₂)—organic derivatives of ammonia (NH₃) with 1 or more of the hydrogens replaced with an R group
A. Types of amines
1. Primary amine

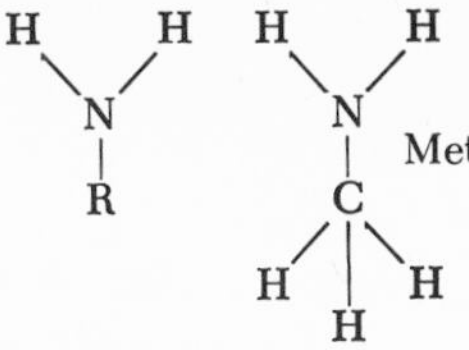

2. Secondary amine

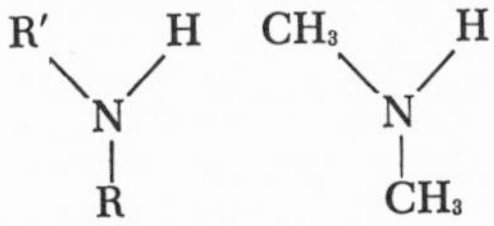

3. Tertiary amine

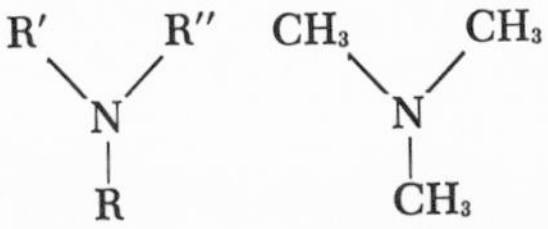

B. Reactions of the amines
1. Amines give a basic reaction in water solution

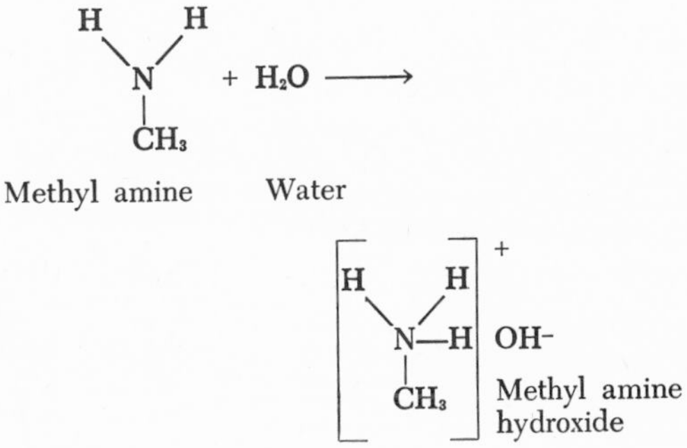

2. Amines react like a base with acids, forming complex ions

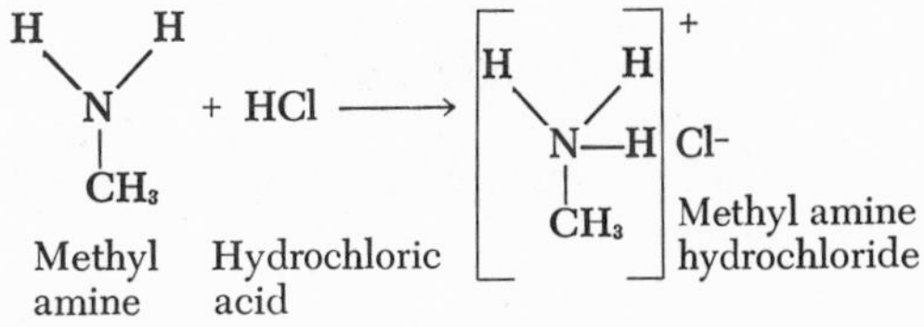

C. Important amines
1. Dimethyl amine—used in processing of leathers, in production of liquid fuel for rocket propulsion, and in making ion exchange resins
2. Trimethyl amine—preparation of ion exchange resins
3. In general, amines are used in dyes, drugs, soaps, disinfectants, insecticides
4. Para-amino phenol—used in photographic developers and for making analgesic drugs
5. Aniline—used in the manufacture of dyes, rubber, drugs, antioxidants
6. Acetanilid—antipyretic and analgesic drug
7. Sulfanilamide—an important sulfa drug

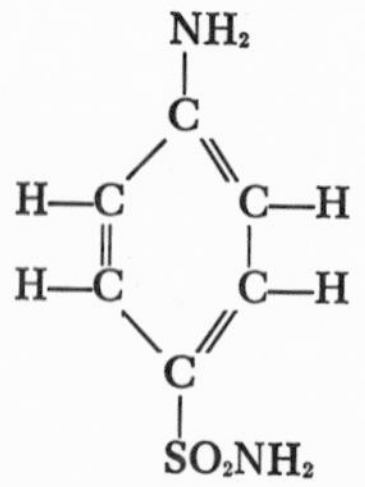

8. Sulfathiazole and sulfadiazine—important sulfa drugs
12. Amino acids—possess 2 functional groups: an amine ($-NH_2$) group and an acid ($-\overset{\overset{O}{\|}}{C}-O-H$), or carbonyl, group
The general formula for an amino acid and an example:

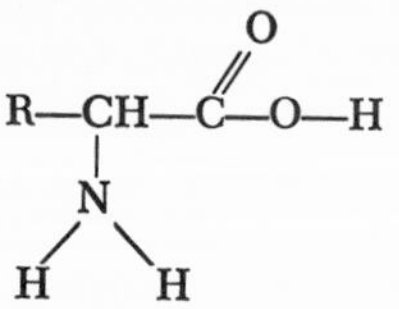

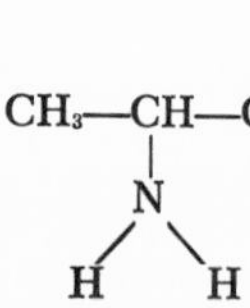

A. Reactions of amino acids
1. Amino acids are able to act as an acid and as a base (amphoteric character)

a. As a base

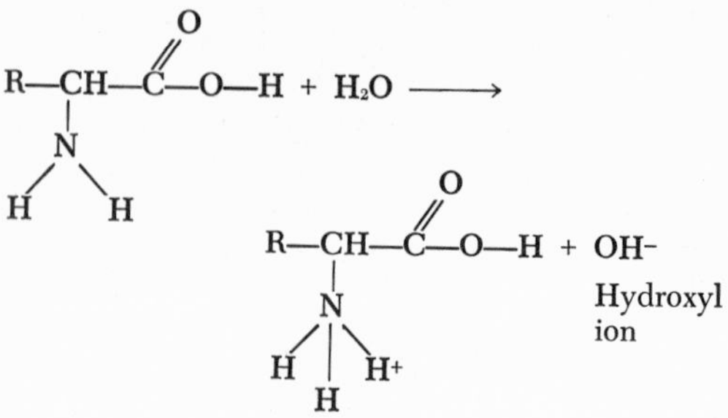

Hydroxyl ion

b. As an acid

Hydronium ion

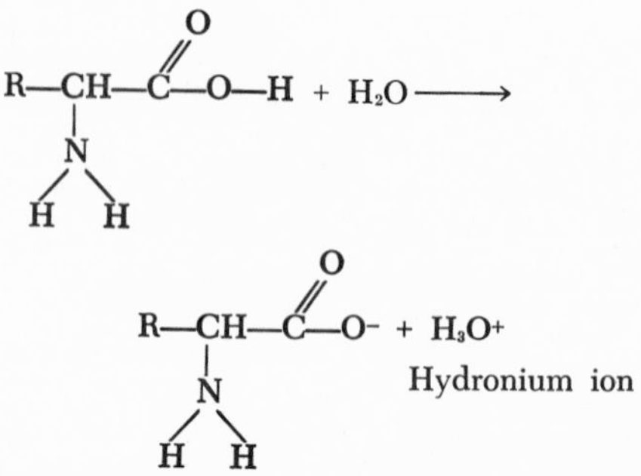

2. Condensation via peptide bond to form proteins

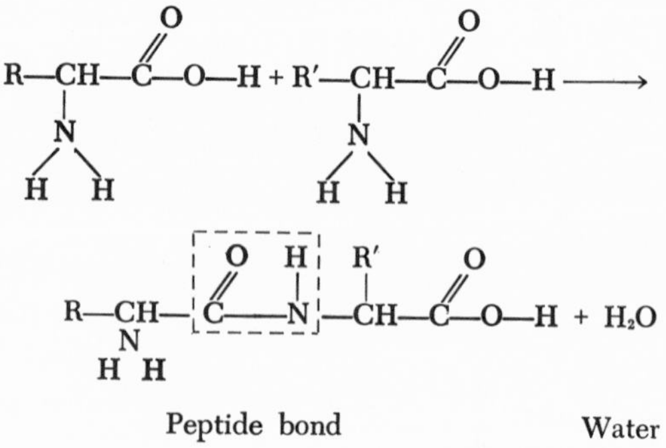

Peptide bond   Water

TABLE 3-4
AMINO ACIDS FOUND IN PROTEINS

Essential (needed in diet)	Nonessential (body can synthesize)
Arginine	Alanine
Histidine	Aspartic acid
Isoleucine	Cysteine
Leucine	Cystine
Lysine	Glutamic acid
Methionine	Glycine
Phenylalanine	Hydroxyproline
Threonine	Proline
Tryptophan	Serine
Valine	Tyrosine

B. Essential amino acids cannot be synthesized well enough in the body to maintain health and growth and must be supplied in the food (Table 3-4)

13. **Heterocyclic compounds—cyclic compounds containing other than carbon atoms**

A. Five-membered rings
   1. Furan

   2. Furfural—an aldehyde derivative of furan; used as a solvent, in manufacture of nylon, and in clinical test for sugars

   3. Pyrrole—constituent of porphyrins that make up hemoglobin, chlorophyll, cytochromes, and the amino acid tryptophan

   4. Imidazole—found in the purines of nucleic acids and in the amino acid histidine

   5. Thiazole—found in penicillin and in the structure of the vitamin thiamin

B. Six-membered rings
   1. Pyridine—important to formation of members of the vitamin B complex of vitamins

   2. Purine—found in nucleic acids, uric acid, stimulants such as tea and coffee, and in Dramamine (motion sickness–relieving drug)

   3. Pyrimidine—used to synthesize nucleic acids, the vitamin thiamin (B_1), and barbiturates (phenobarbital, Amytal, Seconal, etc.)

14. **Alkaloids—nitrogen-containing organic materials extracted from plants**

A. Nicotine—alkaloid in tobacco; used in manufacture of insecticides
B. Atropine—derived from belladonna plant; dilates pupil of eye, used to make cocaine, and is local anesthetic
C. Cocaine—found in cocoa plant; local anesthetic and nerve stimulant
D. Quinine—from cinchona bark; antimalaria drug
E. Atabrine—synthetic drug; similar in action to quinine
F. Morphine—derived from a type of poppy (raw material opium); central nervous system depressant
G. Codeine—opium derivative; central nervous system depressant
H. Demerol—synthetic compound; similar in action to morphine

CARBOHYDRATES

1. **Aldehyde or ketone derivatives of single oxidation of polyhydric alcohols, or com-**

pounds yielding these aldehyde or ketone derivatives upon hydrolysis

```
     H
     |
 H—C—OH
     |        [O]
 H—C—OH   ——→
     |
 H—C—OH
     |
     H
  Glycerol
```

```
          O                      H
          ‖                      |
          C—H              H—C—OH
          |                      |
    H—C—OH      or         C=O        + H₂O
          |                      |          Water
    H—C—OH              H—C—OH
          |                      |
          H                      H
  Glyceraldehyde   Dihydroxyacetone
```

A. Include simple sugars, starches, celluloses, gums, and resins
  1. Widespread in plant and animal tissue
  2. Contain carbon, hydrogen, and oxygen with the hydrogen and oxygen present in approximately the ratio of 2 to 1
B. Synthesis—plants synthesize carbohydrates from carbon dioxide and water with the aid of the green pigment chlorophyll (which acts as an enzyme) and the solar energy of the sun; example:

$$\text{Sunlight} + 6CO_2 + 6H_2O \longrightarrow C_6H_{12}O_6 + 6O_2$$
$$\text{Simple sugar}$$

This process is called *photosynthesis*

2. Classification
A. By functional group
  1. Carbohydrates having the aldehyde group are called *aldoses*
  2. Carbohydrates having the ketone group are called *ketoses*
B. By complexity of the molecule
  1. Carbohydrate having a single ketose or aldose molecule is called a *monosaccharide*—a *simple sugar*
  2. Carbohydrate formed by combining 2 aldose molecules or an aldose and a ketose molecule is called a *disaccharide*
  3. Carbohydrate having more than 2 simple sugars joined in a molecule is called a *polysaccharide*
C. Monosaccharides are subclassified by the number of carbons they contain
  1. Diose—2
  2. Triose—3
  3. Tetrose—4

  4. Pentose—5
  5. Hexose—6

3. Reactions of carbohydrates
A. Aldoses can change to ketoses and vice versa through formation of intermediate *enediol* compound

```
      O                 H—C—OH              H
      ‖                     ‖                |
      C—H                   C—OH         H—C—OH
      |                     |                |
  H—C—OH               HO—C—H            C=O
      |        ⇌         |        ⇌        |
  HO—C—H               H—C—OH         HO—C—H
      |                     |                |
  H—C—OH               H—C—OH          H—C—OH
      |                     |                |
  H—C—OH               H—C—OH          H—C—OH
      |                     |                |
  H—C—OH               H—C—OH          H—C—OH
      |                     |                |
      H                     H                H
   Aldose               Enediol           Ketose
```

```
      O                 H—C—OH                   H
      ‖                     |                    |
      C—H               H—C—OH               H—C—OH
      |                     |                    |
  H—C—OH               HO—C—H                    C—O
      |                     |           O    H /  |  \
  HO—C—H                H—C—OH    or    C    |/   |   H
      |        ⇌         |                  |\   OH   |
  H—C—OH               H—C—OH          OH\  C—C
      |                     |                    |   |
  H—C—OH               H—C—
      |                     |                    H   O
  H—C—OH               H—C—OH
      |                     |
      H                     H
   Glucose            Ring form of glucose
```

B. Reducing action—enediols act as reducing agents to metal ions causing a loss in positive valence; example:

$$\begin{array}{c}\text{Aldose}\\ \text{or} \\ \text{ketose}\end{array} + \begin{array}{c}OH^-\\ \text{Base}\end{array} \longrightarrow \text{Enediol} + \underset{\text{(blue)}}{2Cu^{++}} \longrightarrow$$

$$\underset{\text{(yellow)}}{Cu_2O + \text{Organic acid}}$$

  1. Benedict's test and Clinitest tablets use copper (II) ions in basic medium—show presence of sugar in urine by change in color
  2. Positive reaction gives colors from green (very little sugar) to brick red (more than 2 gm. of sugar per 100 ml. of urine)
  3. Iron ions ($Fe^{+++} \longrightarrow Fe^{++}$) and silver ions ($Ag^+ \longrightarrow Ag^0$) can be used instead of copper to give a test for sugar
  4. Most monosaccharides and disaccharides (except sucrose) are reducing sugars

C. Fermentation—in presence of a yeast enzyme, *zymase*, many carbohydrates are converted to alcohol and carbon dioxide; example:

$$\text{Glucose} \xrightarrow{\text{(zymase)}} \text{Ethyl alcohol and } CO_2$$

D. Oxidation—strong oxidation will cause carbohydrates to burn, forming CO_2, H_2O, and energy
   1. Cellular oxidation of carbohydrates—source of energy for body functions
   2. Mild oxidation causes aldoses to form acids; example:

$$\text{Glucose} + O_2 \longrightarrow \text{Gluconic acid}$$

E. Ester formation—hydroxyl groups in carbohydrates can form esters with acids; example:

$$\text{Cellulose} + \text{Acetic acid} \longrightarrow \text{Cellulose acetate (important synthetic)}$$

F. Ring formation—many monosaccharides will attain cyclic formation, an interior hemiacetyl (see above)

G. Condensation or polymerization—monosaccharides react together forming disaccharides and polysaccharides with the splitting out of water molecules

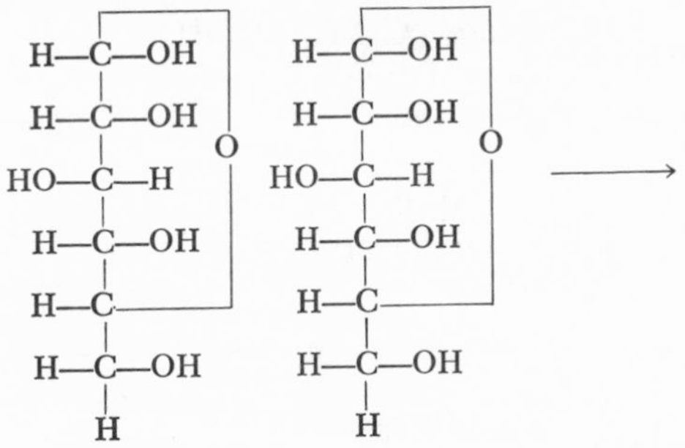

Two glucose molecules

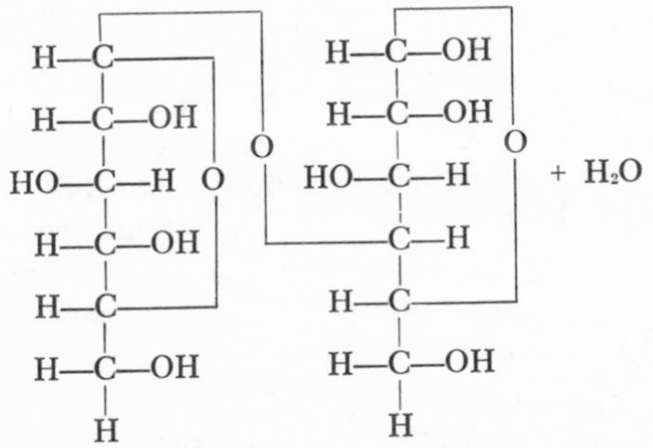

Maltose   Water

H. Hydrolysis—disaccharides and polysaccharides can be broken into monosac-

charides by the addition of water molecules at ester bonds; this can be effected by
   1. Acid hydrolysis
   2. Basic hydrolysis
   3. Enzymatic hydrolysis

4. Important carbohydrates

A. Glycerose and dihydroxyacetone—triose intermediates in cellular metabolism of carbohydrates

B. Ribose and deoxyribose—pentose constituents in nucleic acids

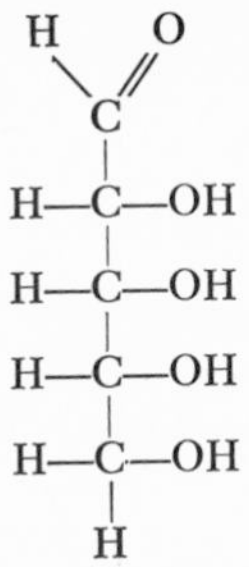

Ribose 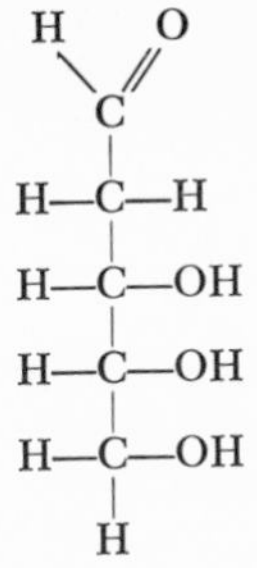   Deoxyribose

C. Glucose (dextrose)—hexose monosaccharide; normal sugar of blood, body fluids, fruits, and vegetables; needs hormone *insulin* for proper utilization in body

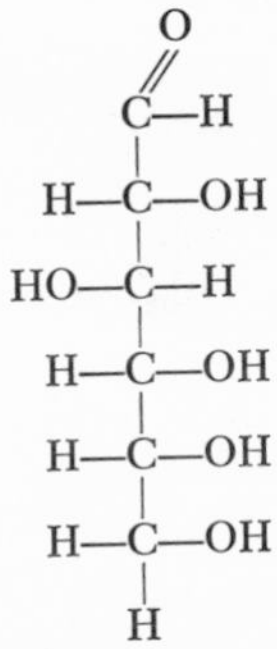

D. Fructose (levulose)—ketose monosaccharide; found in fruits and honey, sweetest sugar known; important intermediate in cellular metabolism of carbohydrates

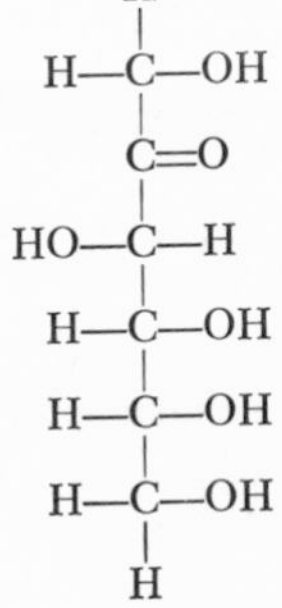

E. Galactose—hexose monosaccharide; present in brain and nervous tissue

$$
\begin{array}{c}
\overset{\displaystyle O}{\underset{\displaystyle }{\overset{\displaystyle \diagup\!\diagup}{C}}}\!\!-\!\!H \\
|\\
H\!\!-\!\!C\!\!-\!\!OH \\
|\\
HO\!\!-\!\!C\!\!-\!\!H \\
|\\
HO\!\!-\!\!C\!\!-\!\!H \\
|\\
H\!\!-\!\!C\!\!-\!\!OH \\
|\\
H\!\!-\!\!C\!\!-\!\!OH \\
|\\
H
\end{array}
$$

F. Lactose (milk sugar) disaccharide of glucose and galactose molecules; bacterial fermentation of lactose to lactic acid causes milk to sour

G. Sucrose (cane sugar)—disaccharide of glucose and fructose molecules; nonreducing sugar, common table sugar used in sweetening and baking

H. Maltose—disaccharide of 2 glucose molecules; found in grains and malt

I. Starch—mixed polysaccharide of glucose molecules found in plants
   1. Amylose—straight-chained glucose polymer
   2. Amylopectin—branched-chain glucose polymer
   3. Chief food carbohydrate in human nutrition
   4. Starch polymers react with iodine to form a blue colored complex; used as a test for starch
      a. Test becomes colorless as starch is hydrolyzed
      b. Starch (blue) ⟶ amylodextrin (purple) ⟶ erythrodextrin (red) ⟶ achroodextrin (colorless) ⟶ maltose (colorless) ⟶ glucose (colorless)

J. Glycogen—polysaccharide polymer of glucose molecules found in human and animal tissue; storage compound in body; hydrolyzes to glucose, maintaining blood glucose levels

K. Cellulose—polysaccharide polymer of glucose found in plants; not digestible by humans; important in manufacture of cotton cloth, paper, and cellulose acetate synthetics

L. Inulin—polysaccharide polymer of fructose, used in kidney function test (inulin clearance test)

M. Agar-agar—polysaccharide polymer of galactose used as a solid medium for bacteriologic studies

LIPIDS

Organic substances essentially insoluble in water but soluble in organic solvents (ether, chloroform, acetone, etc.)

1. **Fatty acids—important constituents of all lipids (except sterols)**
A. Usually straight-chained carboxylic acids
B. Naturally occurring fatty acids contain even numbers of carbon atoms
C. Saturated fatty acids—have no double bonds (points of unsaturation) between their carbon atoms
D. Unsaturated fatty acids—have 1 or more points of unsaturation ($-\overset{|}{C}=\overset{|}{C}-$) between their carbon atoms
E. Essential fatty acids—cannot be synthesized by body; must be taken in by diet; examples:

   1. Linoleic ($C_{17}H_{31}\overset{\displaystyle O}{\overset{\diagup\!\diagup}{C}}-OH$)

   2. Linolenic ($C_{17}H_{29}\overset{\displaystyle O}{\overset{\diagup\!\diagup}{C}}-OH$)

   3. Arachidonic ($C_{19}H_{31}\overset{\displaystyle O}{\overset{\diagup\!\diagup}{C}}-OH$)

2. **Classification of lipids**
A. Simple lipids—esters of fatty acids and alcohols
   1. Fats—the alcohol of fats is the trihydric alcohol *glycerol*

$$
\begin{array}{c}
H \\
|\\
H\!\!-\!\!C\!\!-\!\!OH \\
|\\
H\!\!-\!\!C\!\!-\!\!OH \\
|\\
H\!\!-\!\!C\!\!-\!\!OH \\
|\\
H
\end{array}
$$
Glycerol

      a. Solid fats—fats that are solid at room temperature contain long-chained, saturated fatty acids
      b. Liquid fats (oils)—fats that are liquid at room temperature contain short-chained, unsaturated fatty acids
   2. Waxes—esters of long-chained fatty acids and an alcohol other than glycerol; lanolin, a mixed wax from wool, is used in creams and salves
   3. Reactions of simple lipids
      a. Hydrolysis—splitting into fatty

acid(s) and alcohol by breaking ester bond, is effected by acid, base, or enzymatic action

b. Saponification—basic hydrolysis; *soap* is formed from organic salts of fatty acid and metal ion of base; example:

H   O
| ‖
H—C—O—C—R
   |
   O
   ‖
H—C—O—C—R + 3NaOH —Heat→
   |
   O
   ‖
H—C—O—C—R
   |
   H

Fat   Base

H
|
H—C—OH   O
| ‖
H—C—OH + 3Na—O—C—R
|
H—C—OH
|
H

Glycerol   Soap

c. Addition—fats containing unsaturated fatty acids will form addition products at points of unsaturation

(1) Addition of oxygen will cause fat to become rancid; antioxidants slow this reaction in packaged foods

(2) Unsaturated oils used in paints add oxygen and become hard and glossy

(3) Hydrogenation—liquid fats can form solid fats by adding in hydrogen at double bonds; example:

Vegetable oil + H₂ —Nickel catalyst→ Solid fat (Crisco, Spry, etc.)

(4) Halogen (iodine) adds into double bonds—a test for unsaturation

B. Compound lipids—fats containing chemical substances other than fatty acids and alcohols

1. Phospholipids—contain alcohol, fatty acids, phosphoric acid, and a nitrogenous base (or inositol)

a. Lecithins—contain the alcohol glycerol, fatty acids, phosphoric acid, and the nitrogenous base *choline;* are found in brain and nervous tissue; in blood, lecithin serves to render fats soluble in plasma (a *lypotropic* agent)

b. Cephalins—similar in structure to lecithin except base is *ethanolamine* (—CH₂—CH₂—NH₂); important in brain and nerve tissue; help blood-clotting mechanism

c. Sphingomyelins—made from amino alcohol (sphingosinol), a fatty acid, phosphoric acid, and choline; important in brain and nerve tissue

2. Cardiolipids—made from unsaturated fatty acids, glycerol, and phosphoric acid; found in heart tissue

3. Glycolipids (cerebrosides)—structure contains the monosaccharide galactose, amino alcohol (sphingosinol), and a fatty acid; found in brain tissue and the myelin sheaths of nerves

C. Steroids—complex monohydroxy alcohols found in plant and animal tissues—basic structure, the phenanthrine structure plus a cyclo-pentane ring; characteristic side chains determine specific steroids

Steroid nucleus

1. Cholesterol—a sterol found in human and animal tissues, chiefly in brain and nerve tissue; found in blood in varying amounts; high blood cholesterol seems associated with coronary thrombosis

2. Egosterol—a plant sterol that can be converted to vitamin D by ultraviolet light

3. Bile acids—sterols that aid in digestion and absorption of fats

4. Steroid hormones—sex and adrenal gland hormones

5. Vitamin D—steroid controlling calcium metabolism

PROTEINS

1. Polymers of alpha amino acids connected by peptide bonds

A. Characteristics of proteins
  1. Protein molecules are very large, with molecular weights equal to or greater than 10,000 a.w.u.
  2. Proteins form colloid particles in solution
  3. Synthesis of proteins is in ribosomes of cell, according to specific genetic patterns under direction of the nucleic acids DNA and RNA
  4. Structure patterns of proteins are extremely specific; proteins differ from species to species, individual to individual, organ to organ; present problems for transplant operations
  5. Proteins are the tissue builders of the body

B. Classification of proteins
  1. Simple proteins—give amino acids on hydrolysis
    a. Albumins—water-soluble, coagulated by heat; examples: lactalbumin (milk), serum albumin (blood), egg white
    b. Globulins—insoluble in water, soluble in dilute salt solutions, coagulated by heat; examples: lactoglobulin (milk), serum globulin (blood), gamma serum globulin—form antibodies of blood
    c. Glutelins—soluble in dilute bases or acids, insoluble in neutral solutions; coagulated by heat; example: glutenin (wheat)
    d. Albuminoids—soluble in water; examples: collagen (connective tissue), elastin (ligaments)
    e. Histone—water-soluble; example: globin (hemoglobin)
    f. Prolamines—insoluble in water, soluble in 70% to 80% alcohol; examples: gliadin (wheat), zein (corn)
    g. Protamines—water-soluble; example: protamine (fish spermatozoa)
  2. Compound proteins—contain other molecules than amino acids
    a. Chromoproteins—proteins containing a colored molecule; examples: hemoglobin, flavoproteins
    b. Glycoproteins—proteins containing carbohydrate molecule(s); example: mucopolysaccharide of synovial fluid
    c. Lipoproteins—simple proteins combined with lipid substances; example: lipovitellin in egg yolk
    d. Nucleoproteins—proteins containing nucleic acids; examples: DNA and RNA
    e. Metalloproteins—proteins containing metal ions; example: ferritin (iron transport compound of plasma)
    f. Phosphoproteins—proteins containing phosphoric acid radical; example: casein of milk
  3. Derived proteins—are also called "denatured" proteins; treatment with acids, bases, heat, x-rays, ultraviolet rays, and many other agents causes proteins to alter their molecular arrangements

C. Reactions of proteins
  1. Amphoteric properties—like the amino acids forming them, proteins can act as acid or base in solutions; can act as *buffers*
  2. Hydrolysis—acid, base, or enzyme hydrolysis splits peptide bond; yields proteose ⟶ peptones ⟶ peptides ⟶ amino acids
  3. Denaturation—change in structure renders the protein less soluble, leads to coagulation of protein
    a. Heat—protein and heat ⟶ coagulated protein; examples: cooked egg white, cooked meat, etc.
    b. Salts of heavy metals—silver, lead, mercury, etc.; taken internally, poison because they denature the enzymes of the cells, which are protein in nature
    c. Acetone and alcohol—both harden skin proteins
    d. Inorganic acids and bases—coagulate and hydrolyze proteins
    e. Alkaloids and organic acids—tanning of hides, precipitation of blood proteins for clinical tests
    f. Rays—x-rays, infrared rays, ultraviolet rays—long exposure can cause cataracts (precipitation of lens protein in eye)
  4. Salting out—concentrated salt solutions render soluble proteins insoluble
  5. Color reactions
    a. Xanthoproteic test—protein having benzene ring (as found in the amino acids tyrosine and phenyl-

alanine) will turn yellow on addition of concentrated nitric acid; heat and a second addition of sodium hydroxide will turn the yellow to orange
   b. Millon's test—protein having a phenolic ring (as found in the amino acid tyrosine) will form red precipitate on addition of a mixture of mercuric and mercurous nitrates
   c. Biuret test—test for the peptide bond; violet color appears on addition of a hydroxide and dilute copper sulfate solution; negative for free amino acids (no peptide bond)
   d. Hopkins-Cole test—protein that contains the indole structure (amino acid tryptophan) shows a violet color on addition of glyoxylic acid and concentrated sulfuric acid
   e. Ninhydrin test—test for free amino acids, ninhydrin reagent gives blue color

NUCLEOPROTEINS

1. **Specific proteins found in cells, made of large and complex molecules having important functions**
A. Composition of nucleoproteins
   1. Hydrolysis of nucleoproteins results in nucleic acids and protein
   2. Hydrolysis of nucleic acid yields
      a. Phosphoric acid—H_3PO_4
      b. Pentose sugars—ribose or deoxyribose
      c. Purine or pyrimidine bases
         (1) Purine bases—adenine, guanine
         (2) Pyrimidine bases—cytosine, uracil, thymine
   3. Combination of a purine or pyrimidine base with either ribose or deoxyribose forms a *nucleoside*
   4. Addition of phosphoric acid to a nucleoside forms a *nucleotide*
   5. Polymerization of nucleotide molecules via ester bonds yields a nucleic acid—the shape of DNA is that of a *double helix* (Fig. 3-5)
B. Two main forms of nucleic acid: RNA and DNA (*ribose nucleic acid* and *deoxyribose nucleic acid*)
   1. RNA yields the following on hydrolysis: adenine, guanine, cytosine, uracil, ribose, phosphoric acid

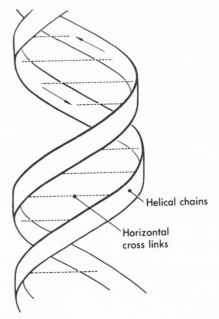

FIG. 3-5
Double helix.

Helical chains

Horizontal cross links

   2. DNA yields the following on hydrolysis: adenine, guanine, cytosine, thymine, deoxyribose, phosphoric acid
C. Role of DNA and RNA in protein synthesis
   1. DNA appears chiefly in the chromatin material of the nucleus of cells
      a. Chromatin material contains the chromosomes, which in turn hold the genes
      b. DNA seems to hold the coded genetic information of the genes
   2. RNA is found both inside the nucleus and in the cytoplasm of cells
   3. RNA occurs in three forms: messenger RNA (mRNA), transfer RNA (tRNA), and ribosomal RNA (rRNA)
      a. mRNA's function is to transmit the coded genetic information from the DNA molecules in the cellular nucleus to the rest of the cell to effect the genetic regulation of protein synthesis
      b. In the ribosomes of the cell, the mRNA effects the synthesis of tRNA
      c. The mRNA, rRNA, and tRNA direct the synthesis of proteins in the ribosomes from amino acids, according to coded genetic information originally found on DNA

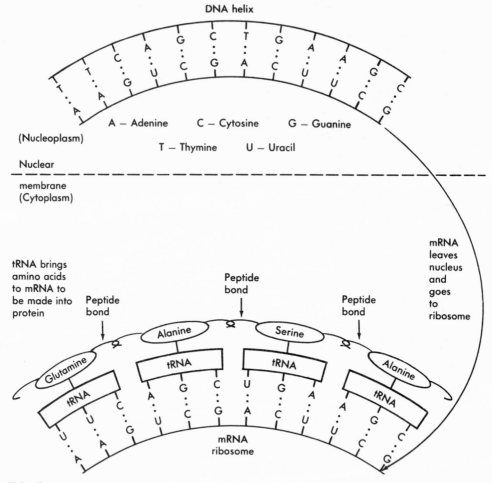

FIG. 3-6
Protein synthesis under DNA direction.

4. It is due to the activity of DNA and RNA that protein structure in species, individual, and organ is specific in so many cases (Fig. 3-6)
D. Other important related compounds
   1. ATP and ADP (adenosine triphosphate and adenosine diphosphate) are energy-storing compounds in cells
   2. NAD (nicotinamide adenine dinucleotide) and NADP (nicotinamide adenine dinucleotide phosphate) are important in hydrogen transport in the metabolism of foods

ENZYME ACTION

A. Enzymes—organic catalysts—enter into reaction; are re-formed at end of reaction, needed in minute amounts

B. Enzymes are protein in nature and are inactivated by all things denaturing proteins
C. Substrate—the substance acted upon by an enzyme
D. Names of enzymes—usually have ending "ase" added on name of substrate; example: sucrase, enzyme hydrolyzing sucrose; also have ending "ase" added to action of enzyme; example: lactic acid dehydrogenase, an enzyme removing hydrogen from lactic acid
E. Specificity of enzymes—being proteins, enzymes usually quite specific
   1. Temperature—enzyme activity high at temperature specific for that enzyme; low at all others
   2. pH—activity high at the pH specific

TABLE 3-5
CHEMISTRY OF DIGESTION

Secretion	Gland of secretion	Enzyme	Optimum reaction	Substrate	Example	End product
Saliva	Sublingual Submaxillary Parotid	Ptyalin (salivary amylase)	pH 6.7-7.2	Carbohydrates	Bread Potatoes	Maltose Dextrin
Bile	Liver	Action due to salts	pH 7.5-8.2	Fats	Butter	Emulsified fats
Pancreatic juice	Pancreas	Trypsin Chymotrypsin Amylopsin (amylase) Steapsin Maltase Carboxypeptidase	pH 6.0-9.0 pH 6.0-10.0 pH 7.5-8.2 pH 7.5-8.2 pH 7.5-8.2 pH 7.5-8.2	Protein Protein Carbohydrates Fats Maltose Peptides	Meat Beans Bread, starch, flour Fat meat, ham, butter	Proteoses, peptones, polypeptides Maltose Fatty acids and glycerol Glucose Amino acids
Succus entericus (intestinal juice)	Glands of intestinal wall Brunner's glands Lieberkühn's glands	Aminopeptidase Dipeptidase (erepsin) Maltase Lactase Sucrase (invertase) Nuclease Phosphatase Nucleosidase	pH 7.0-9.0 pH 7.0-9.0 pH 7.0-9.0 pH 7.0-9.0 pH 7.0-9.0 pH 7.0-9.0 pH 7.0-9.0 pH 7.0-9.0	Peptides Dipeptides Maltose Lactose Sucrose Nucleic acid Mononucleotides Nucleosides		Amino acids Amino acids Glucose Glucose and galactose Glucose and fructose Mononucleotides Nucleosides, phosphates Pentoses, purines, and pyrimidines
Gastric juice	Glands of stomach mucosa (chief cells)	Pepsin Rennin Lipase	pH 1.5-1.8 pH 5.0	Protein Milk casein Fats, oils	Meat, beans, legumes Milk Butter, cocoa oil, olive oil	Proteoses, peptones, peptides Paracasein + Ca^{++} Fatty acids and glycerols

for the enzyme; low at all other pH values

3. Substrate—usually one enzyme will catalyze only one reaction

F. Activators and inhibitors—certain inorganic ions act to speed up or slow down enzyme activity

G. Coenzymes—some enzymes exist in two parts: an *apoenzyme* and a *coenzyme*
1. The two together—called a *holoenzyme*
2. Apoenzyme—protein in nature
3. Coenzyme—nonprotein in nature; example: certain B vitamins are coenzymes in metabolism

CHEMISTRY OF DIGESTION

A. Digestion is carried on by a series of reactions
B. These reactions are hydrolytic in nature
C. The catalysts in digestion are enzymes—the digestive enzymes
D. Purpose of enzymatic hydrolysis of digestion is to render food small enough to be absorbed into body
E. The digestive process is summarized in Table 3-5

VITAMINS

1. **Materials needed in minute quantities in diet; body cannot synthesize** (Table 3-6)

TABLE 3-6
VITAMINS

Name	Chemical name	Deficiency causes	Occurrence
Fat-soluble vitamins			
Vitamin A	Retinol	Xerophthalmia, keratomalacia	Fish liver oils, liver, oils, eggs, vegetables
Vitamin D	Calciferol, 7-de-hydrocholesterol	Rickets, poor teeth	Fish liver oils, liver oils; skin oils plus sunlight
Vitamin E	Tocopherols	Muscular weakness, sterility	Egg yolk, wheat germ
Vitamin K	Naphthoquinones	Reduced prothrombin, excessively long bleeding and clotting times	Egg yolk, wheat germ, green leafy vegetables
Water-soluble vitamins			
Vitamin B_1	Thiamin	Beri-beri, anorexia, neuritis	Yeast, whole grain cereals
Vitamin B_2	Riboflavin	Sore lips, photophobia, inflammation of cornea	Milk, liver, eggs
Vitamin B_3	Pantothenic acid	Human deficiency rare	Many food sources
Vitamin B_6	Pyridoxine	Sore and swollen tongue, nervousness	Liver, eggs, whole grain cereals
Vitamin B_7	Biotin	Human deficiency rare	Many food sources
Niacin	Nicotinamide, nicotinic acid	Pellagra	Liver, meat, whole grain cereals
PABA	Para-aminobenzoic acid	Growth retardation, gray hair	Liver, yeast, whole grain cereals
Folic acid (vitamin B_c)	Pteroylglutamic acid (PGA)	Macrocytic anemia	Yeast, liver, green leafy vegetables
Vitamin B_{12} (extrinsic factor)	Cobalamin	Macrocytic anemia, growth retardation, loss of nerve function	Many food sources Deficiency caused by faulty absorption, lack of "intrinsic factor"
Vitamin C	Ascorbic acid	Scurvy	Citrus fruits, green leafy vegetables, tomatoes, peppers

2. Many have coenzyme roles in metabolism
3. **Classification**
A. Fat-soluble
 1. Vitamin A—maintains cells and tissue in healthy state; needed for vision in dim light
 2. Vitamin D—regulates calcium metabolism
 3. Vitamin E—antioxidant
 4. Vitamin K—prothrombin synthesis for proper blood clotting
B. Water-soluble
 1. Vitamin B complex—many are coenzymes in metabolism
 2. Vitamin B_{12} is *extrinsic factor* necessary to prevent pernicious anemia
 3. Folic acid (vitamin B_c)—normal maturation of erythrocytes (red blood cells)
 4. Ascorbic acid (vitamin C)—maintains connective tissue in normal state
4. **Other essential food factors—not strictly vitamins**
 Appear to be needed in small amounts in diet for health
A. Choline—used in synthesis of lecithin; widely distributed in foods so human deficiency is rare; seems to prevent fatty livers
B. Inositol—importance in human nutrition still under investigation; possible role in carbohydrate metabolism suggested; widely distributed in foods
C. Bioflavonoids—lack in diet causes increased capillary permeability and fragility; exact role in human nutrition under investigation; found in citrus fruits, other fruits and vegetables
D. α-Lipoic acid—role in human nutrition under investigation; possible enzymatic role in carbohydrate and protein metabolism indicated; found in yeast and liver

CHEMISTRY OF BLOOD, URINE, AND HORMONES
Blood

1. **Circulating tissue**
A. Fluid—plasma
B. Cells—erythrocytes (red cells), leukocytes (white cells), platelets
2. **Chemical nature**
A. Water
B. Proteins
C. Amino acids
D. Glucose
E. Liquids
F. Inorganic salts
G. Vitamins
H. Waste products—urea, uric acids, etc.
I. Hormones
J. Enzymes
3. **Function**
A. Transport of food materials
 1. From intestinal tract to tissues
 2. From storage tissues to metabolizing cells
B. Transport of gases
 1. Oxygen from lungs to cells
 2. Carbon dioxide from cells to lungs
C. Transport of waste materials from cells to organs of excretion
D. Distribution of hormones, antibodies, and certain enzymes
E. Defense against infection, by action of antibodies and leukocytes
F. Wound healing through clot formation
G. Regulation and distribution of body temperature
H. Regulation of body acid-base balance through blood buffers
4. **Formation of blood clot—coagulation**
A. Function—prevention of blood loss and promotion of wound healing
B. Mechanism
 1. Blood contains prothrombin, calcium salts, fibrinogen
 2. Blood platelets and tissues contain thromboplastin
 3. Injury causes blood platelets and tissue to break and blood vessels to rupture, mixing blood and thromboplastin

$$\text{Prothrombin} \xrightarrow{\text{Thromboplastin, Ca}^{++}} \text{Thrombin}$$

$$\text{Fibrinogen} \xrightarrow{\text{Thrombin}} \text{Fibrin}$$

$$\text{Fibrin fibers + Blood cells} \longrightarrow \text{Clot}$$

 4. Calcium ions necessary for clotting, chemicals that bind up calcium act as anticoagulants outside of body; example: potassium oxalate
 5. Heparin blocks the conversion of prothrombin to thrombin; is used in and out of body to prevent clotting
 6. Antithrombin in blood dissolves clots, helps prevent clots in the body
 7. Vitamin K necessary for synthesis of prothrombin in liver
5. **Blood buffers**
A. Proteins, amino acids, bicarbonates, phosphates—resist change in the pH of the blood

B. Without blood buffers, changes in pH would be incompatible with life
6. **Changes in composition of blood reflect changes brought about by disease**
7. **Blood gases**
A. Oxygen transported by blood chiefly through combination with hemoglobin of red blood cells
B. Carbon dioxide transported by blood as bicarbonates and dissolved in plasma
C. Carbonic anhydrase, an enzyme in the red blood cells, aids in converting carbon dioxide to bicarbonates

$$CO_2 + H_2O \xrightarrow{\text{Carbonic anhydrase}} H^+ + HCO_3^-$$

Bicarbonate ion

Urine

1. **Water solution of inorganic salts and organic compounds**
2. **Important in excretion**
3. **Analysis yields information of physical condition in health and disease**
4. **Normal urine**
A. Amount—800 to 1,800 ml. per 24 hours
B. Color—light yellow to dark brown, due to pigments (urobilin, urochrome, etc.)
C. Odor—aromatic (fresh); food and drugs alter odor
D. Sediment—varies; due to diet and other normal changes
   1. Few blood cells
   2. Few epithelial cells
   3. Phosphates
   4. Urates
   5. Uric acid crystals
   6. Calcium oxalate
E. Specific gravity (1.008 to 1.025) varies greatly, depending on fluid intake
F. Reaction—usually acid (pH 5 to 7 average normal); alkaline immediately after meal
G. Proteins—negative; protein in urine usually associated with pathology
H. Sugar—trace to negative; presence of urinary carbohydrate usually pathologic
I. Ketone bodies—negative; ketone bodies in urine appear in metabolic disorders
J. Indican—negative; positive results indicate intestinal putrefaction
K. Bile—negative; positive results indicate liver or gallbladder dysfunction
L. Blood—trace to negative; positive results indicate bleeding in renal organs

Hormones

1. **Produced by glands of internal secretion —endocrine glands**
2. **Discharged into blood**
3. **Carried by blood to site of activity**
4. **Regulate functioning of body**
5. **Some important hormones**
A. Thyroid hormone (thyroxine)—regulates metabolism
B. Parathyroid hormone—regulates calcium metabolism
C. Pancreatic hormone (insulin)—regulates carbohydrate metabolism
D. Anterior pituitary hormones
   1. Growth hormone—influences growth, maintains tissues and bones
   2. Gonadotropic hormone—regulates sexual growth and function
   3. Thyrotropic hormone—regulates thyroid gland
   4. Adrenocorticotropic hormone (ACTH) —maintains adrenal gland function
E. Posterior pituitary gland hormone
   1. Oxytocin—stimulates smooth muscle
   2. Vasopressin—antidiuretic hormone— diminishes water excretion by kidneys
F. Cortical adrenal gland hormones
   1. Regulate salt balance
   2. Regulate carbohydrate and protein metabolism
G. Medullary adrenal gland hormones
   1. Epinephrine—regulates
      a. Heart rate and cardiac output
      b. Blood pressure; acts as a vasoconstrictor
      c. Muscle constriction
      d. Conversion of glycogen to glucose; thereby affects blood sugar
   2. Norepinephrine
      a. Acts as vasoconstrictor
      b. Regulates and raises blood pressure
H. Sex hormones
   1. Male and female hormones are produced by gonad tissues
   2. Chemically these hormones are related to cholesterol
   3. These hormones determine primary and secondary sex characteristics, regulate sexual function, pregnancy, and lactation in the female
   4. Chief female sex hormones are the estrogenic hormone and progesterone
   5. Chief male sex hormones are androsterone and testosterone
   6. Increase in urinary estrogenic and

gonadotropic substances in early pregnancy is the basis of pregnancy tests

I. Gastrointestinal hormones function to regulate digestive functions
1. Gastrin—stimulates flow of gastric juices
2. Enterogastrone—inhibits flow of gastric juices
3. Secretin—stimulates flow of pancreatic juices and bile
4. Pancreozymin—stimulates flow of pancreatic juice
5. Cholecystokinin—stimulates contraction of gallbladder
6. Enterocrinin—stimulates flow of intestinal juice

METABOLISM OF CARBOHYDRATES, FATS, AND PROTEINS

1. Breakdown products of digestion utilized for energy and tissue synthesis in body
2. Glycolysis
A. Enzymatic anaerobic process; no oxygen necessary
B. Quickly converts simple sugars to energy
C. End products, pyruvic and lactic acids

$$C_6H_{12}O_6 \longrightarrow \underset{\text{Pyruvic acid}}{\overset{\text{COOH}}{\underset{\text{COOH}}{\overset{|}{C=O}}}} \overset{[H]}{\longrightarrow} \underset{\text{Lactic acid}}{\overset{\text{COOH}}{\underset{\text{COOH}}{\overset{|}{CHOH}}}}$$

Simple sugar

3. Citric acid cycle
A. Main oxidative pathway of metabolism
B. Releases more energy than glycolysis
C. Enzymes catalyze each step of process
D. Energy produced from metabolism stored in energy storage compounds adenosine di- and tri-phosphates (ADP, ATP)

REVIEW QUESTIONS FOR CHEMISTRY
Multiple choice

Read each question carefully and consider all possible answers; when you have decided which answer is best, blacken in the corresponding space on the answer sheet. There is only one best answer for each question (or implied question).

1. A substance that conducts an electric current when in solution is called
   1. A colloid
   2. An alkali
   3. An electrolyte
   4. An insulation
2. A solution containing 1 gram-equivalent weight of solute in 1 liter of solution is called
   1. An isotonic solution
   2. A normal solution
   3. A molar solution
   4. A saturated solution
3. A homogeneous mixture of 2 or more substances is
   1. A suspension
   2. A solvent
   3. A hydrate
   4. A solution
4. Two substances having the same osmotic pressure are said to be
   1. Isotonic
   2. Hemolyzed
   3. Hypotonic
   4. Hypertonic
5. A group of 2 or more elements chemically united in definite proportions as to weight and having different properties than when standing alone is
   1. An element
   2. A mixture
   3. An atom
   4. A compound
6. The law that states that in an ordinary reaction matter can neither be created nor destroyed but may be changed in form is
   1. The law of conservation of energy
   2. The law of conservation of matter
   3. The law of combining weights
   4. The law of definite composition
7. The process by which oxygen is being constantly returned to the air is
   1. Hydrogenation
   2. Photosynthesis
   3. Hydration
   4. Saponification
8. The best first-aid treatment for acid burns on the skin is to wash them with water and then apply a solution of
   1. Sodium hydroxide
   2. Sodium chloride
   3. Sodium bicarbonate
   4. Sodium sulfate
9. An increase in positive valence or a loss of electrons by an element is called
   1. Combustion
   2. Photosynthesis
   3. Reduction
   4. Oxidation
10. An atom having in the nucleus a different number of neutrons than other atoms of that same element is
   1. An ion
   2. An isotope
   3. A neutron
   4. An allotrope
11. If a sample of hard water can be softened by boiling, it may originally have contained
   1. $MgCl_2$
   2. $MgCO_3$
   3. $Mg(HCO_3)_2$
   4. $MgSO_4$
12. A substance that influences the speed of a reaction but is not itself altered in the reaction is
   1. A catalyst
   2. A dehydrating agent
   3. An oxidizing agent
   4. A reducing agent
13. A salt whose water solution will turn blue litmus paper red is
   1. Sodium chloride
   2. Silver nitrate
   3. Sodium acetate
   4. Ammonium chloride
14. A solution of sodium hydroxide would be expected to have a pH of
   1. 3
   2. 7
   3. 6
   4. 10
15. The number of ions resulting from the dissociation of 1 molecule of Na_2CO_3 is
   1. 5
   2. 2
   3. 3
   4. 6
16. The boiling point of a concentrated solution of sodium chloride is

1. Higher than pure water
2. Lower than pure water
3. The same as pure water

17. In water the ratio of oxygen to hydrogen by volume is
    1. 8 to 1   3. 2 to 1
    2. 1 to 9   4. 1 to 2

18. Substances that will not pass through a semi-permeable membrane when in solution are
    1. Acids   3. Colloids
    2. Hydrates   4. Crystalloids

19. In water the ratio of the weight of hydrogen to the weight of oxygen is
    1. 9 to 1   3. 1 to 2
    2. 1 to 8   4. 2 to 1

20. A patient of yours has a temperature of 99.8° F. This is the same as a temperature of
    1. 37.67° C.   3. 37.0° C.
    2. 38.19° C.   4. 36.5° C.

21. After being heated strongly a dry crystal was observed to weigh less; the crystal
    1. Must have contained water of crystallization
    2. May have been a carbonate
    3. Was deliquescent
    4. Was hygroscopic

22. If 4 gm. of H_2 are burned in an excess of oxygen, the number of grams of water formed is
    1. 32   3. 36
    2. 2   4. 4

23. The formula of hypochlorous acid is
    1. HClO   3. $HClO_3$
    2. $HClO_2$ 4. HCl

24. Acetic acid is classed as a weak acid because
    1. It lacks hydrogen
    2. It is poorly ionized
    3. It contains oxygen
    4. It contains carbon

25. A good first-aid treatment for an alkali (base) burn is to wash it with water and then flood it with
    1. A weak acid   3. A solution of salt
    2. A weak base   4. Alcohol

26. As one of its products, the reaction 2K + 2 HCl yields
    1. An acid   3. A salt
    2. A base   4. Water

27. When 1 gram-equivalent weight of HCl is added to 1 gram-equivalent weight of NaOH in a water solution, the resulting mixture has a pH of
    1. 3   3. 8
    2. 7   4. 10

28. A true solution is always
    1. Cloudy   3. Clear
    2. Colored

29. Water can be made chemically pure by
    1. Boiling   3. Distillation
    2. Filtration

30. Boiling germ-laden water makes it
    1. Better flavored
    2. Chemically pure
    3. Safe for drinking purposes

31. A crystal of ammonium chloride dropped into a supersaturated solution of ammonium chloride will
    1. Cause NH_4Cl crystals to separate from the solution

2. Cause no change in the solution
3. Dissolve in the solution

32. Neutralization reactions go to completion because
    1. Undissociated water is formed
    2. A salt is always formed
    3. A soluble gas may be formed
    4. Water may be present

33. A binary salt is
    1. $NaHCO_3$ 3. $(NH_4)_2SO_4$
    2. $MgBr_2$ 4. $KClO_3$

34. The reaction between hydroxyl ions and hydrogen ions is called
    1. Hydrolysis   3. Decomposition
    2. Neutralization   4. Fusion

35. A sugar solution will not conduct electricity because it lacks
    1. Electricity   3. Electrons
    2. Ions

36. An acid
    1. Turns litmus blue
    2. Contains the OH group
    3. Neutralizes other acids
    4. Tastes sour

37. The slippery feel and bitter taste that characterize solutions of soda, borax, soap, and lye are due to the presence of
    1. The acid   3. The sodium ion
    2. The hydrogen ion 4. The hydroxyl ion

38. NH_4^+ is a
    1. Compound   3. Liquid
    2. Gas   4. Radical

39. The reaction between NH_3 and H_2SO_4 yields
    1. NO and H_2S 3. $(NH_4)_2SO_4$ and H_2
    2. $(NH_4)_2SO_4$ 4. HNO_3 and S

40. Sodium acetate is a salt of a
    1. Strong base and a strong acid
    2. Strong base and a weak acid
    3. Weak base and a strong acid
    4. Weak base and a weak acid

41. Which compound makes water permanently hard?
    1. $CaCO_3$ 3. $MgSO_4$
    2. $Ca(HCO_3)_2$ 4. Na_2SO_4

42. A weak base is
    1. $CaCO_3$ 3. KOH
    2. $Ca(OH)_2$ 4. NH_4OH

43. Plaster of Paris is composed mainly of calcium
    1. Hydroxide   3. Phosphate
    2. Dichromate   4. Sulfate

44. The element with the atomic number 2
    1. Has a valence of +2   3. Is inert
    2. Is amphoteric   4. Is a metal

45. The gram-molecular weight of Na_2CO_3 is
    1. 80 gm.   3. 44 gm.
    2. 106 gm.   4. 60 gm.

46. The valence of sulfur in H_2SO_4 is
    1. 0   3. 6
    2. 2   4. 4

47. An unsaturated hydrocarbon contains
    1. C—OH groups
    2. C=C groups
    3. C—C groups
    4. C—H groups

48. Identify the formula of a fat
    1. CH_3—O—C_2H_5
    2. CH_3

       $\underset{\underset{CH_3}{|}}{C}$=$CH$ CH_3

    3. $C_3H_5(OH)_3$
    4. $C_3H_5(OOC$—$C_{15}H_{33})_3$

49. Identify the aldehyde
    1. CH_3—O—CH_3 3. CH_3 $CHOHCH_3$
    2. CH_3COCH_3 4. CH_3COH

50. Identify the peptide bond
    1. CH_3 OCH_3
    2. CH_3 CNH_2 $CONH$ CCH_3 $COOH$
    3. CH_3 $COOCH_2$ CH_3
    4. CH_3 CH_2 $COCH_3$

51. Identify the enzyme
    1. Fructose   3. Fructase
    2. Glucose   4. Maltose

52. Identify which one of the following is an ester

    1.

    H—C$\overset{\overset{H}{|}}{C}$C—CH$_2$OH
    H—C   C—H
       C
       |
       H

    2.

    H—C$\overset{\overset{H}{|}}{C}$C—COOCH$_3$
    H—C   C—OH
       C
       |
       H

    3. CH_3—CH_2—CH_3

    4.

    H—C$\overset{\overset{H}{|}}{C}$C—OH
    H—C   C—H
       C
       |
       H

53. Hydrolysis is involved in (a) digestion of fats, (b) digestion of proteins, (c) digestion of carbohydrates, (d) the breakdown of glycogen to glucose in the liver
    1. a and b   3. b, c, and d
    2. a, c, and d   4. All of them

54. $NaHCO_3 + H_2O \longrightarrow$
    1. $Na_2CO_3 + H_2O + H_2$
    2. $NaOH + H_2CO_3$
    3. $NaHCO_3 + H_2O$
    4. $Na + H_2O + CO_2$

55. Radium is stored in lead containers because
    1. Considerable heat is produced when radium disintegrates
    2. The lead absorbs the harmful radiations

    3. Radium is a heavy substance
    4. Lead prevents disintegration of the radium

56. Being able to act as a base or an acid depending on circumstances (having amphoteric properties) is characteristic of
    1. Fats   3. Carbohydrates
    2. Amino acids   4. Lecithins

57. The basis for Benedict's test is
    1. Aldehyde + Copper II oxide $\longrightarrow$ Acid + Copper I hydroxide
    2. Acid + Copper II oxide $\longrightarrow$ Aldehyde + Copper I hydroxide
    3. Acid + Copper II hydroxide $\longrightarrow$ Aldehyde + Copper I oxide
    4. Aldehyde + Copper II hydroxide $\longrightarrow$ Acid + Copper I oxide

58. Identify the organic acid
    1. CH_3CH_2OH 3. CH_3CH_2COH
    2. CH_3COOH 4. CH_3COCH_3

59. In the accompaning picture
    1. The cell will swell
    2. The cell will shrink
    3. The cell will rupture
    4. The cell will show no change

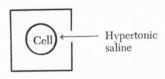

Hypertonic saline

60. The name for an organic catalyst in the body is
    1. Polypeptide   3. Phospholipid
    2. Enzyme   4. Emulsifier

61. Amino acids that cannot be synthesized by the body are called
    1. Balanced amino acids
    2. Acid amino acids
    3. Basic amino acids
    4. Essential amino acids

62. Butane has the formula
    1. C_4H_{10} 3. C_4H_9COOH
    2. C_8H_{18} 4. C_2H_4

63. One of the products of the following reaction $CH_3CH_2OH + CH_3COOH \longrightarrow$ is
    1. An ester
    2. An alkyl halide
    3. A phenol
    4. An alcohol

64. Identify the alcohol
    1. CH_3CH_2OH
    2. CH_3COOH
    3. CH_3COH
    4. CH_3COCH_3

65. A substance that acts as a coenzyme is
    1. Ascorbic acid   3. Vitamin K
    2. Vitamin B_1 4. Vitamin D

66. The fermentation of $C_6H_{12}O_6$ yields carbon dioxide and
    1. C_2H_2 3. $C_3H_5(NO_3)_3$
    2. C_2H_6 4. C_2H_5OH

67. An example of a buffer system is a mixture of
    1. Acetic acid and carbonic acid
    2. HCl and NaOH
    3. Acetic acid and potassium acetate
    4. Carbonic acid and KOH

68. Identify the phenol

1.

$$\begin{array}{c} H \quad H \\ | \quad | \\ C-C \\ // \quad \backslash \\ H-C \quad \quad C-OH \\ \backslash \quad // \\ C=C \\ | \quad | \\ H \quad H \end{array}$$

2.

$$\begin{array}{c} H \quad H \\ | \quad | \\ C-C \\ // \quad \backslash \\ H-C \quad \quad C-COOH \\ \backslash \quad // \\ C=C \\ | \quad | \\ H \quad H \end{array}$$

3.

$$\begin{array}{c} H \quad H \\ | \quad | \\ C-C \\ // \quad \backslash \\ H-C \quad \quad C-COH \\ \backslash \quad // \\ C=C \\ | \quad | \\ H \quad H \end{array}$$

4.

$$\begin{array}{c} H \quad H \\ | \quad | \\ C-C \\ // \quad \backslash \\ H-C \quad \quad C-CH_2OH \\ \backslash \quad // \\ C=C \\ | \quad | \\ H \quad H \end{array}$$

69. Identify the amino acid
    1.
    $$\begin{array}{c} CH_3 \\ \backslash \\ CNH_2CH_3 \\ / \\ CH_3 \end{array}$$
    2. $H_2NCH_2CH_3$
    3. $CH_3CH_2CHNH_2COOH$
    4. CH_3COOH

70. The formula

$C_3H_5(OOC-C_{15}H_{33})_3 \xrightarrow{\text{Enzyme}}$
$3C_{15}H_{33}COOH + C_3H_5(OH)_3 + 3H_2O$
represents
1. The formation of a soap
2. Digestion of protein
3. Hydrolysis of a fat
4. Hydrolysis of starch

71. The pH of the blood is maintained by
    1. Fatty acids
    2. Glucose
    3. Buffers
    4. Phosphatase

72. Enzymes have a chemical structure similar to
    1. Fats
    2. Carbohydrates
    3. Sterols
    4. Proteins

73. Many hormones of the body have a chemical structure similar to
    1. Fats
    2. Amino acids
    3. Sterols
    4. Glucose

74. An example of an unsaturated straight-chain hydrocarbon is

1. CH_4
2. C_2H_6
3. C_2H_4
4. C_3H_7OH

75. Proteins are
    (a) Amphoteric
    (b) Made of hydrogen, carbon, nitrogen, and oxygen
    (c) Precipitated by heavy metals (mercury, etc.)
    (d) Hydrolyzed by dilute acid
    (e) Found in plants and animals
    1. a, c, and e
    2. b, d, and e
    3. a, b, and c
    4. All of them

76. Lipids
    (a) Are found in plants and animals
    (b) Are soluble in water
    (c) Will burn as a fuel
    (d) Will make soap with an alkali
    (e) Contain hydrogen and oxygen and nitrogen
    1. a, c, and d
    2. All of them
    3. b, d, and e
    4. b, c, and d

77. Carbohydrates
    (a) Are found in plants and animals
    (b) Contain carbon, hydrogen, and oxygen
    (c) Provide energy in the body
    (d) Are originally made by animals
    (e) Are inorganic compounds
    1. a, b, and c
    2. a, c, and e
    3. All of them
    4. b, d, and e

78. Substances used in anesthesia are
    (a) Methyl chloride
    (b) Chloroform
    (c) Oxygen
    (d) Ethyl chloride
    (e) Iodoform
    1. All except e
    2. b, d, and e
    3. a, c, and e
    4. All of them

79. A colloid
    (a) Is able to pass through animal membranes
    (b) Has large molecules
    (c) Is able to adsorb electric charges on its molecules
    (d) Can form an emulsion
    (e) Is always ionic in form
    1. a, b, and c
    2. b, c, and e
    3. b, c, and d
    4. None of them

80. An acid
    (a) Turns litmus blue
    (b) Has a sour taste
    (c) Has a pH of over 8.0
    (d) Ionizes in solution
    (e) Reacts with a metal, releasing hydrogen gas
    1. a, b, and d
    2. a, c, and d
    3. All of them
    4. b, d, and e

81. An electrolyte is a substance that
    (a) Conducts an electric current
    (b) Is a nonmetal
    (c) Has a blue color
    (d) Can be used in storage batteries
    (e) Is ionic in form at all times
    1. a and d
    2. c, d, and e
    3. a, c, and e
    4. All of them

82. A solution
    (a) Is always made of water
    (b) May have alcohol as a solvent
    (c) Must be a liquid
    (d) Is a homogeneous mixture

(e) Is made up of varying amounts of a solute and a solvent
   1. a, d, and e   3. b, d, and e
   2. a, b, and e   4. None of them

83. Hydrolysis is the
   1. Reaction of a salt with water to form an acid and a base
   2. Reaction of an acid and a base
   3. Reaction of water with any substance
   4. Loss of valence in a reaction

84. The factors that influence enzyme action are the
   (a) Amount of substrate present
   (b) Acidity of the medium
   (c) Appetite of the person
   (d) Size and posture of the individual
   (e) Temperature of the solution
   1. a, c, and e   3. All of them
   2. b, c, and e   4. a, b, and e

85. An ion is
   1. One particle of hydrogen
   2. An atom or groups of atoms with an electric charge
   3. One molecule of water
   4. One pole of a battery

86. Iron salts are necessary in the body to
   1. Give the muscles strength
   2. Form hemoglobin
   3. Maintain the acid-base level of the blood
   4. Maintain normal osmotic pressure in the blood

87. An example of a physical change is
   1. Melting of ice
   2. Burning of wood
   3. Souring of milk
   4. Tarnishing of silver

88. An example of a chemical change is
   1. Shattering of glass
   2. Freezing of water
   3. Fermentation of fruit
   4. Hardening of gelatin

89. The chemical name for aspirin is
   1. Salicylic acid
   2. Sal soda
   3. Acetylsalicylic acid
   4. Sodium salicylic acid

90. Valence
   1. Is the combining capacity of an element
   2. Is the plus or minus sign of an element
   3. Has to do with the weight of a substance
   4. Balances a formula

91. The structural unit of a compound is
   1. A molecule   3. An ion
   2. An atom   4. A neutron

92. The fact that a compound always contains the same elements, in the same proportion by weight and united in the same manner, is called the law of
   1. Conservation of energy
   2. Definite composition
   3. Conservation of mass
   4. Multiple composition

93. A calorie is a unit of
   1. Heat   3. Mass
   2. Weight   4. Light

94. Ozone is an allotropic form of
   1. Hydrogen   3. Oxygen
   2. Water   4. Carbon

95. With respect to human blood cells, sodium chloride solution of 0.85% strength is
   1. Isotonic   3. Hypotonic
   2. Hypertonic   4. Isomeric

96. By addition of more hydrogen to an unsaturated fat the
   1. Substance is changed to a protein
   2. Caloric value is decreased
   3. Molecular weight is increased
   4. Fat is made more digestible

97. Buffers
   (a) Must be acid salts
   (b) Must be basic salts
   (c) Are amphoteric
   (d) Protect the body fluids against excess acid or base
   (e) Are normal salts
   1. c, d, and e   3. d and e
   2. a, b, and c   4. c and d

98. The hydrogen ion content of a solution can be shown by
   (a) Litmus paper
   (b) Sodium chloride solution
   (c) Methyl orange
   (d) Hydrogen peroxide
   (e) Phenolphthalein
   1. a, c, and e   3. a, b, and c
   2. c, d, and e   4. a, b, c, and e

99. Properties of colloids that help to differentiate them from crystalloids are
   (a) Small molecules
   (b) Nonpassage through filters
   (c) Adsorption of substances on molecular surfaces
   (d) Electrically charged particles
   (e) Low osmotic pressure
   1. c, d, and e   3. All of them
   2. b, c, and e   4. b, d, and e

100. Oxygen has many uses; some are
   (a) In anesthesia
   (b) As a disinfectant
   (c) To fill light bulbs
   (d) In cardiac failure
   (e) In respiratory diseases
   1. a, b, and e   3. b, d, and e
   2. All except c   4. All except a

101. The constant source of glucose for maintaining blood glucose at normal levels at all times is
   1. Ingested food
   2. Intestinal hydrolysis
   3. Liver glycogen
   4. Gluconeogenesis

102. Excessive loss of gastric juice due to gastric lavage or pernicious vomiting can lead to
   1. Acidosis
   2. Alkalosis
   3. Loss of osmotic pressure of the blood
   4. Loss of oxygen from the blood

103. Oxyhemoglobin is used by the body chiefly as a means of
   1. Catalytic action
   2. Oxygen transport
   3. Nitrogen transport
   4. Fat transport

104. The crossroad of metabolism where all metabolic paths meet in a common oxidation pathway is called
   1. Citric acid cycle
   2. Glycolysis
   3. Ornithene cycle
   4. Positive nitrogen balance

105. Which of the following are not found in normal urine?
     (a) Urea
     (b) Protein
     (c) Uric acid
     (d) Glucose
        1. a and b   3. b and d
        2. a and c   4. All of them
106. Fats in the body are rendered easy to digest due to the emulsifying action of
     1. Hydrolysis   3. Enzymes
     2. Bile salts   4. Proteins
107. Ammonia is produced by the kidney cells. This is excreted and helps maintain
     1. Blood clotting
     2. Osmotic pressure of the blood
     3. Acid-base balance of the body
     4. Normal red blood cell production
108. Ketone bodies appear in the blood and urine when fats are being oxidized in great amounts. This condition is associated with
     (a) Starvation
     (b) Diabetes
     (c) Positive nitrogen balance
     (d) Bone healing
        1. a and b   3. b and d
        2. a and c   4. All of them
109. Glucose $\longrightarrow$ Glycogen (in the liver); the hormone that aids this reaction is
     1. Insulin   3. Enterogastrone
     2. Epinephrine   4. Estrogen
110. Glycogen $\longrightarrow$ Glucose (in the liver); the hormone that aids this reaction is
     1. Insulin   3. ACTH
     2. Epinephrine   4. Estrogen
111. An enzyme important in carbon dioxide transport is
     1. Phosphatase
     2. Zymase
     3. Trypsin
     4. Carbonic anhydrase
112. Poor bone formation results from the lack of
     (a) Calcium
     (b) Phosphorus
     (c) Vitamin D
     (d) Parathyroid hormone
        1. a and b   3. b and d
        2. b and c   4. All of them
113. Urea is formed from the breakdown of
     1. Purines   3. Carbohydrates
     2. Proteins   4. Fats
114. An overexercised muscle that has too little oxygen supply may become sore resulting from a buildup of
     1. Butyric acid
     2. Lactic acid
     3. Aceto-acetic acid
     4. Acetone
115. A substance that acts as a poison because it unites with the iron of hemoglobin and prevents it from combining with oxygen is
     1. H_2CO_3 3. CO_2
     2. CO   4. $NaHCO_3$
116. Energy stored as ATP, ADP, and other high-energy compounds is formed chiefly by
     1. Oxidation of glucose
     2. Hydrolysis of fats
     3. Respiration
     4. Peptidation

117. An ion that acts as a catalyst in blood clotting is
     1. Fe^{+++} 3. F^-
     2. Ca^{++} 4. Cl^-
118. Thromboplastin is found in
     1. Plasma   3. Platelets
     2. Erythrocytes   4. Bile
119. A vitamin necessary for the synthesis of prothrombin by the liver is
     1. Vitamin K   3. Vitamin D
     2. Vitamin B_{12} 4. Vitamin C
120. Glycolysis
     (a) Is an anaerobic process
     (b) Converts sugars to energy
     (c) Can produce lactic acid as an end product
     (d) Releases more energy than the citric acid cycle
        1. a and b   3. a, b, and c
        2. b and d   4. All of them
121. A hormone that influences growth and maintains tissues and bones is
     1. Thyroxine   3. Heparin
     2. Insulin   4. Growth hormone
122. A hormone that regulates sexual growth and function is
     1. Oxytocin
     2. Vasopressin
     3. Gonadotropic hormone
     4. Insulin
123. Carbohydrate metabolism is regulated by
     1. Insulin
     2. Parathyroid hormone
     3. Gonadotropic hormone
     4. Oxytocin
124. Flow of gastric juices is stimulated by
     1. Enterogastrone
     2. Secretin
     3. Gastrin
     4. Enterocrinin
125. Hormones that stimulate the flow of pancreatic juice are
     (a) Cholecystokinin
     (b) Enterocrinin
     (c) Enterogastrone
     (d) Pancreozymin
     (e) Secretin
        1. a and b   3. d and e
        2. c and d   4. All of them
126. Epinephrine regulates
     (a) Heart rate
     (b) Cardiac output
     (c) Blood pressure
     (d) Muscle constriction
     (e) Blood sugar
        1. a and c   3. c, d, and e
        2. b, c, and e   4. All of them
127. Blood contains
     (a) Plasma
     (b) Erythrocytes
     (c) Leukocytes
     (d) Platelets
     (e) Enzymes
        1. a and b
        2. b and d
        3. b, c, d, and e
        4. All of them

Completion

Place the proper word or words in the space provided to complete the statement.

128. Energy is defined as _____.
129. A calorie (cal.) is _____
_____.
130. One atomic weight unit of mass (a.w.m.) is approximately equal to _____.
131. Enzymes are _____.
132. Hydrogenation of a liquid fat results in _____
133. Oxidation means
   a. _____.
   b. _____.
134. Because of its _____, water is an excellent solvent for ionic or slightly ionic substances.
135. An electrolyte is a substance that _____ and allows _____.
136. NaHCO₃ in solution would be (acid, basic, neutral) in reaction.
137. Protection from radiation is effected by
   a. _____.
   b. _____.
   c. _____.
138. Organic acids produced from hydrolysis of fats are called _____.
139. _____, _____, and _____ cannot be synthesized well enough in the body to maintain health and growth and must be taken in via the diet.
140. _____ are aldehyde or ketone derivatives of a single oxidation of polyhydric al-

cohols or compounds yielding these aldehyde or ketone derivatives upon hydrolysis.
141. _____ are polymers of alpha amino acids connected by peptide bonds.
142. A positive Benedict test shows the presence of a _____.
143. A polysaccharide polymer of glucose found in human and animal tissue is _____.
144. The main classifications of proteins are _____
145. Nucleoproteins have the following composition:
   a. _____.
   b. _____.
   c. _____.
   d. _____.
146. Enzymes are _____ in nature.
147. The purpose of digestion is _____
_____.
148. Vitamins are classified as _____.
149. The class of foods that builds body tissue is _____.
150. Carbon, hydrogen, oxygen, and nitrogen are found in _____.
151. Name the end products of protein digestion _____.
152. Name end products of carbohydrate digestion _____.
153. Name end products of fat metabolism _____.
154. Intravenous medications should be _____ to blood.

SCORES

1	5
2	6
3	7
4	8

NAME _____ DATE _____
LAST   FIRST   MIDDLE

SCHOOL _____ CITY _____

DATE OF BIRTH _____ AGE _____ SEX ___ M OR F

GRADE OR CLASS _____ INSTRUCTOR _____

NAME OF TEST _____ PART _____

DIRECTIONS: Read each question and its numbered answers. When you have decided which answer is correct, blacken the corresponding space on this sheet with the special pencil. Make your mark as long as the pair of lines, and move the pencil point up and down firmly to make a heavy black line. If you change your mind, erase your first mark completely. Make no stray marks; they may count against you.

SAMPLE:

1. Chicago is
1—1 a country
1—2 a mountain
1—3 an island
1—4 a city
1—5 a state

BE SURE YOUR MARKS ARE HEAVY AND BLACK.
ERASE COMPLETELY ANY ANSWER YOU WISH TO CHANGE.

Printed by the International Business Machines Corporation, Endicott, N. Y., U. S. A.   IBM FORM I.T.S. 1000 B 108

(Answer grid numbered 1–150, columns 1 2 3 4 5)

THE SOCIAL SCIENCES AND HISTORICAL BACKGROUND FOR NURSING

The social sciences

History and trends of nursing with emphasis on

twentieth century

THE SOCIAL SCIENCES

Arnold, M. B.: Feeling and emotion, New York, 1970, Academic Press, Inc.

Beadie, M.: A child's mind, how children learn during the critical years from birth to age five, Garden City, N. Y., 1971, Doubleday & Co., Inc.

Bernard, J., and Thompson, L.: Sociology: nurses and their patients in a modern society, ed. 8, St. Louis, 1970, The C. V. Mosby Co.

Birenbaum, W. M.: Overlive, power, poverty and the university, New York, 1969, Dell Publishing Co., Inc.

Brown, E. L.: Newer dimensions in patient care, New York, 1965, Russell Sage Foundation.

Carlson, C. E.: Behavioral concepts and nursing intervention, Philadelphia, 1970, J. B. Lippincott Co.

Carp, F. M.: A future for the aged, Austin, Tex., 1966, University of Texas Press.

Clemence, Sister M.: Existentialism: a philosophy of commitment, American Journal of Nursing 66:500, 1966.

Devries, E.: Man in rapid social change, Garden City, N. Y., 1961, Doubleday & Co., Inc. (published for the World Council of Churches).

Dobzhansky, T.: The biological basis of human freedom, New York, 1956, Columbia University Press.

Facts about nursing: a statistical summary, New York, American Nurses Association (published annually).

Fishman, J. A.: Sociolinguistics, a brief introduction, 1970, Newbury House, Publishers.

Gorton, J. V.: Behavioral components of patient care, New York, 1970, The Macmillan Co.

Growing up poor, U. S. Welfare Administration Pub. no. 13, Washington, D. C., 1966, U. S. Government Printing Office.

Heckel, R. V., and Jordan, R. M.: Psychology: the nurse and the patient, ed. 2, St. Louis, 1967, The C. V. Mosby Co.

Hoffer, E.: The ordeal of change, New York, 1963, Harper & Row, publishers.

Madigan, M. E.: Psychology: principles and applications, ed. 5, St. Louis, 1970, The C. V. Mosby Co.

Matheney, R. V., and Topalis, M.: Psychiatric nursing, ed. 5, St. Louis, 1970, The C. V. Mosby Co.

May, R., editor: Existential psychology, New York, 1967, Random House, Inc.

Mead, M.: Cultural patterns and technical change, Paris, 1953, United Nations Educational, Scientific, & Cultural Organization.

Rasmussen, S.: Technical nursing, dimensions and dynamics, Philadelphia, 1972, F. A. Davis Co.

Roger, C. R.: Client-centered therapy, Boston, 1951, Houghton Mifflin Co.

Roger, C. R.: On encounter groups, New York, 1970, Harper & Row, Publishers.

Schwartz, L. H., and Schwartz, J. L.: The psychodynamics of patient care, Englewood Cliffs, N. J., 1972, Prentice-Hall, Inc.

Silberman, C. E.: Crisis in the classroom. The remaking of American education, New York, 1971, Vintage Books, Inc., Division of Random House.

The social sciences deal with human behavior and the consequences of human behavior

1. **Social science disciplines**
A. History
B. Political science
C. Economics
D. Anthropology
E. Sociology
F. Psychology
G. Others with social application
2. **The study of social sciences and their interrelationships is a part of traditional nursing**

WHY IS ANTHROPOLOGY IMPORTANT TO NURSES?

1. **Anthropology contributes through the study of man, his culture, and interrelationships**

2. **Applies many psychological and sociologic principles in the study of culture**
A. Physical anthropology is study of the biologic origins of man and variations in species
B. Social and cultural anthropology studies the way of life of various communities and analyzes their culture

WHY IS SOCIOLOGY IMPORTANT TO NURSES?

1. **Because nurses work in social organizations**
A. Hospitals
B. Public health agencies
C. Clinics and doctors' offices
D. Extended care facilities
E. Industrial organizations
F. Schools
G. Other agencies and institutions
2. **Because doctor-nurse-patient relationships are social processes**
3. **Because professional nursing is a social system**
4. **Because nurses need to understand the world in which they live**
A. Man's behavior in his social environment
B. His values, attitudes, beliefs, and self-images
C. The social factors that affect man's behavior
   1. Similarities and differences among ethnic groups
      a. Language
      b. Religion
      c. Education
      d. Nationality
   2. Biologic differences
      a. Race
      b. Sex
      c. Age
      d. Heredity
   3. Sociocultural differences
      a. Learned behavior and its transmission

CONTRIBUTIONS OF SOCIOLOGY

1. **Sociology is social science about 100 years old, having many definitions**
2. **It is a scientific study of human group life and the results of group life**
3. **Way in which sociology can contribute to nursing education**
A. Study of social roles
B. Analysis of attitudes

C. Study of effect of group influences on the individual
D. Study of the emerging personality in social interaction
4. **Some specialized fields of sociology**
A. Family life
B. Population analysis
C. Social gerontology
D. Medical sociology
E. Race relationships
F. Criminology
G. Communication

THE SOCIOLOGIST AT WORK

1. **Scientific observation**
2. **Scientific studies (research)**
A. Experiments
B. Statistical studies
C. Questionnaires and interviews
D. Observations

WHY IS PSYCHOLOGY IMPORTANT TO NURSES?

1. **Modern psychological concepts had their origin thousands of years ago in man's efforts to understand the universe in which he lived**
2. **Psychology as a science is a product of the nineteenth century**
A. William James wrote *Principles of Psychology* in 1880; studied the will, memory, and emotions
B. William Wundt established first laboratory for study of conscious experience (Leipzig, 1897)
3. **Early schools of psychology came into existence in twentieth century**
A. Each made some contribution to the science of behavior
B. Many concepts of early schools are no longer accepted or have been modified
C. Some concepts remain controversial

SOME EARLY SCHOOLS OF PSYCHOLOGY

1. **Structuralist**
A. Based on principles that life is made up of sensations, images, feelings
B. Used introspection to learn physiologic and psychological effects of stimuli and sensations resulting from different stimuli
2. **Functionalist**
A. Used introspection
B. Expanded to include behavior and ad-

justment and to learn how man adjusts to his environment

3. Behaviorist
A. Used study of overt behavior
B. Believed behavior to be determined by stimulus and response

4. Gestaltist
A. Gestalt means "whole"
B. Emphasized idea that the whole of behavior is more important than its parts; theory formed basis for later concept of study of whole person

5. Psychoanalytic
A. Techniques of psychoanalysis were developed under leadership of Sigmund Freud, Viennese physician and psychiatrist
B. Based on belief in unconscious mental processes that influence behavior
C. Primary interest was in treatment of unstable individual (see Psychiatric nursing, Chapter 12)

CONTEMPORARY PSYCHOLOGICAL PHILOSOPHY

1. Neo-Freudian philosophy
A. The "real self"
  1. Individual has biologic potential for growth
  2. Possesses feelings, thoughts, gifts, capacities to develop real self
  3. Only the individual can accomplish this
B. The "idealized self"
  1. Indicates what the person believes he should be
  2. Thwarts development of real self
  3. Develops neurotic image of what the person thinks he should be
C. The "actual self"
  1. Includes everything that the individual is at any precise moment
D. Philosophy indicates that both the individual and the environment contribute to development of the personality and the real self

2. Existential philosophy of psychology
A. Originated in France
B. Gained importance in the United States after World War II
C. Seeks to understand man's behavior and experiences and the nature of the man who experiences
D. Places emphasis on "the emerging becoming human being" and on the idea that man is forever becoming

E. Holds that man exists in a purposeless world and that he must oppose his environment by exercising his free will
F. Stresses the worth of the individual and believes in the responsibility of the individual for shaping his own self
G. There is a wide divergence of opinion concerning philosophy, and it has many adaptations
H. Exerts considerable influence on counseling process and psychotherapy

EXPERIENTIAL LIVING*

A social movement with emphasis on social health and welfare—impact of the movement is being felt in many aspects of contemporary society, resulting in social change

1. Institutions affected by the movement
A. The family
B. Occupations and professions
C. Educational units
D. Medical care facilities
  1. Hospitals
  2. Health centers
  3. Health departments

2. Individuals affected by the movement
A. The sick person, who must share responsibility for his care and treatment and assume role of becoming well
B. Youth, seeking the meaning of life through new experiences
  1. Psychomimetic drugs
    a. Marijuana
    b. Amphetamines
    c. Lysergic acid diethylamide (LSD)
  2. Hypnosis
  3. Other means

THE PSYCHOLOGIST AT WORK

1. Studies human behavior
2. Applies psychological principles in helping individuals with problems faced in life situations
3. Nature of position determines specific duties of psychologist
A. Clinical psychology—specialty is concerned with problems of maladjustive behavior: diagnosis and, through techniques of psychotherapy, helping individual with adjustment problems
B. Abnormal psychology—is closely related to clinical psychology; applies psycho-

---

*Term used by Folta, J. R., and Deck, E. S., editors: A sociological framework for patient care, New York, 1966, John Wiley & Sons, Inc., p. 49.

logical principles for the understanding of abnormal behavior

C. Counseling psychology—helps normal persons with problems
1. Educational
2. Vocational
3. Marital
4. Other

D. Industrial psychology—uses techniques of interviewing and counseling; works with individuals or groups in social organizations
1. Business
2. Industry
3. Government agencies
4. Civic groups

COMMUNICATION AND HUMAN INTERACTION

1. **Communication—a sharing of meaningful experience through mutual response**
A. The medium of social interaction

2. **Some principles of communication**
A. Satisfaction is reduced when communication is impeded
B. Work efficiency is reduced by poor communication
C. Status may affect freedom of communication
D. Social interaction can increase liking; the more frequent interaction, the better liking
E. Full, free communication important in group decision-making
F. The language and channel of communication must be adapted to the person for whom it is intended
G. Feedback is necessary to evaluate the effectiveness of communication and guide the conversation

3. **Some barriers to effective communication**
A. Differences in language
1. Too technical for one of participants
2. Ethnic background differences
B. Lack of clarity
C. Feelings of hostility
D. Role conflict as to who does what and when
E. Failure to listen
F. Improper interpretation
G. Differences in social and educational status
H. Age
I. Variation in cultural experience

1. Social interaction with well-educated, well-traveled persons results in
a. New ideas
b. New role models
c. New skills
d. New knowledge
e. Increased confidence

4. **Contemporary media of mass communication**
A. Increase in growth and variety mass media of communication
1. Commercial television—profound influence on mass behavior of people
a. Education
b. Religion
c. Recreation
d. Health
e. Politics
f. Foreign affairs
g. Social unrest
h. Propaganda
2. Radio—8 of 10 persons listen to radio
3. Newspapers—9 of 10 persons read a newspaper at some time
4. Magazines, books, other periodicals
5. Movies
6. Person-to-person speech

5. **Doctor-nurse-patient communication**
A. Full and free communication affected by many factors
1. Cultural
2. Psychological
3. Sociologic
B. Doctor may view nurse only as technical assistant; example: doctor to nurse —"give Mr. Smith 1,000 ml. of 5% glucose solution"
C. Doctor may view nurse as administrative assistant; example: doctor to nurse—"get Mr. Smith's old record"
D. Nurse-patient communication may be impeded because of role conflict; example: patient to nurse—"why do I have to have this glucose?" and nurse to patient—"I don't know; you'll have to ask the doctor"
E. Social status of members of health team may be barrier to communication
F. Traditionally nurse taught to avoid patient involvement
G. Doctor and nurse too busy to listen to patient
H. Failure to recognize nonverbal communication

6. **Nonverbal communication**
A. May be as important as verbal communication

B. May indicate patient's distress and need for assistance
  1. Does not always indicate need for relief of *physical* distress
C. Kinds of nonverbal behavior
  1. Expressions of anxiety, pain, tension, fear
  2. Posture, gestures
  3. Irritability
  4. Uncommunicative attitude
  5. Smiling
D. Nurse is exhibiting nonverbal behavior when she
  1. Has brisk manner
  2. Ignores patient's questions
  3. Avoids question or gives short, quick, nonspecific answer

7. **Verbal behavior may indicate underlying problems**
A. Everyone has problems; patients are people with special kinds of problems
B. Patient sometimes expresses dissatisfaction about
  1. Noise
  2. Lack of nursing care
  3. Food (may show nonacceptance of diet)
  4. Pain
  5. Trivial matters
C. Patient sometimes plays role of "good patient"
  1. Creates no verbal or nonverbal evidence of problems
  2. May have numerous psychological problems
  3. Amount of nursing care patient believes he should have is determined by how he views his illness

INTERVIEWING AND COUNSELING

1. **Recognized as branch of psychology**
2. **Has a number of definitions**
A. May be considered a verbal dialogue between two persons for the purpose of changing or modifying behavior
3. **Techniques of interviewing and counseling**
A. Directive
  1. Interviewer accepts the major responsibility and determines the goals and the direction of the interview
  2. Purposes
    a. To secure information
    b. To give information
    c. To motivate or influence behavior
  3. Some basic principles
    a. Know what you wish to accomplish
    b. Avoid personal prejudice
    c. Provide for privacy
    d. Gain confidence and establish pleasant association with interviewee
    e. Develop art of listening, but keep control of interview
    f. Avoid suggesting answers to client
    g. Avoid negative questions
  4. The directive interview may be used by nurses for
    a. Taking patient's history (securing information)
    b. Teaching patient to administer his own insulin (giving information)
    c. Telling mother importance of immunization and encouraging her to bring child to clinic—as done by public health nurse (motivating or changing behavior)
B. Nondirective
  1. Client-centered; the client does the talking and is free to explore his problem
  2. Technique developed by Carl Rogers
    a. Assumes that each individual has the right to be psychologically independent and has the right to select his own goals
  3. Some basic principles
    a. Not satisfactory in all counseling situations
    b. The client has the right to his own feelings and beliefs
    c. The counselor must be able to listen
    d. Counselor must accept the whole individual
  4. The counseling process—basic attitudes required of counselor
    a. Acceptance—positive attitude toward client and his right to make decisions
    b. Permissiveness—allowing client the right to direct the interview, the right to reveal or withhold whatever he desires
    c. Confidence in the ability of the client for self-direction
  5. Techniques in nondirective counseling
    a. Establishment of rapport
    b. Reflection of feeling; counselor tries to understand feeling and attitude expressed by client
    c. Acceptance; any response should

indicate that the counselor understands, set stage for client to continue talking
  d. Counselor maintains silence; client,
     as he talks, gains insight into prob-
     lem and understanding of self
  e. Open-ended question
  f. Paraphrasing

SIMILARITIES AND DIFFERENCES AMONG ETHNIC GROUPS

1. **Language**
A. From earliest times man has sought to
   communicate with fellowmen
   1. First attempts used sounds and signs
   2. Then came spoken language
   3. Long-range communication was by
      smoke or sound of tom-tom
      a. Today communication is indicated
         by flag at half mast, siren, whistle
B. Language the means by which communication and interaction occur among all
   people
C. Language the product of the culture
   with which it evolves and the environment in which it is used
   1. Immigrants often cling to native
      language and may form cultural is-
      lands or subculture groups
   2. English-speaking people believe ev-
      eryone should speak English
   3. English-speaking people have difficul-
      ty understanding bilingualism and bi-
      culturalism
   4. People are considered civilized when
      they have a written language
   5. Translation of words may be barrier
      to individual or international under-
      standing
   6. Variations of some language are found
      among members of same nationality or
      ethnic group
D. Language the medium by which men
   attain
   1. Educational goals
   2. Scientific knowledge and skills
   3. Political ambitions
   4. Working relationships and understand-
      ing of fellowmen
   5. Through language, doctor-nurse-pa-
      tient relationships are facilitated
   6. Language the medium for patient
      teaching
E. Language the medium through which
   1. Emotional feelings—love, hate, etc.—
      are transmitted

2. Man is warned of danger or hazards
3. Thinking is stimulated, and ideas and
   concepts are transmitted
F. Patients may not understand or may mis-
   interpret the language of doctors and
   nurses
   1. May lead to anxiety, worry, and
      frustration in patients
G. Ethnic groups may speak different language from that of doctor and nurse
   1. Patient then is unable to make his
      needs known

2. **Religion**
A. The religious foundations are, in part, in
   the psychosocial personality
B. Religious beliefs in some form have existed in every culture
C. Religious leaders who met the spiritual
   needs of people have arisen in all cultures: Moses, Buddha, Jesus, Mohammed
D. Religion is universal in twentieth century
   1. Rituals, emotions, beliefs, religious be-
      havior varied
E. Evolution of modern denominations
   1. Religious protest groups formed move-
      ments
      a. Early Christian groups
      b. Protestant reform of Middle Ages
      c. Pentecostal movement of early pio-
         neer days
   2. Formation of sects by religious groups
      who were in conflict with society
      a. Became more cohesive and perma-
         nent
      b. Established code of moral ethics
   3. Denomination result of increasing
      adaptation of sect
      a. Modern denominations more co-
         operative and unite in planning for
         community religious needs
         (1) National Conference of Chris-
             tians and Jews; Catholics first
             admitted in 1968
         (2) National Council of the
             Churches of Christ in the
             United States of America
   4. Major religions of the world
      a. Roman Catholicism
      b. Protestantism
      c. Judaism
      d. Hinduism
      e. Islamism
   5. The church a religious, cultural, edu-
      cational, and social institution

a. Over ⅗ of population in the United States has church membership
b. Positive relationship exists between church membership and socioeconomic status
c. Modern church cooperates with social organizations
d. Plays a dominant role in education of children and youth
   (1) Parochial schools
   (2) Church colleges and universities
   (3) Programs of nursing
   (4) Lectures, forums, classes, etc.
e. Clergy is trained for greater role in dealing with problems
   (1) Marriage counseling
   (2) Problems of alcoholism
   (3) Problems of delinquency
   (4) Specialized training for hospital chaplains
   (5) Chaplains trained to work with youth in colleges and universities
f. Trends in modification and reform are affecting
   (1) Church ritual
   (2) Unification of denominations
   (3) Integration of ethnic and biologically different groups

F. Religion and the seriously ill or dying patient
1. Religious concepts intimately associated with life hereafter
2. Attitudes closely related to religious orientation of individual, his age, and his sex
3. Patient may feel that his illness and suffering is punishment from God
4. May be resentful—"why did God let this happen to me?"
5. May be resigned and accept illness and death as "God's will"
6. May look forward to a new life in hereafter
7. May express concern about family without him
8. May be apprehensive about what will happen in afterlife
9. Feelings about death vary among people—both the religious and the non-religious

G. Doctors and nurses may avoid the dying patient
1. Reminds them of own death and preparation for it
2. Their education emphasizes saving of life
3. Need to understand the psychological and sociologic meaning of death

3. **Education**
A. Informal education
   1. Characteristic of preliterate and primitive cultures
      a. Training for survival
   2. The young learn from their elders
   3. Same skills and crafts are passed from one generation to next
   4. Many nursing skills remain unchanged through decades and pass from one generation to next
   5. Isolated groups in twentieth century continue same skills as ancestors
B. Formal education
   1. Slow development before twentieth century
      a. Transition from training to education
   2. Formal education available only to upper social class, sexes segregated
   3. Industrial revolution required more specialized training
   4. Early schools of nursing used apprenticeship type of training
   5. Expansion of state-supported schools
   6. Federal government support to schools
      a. Elimination of racial segregation in schools
   7. Annual increase in enrollment through postgraduate level
   8. Adult education
      a. Basic academic skills
      b. Vocational skills
      c. Continuing education
   9. Transition of nursing education into academic institutions
      a. Development of postgraduate curricula in nursing
      b. Inservice and continuing education for nurses
      c. Clinical specialization on postgraduate level
C. Education and the social process
   1. Ranks individuals from high to low
   2. Determines success and failure
   3. Provides for social stratification
   4. Status-sifting, through
      a. Dean's list
      b. Honors program
      c. Special awards and scholarships

4. **Nationality**
A. Nation the unit of social organization

B. Characteristics of nationalism
  1. Strong feelings of loyalty and pride
  2. Support of country "right or wrong"
  3. Collective identity
  4. Sharing a common fate
  5. Ability to develop great economic and military efforts
C. Strength of nationalism varies among nations
  1. Variation in same country at different times
D. Ethnic groups differentiated by
  1. Common culture
  2. Strong group feeling
  3. Geographic location
  4. Common religion, language, or nationality
  5. All minority groups—Negroes, Jews, Mexicans, Cubans, etc.—are ethnic groups
E. Ethnic group structure in the United States
  1. National origin from other countries
    a. Formation of subcommunities
  2. From rural to urban
    a. Categorized as "country hick," "greenhorn," "city slicker"
  3. From slums and ghettos to middle-class living
    a. New York City stereotyped "melting pot of world"
F. Ethnic groups and nursing
  1. Within hospital
    a. Variation in reaction to illness and handicap
    b. Language barriers
    c. Family cohesiveness in illness
    d. Response to pain
    e. Superstition
    f. Racial factors
    g. Diet
      (1) Patient may have difficulty understanding use of special diets
  2. Nurse will need to understand differences and similarities among ethnic groups
    a. Provide comprehensive nursing care without regard to race, creed, or national origin
    b. Be familiar with social organizations that provide services to special ethnic groups

BIOLOGIC DIFFERENCES

1. **Race—a group having same distinctive combination of physical traits**

A. Skin color, color and texture of hair, eye fold, shape of nose, lips, contour of head, and body build
B. Primary racial stocks
  1. Mongoloid—yellow and brown
  2. Negroid—black
  3. Caucasoid—white
C. All other groupings, not as race but as social entity
D. Racist society—dominated by one group
E. Equalitarian society—all groups treated equally
F. Patterns of racial discrimination
  1. Annihilation of Jews by Nazis
  2. Genocide—ethnic group eliminated by slaughter and destruction of their culture
  3. Expulsion and partition
    a. Ethnic groups moved to Siberia by Russia
    b. United States moved Japanese to concentration camps during World War II
    c. Urban renewal—expulsion and resettlement of people
  4. Segregation and discrimination
    a. Black dominated by whites in United States
    b. Indians forced to live on reservations
    c. Caste system of India
G. Racism, discrimination, and reform movements
  1. Rise of protest groups
  2. Most modern efforts largely by blacks and Indians
  3. Characteristics of movement
    a. Political and economic pressure
    b. Demonstrations
    c. Voter registration
    d. Marches
    e. Court litigation
    f. Publicity
  4. Educational groups seeking greater control of education
H. Federal legislation to promote integration of minority groups
2. **Sex—the foundation of family life**
A. Biologic differences
  1. Conceptions—males outnumber females
  2. Abortions and stillbirths—more males lost
  3. Sex ratio greater at birth for males
  4. Infant mortality greater for males

5. Life expectancy greater at birth for females
6. Increase of females over males 33.5 million to 35.5 million by 1980
B. Predisposition to disease
1. Males more susceptible to
a. Heart attacks
b. Ulcers
c. Gout
d. Some neurologic disorders
C. Behavior problems
1. More problems related to males, in
a. Alcoholism
b. Juvenile delinquency
c. Drug addiction
d. Incorrigibility
e. Serious crimes
f. Suicide
D. Sex and changing family patterns
1. Marriage
a. In 82% of husband-and-wife families, 92.1% of husbands and wives are ages 14 to 24 years
b. Increase in marriage rates
c. Women marrying younger
d. More married students in high school
e. 25% of college students married
f. Programs of nursing admitting married students
g. Increase in sharing of responsibility in home
h. Marriage as joint career
i. Planning for parenthood
j. Legalized abortions
2. Decrease in size of family
a. Most children born before mother 30 years of age
b. Children considered an economic liability
c. Contributing factors
(1) Urbanization
(2) Increased emphasis on recreation
(3) Social mobility
(4) Increased educational aspirations
d. Contraception—a technique for limiting size of family
E. Emancipation and prejudice
1. Rights for women began in 1800
2. Women's suffrage, 1920
3. Nurses given rank and privileges in Armed Forces
4. More than 50% of women were in labor force by 1970

5. Many professions and occupations open only to men, or have only limited opportunity for women
a. Medicine
b. Law
c. Clergy
d. Commercial aviation
e. Prestige jobs in government
f. College administration
g. Hospital administration
6. Half of employed women in menial jobs or in jobs directed by men
7. More women than men in nursing
3. **Age**
A. Heavy dependency at extremes of age range
1. High birth rate and high death rate result in young population
B. American culture places value on children
1. White House Conference on Children and Youth every ten years
2. Community activities with accent on children
a. Education
b. Child study groups
c. Summer camps
d. Recreational programs
e. Health programs
f. Character building organizations
g. Others
C. Little emphasis on the aged prior to 1961
1. Some characteristics of the aged
a. More aged women than men
b. Most have limited financial resources
c. About ⅔ receive federal or state aid
d. Problems of housing, recreation
e. Many with chronic disease
D. 1971 White House Conference on Aging
1. Fourteen Conference Sections and seventeen Special Concerns Sessions made a good many overlapping, similar, and even almost identical recommendations
2. Principal recommendation: financial aid for elderly homeowners and renters
a. Property tax relief
b. Rent supplement
c. Maintenance and rehabilitation of property
d. Rent control
4. **Heredity**
A. Result of interaction of genes

1. Union of male sperm and female ovum
   a. Division of chromosomes—23 from male and 23 from female
   b. About 72,000 genes from each parent
   c. Genes from each parent paired
      (1) Combinations unlimited
   d. Traits and characteristics carried in genes
2. Matching of dissimilar genes results in intermediate characteristic
   a. One gene may prevail—*dominant*
   b. Other gene, concealed—*recessive*
      (1) May be matched with recessive gene in next generation
3. Traits and characteristics of individual result from
   a. Genes that are combined at time of fertilization
   b. Interactions of genes
   c. Environmental factors
4. Genetically, child born with potential for physiologic and psychological growth and development
B. Physical traits inherited under normal conditions
   1. Skin coloring
   2. Color and texture of hair
   3. Shape of face and head
   4. Eye color
   5. Body build
   6. Sex
   7. Brain patterns
   8. Predisposition for emotional reaction according to environmental conditions
C. Everyone carries defective genes
   1. Conditions believed to result from defective genes
      a. Hemophilia
      b. Color blindness
      c. Mental retardation
      d. Cystic fibrosis
      e. Galactosemia
      f. Phenylketonuria
   2. Environmental factors and heredity
      a. During gestation
         (1) Syphilis in mother
         (2) Rubella during pregnancy
         (3) Others being studied—mumps, hepatitis, influenza
      b. During neonatal period and infancy
         (1) Any condition resulting in structural and functional change

D. Many questions unanswered about heredity and inheritance
E. Potential for growth and development exists at birth
F. What happens after birth concerns environmental influence

SOCIOCULTURAL DIFFERENCES

Affecting any socioculture are both the social system and the concept of culture involved

1. **The social system**
A. Establishes standards for social behavior
   1. Variation among ethnic and nationality groups
      a. Some common elements
B. Regulates behavior through system of sanctions, which forms the basis for social control of behavior
   1. Positive sanctions
      a. Approval
      b. Recognition
      c. Praise
      d. Prestige
      e. Honors
   2. Negative sanctions
      a. Criticism
      b. Ridicule
      c. Legal punishment
2. **The concept of culture**
A. Lack of agreement on specific definition
B. May be considered as a system of behavior shared by a group of people
   1. Society consists of groups of people
   2. Culture—the ways in which people model their behavior, including their ideas and values
C. Folkways result from experience and are passed from one generation to next
   1. Differences between ethnic and cultural groups, and some commonalities
   2. Have weak sanctions
   3. Strong resistance to deviation
   4. Customary ways of doing things, accepted by the group and society
D. Mores—obligatory behavior
   1. Strong sanctions
      a. Condemn behavior believed wrong
      b. Equally strong in upholding what is believed right
      c. Often regulated by laws
         (1) Punishment for violation, as in murder
E. Culture-change in modern society
   1. Requires immediate handling of new situations not covered by mores

a. Regulations and ordinances
F. Subculture, a group of people set apart from the rest of society
1. May be social class—rich or poor
2. Nationality—cultural islands
3. Age—young or old
4. Ethnic groups

SOCIETY AND HEALTH CARE INSTITUTIONS

1. **Society places value on protecting selected members of its citizens in health and illness**
A. Provides for individual membership through
   1. Tax-supported and voluntary health care facilities
   2. Family welfare services
   3. Prevention and control of disease and illness
   4. Unemployment insurance
   5. Workmen's Compensation
   6. Social Security
   7. Protection of food, water, and drug supplies
   8. Public education
   9. Hospital and medical insurance
   10. Scholarships, grants, etc. for health education and training
   11. Research
   12. Medicare and Medicaid for the aged
2. **The hospital as a social institution**
A. Has a unique social structure
   1. Characteristics
      a. Formal hierarchy of authority
      b. Policies, rules, and regulations
      c. Interpersonal behavior
      d. Struggle for prestige
      e. Bureaucratic
      f. Becoming more specialized
B. Functions of the hospital
   1. Primary function
      a. Care of the sick person
      b. Physician responsible for cure of illness
      c. Increasing emphasis on medical team
   2. Secondary functions
      a. Research
      b. Teaching
      c. Acquisition, maintenance, and housing of equipment to carry out above functions
C. Culture of the hospital
   1. Sets standards for behavior of employees

a. Written policies, job analyses, etc.
   2. Sets standards for behavior of patient, who
      a. Loses customary role
      b. Is relieved of identity with larger society
      c. Has activities planned for him by others
      d. Follows time schedules not his own
      e. Is expected to conform to passive role
   3. Sets standards for family and visitors
      a. Visiting hours
      b. Rules of conduct
   4. Folkways of hospital—customary ways of doing things: nursing procedures, keeping records, etc.
   5. Mores of hospital—prohibitions and obligations
      a. May prohibit smoking on duty
      b. Include obligation to be on duty on time
   6. May apply positive or negative sanctions

SOCIALIZED HEALTH BEHAVIOR

1. **Perceptions of health or illness vary among individuals, ethnic groups, and cultures**
A. Stigma may be attached to certain illnesses
   1. Tuberculosis
   2. Venereal disease
   3. Cancer
   4. Mental illness
B. Religious subculture groups may vary in beliefs, attitudes, and practices in health and illness
C. Pain—groups show differences in perception, judgment, and response
2. **The individual views his health and illness as intimate and private**
A. May be reluctant to discuss his health problems
B. Anxiety may interfere with communicating health problem
C. Denies symptoms if threatened by
   1. Loss of member—breast or extremity
   2. Altered physical function—as in colostomy
   3. Disfigurement
3. **Stress and physiologic reactions**
A. Environmental stress results in strain on organism, in
   1. Reactivating tuberculosis infection
   2. Peptic ulcer

3. Coronary artery disease
4. Neurodermatoses
5. Ulcerative colitis
6. Psychic vomiting
7. Psychoneurotic symptoms
8. Excessive smoking and alcoholism

B. During serious illness, individual is concerned with survival
  1. Postoperative patients may react to stress by overt behavior, being
    a. Resentful
    b. Complaining
    c. Irritable
    d. Uncooperative
    e. Angry
  2. Anticipatory behavior in preoperative patient is factor in postoperative behavior
    a. Emotional reaction greater
      (1) When preoperative level of fear is low
      (2) When preoperative level of fear is unusually high
    b. Fear may have origin in repressed childhood fear
      (1) Reassurance by nurse may be ineffective
C. Psychological approach may teach individual how to handle stress situations

GROWTH AND DEVELOPMENT

1. **All growth and development integrated and coordinated; overall rate throughout life-span reflects interplay of heredity and environment**
A. Physical growth and development
  1. Begins with conception
  2. Major physical growth complete by age 18 to 21, although anatomic and physiologic changes are lifelong process
  3. Is both quantitative and qualitative
  4. May be affected by intrinsic and extrinsic factors
  5. May be characterized by acceleration, regression, quiescence, peaks, and plateaus
  6. Sequence is usually predictable
B. Maturation directed toward total integration of self
  1. Begins with conception
  2. Continuous throughout life
  3. Determines or influences individual behavior
  4. Emphasizes intrinsic factors
C. Maturation and learning

  1. Infant learns to creep, crawl, stand, walk, run, jump
  2. Stage of maturation determines readiness for learning
  3. Neuromuscular development proceeds from simple to complex
  4. Intellectual and psychosocial developments also proceed sequentially
2. **Early responses of infant**
A. Violent stimuli at birth result in distress, evidenced by crying
B. Relief from frustration, tension, and discomfort sought by
  1. Crying
    a. Brings security, soothing emotions, protection
  2. Sucking—source of pleasure and satisfaction
    a. Provides relief from tension
    b. Relieves pain
    c. Physiologic need greatest in first 3 or 4 months
C. Startle or Moro response—an emergency reaction
  1. Results in physical activity: kicking, crying, muscular contraction of fingers, etc.
  2. Infant may learn fear, anger, or need for caution
D. Gradual substitution of emotions
  1. Smiling, for crying
  2. Delight, for emergency reaction
E. Mother provides first emotional climate for infant
F. Social development evident at about 1 month when infant distinguishes self and non-self; recognizes mother
3. **The young child**
A. Is at age of emotional disturbances
  1. Marked by frustration, conflict, aggressiveness, fear, temper tantrums, jealousy, and anxiety
B. Seeks to be independent
C. Wants approval and acceptance by family
D. Begins to establish social contacts outside family
E. Develops sense of right and wrong
F. Through maturation, child increases degree of
  1. Responsibility
  2. Self-direction
  3. Self-control
G. Factors contributing to social growth and development
  1. Emotional environment of home

2. Socioeconomic status
3. Culture
4. Parental maturity
5. Parental expectations
6. Parental acceptance or rejection

4. **The older child**
A. Socialization accelerated
   1. Social contacts of same sex
   2. Stability of friendships
   3. Competitive interests
   4. Common interests in groups and gangs
   5. Increase in frustration
      a. Outbursts of anger
      b. Frequent quarrels
      c. Increased desire for independence

5. **Preteen period**
A. Changes in social behavior patterns
   1. Increase in romantic interests
   2. Less rejection of opposite sex
   3. Changing patterns result from
      a. Overlapping and flexibility of sex roles in modern society
B. Common interests developing from increased social interaction, in
   1. Schools
   2. Churches
   3. Community organizations
C. Increased emphasis on equality between sexes
   1. Socioeconomic status
   2. Education
   3. Occupational opportunity
D. Strong desire for conformity
E. Increase in social pressures

6. **Adolescence—arbitrary grouping within total life-span**
A. Earlier, emphasis placed on psychology of period
   1. Adjustment to physiologic changes
   2. Adjustment and adaptation to accepted mores established by society
B. Contemporary trend directed toward sociologic factors of period
   1. Individual considered as inexperienced adult
   2. Qualified for full participation in society
      a. Needs to gain experience while participating
C. Adolescent given minority status in contemporary society; is age-separated and age-segregated
   1. Lack of economic opportunity
      a. Stereotyped as inexperienced and irresponsible
      b. Rejected as unsuitable for adult status in economic society
   2. Legal restrictions about
      a. Driving an automobile
      b. Voting
      c. Attending public school
   3. High school and college keep individual out of economic competition
D. Attitudes toward authority often hostile and rebellious
E. More willing to break with traditional social norms
F. Develops many attitudes, often inconsistent
   1. Attitudes develop from and out of social environment
G. Religious concepts change
H. Group membership usually with those of same economic status
I. Some results of faulty socialization
   1. Delinquency
   2. Crime
   3. Dropping out of school
   4. Subculture groups
   5. Mental illness

7. **Maturity (adulthood)**
A. Basic status and concerns
   1. Physical growth complete
   2. Vocational choice, capability, and adjustment
   3. Pairing, marriage, or other arrangements
   4. Goals and sense of values
   5. Utilizing potential to best advantage
   6. Making discriminating choices
   7. Having confidence and being socially adequate
B. Emotional maturity
   1. Is less troubled by stress situations
      a. Recovers from stress more readily
   2. Can face life and problems realistically
   3. Exercises restraints and directs feelings into acceptable channels
   4. Makes independent decisions
   5. Accepts self and others
   6. Recognizes needs of others
   7. Has ability to make long-term plans
   8. Lives in harmony with mores of society

8. **Subculture of aged in American culture**
A. Definition—subculture is group having
   1. Commonalities among members
   2. Little or no interaction with other groups

B. Characteristics of subculture of aged
1. Social alienation
   a. Limited interaction with children and young people
   b. Many believe society only for young people
   c. Families tend to place aged in nursing homes or institutions
2. Disengagement
   a. Solitude
   b. Social isolation
   c. Loneliness
3. Segregation
   a. Increasing number of nursing homes, retirement homes, housing projects, senior citizens groups, organizations, etc.
      (1) Set individual apart from larger society
4. Social welfare and the aged as a social problem
   a. Society not ready for large numbers of aged
      (1) Problems with society, not with aged
      (2) Chronic health and illness
      (3) Government assistance programs for aged
   b. Aging group—individual's consciousness
      (1) Is aware of being or becoming old
      (2) Recognizes deprivation he is subject to
      (3) Feels positive relationship with age group because of deprivation
      (4) In self-evaluation, compares self with others in age group under similar conditions
C. Ways aged may meet stress
1. Defend self from devaluation by withdrawing from society
2. Defend self by paranoid thinking
   a. Interpret social process as important to his personal interests
3. Feel increased psychological tensions, with resultant
   a. Psychosomatic illness
   b. Increasing difficulty in adaptation
   c. Changes in attitude—become self-assertive and domineering or feel loss of self-confidence and self-worth
   d. Increase in commitment to mental hospitals

4. Many persons adapt to age and social change and make valuable contributions to society

SUBNORMAL GROWTH AND DEVELOPMENT

1. Mental retardation
A. Classification
   1. Profound
   2. Severe
   3. Moderate
   4. Mild
B. Characteristics
   1. Reduced intellectual functioning
   2. Impaired ability to adapt to social environment
   3. Decreased rate of maturation
   4. Impaired learning potential
C. Causes
   1. Genetic factors
   2. Chromosome anomalies
   3. Environmental factors
      a. Fetal life
         (1) Congenital deformities
         (2) Hydrocephalus
         (3) Microcephalus
      b. Maternal infection
         (1) Syphilis
         (2) Rubella
         (3) Toxoplasmosis
      c. Toxic agents
         (1) X-ray therapy
         (2) Lead poisoning
         (3) Hemolytic jaundice, resulting from blood transfusion with incompatible blood
      d. Birth injury
         (1) Cerebral injuries
         (2) Anoxia and asphyxia at birth
      e. Premature birth, because of
         (1) Toxemia of pregnancy
         (2) Hemorrhagic complications of pregnancy
      f. Vitamin deficiency during early pregnancy
      g. Hormonal diseases
         (1) Diabetes
         (2) Hypothyroidism
      h. Socioeconomic deprivation
D. Retardation types, arbitrarily based on IQ
   1. Profound—IQ below 20
   2. Severe—IQ 20 to 35
   3. Moderate—IQ 36 to 52
   4. Mild—IQ 53 to 68
E. Increased interest in mental retardation

1. Construction of centers for research
   a. Federal government support
2. Training of professional persons—physicians, nurses, teachers—to work with retarded
3. Programs through Social and Rehabilitation Service for training in skills
4. Prevention and treatment of infectious diseases that injure fetus
5. Programs for improved socialization, dependent upon degree of retardation

F. No medical treatment to increase intellectual growth

REVIEW QUESTIONS FOR THE SOCIAL SCIENCES
Multiple choice

Read each question carefully and consider all possible answers. When you have decided which answer is best, blacken in the corresponding space on the answer sheet. There is only one best answer for each question.

Note: Social sciences are not pure sciences, as chemistry is. Therefore, the outcome may not be predictable in dealing with human behavior. What may appear as a correct solution in one situation may be totally wrong in another or under different circumstances.

Situation: Janet, age 14, was the youngest of 10 children. Standard intelligence tests indicated that she was mildly retarded. Her mother had a violent temper and dominated the family. Her father had had a criminal record. Both parents quarreled a great deal. Janet attended regular school. She had a tendency to daydream and was more or less tolerated by the teacher and the other children. She was unable to keep up with her classwork, and nothing was expected of her. Her mother felt that school was a waste of time anyway, which kept Janet from helping with household chores. It was discovered that Janet had broken a window and entered the home of wealthy people who were traveling abroad. Each evening when she entered the home she dressed herself in the evening gowns and other bits of finery, paraded before the mirrors, and reposed on the luxurious furniture. She then carefully replaced everything and slipped out of the home. See following questions.

1. Some conclusions that might be drawn from the situation are that Janet
   1. Had inherited criminal tendencies from her father
   2. Was indulging in fantasy play normal for a child her age
   3. Showed signs of mental, emotional, and social deprivation
   4. Tried to learn through experience how people of high socioeconomic background live

2. Characteristic behavior of normal children in Janet's age group includes
   1. Resentment and total rejection of parental authority
   2. Eagerness to please
   3. Lack of understanding of right and wrong
   4. Desire for independence, coupled with need for parental guidance

3. If Janet is admitted to the hospital as a result of her behavior pattern, the nurse may expect that she will predominantly show signs of
   1. Withdrawal   3. Gregariousness
   2. Aggression   4. Hostility

4. In terms of the mild mental retardation exhibited by Janet, it is likely that
   1. The symptoms are irreversible
   2. She will need to be institutionalized
   3. Drug therapy will increase her capabilities
   4. Placing her into a stimulating, loving environment may increase her capabilities

5. Daydreaming is indulged in by
   1. Mentally ill individuals only
   2. All people from time to time
   3. People who have adapted to a poor environment
   4. Children, primarily

6. Because of the climate in Janet's home, Janet's behavior may be a sign of need for
   1. Relaxation of discipline
   2. Increasing discipline
   3. Acceptance
   4. Educational stimulation

7. It can be assumed that, without alteration in Janet's home environment, Janet at 21 will show
   1. Complete adjustment to her environment
   2. Regression to level of a 6-year-old
   3. Continued impaired ability to function on her age level
   4. Rapidly increasing ability to master intellectual skills

8. The environment in the classroom has contributed in which manner to Janet's development? It has
   1. Provided encouragement of growth by special attention
   2. Increased her learning ability by allowing her to pursue her daydreams
   3. Developed her scholastic ability by recognition of achievement
   4. Inhibited her learning potential by ignoring her

9. Mental retardation is due to
   1. Hereditary influences only
   2. Environmental influences only
   3. A mixture of genetic and environmental influences
   4. A variety of causes, among which both heredity and environment play a part

10. A major aspect in treatment of persons who are mildly to moderately retarded is to
    1. Place the individual in an institution with people of similar ability
    2. Provide intensive psychotherapy
    3. Provide opportunity for socialization with normal individuals
    4. Provide group therapy, using nondirective techniques

11. Schools of theology are placing increasing emphasis on the psychosocial functions of clergymen. All of the following are included except
    1. Marriage counseling
    2. Work as hospital chaplain
    3. Counseling psychology
    4. Organizing church schools of nursing
12. Doctor-nurse communication is often impeded by
    1. Role conflict
    2. Trivial matters
    3. Social status
    4. Religious affiliation
13. Barriers to doctor-patient communication may result from all of the following except
    1. Technical language
    2. Economic difference
    3. Ethnic background
    4. Educational status
14. Lack of communication between nurse and patient may be the result of
    1. The hospital social system
    2. Patient thinks nurse doesn't know
    3. Nurse responds only to doctor
    4. Patient feels nurse is too busy to listen to him
15. The hospital is a social institution. Its primary function is
    1. Research
    2. Training nurses
    3. Training doctors
    4. The care of sick people
16. Nurses need to understand the world in which they live. Understanding may be acquired through all the following, except
    1. Attending a university school of nursing
    2. Interest and participation in the creative arts
    3. Travel
    4. The culture of other hospitals
17. This decade has been considered a crucial period in American society. Some of the reasons for this are listed. Which is the one exception?
    1. Anti-Vietnam war movements
    2. Leadership of youth in Civil Rights
    3. The "hippie" movement
    4. The conservative elements in politics

Situation: Oweenee, an American Indian woman, age 34, believed to belong to the Cherokee tribe, was admitted to the Indian hospital. She appeared to be quite ill and the doctor wanted to question her about her illness. The doctor and the nurses asked Oweenee numerous questions, to which she made no reply. She remained completely silent and did not indicate that she even understood what was being said to her. Finally the doctor brought a Cherokee Indian interpreter to the bedside. It was then discovered that Oweenee was not Cherokee but belonged to the Creek tribe. The Cherokees and the Creeks do not speak the same language and do not understand each other. Frequently they do not learn the English language, and the English-speaking people rarely learn the Indian language. Questions 18 through 24 are related to this situation.

18. Sociologic concepts that may be drawn from the above situation include
    1. American Indians are an ethnic group
    2. They are always bilingual
    3. Their numbers are decreasing
    4. Because of their skin color they belong to the Negroid race
19. In general, the American Indians may be considered a
    1. Distinct race, economically deprived, segregated
    2. Distinctive, economically deprived group, having high crime rate
    3. Minority group, having high crime rate, segregated
    4. Minority group, segregated, socioeconomically deprived
20. Factors that affect Oweenee's hospitalization include her
    1. Belonging to a different culture
    2. Language as barrier to communication
    3. Hostility toward the doctor
    4. Genetic characteristics
21. The number of American Indians in the United States was placed at 524,000 in 1960. Indications are that their number is
    1. Remaining stable
    2. Decreasing
    3. Disappearing through intermarriage
    4. Increasing faster than that of the general population
22. When a patient from a minority and socially deprived economic group is admitted to the hospital, the nurse may expect that
    1. Patient will be demanding
    2. Anxiety and fear will be present
    3. Behavior will be passive
    4. Patient is probably mentally retarded
23. Oweenee's inability to understand the Cherokee language is an example of
    1. Variation of language among the same ethnic groups
    2. Subculture of ethnic groups
    3. The translation barrier
    4. Lack of education
24. Oweenee's language is the product of her culture and is
    1. An example of bilingualism
    2. Combined with the effect of domination of one cultural group over another
    3. Combined with the influence of a common culture
    4. Influenced and changed by culture of the country
25. The predisposition toward emotional behavior is
    1. Inherited
    2. The result of environmental influences
    3. Based on the specific social system
    4. Fashioned by genetic and environmental forces
26. All of the following are examples of ways in which society protects the health of its citizenry except
    1. Control of food and drugs
    2. Provision of health care facilities
    3. Financial assistance to institutions of higher education

4. Support of programs to educate health care workers
27. In the nondirective technique of counseling, the counselor recognizes that he must
    1. Control the interview
    2. Allow the client to direct the interview
    3. Do most of the talking
    4. Be concerned only with attitudes
28. The psychological reaction of a patient to a nursing procedure may be affected by the timing of instruction given to the patient. Anxiety and stress is lessened if information is given
    1. Several hours before the procedure
    2. After the procedure
    3. Just before the procedure
    4. At no time
29. The predisposition for emotional behavior may be described by all the following except
    1. Totally dependent upon the environment
    2. An inherited trait
    3. The result of the social system
    4. Caused by negative sanctions
30. The extent to which society seeks to protect the health of its citizens is evidenced by all except one of the following
    1. Economic services to depressed families
    2. Assistance programs for the aged
    3. Provision of medical care facilities
    4. Limiting consumer control
31. Characteristics of the modern hospital may include all the following except one
    1. Membership in APHA
    2. Hierarchy of authority
    3. Training student nurses
    4. Bureaucratic
32. The hospital is a social organization and the following statements are correct except for
    1. Has its own culture
    2. Has its own folkways and mores
    3. Controls the cure of illness
    4. Establishes negative and positive sanctions
33. The behavior of the hospitalized patient may be affected by all except
    1. Ethnic differences
    2. Biologic differences
    3. Socioeconomic differences
    4. Psychosocial growth and development
34. Doctor-nurse interaction may be impeded because of all except one of the following
    1. Role conflict
    2. Age
    3. Social status
    4. Educational background

Situation: Mrs. H had been scheduled for surgery. She received a bedtime sedative to be repeated at 6:00 A.M. When the nurse went in at 6:00 A.M. to administer the medication, Mrs. H stated "I haven't slept all night." The nurse had checked several times during the night and each time had found Mrs. H sleeping.

35. The nurse should recognize Mrs. H's statement as
    1. Indicating an underlying problem
    2. A deliberate fabrication
    3. A sign of her wanting sympathy
    4. A sign of her being afraid she will die
36. The situation could be handled best by

1. Calling her religious counselor
2. Leaving the room without comment
3. Guiding and directing the conversation
4. Providing a climate in which Mrs. H may continue talking
37. The basis for nondirective counseling was the work done by
    1. Sigmund Freud   3. William Wundt
    2. Carl Rogers   4. Karen Horney

Situation: Agnes wrote the following in her autobiography. The socioeconomic status of my family is middle class and my family is dominated by my mother. My parents argue a great deal which makes me feel very insecure because I don't know whom to take sides with. I have a feeling of frustration and resentment and sometimes I feel as though I can't stand any more of it. During my early childhood I had few playmates and my first social contacts outside of my family were made in church and Sunday school. I gained prestige and status by playing the piano for Sunday school. While in high school I wanted to play basketball but had to accept the fact that I did not have the ability to play. I became resentful and utilized escape mechanisms. I have never been able to completely adjust to that situation. Although I am in college now, I fear new experiences and become frustrated.

38. Quarreling in the home frequently is the result of
    1. Problems in authority
    2. Difference in social status
    3. Unemployment
    4. Emotional instability
39. Society is competitive. All human beings compete in one way or another. Through competition, Agnes had hoped to
    1. Avoid conflict with peer groups
    2. Develop the "real self"
    3. Develop a feeling of security
    4. Achieve status
40. Cooperation is psychologically important to each individual. When cooperation and competition are in conflict, emotional behavior results. Agnes displayed emotional behavior by
    1. Seeking new ways of competing
    2. Becoming resentful of others
    3. Dropping out of school
    4. Daydreaming
41. It may be assumed that the fear, frustration, and insecurity that Agnes admits resulted, in part, from
    1. Apparent immaturity
    2. Social conflict in the home
    3. Socioeconomic status of her family
    4. Lack of educational goals
42. To help Agnes overcome her feelings of fear and frustration she might
    1. Play basketball in college
    2. Be referred for counseling
    3. Get a job and make new friends
    4. Live in a college dormitory
43. Apparently one of the most satisfying experiences in Agnes' life was playing the piano in Sunday school. Satisfaction was felt because this
    1. Gave her status and prestige

2. Provided an escape from competition
3. Helped develop the "idealized self"
4. Provided an escape from home

44. Fear and apprehension among hospital patients may result from all of the following except
   1. Fear of incurable disease
   2. Ability to adjust to reality
   3. Worry over conversation between doctors and nurses
   4. The impersonal attitude of nurses

45. Social change in education is evidenced by all of the following except
   1. Increase in school dropouts
   2. Transition of nursing education into colleges
   3. Decreased emphasis on adult education
   4. Elimination of racially segregated schools

46. The nurse in the hospital may expect to find the following among different ethnic groups except
   1. Difference in response to pain
   2. The same psychological reaction to illness
   3. Language barriers
   4. Difference in skin coloring

47. Social protest groups have existed throughout history. They have differed in cause, composition, and methods. Some early protest movements were among
   1. Agricultural workers
   2. Religious groups
   3. Universities
   4. Subculture groups

48. Many modern protest groups have arisen because of conflict among
   1. Religious groups
   2. Races
   3. Court decisions
   4. Educational backgrounds

49. The birth rate in the United States is declining. One general reason for this is
   1. Increase in abortions
   2. Use of contraceptives
   3. Planned parenthood clinics
   4. Children being considered an economic liability

50. When birth and death rates are low, we may expect
   1. An increase in the number of elderly persons
   2. An increase in the number of persons of age 15 to 25
   3. A stable population
   4. More marriages at young age

51. Biologic differences between sexes indicate that
   1. Males at age 25 outnumber females
   2. Life expectancy at birth is greater for females
   3. Life expectancies at birth are equal
   4. Infant mortality is greater for females

52. Studies indicate that family patterns are changing. The only one of the following not revealed is
   1. Husband and wife are younger
   2. Decrease in social mobility
   3. Women marrying younger
   4. Increase in marriage rates

53. Although more male than female infants are born, there are differences in longevity that may in part be attributed to all of the following except

1. Increased mortality rate among males
2. Males' predisposition to certain diseases
3. More suicide among males
4. Increase in technology

54. During periods of anger or fear the following physiologic changes may be expected to occur, except for which one?
   1. Increase of glucose in the blood
   2. Autonomic nervous system in control
   3. Disturbance of homeostasis
   4. Lower metabolic rate

55. Anger results from
   1. Jealousy   3. Frustration
   2. Conditioning   4. Internal stimuli

56. John, age 4 years, while visiting with a neighbor talked at length about a big black bear that lived in the woods back of his house. The neighbor knew that no bear lived in the woods. John's imagination about the bear is
   1. An example of lying
   2. Due to lack of intelligence
   3. Probably due to conditioning
   4. Normal for his age

57. Fears among school age children are least related to which of the following?
   1. Failure in school   3. Physical danger
   2. Ridicule   4. Family mobility

58. How a person feels about death may be least related to
   1. His age and sex
   2. His socioeconomic status
   3. The church he belongs to
   4. His ethnic group

59. The seriously ill or dying patient may exhibit the following types of behavior, except for
   1. Resentment   3. Apprehension
   2. Resignation   4. Euphoria

60. If similar genes are matched at the time of fertilization, the characteristic in the offspring will be
   1. Dominant
   2. Recessive
   3. Intermediate
   4. Determined by fetal environment

61. Defective genes may be carried by
   1. The female only
   2. The male only
   3. Mentally retarded persons only
   4. Everyone

62. The psychophysiologic reactions to stress may contribute to all except which one of the following?
   1. Peptic ulcer
   2. Juvenile delinquency
   3. Coronary artery disease
   4. Reactivation of tuberculosis

63. Immaturity in adulthood may be evidenced through
   1. Inability to make decisions
   2. Ability to make long-range plans
   3. Self-confidence
   4. Mental illness

64. A mature adult will have the feeling of
   1. Social restraints
   2. Social isolation
   3. Social adequacy
   4. Psychosocial problems

65. Social trends that have tended to categorize the elderly as a subculture include all except

1. Senior citizens groups
2. Increase in number of aged women
3. Isolation in nursing homes
4. Segregation in housing projects
66. Social factors that may tend to counteract subculture of the aged include all of these except
    1. Increased interaction with family
    2. Employment
    3. Active resistance toward aging
    4. More old-timers clubs
67. Organizations such as senior citizens groups and golden age clubs tend to
    1. Provide job placement
    2. Be controlled by power structure
    3. Stereotype the elderly person
    4. Emphasize "grandparent" role
68. One of the *most crucial* psychosocial adjustments that the elderly person must make is adjustment to
    1. Occupational retirement
    2. Increased family responsibilities
    3. Social embarrassment
    4. Racial integration
69. A subculture is always one in which members have the following characteristics
    1. Are of the same nationality
    2. Have little or no interaction with other groups
    3. Are persons of the same economic status
    4. Are persons of the same ethnic patterns
70. The aged person may react negatively to a stress situation by
    1. Withdrawing from society
    2. Accepting deprivation

3. Identifying with age group
4. Developing leisure activities
71. When an elderly person is placed in a nursing home, he is likely to
    1. Join a golden age club
    2. Feel more secure
    3. Achieve status
    4. Undergo depersonalization
72. In the school of nursing, the nursing student will be introduced to the study of human behavior through the study of all the following except
    1. Psychology
    2. Psychiatric nursing
    3. Sociology
    4. Anatomy and physiology
73. The psychosocial health behavior of some persons may be affected by all of these except
    1. Economic deprivation
    2. Feelings of stigma
    3. Mores of the culture
    4. Hospital visiting hours
74. Mortality from breast cancer may result, in part, from
    1. Denial of symptoms   3. Anxiety
    2. Response to pain   4. Overt behavior
75. The preoperative patient who shows little or no fear of the surgical procedure may be expected to
    1. Show no postoperative fear
    2. Require more assurance from the nurse
    3. Have a greater postoperative emotional reaction
    4. Develop involutional psychotic reaction

SCORES

1	5
2	6
3	7
4	8

NAME _____ AGE _____ SEX _____ M OR F

LAST   FIRST   MIDDLE   DATE _____

DATE OF BIRTH _____

SCHOOL _____ CITY _____

GRADE OR CLASS _____ INSTRUCTOR _____

PART _____

NAME OF TEST _____

DIRECTIONS: Read each question and its numbered answers. When you have decided which answer is correct, blacken the corresponding space on this sheet with the special pencil. Make your mark as long as the pair of lines, and move the pencil point up and down firmly to make a heavy black line. If you change your mind, erase your first mark completely. Make no stray marks; they may count against you.

SAMPLE:

1—1 a country
1—2 a mountain
1—3 an island
1—4 a city
1—5 a state

1. Chicago is

BE SURE YOUR MARKS ARE HEAVY AND BLACK.
ERASE COMPLETELY ANY ANSWER YOU WISH TO CHANGE.

Printed by the International Business Machines Corporation, Endicott, N. Y., U. S. A.

IBM FORM I. T. S. 1000 B 108

5

HISTORY AND TRENDS OF NURSING WITH EMPHASIS ON TWENTIETH CENTURY

Abdellah, F. G., Beland, I. L., Martin, A., and Matheney, R. V.: Patient-centered approaches to nursing, New York, 1960, The Macmillan Co.

American Nurses Association: First position paper on education for nursing, American Journal of Nursing 65:106, 1965.

Anderson, B. E.: Nursing education in junior colleges, Philadelphia, 1966, J. B. Lippincott Co.

Bixler, R. W., and Bixler, G. K., editors: Administration for nursing education in a period of transition, New York, 1954, G. P. Putnam's Sons.

Bridgeman, M.: Collegiate education for nursing, New York, 1953, Russell Sage Foundation.

Bridges, D. C.: A history of the International Council of Nurses: the first sixty-five years—1899-1964, Philadelphia, 1967, J. B. Lippincott Co.

Bullough, V. L., and Bullough, B.: The emergence of modern nursing, ed. 2, New York, 1969, The Macmillan Co.

Cafferty, K. W., and Sugarman, L. K.: Stepping stones to professional nursing, ed. 5, St. Louis, 1971, The C. V. Mosby Co.

Committee on the Grading of Nursing Schools: Nursing schools today and tomorrow, New York, 1937, National League for Nursing.

Griffin, G. J., and Griffin, J. K.: Jensen's history and trends of professional nursing, ed. 6, St. Louis, 1969, The C. V. Mosby Co.

Haynes, I.: N.L.N. at ten, Nursing Outlook 10:372, June, 1962.

MacDonald, G.: Development and accreditation in collegiate nursing education, Philadelphia, 1965, J. B. Lippincott Co.

Marshall, H. E.: Dorothea Dix: forgotten samaritan, New York, 1967, Russell Sage Foundation.

Matheney, R.: Can nursing live with open admissions? American Journal of Nursing 70:2561, 1970.

Montag, M.: Cooperative research project in junior and community college education for nursing, New York, 1952, McGraw-Hill Book Co., Inc.

Montag, M.: Community college education for nursing, New York, 1959, McGraw-Hill Book Co., Inc.

National Commission for Study of Nursing and Nursing Education, J. P. Lysaught, director: An abstract for action, New York, 1970, McGraw-Hill Book Co.

National League for Nursing: Criteria for the evaluation of educational programs in nursing leading to an associate degree, New York, 1962, The League.

Nursing and nursing education in the United States, report of the Rockefeller Committee for the Study of Nursing Education, New York, 1923, The Macmillan Co.

Olson, E. V.: Education—for what? American Journal of Nursing 70:1508, 1970.

Roberts, M. M.: American nursing, New York, 1954, The Macmillan Co.

Roberts, M. M.: American nursing history and interpretation, New York, 1961, The Macmillan Co.

Rogers, M. E.: Reveille in nursing, Philadelphia, 1964, F. A. Davis Co.

Smith, D. W.: Some problems of baccalaureate programs, American Journal of Nursing 70:120, 1970.

Spalding, E. K., and Notter, L. E.: Professional nursing, ed. 8, Philadelphia, 1970, J. B. Lippincott Co.

Walsh, M. E.: N.L.N. faces the seventies (editorial), Nursing Outlook 18:27, March, 1970.

Wilson, A. V.: A nurse in the Yukon, New York, 1966, Dodd, Mead & Co.

ABBREVIATIONS

ANA	American Nurses' Association
AAIN	American Association of Industrial Nurses
ACSN	Association of Collegiate Schools of Nursing
ARC	American Red Cross
ICN	International Council of Nurses
NLN	National League for Nursing
NLNE	National League of Nursing Education
NOPHN	National Organization of Public Health Nursing
NSNA	National Student Nurses' Association
USPHS	United States Public Health Service
WHO	World Health Organization

CURRENT TRENDS AFFECTING NURSING

1. **Changes in nursing**
A. Legal changes in definition of nursing practice
   1. Nurses require improved preparation and continued education
      a. Eventually all nursing education will be under aegis of educational institutions
      b. Nurses make independent, critical decisions
      c. Increasing emphasis is placed on psychological, sociologic, and rehabilitative factors in nursing
   2. Nurses must understand wide range of new drugs and treatments, and the operation of mechanical equipment
B. Impact of *ANA position paper* reflects change in preparation
   1. Many diploma schools closing
   2. Increase in associate degree and baccalaureate programs
   3. Steady increase in master's and doctoral programs
C. Economic factors
   1. Nurses more assertive; are seeking
      a. Improvements in patient care opportunities

b. Improved working conditions
   2. Collective bargaining attempted through professional organizations
   3. Efforts by unions to organize nurses, health workers
   4. Economics of professional education, scholarships, government subsidy
D. Research
   1. More nurses engaged in research in nursing
   2. Results of research being implemented in nursing education and in improvement of patient care
E. Technology and effects in nursing
   1. Electronic monitoring and computers
   2. Specialized care units, such as
      a. Cardiopulmonary units
      b. Intensive care units
      c. Inhalation therapy units
   3. Aerospace nursing
2. **Changes in medical practice**
A. Proportional decrease in physicians in general medical practice
   1. Change in medical school curricula
   2. Many enter full-time research, teaching, and administration
   3. Increase in medical specialization
B. Progress in preventive medicine and health care
   1. Immunizing agents for infectious disease
   2. Immunosuppressive drugs and radiation
   3. Increase in knowledge of human physiologic function during health
C. More knowledge about prolonged illness and chronic disease
   1. Dialyzing techniques
   2. Organ transplants
   3. Impact of such illness on person and on family
D. Progress in surgery
   1. Safer anesthesia
   2. More extensive complex surgery
E. Technical and professional advances in aerospace medicine increase knowledge of human function under stress
F. Greater variety of paraprofessionals
3. **Social change**
A. Increase and change in population
   1. Number of persons age 65 and older increasing
   2. Decrease in mortality during infancy and childhood
   3. Decline in birth rate in many areas
B. Demand for improved health care

1. Increase in number of hospital beds and health centers
C. Urbanization and ecologic shifts intensify health problems
D. Current trends likely to continue for some time, with intensification possible

SOME EARLY NURSING HISTORY
1. **Linked to social and cultural structure**
A. Graeco-Roman and Medieval Periods
   1. Major influences
      a. Religious
      b. Military
B. Post-Reformation Era: status of women very low
C. Period of early social reforms
   1. Early influences in nursing
      a. Protestant nursing sisters
      b. Sisters of Mercy
      c. Deaconess movement started in 1836 at Kaiserswerth, Germany
      d. Work of Florence Nightingale had profound effect on nursing
   2. Industrial Revolution and social reforms
   3. Scholars sought to understand the human body and the cause of diseases
2. **Early schools of nursing in the United States**
A. New England Hospital for Women and Children, 1872
   1. Under direction of Dr. Susan Dimock and Dr. Marie Zakrzewski
   2. Linda Richards, first graduate
B. Three schools organized in 1873
   1. Bellevue, New York
   2. Connecticut Training School, New Haven; later gave way to Yale School of Nursing
   3. Boston Training School; later became Massachusetts General Hospital Training School
C. Johns Hopkins Hospital School of Nursing, 1889; Isabel Hampton, director
D. Illinois Training School for Nurses, Chicago, 1880; autonomous school; closed in 1929 when Cook County Hospital School of Nursing came into existence
E. By 1880, there were 15 schools in the United States

NURSING LEADERSHIP—PAST AND PRESENT
Hundreds of women, both nurses and laywomen, have contributed to the progress of nursing; only a few can be mentioned.

1. **Florence Nightingale (1820-1910)**
A. Laid the foundations for reform in nursing
   1. Recognized the value in education for nursing
   2. Believed that
      a. Nurses should be trained in hospitals
      b. Students' records should be kept
      c. Doctors should be paid for teaching
      d. There should be correlation of theory and practice
      e. Licensing of nurses should be opposed
   3. Helped to improve the status and emancipation of women
B. Was best known for work in Crimea
C. Nightingale Fund ($220,000) collected as a tribute to her, to be used to further nursing education; used to establish school of nursing at St. Thomas Hospital, London, 1860
D. Florence Nightingale Foundation established in 1912; provides scholarships in public health, administration and teaching, and social work
E. National Hospital Day established on the hundredth anniversary of Miss Nightingale's birth
F. Wrote extensively and was expert on many subjects; her advice was often sought
(For more information on Miss Nightingale refer to references)
2. **Linda Richards (Melinda Ann Judson Richards)**
A. America's first trained nurse
   1. Graduated from New England Hospital for Women and Children, 1873
   2. Following graduation became night supervisor at Bellevue; soon accepted the position of superintendent of nurses at Massachusetts General Hospital
   3. Aided in organizing schools of nursing
      a. Massachusetts General Hospital
      b. Boston City Hospital
      c. St. Luke's International Medical Center in Tokyo
      d. Founded first school of nursing in Japan (Kyoto, 1885)
   4. President of NLNE, 1894
3. **Isabel Hampton Robb—educator, administrator, author**
A. Graduated from Bellevue, 1883

B. Superintendent of nurses, Illinois Training School for Nurses, 1886
  1. Arranged graduate course of clinical experience and classwork
  2. Arranged affiliations for students at other hospitals
C. Became first principal of School of Nursing at Johns Hopkins, 1889
D. First president of Nurses' Associated Alumnae of the United States and Canada (later ANA), 1896 to 1901
E. President of NLNE, 1908
F. A founder and original stockholder of American Journal of Nursing Company
G. Helped to establish Chair of Nursing and Health at Teachers College, Columbia University

4. **Mary Adelaide Nutting**
A. Graduated with first class at Johns Hopkins Hospital School of Nursing
B. Succeeded Mrs. Robb as superintendent of nurses at Johns Hopkins, 1894
C. Established reforms in nursing education
  1. Preclinical period
  2. 8-hour day
  3. Lengthened course, to 3 years
  4. Abolished monthly allowance for students
D. President of NLNE, 1896
E. Instructed during creation and development of Department of Nursing and Health at Teachers College, Columbia University
F. First professor of nursing, 1907 to 1925, at Teachers College, Columbia University
G. Coauthor of four-volume *History of Nursing*

5. **Clara Barton**
A. Volunteer nurse during Civil War
B. Organized American Red Cross in 1882; was first president
C. Established reserve of Red Cross nurses to serve in case of national disaster, 1893

6. **Lillian Wald (1867-1940)**
A. Graduate of New York Hospital School of Nursing, 1891
B. Founder of Henry Street Settlement
C. Lecturer, Department of Nursing Education, Columbia University
D. First president of NOPHN
E. Helped in establishment of Children's Bureau, Metropolitan Life Insurance Company nursing service, and American Red Cross nursing service

7. **Mary M. Roberts**

A. Editor of *American Journal of Nursing*, 1921-1949; appointed editor emeritus on retirement
B. Author of *American Nursing—History and Interpretations*

8. **Annie Warburton Goodrich (1876-1955)**
A. One of most outstanding nurse educators of twentieth century
  1. Superintendent of nurses at several New York hospitals
  2. State inspector of nurses' training schools in New York
  3. Director of visiting nursing at Henry Street Settlement
  4. Dean of Army School of Nursing, 1918
  5. Dean of Yale University School of Nursing
  6. Helped to establish Vassar Training Camp program
  7. President of International Council of Nurses

9. **Isabel Maitland Stewart (1878-1966)**
A. Nurse educator, author, teacher
B. First nurse to receive a master's degree from Columbia University
C. Active on numerous committees
  1. Education Committee of NLNE
  2. Chairman, Educational Policies and Resources of National Nursing Council for National Defense
  3. First editor of Department of Nursing Education of *American Journal of Nursing*
D. Active participation in organizations
  1. ACSN
  2. NLNE
  3. ICN
  4. Florence Nightingale Foundation
E. Author
  1. *Education of Nurses*
  2. Coauthor of *Short History of Nursing*
  3. *The Educational Program of the School of Nursing*
  4. Numerous articles for journals

10. **Mary Eliza Mahoney (1845-1926)**
A. Graduate of New England Hospital for Women and Children, 1879
  1. First Negro professional nurse in United States
  2. Mary Mahoney Award established by National Association of Colored Graduate Nurses in 1949; presently awarded by ANA

11. **Lucile Petry Leone (1903-   )**
A. Graduate of Johns Hopkins School of Nursing, 1927

B. Teaching positions
1. Yale University School of Nursing
2. University of Minnesota
3. Dean of New York Hospital School of Nursing, 1941
4. Texas Woman's University, 1961
C. Consultant for USPHS on nursing problems of school of nursing enrollments, 1941
D. Director of Nursing Education of USPHS, to administer Cadet Nurse Corps Program
E. Chairman of Joint Committee on Unification of Accreditation Activities
F. Technical expert on nursing at second assembly of WHO in Geneva, 1948
G. Chief Nurse Officer and Assistant to Surgeon General of USPHS, 1949; attained rank of Brigadier General—first woman in United States to hold the rank
H. Lucile Petry Leone Award established by USPHS, 1966

12. Mildred Montag (1908-   )
A. Graduate of the University of Minnesota
1. Wrote *The Education of Nursing Technicians* as a doctoral dissertation at Teachers College, Columbia University
2. Headed the cooperative research project for nursing, 1952, that helped to implement her dissertation in junior and community colleges, 1952 to 1957
3. Revolutionized present-day nursing education
   a. There are now over 500 associate degree programs in nursing

13. Mrs. Lulu Wolf Hassenplug—now retired
A. Graduate of Army School of Nursing, Washington, D. C.
B. Bachelor's degree from Teachers College, Columbia University
C. Master's degree in public health from Johns Hopkins University, Baltimore
D. Professor and dean, emeritus, of the School of Nursing, University of California, Los Angeles
E. Formerly chairman of NLN's Council of Baccalaureate and Higher Degree Programs
F. Received NLN's Mary Adelaide Nutting Award in 1965, for a quarter of a century of creative, constructive devotion and outstanding contribution to the development of nursing as a professional discipline within the American system of higher education

G. Received honorary doctorate of science from the University of New Mexico and Bucknell University
H. Western Interstate Commission on Higher Education has cited her for distinguished service
I. Named Los Angeles Woman of the Year in Education in 1958 by the Los Angeles Times
J. Sigma Theta Tau made her an honorary member in recognition of her outstanding service in nursing through leadership in nursing education
K. Alpha Tau Delta gave her its Gold Key Award, for outstanding service to nursing
L. Served as consulting editor to the Bulletin of Sociology published by the National Institute of Mental Health
M. Appointed by Governor Ronald Reagan to serve for four years (1971-1975) on the Advisory Committee on Physician's Assistant Programs to the California Medical Board
N. Was a member of the Surgeon General's Consultant Group on Nursing that issued the 1963 report, *Toward Quality in Nursing: Needs and Goals;* this report formed the basis for the Nurse Training Act of 1964, which granted federal aid to nursing education
O. Served as civilian nursing consultant to the Sixth United States Army as part of the Nursing Advisory Committee of the National Institute of Mental Health
P. Served as chairman of the Western Council on Higher Education for Nursing and as a member of the Defense Advisory Committee on Women in the Services
Q. Was professor of nursing at Vanderbilt University, Nashville
R. Was associate professor, Medical College of Virginia, Richmond
S. Was educational director of the School of Nursing, Jewish Hospital, Philadelphia
T. Was instructor in nursing at Piedmont Hospital, Atlanta

14. Dr. Helen Nahm—now retired
A. Recently retired as dean, School of Nursing, University of California, San Francisco Medical Center
B. Graduate of the University of Missouri School of Nursing
C. Master's and doctoral degrees received from the University of Minnesota
D. Served on board of directors at NLN, 1959 to 1967

E. Was NLN second vice-president from 1959 to 1963

F. Was director, Division of Nursing Education, for 4 years at NLN

G. Was first director of the National Nursing Accrediting Service, which became a program of the NLN upon its founding in 1952

H. Was awarded NLN's Mary Adelaide Nutting Award for outstanding leadership and achievement in nursing in 1967

I. Cited specifically for her efforts in creating a national accrediting service for schools of nursing

J. Has been the recipient of many other honors and awards, among them honorary doctoral degrees from the Universities of Missouri, California, and Cincinnati

K. Received a Citation of Merit from the University of Missouri and a Distinguished Service Award from the University of Minnesota

L. Has served on the American Nurses' Association Commission on Nursing Education and is a member of the American Psychological Association

15. Dr. Martha E. Rogers

A. Graduate of Knoxville General Hospital School of Nursing, Knoxville, Tennessee, in 1936

B. Received B.S. degree in 1937 from George Peabody College, Nashville, Tennessee

C. Received M.A. in 1945 from Teachers College, Columbia University, New York

D. Received M.Ph. degree in 1952 from Teachers College, Columbia University

E. Received doctoral degree in 1954 from Johns Hopkins University, Baltimore, Maryland

F. Is at present time professor and head, division of Nurse Education, New York University, New York

G. Research assistant at Johns Hopkins University, from 1953 to 1954

H. Executive director, Visiting Nurse Service, 1945 to 1951, in Phoenix, Arizona

I. Assistant educational director and assistant supervisor at Visiting Nurse Association, Hartford, Connecticut, 1940 to 1945

J. Staff nurse and rural public health nurse at Children's Fund of Michigan, 1937 to 1939

K. Member of NLN Commission on Historical Source Materials in Nursing

L. Was president of New York State League for Nursing

M. Was secretary of Arizona State League for Nursing

N. Received award for inspiring leadership in intergroup reaction

O. Received alumni award from New York University, for outstanding contribution to nursing, 1965

P. Editor of *Nursing Science Journal*, 1963 to 1966

Q. Author of *Educational Revolution in Nursing*, 1966, *Reveille in Nursing*, 1964, and numerous articles

16. Dr. R. Louise McManus—now retired

A. Received her nursing degree at Massachusetts General Hospital

B. Received B.S., M.A., and Ph.D. at Columbia University, New York

C. Was active in nursing for 45 years and recognized as the designer of the first national testing service for the nursing profession—the second largest educational testing program in the country

D. Had a major role in initiating experiments that led to team nursing, introduced in 1949 and now widely used in hospitals throughout the country

E. Was one of the earliest advocates of experimentation for a 2-year academic program in nursing in junior and community colleges and spearheaded the movement for such programs by arranging for the establishment of a national cooperative research project at Teachers College in 1952—both to assist junior and community colleges in developing programs in nursing and to carry out research to test the quality of the programs

F. Worked to establish the Institute of Research and Service in Nursing Education at Teachers College, which carries on research and serves as a training center for research workers in nursing

G. Was consultant to the Department of Nursing at Walter Reed Army Institute of Research in Washington

H. Was honorary consultant to the Bureau of Medicine and Surgery of the U. S. Navy, the Dean's Committee of the Veterans Administration, and advisor to the Surgeon General in the National Advisory Health Council

I. Served on the Defense Advisory Committee on Women in the Services

J. Was chairman of the Nursing Council of the Florence Nightingale International Foundation, an affiliate of the International Council of Nurses

K. Has written extensively for nursing journals and is author of *The Effect of Experience on Nursing Achievement* and coauthor of *The Hospital Head Nurse*

L. Served as director of the Department of Nursing Education, Teachers College, Columbia University

M. Prior to serving as director at Teachers College, she served in the department as research assistant, instructor, and executive officer

N. Was director of nurses at Waterbury (Conn.) Hospital School of Nursing before going to Teachers College

17. Dr. Eleanor C. Lambertsen

A. Is now dean, Cornell University–New York Hospital, and professor of nursing

B. Received her nursing degree from Overlook Hospital School of Nursing, Summit, New Jersey

C. Received B.S., M.A., and Ed.D. from Columbia University, New York

D. Was chairman, Department of Nursing Education, at Teachers College, Columbia University, 1961-1970

E. Evaluated Israel's first baccalaureate degree program in nursing at the University of Tel Aviv

F. Serves on the Nursing Advisory Committee for the U. S. Department of Defense, the Health Task Force of Urban Coalition, the Commission on Nursing Service of the American Nurses' Association

G. Serves on the board of directors and the Education Committee of the Visiting Nurse Service of New York City and on the Expert Advisory Panel of the World Health Organization

H. Has received innumerable honors and awards from organizations and learned societies

18. Pearl Parvin Coulter—now retired

A. Former dean, University of Arizona, College of Nursing, Tucson, Arizona

B. Received A.B. at University of Denver in 1926 and M.S. in 1927; attended University of Colorado School of Nursing, 1935; received certificate in PHN, George Peabody College, 1936

C. Was associate professor at University of Colorado School of Nursing, 1943 to 1948, and professor, 1948 to 1957

D. Was associate professor of nursing, 1942 to 1943 at University of Wisconsin School of Nursing; was instructor, assistant professor, and associate professor, 1937 to 1941, Peabody College

E. Educational director, PHN, Nashville Health Department, 1939 to 1941

F. Formerly president, Arizona State Board of Nursing

G. Formerly board member of Arizona League for Nursing

H. Formerly member of NLN Task Force and member of NLN Bylaws Committee

I. Formerly president, Colorado League for Nursing, and Colorado State Nurses Association

J. Formerly board member of American Journal of Nursing Company

K. Formerly chairman of Mary Roberts Scholarship Committee

L. Formerly member of the board of directors at NLN

M. Received Public Health Nurse of the Year Award in 1962, given by ANA

N. Author of *The Nurse in the Public Health Program*, 1954

O. Author of *The Winds of Change*, a progress report on regional cooperation in collegiate nursing education in the West, 1962; also wrote many magazine articles

19. Mrs. Judith G. Whitaker

A. Former executive director of American Nurses' Association, 1958 to 1969

B. Received nursing degree from Nebraska Methodist Hospital School of Nursing in Omaha

C. Received B.S. and M.A. degrees from Columbia University, New York

D. During her tenure as executive director at ANA the association increased its membership, more than doubled its staff and operating budget, and effected a basic reorganization to extend its activities and functions in behalf of nursing in the public interest

E. Mrs. Whitaker has visited and worked with the constituent associations in 50 states and has served on a variety of national and international commissions dealing with every aspect of nursing

20. Dr. Faye G. Abdellah

A. Chief Nurse Officer, U. S. Public Health Service

B. Was nurse researcher in the government office in New York City in 1919

C. Graduated as R.N. at Fitkin Memorial Hospital School of Nursing, Neptune, N. J., 1942

D. Received B.S. in 1945 at Columbia University, M.A. in 1947, and Ed.D. in 1955

E. Received LL.D., Western Reserve University, 1967

F. Director of health education, Child Education Foundation, New York City, 1943 to 1945

G. Faculty, Yale School of Nursing, 1945 to 1948

H. Research fellow and faculty member, Teachers College, Columbia University, 1948 to 1949

I. Chief, Nursing Education Bureau, Division of Nursing Resources, USPHS, Department of Health, Education, and Welfare, Washington, D. C., 1949 to 1959

J. Senior consultant, nursing research, 1959 to 1962

K. Chief, Research Grants and Fellowship Bureau, 1962

L. Consultant, Western Interstate Commission for Higher Education

M. Recipient, Federal Nursing Service awards, 1964

N. Fellow, American Psychological Association

O. Member, American Nurses' Association and NLN

P. Member, American Academy of Arts and Sciences

Q. Author of *Patient-Centered Approaches to Nursing,* 1960, and *Better Patient Care Through Nursing Research,* 1965; also many articles in the field of nursing

R. Is recognized as one of the ablest nurse researchers in the nation

S. Was one of the first two women to receive the commission of Admiral in the USPHS

21. Dr. Ruth B. Freeman—now retired

A. Graduate of Mt. Sinai Hospital School of Nursing, New York

B. Professor of public health administration, School of Hygiene and Public Health, Johns Hopkins University, Baltimore

C. Served on the board of directors at NLN; elected in 1967

D. Formerly a member of World Health Organization's expert advisory panel on nursing

E. Served as consultant on nursing for the medical and natural sciences program of the Rockefeller Foundation for 1 year

F. Formerly a member of the Committee for the White House Conference on Children and Youth

G. Served as national administrator of the American National Red Cross Nursing Services and as consultant to the National Security Resources Board

H. Awards received
1. M. Adelaide Nutting Award
2. Pearl McIver Public Health Nurse Award
3. Annual nursing award of Department of Nurse Education, New York University

I. Received M.A. and Ed.D. degrees from New York University

J. Was president of National League for Nursing

22. Jessie M. Scott

A. Assistant Surgeon General and Director, Division of Nursing, National Institutes of Health, Bethesda, Maryland

B. Career of almost 30 years in nursing covers experience in many specialty areas

C. Came to Public Health Service in 1955 and has been with the Division of Nursing continuously since that time

D. Consultant to a number of states in the conduct of surveys to define their nursing needs

E. Directed many workshops to teach hospital staff the methods used by the Division of Nursing for studying the activities of various levels of nursing personnel to curtail the loss of professional nurse time

F. Deputy Chief from 1957 until she was appointed Chief early in 1964

G. To assist the Public Health Service in finding new approaches to community health services, she conducted an exploratory study that led to the first federally supported experimental study on progressive patient care

H. Assigned to India to counsel on problems of nursing shortages and education, promote improved utilization of nursing personnel, and help plan for a national survey of nursing needs and resources

I. The only nurse on a five-member joint Public Health Service–American Hospital Association team that made an on-site study of the organization of services for the chronically ill in England and Scotland in 1961

J. Member of a team studying health needs and services in Liberia

K. Counselor and assistant executive secretary of the Pennsylvania Nurses' Association for 6 years

L. Was educational director of Mt. Sinai Hospital (Philadelphia) and taught at Jefferson Medical College Hospital (Philadelphia), St. Luke's Hospital (New York), and the University of Pennsylvania; was visiting lecturer at graduate seminars

M. Member on the Selective Service Commission of Pennsylvania and Philadelphia Citizens' Committee on Public Health

N. Active on numerous Public Health Service committees, including the Service's Committee on Career Development for Nursing

O. Is a member of American Nurses' Association, NLN, and the American Public Health Association

P. Received her nursing diploma from Wilkes-Barre General Hospital School of Nursing in 1936

Q. Studied biologic science at the University of Pennsylvania

R. Received B.S. degree in education at University of Pennsylvania in 1943

S. Received master of arts degree in personnel administration from Teachers College, Columbia University, in 1949

T. Was one of the first two women to receive the commission of Admiral in the USPHS

23. Inez Haynes

A. Graduate of the Scott and White Memorial Hospital School of Nursing in Texas

B. Received bachelor's degree from the University of Minnesota

C. Began her Army career in 1932 as Second Lieutenant, serving as operating room nurse in Texas and the Philippine Islands

D. Advanced to administrative and supervisory positions with the Army in the United States, Europe, and the Far East

E. Was Chief of the Army Nurse Corps, holding rank of Colonel, which was the highest rank for nurses to achieve at the time—1959

F. Vice-president, Citizens Committee for the World Health Organization

G. Member of the board of directors, National Council of Homemaker Services

H. Member of the nursing advisory committee, U. S. Department of Defense, and of executive committee of the National Health Council and the National Assembly for Social Policy and Development

I. Active in the American National Council for Health Education of the Public, Pilots International, Council of Federal Nursing Services, and Sigma Theta Tau

J. Holds the U. S. Legion of Merit, and the Distinguished Service Award of the University of Minnesota

K. Was general director of the National League for Nursing for 10 years, 1959 to 1969

NURSING ORGANIZATIONS

1. National League for Nursing

A. Outgrowth of Nursing Section Meeting at World's Fair, Chicago, 1893

  1. Meeting of Training School Superintendents called for New York, 1894

    a. American Society of Superintendents of Training Schools for Nurses organized, 1894

    b. Renamed National League of Nursing Education, 1912

    c. Reorganization and formation of National League for Nursing, 1952

B. "Task Force" appointed to study structure to better meet issues and demands of modern nursing, 1963

  1. Recommendations and amended bylaws for new structure accepted at annual meeting, 1967

  2. New structure provides for 2 divisions of members: agency and individual

    a. Full membership available for anyone who is not a nurse but is interested in nursing and the work of NLN

  3. Division of agency members—councils

    a. Hospitals and related institutional nursing services

    b. Home Health Agencies and Community Health Services

    c. Associate degree programs

    d. Diploma programs

    e. Baccalaureate and higher degree programs

    f. Practical nursing programs

  4. Community planning

C. Functions of NLN

  1. Identify nursing needs of society and promote programs to meet them

  2. Develop and support services for im-

provement in nursing services and education

3. Work with ANA and other groups in the interest of nursing
4. Provide worldwide leadership in meeting nursing needs of all peoples

D. At 1971 convention, Anne Kibrick was elected president

2. **National League for Nursing and accreditation of nursing programs**

A. In 1939 NLNE took initiative for inspection of nursing schools
   1. Inspection on voluntary basis
   2. Published list of 70 accredited schools in 1941

B. National Nursing Accrediting Service established in 1949
   1. Organizations previously engaged in accrediting services
      a. NLNE, NOPHN, ACSN, and Conference of Catholic Schools of Nursing
      b. Temporary directors of new service, Hazel Goff and Julia Miller, until 1950

C. Subcommittee of Committee for the Improvement of Nursing Services with assistance of USPHS conducted study of basic nursing education, known as *School Data Analysis*
   1. Interim classification of schools of nursing offering basic programs, based on *School Data Analysis,* was published in *American Journal of Nursing,* 1949
   2. *Nursing Schools at Mid-Century* followed and was published in 1950
   3. List of fully accredited schools was published annually from 1949 to 1953 in *American Journal of Nursing;* now published in *Nursing Outlook*

D. NLN developed 5-year plan for temporary accreditation of schools of nursing
   1. Purpose: to work with schools and provide the stimulation and help needed to improve their programs of nursing education
   2. First list of schools receiving temporary accreditation published in 1952
   3. Temporary accreditation terminated Dec. 31, 1957; many schools obtained full accreditation as result of program
   4. Provisional accreditation extended to those schools with potential for becoming fully accredited; provisional accreditation ended Dec. 31, 1959
   5. Only full accreditation now available

E. NLN named the accrediting agency for nursing schools receiving federal assistance under Nurse Training Act, 1964
   1. Recognized by National Commission on Accrediting as an auxiliary accrediting association for associate degree programs in nursing

F. Accreditation team usually includes 2 nurse educators

G. NLN accreditation for schools of practical nursing inaugurated, 1966

H. Preliminary accreditation for public health units for 2-year period

I. Full accreditation for public health units extended to 5-year periods in 1968

3. **American Nurses' Association**

A. Delegates of 10 alumnae associations met in New York in 1896 to plan new organization
   1. Nurses' Associated Alumnae of the United States and Canada organized, 1897 (later became 2 organizations)
      a. One named American Nurses' Association, 1911
      b. Other named Canadian Nurses' Association, 1924

B. Reorganization in 1952

C. Association composed of professional nurses
   1. Federation of constituent state associations
   2. Membership through local and state constituent associations
   3. Programs and policies a function of delegates who are elected by state sections
      a. House of Delegates elects board of directors

D. Eight sections represent occupational groups
   1. Public health nursing
   2. Private duty nursing
   3. General duty nursing
   4. Institutional nursing service administration
   5. Educational administrators, consultants, and teachers
   6. Industrial or occupational health nursing
   7. Office nursing
   8. Special groups—for nurses whose activities place them in groups too small for a section
      a. Executive secretaries
      b. Nurse anesthetists
      c. Occupational therapists (nurses)
      d. Physical therapists (nurses)

e. Nurse editors

f. Recruitment nurses in Armed Services

g. Others

E. Two new conference groups organized, 1962

1. Geriatric nursing practice
2. Medical-surgical nursing

F. Functions of ANA

1. Promote high standards of nursing practice
2. Promote opportunities for nurses and maintain active interest in their welfare
3. Represent nursing interests in the matter of federal legislation that affects nursing

G. Some activities of ANA

1. Economic Security Program
2. Research in nursing
3. Maintenance of a professional counseling and placement service for new graduates

4. National Student Nurses' Association (NSNA)

A. Subcommittee appointed by ANA in 1946 to study feasibility of student organization

1. Two students appointed to subcommittee in 1949
2. Students wished organization of their own, 1950
3. Students voted to form national council of student nurses (NSNA); to have the guidance of ANA and NLN
4. Constitution and bylaws adopted and officers elected by students, 1953
   a. Central office established at ANA headquarters, 1955
   b. Newsletter with limited circulation published
5. Steps taken to incorporate organization and copyright newsletter
6. Newsletter discontinued and new magazine *Imprint* published 4 times a year, beginning in 1968

B. Objectives of NSNA

1. Prepare for membership in professional organizations
2. Provide for a channel of communication between all nurses, on worldwide scale
3. Assist in individual growth, development, and good citizenship

C. Members of organization participate in variety of community and professional activities

5. American Association of Industrial Nurses

A. Organized in 1942

B. In reorganization, 1952, voted to retain identity

C. Purposes of association

1. Improve community health through improving health of worker
2. Develop standards for industrial nursing
3. Provide means of communication among industrial nurses
4. Promote interest and participation in nursing activities

6. Association of Operating Room Nurses

A. Organized in 1957

B. Purposes

1. Provide forum for exchange of ideas
2. Provide for discussion of mutual problems
3. Improve services to patients
4. Improve interpersonal relationships

INTERNATIONAL ORGANIZATIONS

1. World Health Organization, organized in 1946, an agency of the United Nations Organization that was organized in 1945

A. Mrs. Elmira Bears Wickenden, advisor delegate to WHO first assembly

B. Expert Committee on Nursing organized in 1950

1. To promote worldwide development of nursing
2. To advise WHO of nursing needs
3. Mary I. Lambie presided at first meeting of committee
4. Mrs. Lucile Petry Leone, the American representative
5. Reports of Expert Committee published in *Technical Report Series*

C. Publications of WHO

1. *World Health Magazine*
2. *Weekly Epidemiological and Vital Statistics Reports*
3. *Guide for National Studies of Nursing Resources*
4. Reports of meetings of all expert committees

2. International Red Cross

A. Founded by Henri Dunant, a Swiss, in 1829

B. American Red Cross Committee, organized by Clara Barton in 1861

1. National Committee on Red Cross Nursing Service appointed in 1909; Jane A. Delano, chairman

a. To establish and maintain high standards for nurse membership
b. Responsible for recruitment and maintenance of reserve of nurses for military services or disaster until 1947
c. Red Cross reorganized nursing service to meet community needs

C. Some current activities of ARC
1. Disaster nursing
2. Instruction in home nursing and training of volunteer nurses' aides
3. Courses in first aid and lifesaving
4. Services to military personnel and their families
5. Junior Red Cross Societies
6. Blood collection and blood banks
7. Numerous other activities

D. International Red Cross through the Geneva Convention of 1864 facilitates humane treatment of prisoners during war, protection of hospitals and ambulances having emblem of the Red Cross

3. **International Council of Nurses**
A. Began at meeting of the Matrons' Council of Great Britain and Ireland, in London, 1899
1. Provisional committee appointed to formulate plans for organization
   a. Mrs. Robb and Miss Dock from United States appointed to committee
B. Committee met in London and adopted constitution in 1900
1. Mrs. Bedford Fenwick, editor of *British Journal of Nursing,* considered founder and elected first president
C. First meeting held in Buffalo, New York, 1901
D. ICN is a federation of national professional nursing organizations; membership is limited to 1 nursing organization from each participating country or state; the United States is represented by the ANA
1. Fifty-nine countries with membership in 1965
2. Charter members: United States, Germany, and England
E. Objectives of ICN
1. Obtain high standards of nursing
2. Promote the development of nursing as a profession
3. Protect the worldwide socioeconomic welfare of nurses
F. Florence Nightingale International Foundation established in 1934 as an educational trust

1. Maintains a permanent living memorial to Florence Nightingale
2. Provides postgraduate education for selected nurses
3. Maintains and develops facilities for postgraduate education for nurses

G. Headquarters in London
H. Official organ, *International Nursing Review*
I. Margrethe Kruse of Denmark, President, International Council on Nursing

SOME IMPORTANT STUDIES OF NURSING IN THE UNITED STATES

1. **Committee for the Study of Nursing Education**
A. Resulted from conference called by Rockefeller Foundation, 1918
B. Permanent committee formed with Dr. C. E. A. Winslow as chairman; study financed by the Rockefeller Foundation
1. Study directed by Josephine Goldmark
2. Study of entire nursing situation, especially as related to nursing education
C. Report of study, *Nursing and Nursing Education in the United States,* was published in 1923
1. Report was considered radical at first
2. Major areas of nursing were covered in the study
   a. Preparation of nurses for public health nursing
   b. Supply and demand for nursing service
   c. Adequacy of training facilities
3. Emphasized need for university schools of nursing
D. Result of the study—brought into existence 3 endowed university schools of nursing
1. Yale University School of Nursing, endowed by Rockefeller Foundation; after 1937 school awarded the degree of master of nursing (school now closed)
2. Western Reserve University School of Nursing, endowed by Francis Payne Bolton (for whom the school was later named)
3. Vanderbilt University School of Nursing began in 1930 and later received a million-dollar endowment

2. **Committee on the Grading of Nursing Schools**

A. Stimulated by Rockefeller Report of need for classification of nursing schools
B. Sponsored by ANA, NLNE, and NOPHN with representatives from American Medical Association, American Hospital Association, the general public, and the field of education
C. Committee organized in 1925
   1. Dr. William Darrach, chairman
   2. Dr. May Ayers Burgess, director of study
D. Study covered 7 years, and results were published in 3 reports
   1. *Nurses, Patients, and Pocketbooks*
   2. *An Activity Analysis of Nursing*
   3. *Nursing Schools Today and Tomorrow*
E. Actual grading of nursing schools not done by committee, but facts on which future work could proceed were published

3. Structure Study (Rich Report)
A. Raymond Rich Associates (sociologists) conducted study in 1946; study covered structure, resources, and programs of existing 6 nursing organizations
B. Many nurses participated as members of National Structure Study Committees
C. Purpose, for changing the structure of the professional nursing organization
   1. Coordinate work of organizations
   2. Improve services to nurses
   3. Assist in providing more effective nursing service
D. Many meetings held to discuss the report and resolve differences of opinions
E. At biennial convention in 1950, nurses voted to accept 2 national organizations

4. The Brown Report
A. Study made by Esther Lucille Brown; sponsored by Carnegie Foundation and Russell Sage Foundation
B. Results published in 1948 in *Nursing for the Future*
   1. Findings created a movement for educational reform in nursing; workshops were held on state and local levels to study report and how to implement recommendations
   2. Dean Margaret Bridgeman was engaged by Russell Sage Foundation in 1949 to interpret report and advise on nursing education in institutions of higher learning; results of her counseling were published in 1953 as *Collegiate Education for Nursing*

5. Study Committee of NLN
A. Purposes
   1. Review objectives, purposes, goals, and program activities
   2. See how goals are realized
   3. Study continuing communications, with Study Committee on Functions of ANA
B. Findings indicated need for extensive study of NLN structure
C. "Task Force" appointed by NLN board of directors to study structure, 1963
   1. Recommendations of Task Force presented to NLN board of directors, January, 1966
      a. Approved by NLN board of directors, February, 1967
      b. Recommendation of Task Force and amended bylaws accepted by membership at annual convention, 1967
      c. Reviewed in 1971
D. New structural differences
   1. Way in which membership is organized
   2. Strengthening of constituent units
   3. Increase in two-way communication between constituents and national body

6. Other studies contributing to reform in nursing during the period
A. Committee on the Functions of Nursing, sponsored by the Division of Nursing Education, Teachers College, Columbia University
   1. *Program for the Nursing Profession,* published in 1949
B. A democratic approach to the organization and administration of educational programs. In Bixler, R. W., and Bixler, G. K.: *Administration for nursing education in a period of transition,* New York, 1954, G. P. Putnam's Sons.
C. Cooperative research project in junior and community college education for nursing, 1952, directed by Dr. Mildred Montag
D. National Commission for Study of Nursing and Nursing Education (Jerome P. Lysaught, director): *An abstract for action,* New York, 1970, McGraw-Hill Book Co.
   1. The Commission was established in 1967 by the American Nurses' Association and the National League for Nursing to carry out the recommenda-

tion proposed in 1963 by the Surgeon General's Consultant Group in Nursing

2. A study has been made of the present system of nursing education in relation to the responsibilities and skill levels required for high-quality patient care

3. The suggestions for change are based on three main priorities
   a. Increased research into both the practice of nursing and the education of nurses
   b. Enhanced educational systems and curricula based upon the results of that research
   c. Widened financial support for nurses to ensure adequate career opportunities that will attract and retain the number of personnel required for quality health care in the coming years

4. The report examines the nurse's role, functions, goals, and future based on the findings of carefully prepared questionnaires distributed to many thousands of nurse educators. Such questions as "Is there really a nursing shortage?" and "Should diploma schools be phased out?" are discussed in detail

5. Following the publication of its final report and recommendations, *An Abstract for Action*, the National Commission formally switched its emphasis from investigation to implementation

OFFICIAL PROFESSIONAL NURSING PUBLICATIONS IN THE UNITED STATES

1. *American Journal of Nursing*
A. Founded in 1900
   1. Stock sold only to nurses or alumnae associations; Linda Richards purchased first share of stock
   2. J. B. Lippincott Company published magazine for 20 years; now published monthly by American Journal of Nursing Company
   3. First issue published October, 1900
   4. Sophia Palmer, editor in chief for 20 years
   5. In 1912 ANA became owner of all journal stock; elects the board of directors of the Journal Company
   6. Purposes

a. Provide a continuous record of nursing events
b. Provide a means of communication between nurses
c. Interpret nursing to the public
7. Official organ of ANA
8. Thelma M. Schorr, editor

2. *Public Health Nursing*
A. *Visiting Nurse Quarterly* of the Visiting Nurse Association of Cleveland given to NOPHN when it was organized in 1912, and VNA of Cleveland provided for its maintenance for a number of years
B. Renamed *Public Health Nurse* in 1918
C. Name again changed, to *Public Health Nursing*, in 1931
D. Assets transferred to *Nursing Outlook* in 1952

3. *Nursing Outlook*
A. Absorbed assets of *Public Health Nursing* in 1952
B. Magazine owned and published monthly by the American Journal of Nursing Company; representatives of NLN on board of directors of Company
C. First issue published January, 1953
D. Provides information on all aspects of nursing
E. Official organ of NLN
F. First editor, Mildred Hall; present editor, Edith P. Lewis

4. *Nursing Research*
A. Begun as an activity of ACSN in 1952
B. Purposes
   1. Inform members of result of scientific studies in nursing
   2. Stimulate interest in nursing research
C. NLN took over magazine in 1952
D. First published three times a year; since 1968 published bimonthly by American Journal of Nursing Company

5. *Imprint*
A. Official organ of NSNA, published four times a year, 1968
B. Newsletter previously published to be discontinued

6. **Other publications of professional nursing interest**
A. *International Nursing Review*, official organ of ICN
B. *World Health*, published monthly by WHO
C. *Occupational Health Nursing*, official organ of ASIN, 1969

LEGISLATION AFFECTING NURSING

1. **Early efforts directed toward raising standards of schools of nursing and registration of nurses**
A. First state to enact legislation for registration of nurses—North Carolina, 1903; followed by New Jersey the same year
B. First state to provide for inspection of schools of nursing—New York, 1906; Anna Alline, the first inspector
C. New York State first to require two types of licensing—one for professional nurses and one for practical nurses
D. Inspection of schools of nursing and granting of state approval was forerunner of modern accreditation but did not replace state approval
2. **After World War I**
A. Rapid increase in number of schools and number of graduates
B. Increase in number of subsidiary workers in hospitals
3. **Economic depression 1929-1935**
A. Thousands of nurses unemployed; private duty nurses severely affected
B. Depression legislation
   1. Federal Emergency Relief Act, 1933
   2. Works Progress Administration, 1935
      a. 2,600 nurses employed in 31 states in public health field
      b. 1,800 nurses working in other areas, including bedside nursing
   3. National Recovery Act, 1933, did not cover nurses
   4. Private duty nurses began sharing work; changed from 12-hour day to 8-hour day
C. 400 hospitals and 600 schools of nursing closed by 1940; student enrollment down 20%
4. **Threat of war and shortage of nurses**
A. Federal Security Agency Appropriations Act of 1941 included 1.2 million dollars to assist in training nurses for National Defense
   1. Administered by USPHS and Children's Bureau
   2. Appropriation increased to 3.5 million dollars in 1942
      a. 2,000 students received scholarships
      b. 4,200 graduate nurses received refresher courses
5. **Nurse Training Act (Bolton Act), 1943, creating the Cadet Nurse Corps**
A. Lucile Petry Leone appointed director
B. Provided free education, indoor and outdoor uniforms, and monthly stipend for 30 months
C. Additional benefits to participating institutions
D. By 1948, 124,000 students had graduated
6. **Social Security Act, 1935, and its subsequent amendments**
A. Nurses became eligible for old age benefits in 1951
B. Opened new fields of nursing and increased opportunity
C. Provided stipends and tuitions for preparation in public health nursing and in maternal and child health nursing
D. Amendments in 1965 made provisions for hospital and medical care for persons age 65 and older (Medicare)
   1. Has brought increasing numbers of aged persons into hospitals and nursing homes and shown need of home care
7. **Hill-Burton Act (Hospital Construction Act), 1947**
A. Provides assistance to states for construction of hospitals, nursing homes, public health centers, and other health care facilities
8. **Health Amendments Act, 1956, appropriation for 3 years**
A. Provided traineeships for preparation in administration, supervision, and teaching
B. Traineeships for preparation for first-level positions in public health nursing
C. Traineeships program extended for 5 years, during 1959 session of Congress
D. Included grants-in-aid to states for improvement and expansion of practical nurse programs
   1. In 1961 the Practical Nurse Extension Act was passed
9. **Manpower Development and Training Act, 1962**
A. Administered by Department of Labor
   1. Provides funds for practical nurse training in educational institutions under state Departments of Education
   2. Fiscal 1967, 1 million dollars for refresher courses for inactive professional nurses
10. **Health Professions Educational Assistance Act, 1963**
A. Assistance to schools of nursing, for new construction, expansion, modernization of teaching facilities
11. **Nurse Training Act, 1964**
A. Construction grants

B. Teaching and improvement grants
C. Payments to diploma schools
D. Traineeships for professional nurses
E. Loans to student nurses
  1. Application by students for assistance is made to school or institution being attended
12. **Nurse Training Act of 1971 (P.L. 92-158) signed by President Nixon in November, 1971**
A. This Act continues, with modifications, the authorities for nurse training provided in earlier Acts
B. Major features of the new Act include
  1. Extension and amendments of student assistance
  2. Grant and contract authorities for special projects for improvement in nurse training
  3. Start up grants for new nurse training programs
  4. Capitation grants to encourage expansion of enrollment and preparation of nurse specialists

DEVELOPMENT OF MILITARY NURSING

1. **Army Nurse Corps**
A. Established under Army Reorganization Act of 1901, creating "Army Nurse Corps"
  1. Female nurses
  2. Under medical department of the Army
B. American Red Cross maintained reserve of qualified nurses for the Corps until 1947
  1. Nurses had no official status
C. Relative rank given nurses in 1920
  1. Julia C. Stimson the first woman to receive rank of Major
  2. Did not provide same pay schedule or travel allowance as for men
D. Permanent commissioned rank given in 1947
E. Male nurses given commissions in the Reserve in 1955
  1. Commissions in the Regular Corps, 1966
F. Legislation providing for promotion, tenure, and standards same as those for men passed by Congress in 1967
  1. Nurses may hold permanent rank, including Colonel
  2. Promotion based on selection of best-qualified persons
  3. First General appointed in 1971: Annie Mae Hays

G. Student Nurse Program
  1. Students of diploma programs who are enrolled in collegiate baccalaureate degree programs accredited by NLN and approved by Army
    a. Requirements for degree must be completed within 24 months
    b. Six months prior to completion, nurse is commissioned as Second Lieutenant in Army Nurse Corps Reserve
      (1) Placed on salary; corresponding privileges provided by Army
    c. Students receiving benefits of less than 12 months must spend 2 years on active duty with the Army
    d. Students receiving benefits of more than 12 months will spend 3 years on active duty
H. Registered Nurse Program
  1. Nurses who complete degree requirements in less than 12 months
    a. Are commissioned as First or Second Lieutenant
    b. Will remain on active duty 3 years
I. Graduate of 2-year associate degree programs admitted to Army Nurse Corps must be accredited by NLN in 1971
J. Present Chief of Army Nurse Corps, Brigadier General Lillian Dunlap
2. **Navy Nurse Corps**
A. Established by Navy Appropriations Act, 1908
B. Recruitment under Red Cross, same as for Army
C. Permanent commissions given in 1947
D. Navy Nurse Corps Candidate Program
  1. Senior students in basic collegiate programs may apply
E. First Navy nurses assigned to serve on hospital ship, 1920, USS Relief
F. Graduate nurses enrolled in collegiate degree nursing program who will complete degree requirements for B.S. degree in 2 years or less
  1. May receive tuition and salary
  2. For last 6 months receive commission as Ensign
  3. Must serve 2 to 3 years on active duty with the Navy following graduation
G. Present Chief, Captain Veronica M. Bulshelfski
3. **Air Force Nurse Corps**
A. Established in 1949 as a part of Air Force Medical Service

1. Includes flight nurses and nurses serving in Air Force hospitals
2. Flight nurses trained for air evacuation and are members of air evacuation squadron
3. Nurses may retire after 20 years and receive retirement benefits at age 60
4. Corps provides for professional growth
   a. Selected nurses may receive university education leading to a degree, with full pay and allowances
   b. "Operation Bootstrap" provides financial assistance to nurses having 1 year or less toward a baccalaureate or master's degree
   c. Courses offered each year
      (1) Anesthesia
      (2) Aerospace nursing
      (3) Flight nursing
      (4) Nursing service administration
      (5) Obstetric nursing
   d. Associate degree nursing graduates admitted in spring of 1972
5. Appointments may be given, up to rank of General
6. Present Chief of the Corps, Colonel Ethel Ann Hoefly

4. United States Public Health Service

A. Created Division of Nursing Service in 1946; Division now under Community Health, Bureau of States Services
B. Formed commissioned corps of nurses in 1944
   1. Appointments made to Reserve Corps
   2. Regular Corps requires a baccalaureate degree
   3. Grades, rank, pay, retirement and allowances same as in U. S. Army
      a. Titles for same rank different
         (1) U. S. Public Health Service Nurse Officer
         (2) Army Nurse Corps Captain
         (3) Navy Nurse Corps Lieutenant
         (4) Air Force Nurse Corps Lieutenant
   4. Chief Nurse Officer, Dr. Faye G. Abdellah

REVIEW QUESTIONS FOR HISTORY AND TRENDS OF NURSING WITH EMPHASIS ON TWENTIETH CENTURY
Multiple choice

Read each question carefully and consider all possible answers. When you have decided which answer is best, blacken one space on the answer sheet. There is only one best answer for each question.

Situation: Judy, age 18, is a senior in high school. She is an intelligent, bright, alert girl who ranks in the upper 10% of her class. She has always been interested in nursing but has found it difficult to make a definite decision on nursing as a career. Recently the high school held a career day and a professional nurse from one of the hospitals in the city came to the school to talk to the students about nursing. Judy was impressed with some of the things that she learned from the nurse, and she has now decided to become a nurse. Questions 1 through 29 concern Judy as a senior in high school, a student nurse, and a graduate nurse.

1. Among the things the professional nurse told Judy was that
   1. There is still a shortage of nurses in many areas
   2. 850,000 nurses would be needed by 1980
   3. Nursing is very hard, and teaching school would be easier
   4. She would get credit in medical school if she went on
2. Judy has learned that social change has increased the need for nurses and that one of the reasons more nurses are needed is that
   1. Hospitalization insurance is more available
   2. Urban population is migrating to rural areas
   3. Increasing emphasis is placed on mental health
   4. Number of older people is increasing
3. The professional nurse told Judy that there has been an increase in the number of hospital beds because federal money was provided for hospital construction under the
   1. Federal Emergency Relief Act
   2. Works Progress Administration
   3. Hill-Burton Act
   4. Social Security Act
4. Judy decided to write several schools of nursing for school bulletins; she noticed that one of the bulletins stated that the school was accredited by the National League for Nursing; she asked the school nurse what this meant and was told that
   1. It would give her the right to register in any state
   2. Only university schools are accredited by NLN
   3. She would be eligible for a scholarship
   4. The school had met certain standards set by the NLN
5. She asked why all schools are not accredited by NLN and was told that
   1. NLN accreditation is voluntary and is requested by the individual school
   2. NLN accreditation is very costly and most schools cannot afford it
   3. Some schools have temporary accreditation
   4. It is mandatory for university schools of nursing
6. Judy asked where she could find a list of the schools of nursing that are accredited by NLN; the school nurse told her that the list is published annually in
   1. *American Journal of Nursing*

2. *Nursing Research*
3. *Nursing Outlook*
4. *Journal of Nursing Education*

7. Judy was interested in the National League for Nursing and wanted to know who could be a member; she was told that membership is available to
   1. Any person interested in nursing
   2. Professional nurses only
   3. Professional and practical nurses
   4. Professional nurses and hospital administrators

8. After Judy entered a school of nursing, one of the subjects that she studied was history of nursing; she found the subject very interesting and learned that the first trained nurse in the United States was
   1. Clara Barton
   2. Isabel Hampton Robb
   3. Linda Richards
   4. Dr. Susan Dimock

9. She learned that the first major contribution to modern nursing was the work done by
   1. Mary Adelaide Nutting
   2. Lillian Wald
   3. Mary Roberts
   4. Florence Nightingale

10. The first school of nursing outside of the United States that was devoted exclusively to the care of sick people was established at
    1. Kaiserswerth, Germany
    2. St. Thomas Hospital, London, England
    3. International Medical Center, Tokyo, Japan
    4. Kyoto, Japan

11. The first school of nursing in the United States was at
    1. Bellevue Hospital, New York City
    2. Johns Hopkins Hospital, Baltimore
    3. New England Hospital for Women and Children
    4. Charity Hospital, New Orleans

12. The first trained nurse in the United States was a graduate of
    1. Bellevue Hospital
    2. New England Hospital for Women and Children
    3. Illinois Training School for Nurses
    4. Columbia University

13. After becoming a student nurse Judy learned about the National Student Nurses' Association and was happy to know that she could become a member; she learned that one of the objectives of the association was to
    1. Improve teaching in the school
    2. Improve patient care
    3. Promote worldwide development of nursing
    4. Assist each student in individual growth, development, and citizenship

14. Judy learned that she could subscribe to the official organ of the Student Nurses' Association, which is named
    1. *Imprint*
    2. *Nursing Research*
    3. *World Health Magazine*
    4. *International Nursing Review*

15. While in high school Judy belonged to the Junior Red Cross; now she was learning other things about the Red Cross—one of them being that the American Red Cross was founded by

16. Until 1947 the ARC was responsible for the following activity
    1. Recruiting students for schools of nursing
    2. Recruiting and maintaining a nursing reserve for military service and for disaster
    3. Operating schools of nursing to train nurses for disaster
    4. Maintaining an international blood bank

1. Clara Barton
2. Jane A. Delano
3. Henri Dunant
4. Mrs. Bedford Fenwick

17. The first president of ARC was
    1. Mary Roberts
    2. Annie Warburton Goodrich
    3. Clara Barton
    4. Mary Adelaide Nutting

18. Among the current activities of ARC are the following except for
    1. Classes in home nursing
    2. Courses in first aid
    3. Classes in lifesaving
    4. Classes in fundamentals of nursing

19. As a student nurse Judy became aware that there were too few doctors to meet the needs for health care; she learned that some of the reasons are as follows, except for
    1. More doctors are going into research
    2. Not enough doctors are being graduated
    3. Most doctors do only surgery
    4. Medical school enrollments are limited

20. Judy has learned that technology has affected nursing and that nurses must be prepared to function effectively in all the following areas, except for
    1. Cardiopulmonary laboratory
    2. Inhalation therapy units
    3. Dialysis
    4. Intensive care

21. Following graduation Judy, as a professional nurse, should secure membership in the following professional organization
    1. ANA   3. NLNE
    2. NOPHN   4. ACSN

22. When Judy graduated, she realized the need to keep well-informed concerning developments in professional nursing; she decided that the one way to do this was to subscribe to all or to which one of the following?
    1. *Visiting Nurse Quarterly*
    2. *American Journal of Nursing*
    3. *Nursing Outlook*
    4. *Nursing Research*

23. Judy graduated from a 3-year nursing program; she believed that she would like to teach but realized that more education was essential; however, her funds were limited and so she decided to find out about financial assistance; federal funds became available for scholarships and loans to student and professional nurses under the
    1. Nurse Training Act
    2. Manpower Development and Training Act
    3. Health Amendments Act
    4. Social Security Act

24. In order to secure information concerning the possibility of financial assistance Judy should write to the
    1. Surgeon General of the USPHS

2. National League for Nursing
3. Institution that she wishes to attend
4. Department of Health, Education, and Welfare

25. Agnes and Judy were classmates and Agnes is interested in military nursing; if she decides to go into the Army, she may expect to receive all but one of the following
1. A regular commission
2. Officer status
3. A temporary rank
4. Promotion based on qualifications

26. Judy understands that if she enters a baccalaureate nursing degree program and completes the requirements for a degree in less than 2 years she may apply for admission to the Navy Nurse Corps and would be eligible for
1. The Navy Nurse Corps Candidate Program
2. Operation Bootstrap
3. The air evacuation squadron
4. A hospital ship

27. Under the program Judy would receive all of the following except
1. Tuition and salary
2. Pay for attendance at meetings
3. Commission of Ensign, her last 6 months
4. Active duty for 2 or 3 years following completion of her degree program

28. While working toward a degree in nursing Judy learned that many changes in nursing were taking place; all the following are changes except for
1. Transfer of nursing education from hospital to educational institutions
2. Less specialization in nursing
3. Increase in emphasis on nursing research
4. Increase in 2-year associate degree programs

29. Judy was one of several students who were asked to prepare a window display for National Hospital Day; this day is set aside to
1. Give citizens a chance to see the hospital
2. Promote interest in better patient care
3. Commemorate the one hundredth anniversary of the birth of Florence Nightingale
4. Aid in the recruitment of nurses for military service

Situation: Questions 30 through 42 are general and concern factual information about nursing.

30. The interim classification of schools of nursing was published in the *American Journal of Nursing* in
1. 1923   3. 1952
2. 1962   4. 1949

31. Part of the NLN accreditation program provides all of the following except
1. Temporary accreditation
2. Accreditation of diploma schools
3. Accreditation of baccalaureate and higher degree programs
4. Accreditation of associate degree programs

32. Nurses assigned to recruitment for the Army Nurse Corps may join ANA and be members of
1. Any section they choose

2. Office nursing section
3. A special group
4. Medical-surgical conference group

33. A study of nursing in the United States in 1923 emphasized the need for university schools of nursing; this report is known as
1. Nursing and Nursing Education in the United States
2. Committee on the Grading of Nursing Schools
3. The Brown Report
4. The Rich Report

34. The first state to inspect schools of nursing was
1. New Jersey
2. North Carolina
3. New York
4. Mississippi

35. The first state to enact legislation for the registration of nurses was
1. New York   3. Mississippi
2. North Carolina 4. New Jersey

36. An Act passed in 1943 by the United States Congress, providing funds to train nurses, resulted in the establishment of
1. Refresher courses for graduate nurses
2. Traineeships for public health nurses
3. Training programs for practical nurses
4. The Cadet Nurse Corps

37. Legislation enacted in 1962 provides funds for the training of practical nurses and is known as
1. Health Professions Educational Assistance Act
2. Manpower Development and Training Act
3. Health Amendments Act
4. Hill-Burton Act

38. The first corps of trained nurses for military service was established in 1901 and created the
1. Army Nurse Corps
2. Navy Nurse Corps
3. Commissioned Corps of the USPHS
4. Air Force Nurse Corps

39. A nurse who is commissioned as a Nurse Officer in the USPHS may expect that her rank is the same as Lieutenant in the
1. Peace Corps   3. Navy
2. Army   4. None of the above

40. Amendments to the Social Security Act in 1965 provided for what is known as
1. Operation Bootstrap 3. Intensive care
2. Extended care   4. Medicare

41. Federal funds under the Manpower Development and Training Act are administered by
1. Department of the Interior
2. Department of Labor
3. U. S. Public Health Service
4. Children's Bureau

42. The first nurse to hold the rank of Brigadier General in the United States was
1. Isabel Maitland Stewart
2. Annie Mae Hays
3. Veronica M. Bulshelfski
4. Lucile Petry Leone

NAME _____ DATE _____ DATE OF BIRTH _____ AGE _____ SEX M OR F

LAST   FIRST   MIDDLE

SCHOOL _____ CITY _____ GRADE OR CLASS _____ INSTRUCTOR _____

NAME OF TEST _____ PART _____

DIRECTIONS: Read each question and its numbered answers. When you have decided which answer is correct, blacken the corresponding space on this sheet with the special pencil. Make your mark as long as the pair of lines, and move the pencil point up and down firmly to make a heavy black line. If you change your mind, erase your first mark completely. Make no stray marks; they may count against you.

SAMPLE:

1—1 a country
1—2 a mountain
1—3 an island
1—4 a city
1—5 a state

1. Chicago is

BE SURE YOUR MARKS ARE HEAVY AND BLACK.
ERASE COMPLETELY ANY ANSWER YOU WISH TO CHANGE.

Printed by the International Business Machines Corporation, Endicott, N. Y., U. S. A.

IBM FORM I.T.S. 1000 B 108

THREE

PARACLINICAL NURSING

Nutrition and diet therapy

Pharmacology and therapeutics

CHAPTER
6

NUTRITION AND DIET THERAPY

Bogert, L. J., Briggs, G., and Calloway, D.: Nutrition and physical fitness, ed. 9, Philadelphia, 1971, W. B. Saunders Co.

Fredrickson, D. S., and others: Dietary management of hyperlipoproteinemia: a handbook for physicians: types I, II, III, IV, and V, Bethesda, Md., 1970, National Heart and Lung Institute, National Institutes of Health.

Guthrie, H. A.: Introductory nutrition, ed. 2, St. Louis, 1971, The C. V. Mosby Co.

Guthrie, H. A., and Braddock, K. S.: Programmed nutrition, St. Louis, 1971, The C. V. Mosby Co.

Mitchell, H. S., Rynbergen, M. S., Anderson, L., and Dibble, M.: Cooper's nutrition in health and disease, ed. 15, Philadelphia, 1968, J. B. Lippincott Co.

Robinson, C. H.: Normal and therapeutic nutrition, ed. 14, New York, 1972, The Macmillan Co.

Turner, D.: Handbook of diet therapy, ed. 4, Chicago, 1965, University of Chicago Press.

Williams, S. R.: Nutrition and diet therapy, ed. 2, St. Louis, 1973, The C. V. Mosby Co.

Williams, S. R.: Nutrition and diet therapy: a learning guide for students, ed. 2, St. Louis, 1973, The C. V. Mosby Co.

Wohl, M. G., and Goodhart, R. S.: Modern nutrition in health and disease, ed. 3, Philadelphia, 1964, Lea & Febiger.

Periodicals

Journal of the American Dietetic Association
Journal of Nutrition Education
Nutrition Today

NORMAL NUTRITION

1. **Objectives and appreciations**
A. To acquire knowledge and ability to apply principles of nutrition in health and disease

B. To modify nutritional intake and satisfy influence of religion, tradition, social custom, economic status, and emotional, physiologic, and psychological drives on dietary patterns
C. To appreciate that good nutrition is an important factor in
   1. Promoting health
   2. Improving appearance and feeling of well-being
   3. Improving efficiency
   4. Preventing disease or recovering more quickly from disease
D. To appreciate effects of good nutrition upon patient and herself, nurse must know
   1. Function and fate of food nutrients in body
   2. Recommended allowances of each nutrient
   3. Interrelationships of nutrients
E. To distinguish reliable nutrition resources and use consultants effectively
   1. Dietitian, nutritionist, and physician
   2. Organizations and associations
   3. Textbooks, journals, films, pamphlets, charts

2. **Definitions**
A. Nutrition—science that deals with physiologic needs of body in health and disease; combination of processes by which living organism receives and utilizes materials necessary for maintenance of its functions and growth

B. Dietetics—science and art dealing with application of principles of nutrition in feeding individuals or groups
C. Food—substance that will supply heat and energy, build or repair tissue, and/or regulate body processes
D. Nutrients—basic constituents of food, such as protein, fat, carbohydrate, vitamins, minerals, and water
E. Metabolism—refers to chemical changes occurring in body, such as anabolism (building tissue and substances) and catabolism (breaking down tissue and substances); most frequently refers to chemical actions occurring after absorption

3. **Carbohydrates**
A. Definition—organic compounds (saccharides—starches and sugars) composed of carbon, hydrogen, and oxygen; hydrogen to oxygen usually in a ratio of 2 to 1
B. Classification
   1. Monosaccharides ("mono" meaning 1)
      a. Glucose (dextrose)
         (1) Principal form in which carbohydrate is utilized by the body
         (2) Found in fruits and vegetables and formed in the body from starch digestion
      b. Fructose (levulose) found in honey, fruits, and vegetables
      c. Galactose
         (1) Results from breakdown of lactose (milk sugar)
         (2) Does not occur free in nature
   2. Disaccharides ("di" meaning 2)
      a. Sucrose (ordinary table sugar) processed from cane and beet sugar; found in fruits, vegetables, and syrups
      b. Lactose found in milk
      c. Maltose derived from hydrolysis of starch
   3. Polysaccharides ("poly" meaning many)
      a. Starch found in cereals, fruits, and vegetables
      b. Dextrin, intermediate breakdown product of starch
      c. Cellulose, framework of plants, not digested but provides bulk
      d. Glycogen, animal starch, found in meat and seafood
      e. Pectin found in fruit
      f. Agar-agar found in seaweed, provides soft bulk

C. Digestion (Table 6-1)
D. Absorption and metabolism
   1. Simple sugars absorbed at different rates through intestinal wall into bloodstream by diffusion and active transport, mediated by sodium
   2. Simple sugars transported via portal vein to liver where
      a. Galactose converted to glucose
      b. Glucose and fructose converted to glycogen for storage
      c. Glucose converted to protein by transamination
      d. Glucose converted to fat
      e. Glycogen converted to glucose to maintain blood sugar level
      f. Glucose oxidized to carbon dioxide and water
   3. Glucose transported in blood from liver to muscles and tissues of body for energy metabolism
   4. Glucose may be stored as glycogen in muscles
   5. Excess carbohydrate converted to fat and stored as adipose tissue
E. Influences on carbohydrate metabolism
   1. Phosphorus and members of B complex vitamins necessary for carbohydrate metabolism
   2. Insulin, important in formation of glycogen and absorption of glucose into cell, reduces blood sugar level
   3. Epinephrine accelerates production of glucose from glycogen
   4. Pituitary hormone elevates blood sugar
   5. Liver important site of carbohydrate metabolism
F. Functions of carbohydrates in body
   1. Supply heat and energy
   2. Spare protein
   3. Supply bulk
   4. Promote desirable intestinal flora
   5. Protect liver against toxins
   6. Essential for muscle and tissue function and metabolism
   7. Aid in utilization of fat
G. Role of carbohydrates in diet
   1. Carbohydrates supply 40% to 50% of total calories in average American diet
   2. Carbohydrates inexpensive; used in greater amounts by people in lower income brackets and in Oriental countries, providing up to 80% of total calories
   3. Enrichment of bread and cereal prod-

ucts with thiamine, niacin, riboflavin, and occasionally calcium and iron, important advancements in improving American diet

H. Food sources of carbohydrates
1. High—sugar and sweets, breads, cereal and cereal products, dried fruits, bananas, grapes, potatoes, milk
2. Low—most fresh fruits and vegetables
3. Negligible—meat, poultry, fish, eggs, fats

I. Modifications of carbohydrate intake
1. Decreased carbohydrate intake with other dietary modifications may be recommended for patients with obesity, diabetes mellitus, hypoglycemia, dumping syndrome
2. Elimination of carbohydrate foods that adhere to teeth may be recommended to prevent or reduce number of dental caries
3. High carbohydrate intakes may be recommended for patients who have
   a. Liver diseases (with high protein)
   b. Fever (with high calories)
   c. Malnutrition or underweight (with high calories)
4. Low roughage may be indicated for patients with
   a. Diarrhea
   b. Colitis
   c. Peptic ulcer
   d. Diseases and surgery of gastrointestinal tract
   e. Constipation (low or high roughage)
5. Excessive intake may result in
   a. Obesity
   b. Fermentation in lower bowel resulting in diarrhea
   c. Decreased appetite for other necessary foods
6. Increase in sucrose intake associated with rise in blood lipids and cholesterol in some individuals
7. Low carbohydrate intake accompanied by inadequate caloric intake may result in
   a. Loss of weight
   b. Decreased vitamin B intake

4. Proteins
A. Definition—organic compounds that contain carbon, hydrogen, oxygen, and nitrogen (16%); protein molecule composed of different arrangements and numbers of simpler substances known as amino acids

B. Classification
1. Essential amino acids—cannot be synthesized in body (p. 68)
   a. Isoleucine
   b. Leucine
   c. Lysine
   d. Methionine
   e. Phenylalanine
   f. Threonine
   g. Tryptophan
   h. Valine
   i. Histidine—essential for infants
2. Complete protein
   a. Protein that maintains life and promotes growth
   b. Protein that contains all essential amino acids in proper proportion and amount
   c. Examples include proteins found in milk, eggs, meat, fish, cheese
3. Partially complete protein
   a. Protein that will maintain life but will not promote growth
   b. Examples include proteins found in cereals, legumes, nuts
4. Incomplete protein
   a. Protein that will promote neither growth nor maintenance
   b. Examples include zein in corn and gelatin

C. Digestion (Table 6-1)—cooking enhances digestibility of certain proteins (meats, soybeans)

D. Absorption and metabolism
1. Amino acids absorbed through intestinal wall into portal system
2. Abnormally some unaltered protein may be absorbed directly into bloodstream causing allergic response
3. Amino acids may be
   a. Combined to form proteins that are characteristic of tissue or substance of which they become part
      (1) Muscle and glandular tissue
      (2) Blood proteins
      (3) Enzymes
      (4) Hormones
   b. Deaminized in the liver and converted to urea, carbon dioxide, and water
   c. Converted to glycogen (58%) or to fatty acids (46%)
4. All amino acids, which comprise a substance or tissue, must be present concurrently in proper amounts for construction of that tissue or substance—law of "all or none"

TABLE 6-1
DIGESTION OF FOOD

Site	Secretions	Action
Mouth	Saliva Ptyalin or salivary amylase	Food moistened, softened, and partially ground Some starch converted to maltose Taste buds stimulate flow of other digestive juices
Stomach		Thoroughly mixes food and reduces size of food particles
	Gastrin	Stimulates secretion of gastric juices
	Gastric juice	
	Pepsin (activated pepsinogen)	Reduces protein to proteoses and peptones
	Rennin	Coagulates milk (absent in adults)
	Lipase	Limited action on emulsified fats
	Hydrochloric acid	Provides proper pH for enzyme action Destroys harmful bacteria Converts iron compounds to ferrous form for absorption
Small intestine		
	Hormones	Stimulate secretion of pancreatic enzymes
	Pancreatic juices	
	Trypsin and chymotrypsin	Reduce specific proteins to polypeptides and amino acids
	Peptidase	Reduces polypeptides to amino acids
	Amylase	Converts starch to dextrins and maltose
	Lipase (steapsin)	Converts fats to fatty acids and glycerol
	Intestinal juice	
	Sucrase	Reduces sucrose to glucose and fructose
	Maltase	Reduces maltose to glucose and glucose
	Lactase	Reduces lactose to galactose and glucose
	Lipase	Reduces fats to fatty acids
	Peptidases	Reduces proteins to amino acids
	Cholecystokinin	Stimulates secretion of bile
	Bile	Emulsifies fats

5. Maximum utilization of dietary nitrogen depends on adequate caloric intake

E. Influences on protein metabolism
   1. With inadequate intake of calories, protein will be used to produce energy
   2. Protein loss occurs during
      a. Stress, surgery, injury, burns
      b. Steroid therapy
      c. Bed rest, inactivity

F. Functions of protein in body
   1. Build, maintain, and repair tissue
   2. Perform as component part of tissues and substances
      a. Hormones (insulin)
      b. Enzymes (pepsin)
      c. Antibodies
      d. Blood
         (1) Transport nutrients
         (2) Regulate acid-base balance
         (3) Regulate osmotic balance
   3. Form vitamins such as folic acid and niacin

G. Role of protein in diet
   1. 10% to 15% of calories in average diet derived from protein
   2. 33% ingested protein should represent complete protein
   3. Each meal should include a complete protein or food combinations (grains, legumes) to supply all 8 essential amino acids
   4. Essential amino acids may be supplied by supplementation of incomplete proteins
      a. Milk with cereals
      b. Soybeans with rice
   5. Protein foods relatively expensive; people with limited budgets should favor cheese; fish; powdered, concentrated, or evaporated milk; eggs; supplementation with legumes, cereal, and vegetable proteins for sources of complete protein

H. Food sources of protein
   1. Good—meat, poultry, fish, eggs, milk, legumes, nuts

2. Low—fruits, vegetables, cereals
3. Absent—sugar, fats

I. Recommended daily allowance

1. Food and Nutrition Board of National Research Council recommends 0.9 gm. protein per kilogram body weight for adult; additional 10 gm. during pregnancy; additional 20 gm. during lactation; 2.2 to 1.8 gm. per kilogram body weight for infants from birth to 1 year; for children an additional allowance made (over maintenance) for weight increments
2. Protein need may be determined by measuring nitrogen excretion
   a. Nitrogen balance—nitrogen excretion equals nitrogen intake
   b. Positive balance—nitrogen intake exceeds nitrogen excretion
   c. Negative balance—nitrogen intake is lower than nitrogen excretion

J. Modifications of protein intake

1. Low-protein diets may occasionally be recommended for acute stage of glomerular nephritis; always used for hepatic coma
2. High-protein diets recommended for patients with
   a. Diseases of liver
   b. Peptic ulcer
   c. Nephrosis
   d. Malabsorption syndrome
   e. Hypoglycemia
   f. Nutritional anemias
   g. Infections
   h. Fevers
   i. Wound healing
   j. Hyperthyroidism
   k. Surgery
   l. Malnutrition
   m. Protein loss or stress conditions
      (1) Hemorrhaging
      (2) Burns or wounds
      (3) Fractures or injuries
   n. Growth demands
      (1) Infancy through adolescence
      (2) Pregnancy and lactation
3. Protein deficiency may lead to
   a. Edema
   b. Delayed wound healing
   c. Anemia
   d. Impaired gastrointestinal function
   e. Development of liver damage
   f. Impaired growth
   g. Fatigue
   h. Kwashiorkor

5. Lipids (p. 162)

A. Definition—fats, organic compounds composed of carbon, hydrogen, and oxygen chiefly as glycerol esters of fatty acids

B. Classifications of fats and fatty acids

1. Essential fatty acid—linoleic acid
   a. Essential for growth and healthy skin in infants
   b. Converted to active form, arachidonic acid, in the body
   c. Found in soybean, safflower, and corn oils
2. Saturated fatty acids (containing no double bonds) include stearic, palmitic, and butyric acids
3. Unsaturated fatty acids (containing double bonds)
   a. Monounsaturated fatty acid (containing 1 double bond) includes oleic acid
   b. Polyunsaturated fatty acid (containing 2 or more double bonds) includes linoleic, linolenic, and arachidonic acids
4. Neutral fats (simple fats—triglycerides)
   a. Composed of fatty acids and glycerol
   b. Found in tissue and all organs except brain
   c. Include butyric, oleic, palmitic, and stearic acids
5. Lipid compounds and related lipid substances
   a. Phospholipids
      (1) Composed of fatty acids, glycerol, nitrogen, phosphoric acid
      (2) Found in all cells; a fat transport form
      (3) Include lecithin found in egg yolk
   b. Sterols—composed of fatty acids and certain alcohols
      (1) Cholesterol (animal sterol)
         (a) Synthesized in body
         (b) Found in all body cells, in eggs, liver, animal fats
         (c) Important in fat transportation
         (d) Important in formation of bile, some hormones, vitamin D
      (2) Sitosterol (plant sterol) not readily absorbed by body

(3) Ergosterol (plant sterol) converted to vitamin D
  c. Lipoproteins—composed of fat and protein in varying ratios
    (1) Most important vehicle of fat transport in body
    (2) Chylomicrons — heaviest fat load; formed in intestinal wall after absorption
    (3) Pre-beta, beta, and alpha lipoproteins—carry less fat; formed in liver from endogenous fat and carried to tissues for oxidation
C. Digestion (Table 6-1)
D. Absorption and metabolism
  1. Fatty acids, glycerol, monoglycerides, diglycerides, cholesterol, and phospholipids in combination with bile salts absorbed through intestinal wall
  2. Some fatty acids resynthesized to neutral fats in intestinal wall
  3. Fat transported to bloodstream via lymph system and thoracic duct; some (short and medium chain triglycerides) transported via portal system to liver
  4. In liver
    a. Fatty acids resynthesized to neutral fats and phospholipids
    b. Fats released to bloodstream as lipoproteins
    c. Cholesterol synthesized
    d. Bile salts produced from cholesterol
    e. Fats synthesized from carbohydrate and protein
    f. Fats oxidized to carbon dioxide and water
    g. Glycerol converted to glucose
    h. Fats converted to carbohydrate or protein
  5. Fat may be oxidized for energy, heat, or activity needs
  6. Fat may be stored as adipose tissue for reserve fuel
E. Functions of fat in body
  1. Provide energy; most concentrated source of energy, producing 9 calories per gram
  2. Aid in digestion, absorption, and utilization of other nutrients
  3. Provide fat-soluble vitamins and aid in their absorption and utilization
  4. Provide essential fatty acids
  5. Assist in regulation of body temperature

  6. Assist in support and protection of body organs
F. Role of fats in diet
  1. 40% to 60% total calories in average American diet derived from fat
  2. Fats provide palatability and satiety value to diet
  3. Economy in selection of fats would feature margarine instead of butter; corn, cottonseed, or peanut oil instead of olive oil; and evaporated milk instead of cream
G. Food sources of fats
  1. High—butter, margarine, oil, lard, cream, avocado, olives, fatty meats
  2. Low—most fruits, vegetables, breads, and cereal products
  3. High in polyunsaturated fatty acids— English walnuts, safflower oil, corn oil, soybean oil, cottonseed oil, fish oils
  4. High in saturated fatty acids—coconut oil, chocolate, beef fat, butter, lamb fat, pork fat
H. Modifications of fat intake
  1. Low-fat diet may be recommended for
    a. Gallbladder disease
    b. Atherosclerosis; also for arteriosclerosis
    c. Diarrhea
    d. Anorexia nervosa
    e. Pernicious anemia
    f. Idiopathic steatorrhea
  2. Diet high in polyunsaturated fatty acids and low in saturated fatty acids may be recommended for patients with atherosclerosis or multiple sclerosis; decrease in calories, carbohydrate (glucose), and cholesterol may also be indicated
  3. High-fat intake sometimes recommended for
    a. Underweight (with high-calorie diet)
    b. Peptic ulcer
    c. Epilepsy (with low-carbohydrate diet)
    d. Dumping syndrome
  4. Deficient intake of fat may result in loss of weight or feeling of hunger
6. Minerals
A. Iron
  1. Occurrence
    a. Hemoglobin 70%
    b. Storage depots 25%
    c. Enzymes, muscles, and tissues 5%
  2. Principal function of iron in body is

formation of hemoglobin, myoglobin, and oxidative enzymes
3. Utilization and metabolism
   a. About 10% ingested iron absorbed and utilized by body
   b. Hydrochloric acid in stomach and vitamin C promote the reducing of iron from ferric to ferrous salt
   c. Absorption of iron
      (1) Regulated by body's need for iron
      (2) Favored by presence of vitamin C and HCl
      (3) Occurs as iron, in its reduced form (ferrous salt), combines with apoferritin to form ferritin in intestinal wall
      (4) Prevented by phytates, phosphates, oxalates, and carbonates
   d. Copper aids in formation of hemoglobin from iron
   e. Iron stored principally in liver, spleen, and bone marrow
   f. Iron resulting from breakdown of hemoglobin reutilized and little excreted
4. Foods high in iron—egg yolks, liver, organ meats, meat, apricots, bran, legumes, prunes, enriched and whole grain breads and cereals
5. Modifications of iron in diet
   a. High-iron intake, frequently with iron salts, recommended during periods of growth and pregnancy and frequently for
      (1) Prolonged or chronic blood loss
      (2) Peptic ulcer
      (3) Nutritional anemias
   b. Deficiency—anemia resulting
      (1) After gastrectomy
      (2) From deficient intake over long period and during growth periods
      (3) From chronic blood loss
      (4) From malabsorption syndrome
6. Food and Nutrition Board of National Research Council recommends 10 mg. iron per day for men and postmenopausal women; 18 mg. for women of childbearing age; 1.5 mg. per kilogram body weight for infants; 10 to 18 mg. per day for children
B. Calcium
   1. Occurrence

   a. Almost all calcium in body found in teeth and skeleton
   b. 1% calcium in body found in body fluids and tissues
2. Functions of calcium in body
   a. Builds bones and teeth
   b. Aids in blood clotting
   c. Aids in transmitting nerve impulses
   d. Maintains acid-base balance
   e. Activates enzymes
   f. Important for muscle contraction
   g. Important for membrane permeability
3. Utilization and metabolism
   a. 20% to 30% ingested calcium absorbed and utilized by body
   b. Absorption influenced by body's need for calcium
   c. Factors that favor calcium absorption
      (1) HCl in stomach
      (2) Protein
      (3) Body's need for calcium
      (4) Lactose
      (5) Ratio of calcium to phosphorus of 1:1
      (6) Vitamins C and D
   d. Factors that interfere with calcium absorption
      (1) Impaired fat absorption
      (2) Insoluble calcium compounds result from fatty acids, phytic acid, phosphorus, and oxalates in food
   e. Parathyroid hormone regulates calcium-phosphorus levels in blood
   f. Vitamins A, C, and D important for calcium and phosphorus deposition in bone
   g. Inactive or bedridden persons lose body calcium and have decreased ability to absorb and replace calcium
4. Foods high in calcium—milk and milk products, legumes, fish, green leafy vegetables, enriched cereals
5. Modification of calcium intake
   a. High-calcium intake recommended during periods of growth, pregnancy, and lactation
   b. Low-calcium diets sometimes recommended
      (1) For diagnostic test for parathyroid function
      (2) For urinary calculi

c. Deficient intake or poor absorption of calcium may be manifested by
  (1) Tetany
  (2) Muscle spasms
  (3) Delayed blood clotting
  (4) Stunted growth
  (5) Defective bone and tooth formation
6. Food and Nutrition Board of National Research Council recommends 800 mg. calcium per day for men and women; additional 400 mg. during pregnancy and 500 mg. during lactation; 700 mg. for artificially fed infants; 800 mg. for children 1 to 9 years of age; 900 to 1,400 mg. for adolescents
C. Phosphorus
  1. Occurrence
    a. All body cells and fluids
    b. 80% in bones and teeth
    c. Remainder in muscle cells and fluid in combination with carbohydrate, protein, lipids, and other organic compounds
  2. Functions in body
    a. Builds bones and teeth
    b. Promotes growth
    c. Maintains acid-base balance
    d. Aids in calcium utilization
    e. Important in metabolism, absorption, and transportation of carbohydrate, fat, and protein
    f. Important in energy production
  3. Utilization and metabolism
    a. 70% ingested phosphorus absorbed by body
    b. Vitamin D aids in deposition of phosphorus in bones
    c. Parathyroid hormone regulates calcium-phosphorus blood levels
    d. Sex hormones favor bone growth
  4. Intake should be at least equal to that of calcium in diets for children and during pregnancy and lactation
  5. Foods high in phosphorus—milk, milk products, whole grain cereals, meat, fish, legumes, nuts
  6. Modification of phosphorus intake
    a. Low-phosphorus diet may be recommended for phosphate calculi
    b. Deficiency may result in
      (1) Rickets
      (2) Stunted growth
      (3) Poor development of bones and teeth
    c. Results of excess of phosphorus in diet

(1) Increased excretion of calcium
(2) Decreased absorption of calcium
7. Food and Nutrition Board of National Research Council recommends phosphorus equal calcium allowance for all ages except young infant
D. Sodium
  1. Occurrence
    a. In body fluids
      (1) Largest fraction in blood plasma
      (2) Extracellular fluid
    b. In food
      (1) Most sodium chloride (table salt) added in preparation, seasoning, or preservation of food
      (2) Protein foods such as meat, eggs, and milk good sources of natural sodium
  2. Functions of sodium in body
    a. Regulates body fluids
    b. Maintains acid-base balance
    c. Favors muscle contraction
    d. Transmits nerve impulses
  3. Utilization and metabolism
    a. Kidney regulates retention and excretion of sodium
    b. Adrenal cortex hormone regulates sodium chloride excretion
      (1) Deficient excretion of adrenal cortex hormone causes increased sodium chloride excretion
      (2) Excess excretion of adrenal cortex hormone causes sodium chloride retention
  4. Modifications of sodium intake
    a. Average intake per day 2 to 6 gm. (5 to 15 gm. NaCl)
    b. Sodium restriction may be recommended for
      (1) Edema occurring from
        (a) Cardiac disease
        (b) Liver disease
        (c) Renal disease
        (d) Toxemias of pregnancy
        (e) Steroid therapy
      (2) Hypertension
    c. Deficiency results from
      (1) Chronic diarrhea
      (2) Excessive vomiting
      (3) Low-sodium syndrome may occur if patient on low-sodium diet neglects to maintain medical attention

(4) Excessive sweating
5. Food sources of sodium (Table 6-5)
   a. Main source, ordinary table salt used in cooking, seasoning, and commercial processing of food
   b. Baking powder and baking soda
   c. Soups, sauces, gravies, cheese, salted nuts, salted crackers
   d. Protein foods, meat, fish, and milk, relatively high natural sodium content
   e. Beets, carrots, celery, chard, kale, beet greens, dandelion greens, spinach, and regular canned vegetables high in sodium
   f. Bread, bakery products, butter, and margarine all contain added salt
   g. High sodium content in water in some areas
   h. Generally most fresh and frozen vegetables and fruits, cereals (except those with salt added commercially), and oils low in sodium

E. Potassium
   1. Occurrence
      a. Intracellular fluid
      b. Widely distributed in foods such as meats, fruits, and vegetables
   2. Functions of potassium in body
      a. Regulates osmosis
      b. Transmits nerve impulses
      c. Important for muscle contraction
      d. Maintains acid-base balance
      e. Associated with phosphorylation resulting in glycogen deposit
   3. Excretion and retention of potassium regulated by kidney
   4. Average intake of potassium from 4 to 6 gm. per day
   5. Food sources of potassium
      a. High—whole grain cereals and breads, dried fruits, bananas, meat, poultry, fish, nuts, dried beans, greens, coffee, tea
      b. Low—refined cereals and breads, applesauce, peaches, pears, apricots, asparagus, green beans, beets, peas
   6. Modifications of potassium intake
      a. Low-potassium diet may be recommended for patients with renal failure
      b. When excretion of potassium is impaired, excessive intake may be toxic
      c. Deficiency—demonstrated by muscle weakness, heart irregularities,

respiratory disturbances, and mental confusion
      (1) From dietary cause unlikely
      (2) From G.I. loss, excessive diarrhea or vomiting
      (3) From prolonged administration of glucose and saline
      (4) From hormone and drug therapy
   d. High-potassium intake suggested when certain diuretics administered

F. Iodine
   1. Occurrence
      a. In body in thyroid gland and in small but constant amount in blood
      b. In food
         (1) Iodine content of food depends on soil and water where food is grown
         (2) Use of iodized salt provides adequate amounts and should be emphasized during growth and pregnancy
   2. Chief function—regulation of energy metabolism as constituent of thyroxin
   3. Deficiency in children results in stunted growth and cretinism
   4. Deficiency in adults results in simple goiter, myxedema, and perhaps toxic goiter
   5. Food and Nutrition Board of National Research Council recommends 1 mg. iodine per kilogram body weight for adults per day

G. Magnesium
   1. Occurrence
      a. 75% of magnesium in body in the bones
      b. Remainder in soft tissue and body fluids
   2. Magnesium functions as catalyst in energy metabolism
   3. Magnesium deficiency resulting in tetany and convulsions reported in alcoholics and in persons on severe dietary restrictions
   4. Food and Nutrition Board of National Research Council recommends an intake of 350 mg. magnesium per day for adult male and 300 mg. for adult female

H. Fluorine
   1. Occurrence
      a. Skeletal system
      b. Teeth
      c. Drinking water

2. Chief function of fluorine in retarding or preventing dental caries
   a. Small amount, 1 part per million (ppm) in drinking water, reduces number of dental caries
   b. Fluorine functions either by inhibiting bacterial action or by reducing solubility of tooth enamel
3. Excess of fluorine causes mottling of teeth

I. Sulfur
   1. Essential element supplied chiefly by sulfur-containing amino acids, cystine and methionine
   2. Constituent of insulin, biotin, thiamine, and hair, nails, and skin

J. Copper—important in absorption of iron and utilization of iron for hemoglobin formation

7. Vitamins

A. Definitions
   1. Vitamins—organic compounds essential to life and function; in body in very small amounts
   2. Biosynthesis—formation of vitamins in body
   3. Antivitamins—substances that interfere with action of vitamins
   4. Provitamin—substance that can be converted into vitamin

B. Classification (see also p. 168)
   1. Fat-soluble vitamins
      a. Vitamin A
      b. Vitamin D
      c. Vitamin E
      d. Vitamin K
   2. Water-soluble vitamins
      a. Vitamin C
      b. B complex vitamins

C. Vitamin A
   1. Classification
      a. Preformed vitamin A (animal source)
      b. Provitamin A, carotene (vegetable source)
   2. Characteristics
      a. Stable to ordinary cooking methods, acids, and alkalies
      b. Destroyed by oxidation by high temperatures, prolonged heating, and dehydration
   3. Metabolism
      a. Carotene—converted to vitamin A in intestinal wall and liver
      b. Vitamin A—stored in liver
      c. Factors that interfere with or enhance fat absorption also interfere with or enhance vitamin A absorption
      d. Vitamin E prevents oxidation of vitamin A
   4. Functions
      a. Essential for normal vision
      b. Essential for maintenance of epithelial cells
      c. Essential for bone, tooth, and skin development
   5. Good food sources—butter, liver, eggs, fish oils, cream, whole milk, green leafy vegetables, green peppers, carrots, yellow squash, sweet potatoes, apricots
   6. Deficiency
      a. Retarded bone and tooth formation
      b. Nightblindness
      c. Xerophthalmia
      d. Keratomalacia
      e. Keratinization of mucous membranes and skin
   7. Excess (toxic)
      a. Carotenemia (excessive carotene)
      b. Bone fragility
      c. Nausea
      d. Headache
   8. Food and Nutrition Board of National Research Council recommends 5,000 I.U. vitamin A for adults; additional 1,000 I.U. for second and third trimester of pregnancy; additional 3,000 I.U. for lactation; 1,500 I.U. for infants; from 2,000 to 5,000 I.U. for children 1 to 18 years of age

D. Vitamin D group
   1. Classification
      a. D_2 (activated ergosterol, ergocalciferol)
      b. D_3 (activated 7-dehydrocholesterol, cholecalciferol)
   2. Vitamin D stored in liver
   3. Functions—important in absorption and utilization of calcium and phosphorus for bone and tooth formation
   4. Deficiency
      a. Rickets
      b. Osteomalacia
      c. Osteoporosis
      d. Poor teeth and bones
      e. Bow legs and enlarged joints
      f. Bone calcification failure
   5. Excess (toxic)
      a. Headaches
      b. Nausea

c. Calcification of soft tissue
6. Food source—fortified milk
7. Food and Nutrition Board of National Research Council recommends 400 I.U. vitamin D per day for infants, children, adolescents, and during pregnancy and lactation

E. Vitamin E (tocopherols)
1. Found in vegetable oils, wheat germ, and green leafy vegetables
2. Chief function of vitamin E in body as antioxidant
   a. Protects carotene and vitamin A from oxidation
   b. Protects unsaturated fatty acids from oxidation
3. Increased intake of polyunsaturated fatty acids requires more vitamin E
4. Food and Nutrition Board of National Research Council recommends 30 I.U. vitamin E per day for adult male and 25 I.U. for adult female

F. Vitamin K (menadione)
1. Found in alfalfa and green leafy vegetables
2. Synthesized by microorganisms in intestinal tract—partially absorbed
3. Chief function in synthesis of prothrombin in the liver for use in the blood-clotting mechanism
4. Used to prevent hemorrhagic disease of newborn infants
5. Deficiency may result from prolonged antibiotic therapy, faulty absorption, bile deficiency

G. Vitamin C (ascorbic acid)
1. Vitamin C destroyed by oxidation
2. Functions
   a. Forms intercellular, cementlike substances
   b. Important in calcium and iron absorption
   c. Important in utilization of amino acids
   d. Important in conversion of folic acid to citrovorum factor
   e. Important in bone and tooth formation
   f. Important in capillary integrity
   g. Combats and neutralizes toxins
   h. Activates enzymes
   i. Important in oxidation and reduction reactions
3. Good food sources—citrus fruits, green leafy vegetables, broccoli, cabbage, green peppers, melons, strawberries, tomatoes, potatoes
4. Deficiency
   a. Scurvy
   b. Hemorrhage
   c. Faulty bone development
5. Food and Nutrition Board of National Research Council recommends 55 to 60 mg. vitamin C for adults; 65 mg. for pregnancy and 75 mg. for lactation; 25 to 60 mg. from infancy through adolescence

H. Thiamine (B$_1$)
1. Destroyed by heat and alkalies
2. Functions
   a. Essential for growth
   b. Important in carbohydrate metabolism
   c. Important for normal function and maintenance of gastrointestinal tract
   d. Important for maintenance of nervous system
   e. Important in conversion of tryptophan to niacin
3. Good food sources—pork, liver, eggs, milk, legumes, peas, potatoes, enriched cereals and breads, citrus fruits
4. Deficiency
   a. Beriberi
   b. Loss of appetite
   c. Psychic changes
   d. Muscle weakness
   e. Fatigue
   f. Polyneuritis
5. Food and Nutrition Board of National Research Council recommends 0.5 mg. thiamine per 1,000 calories for all ages but not less than 1.0 mg. per day; additional 0.2 mg. during pregnancy

I. Riboflavin
1. Riboflavin stable to ordinary cooking but destroyed by exposure to light
2. Functions
   a. Important in carbohydrate, protein, and fatty acid metabolism
   b. Necessary for conversion of tryptophan to niacin
   c. Essential for growth
3. Good food sources—milk, liver, pork, meat, fish, poultry, enriched breads and cereals
4. Deficiency
   a. Ariboflavinosis
   b. Cheilosis
   c. Stomatitis
   d. Itching and burning eyes

e. Glossitis

f. Dermatitis

g. Photophobia

5. Food and Nutrition Board of National Research Council recommends 0.7 mg. riboflavin per kilogram for adults; additional 0.3 mg. for pregnancy; additional 0.5 mg. for lactation

J. Niacin

1. Stable to heat, light, alkali, acid, oxidation

2. Important in metabolism of carbohydrate, protein, and fat

3. Tryptophan precursor of niacin

4. Good food sources—liver, fish, poultry, meat, peanuts, peas, enriched breads and cereals

5. Deficiency

a. Pellagra (multiple deficiency)

b. Tongue lesions

c. Gastrointestinal upsets

d. Dermatitis

e. Diarrhea

f. Dementia

g. Death

6. Food and Nutrition Board of National Research Council recommendations in terms of niacin equivalents (tryptophan converted to niacin; 60 mg. tryptophan equal to 1 mg. niacin)—6.6 mg. per 1,000 calories for all ages but not less than 13 equivalents; additional 2 mg. for pregnancy; additional 7 mg. for lactation

K. Pantothenic acid—part of coenzyme A; important in metabolism of carbohydrate, fat, and protein

L. Biotin—important in metabolism of carbohydrate, fat, and protein

M. Pyridoxine

1. Important in metabolism of protein, fat, and carbohydrate

2. Important in conversion of tryptophan to niacin

3. Deficiency in infants characterized by hyperirritability and convulsions

4. Used in treatment of nausea of pregnancy, in certain anemias, and in prevention of dental caries

N. Folacin (folic acid)

1. Folacin found in various foods and synthesized by intestinal bacteria

2. Converted to citrovorum factor in body

3. Functions as enzyme in blood formation

4. Important in protein metabolism

5. Used in the treatment of anemias of

a. Sprue

b. Pregnancy

c. Nutritional macrocytic anemias

d. Megaloblastic anemias in infants

6. Food and Nutrition Board of National Research Council recommends 0.4 mg. folacin per day for adults

O. B_{12}

1. Essential for normal function of bone marrow, nervous system, and gastrointestinal tract

2. Important in protein, fat, and carbohydrate metabolism

3. Important in maturation of blood cells

4. A specific for pernicious anemia (extrinsic factor in food)

5. Found in meat, liver, and milk

6. Food and Nutrition Board of National Research Council recommends 5 mg. B_{12} per day for adults

8. **Energy metabolism** (p. 72)

A. Metabolism refers to chemical changes taking place in body

B. Basal metabolism

1. Refers to energy needs of individual at rest without influence of food

2. Influenced by

a. Age and growth

b. Body composition and sex

c. Endocrine glands

d. Climate

e. Body surface—tall and thin individuals have higher rates than short and plump

C. Total metabolic needs influenced by

1. Basal metabolic rate (BMR)

2. Specific dynamic action of food (SDA) —6%

3. Exercise and activity (50%)

D. Calories

1. Definitions

a. Calorie—amount of heat required to raise temperature of 1 kg. water 1° C.

b. Calorie—indication of potential energy or measure of heat resulting from metabolism of food

2. Functions

a. Provide heat and energy

b. Maintain body weight

3. Modifications of calories in diet

a. Caloric intake in excess of needs— overweight or obesity

b. Caloric intake of less than normal requirements—underweight, malnutrition, and starvation

c. High-caloric diets sometimes recommended for
   (1) Prolonged fevers
   (2) Growth periods
   (3) Malnutrition and underweight
   (4) Hyperthyroidism
d. Low-caloric diets frequently recommended for patients who are overweight or obese; for patients who are overweight and have cardiac disease, diabetes, hypothyroidism, arthritis
4. For gross calculation of total energy needs allow 35 to 40 calories per kilogram body weight

9. **Guide for meeting nutritional adequacy —basic 4***
A. Milk group
  1. Includes
    a. Milk—whole, evaporated, skim, dry, buttermilk
    b. Cheese—cottage, cream, cheddar
    c. Ice cream
  2. Recommended intake—whole milk
    a. Children, under 9 years of age, 2 to 3 cups; 9 to 12 years, 3 or more cups
    b. Teen-agers, 4 or more cups
    c. Adults, 2 or more cups
    d. Pregnant women, 3 or more cups
    e. Nursing mothers, 4 or more cups
  3. Calcium equivalents
    a. 1-inch cube cheddar cheese—½ cup milk
    b. ½ cup cottage cheese—⅓ cup milk
    c. 2 tbsp. cream cheese—1 tbsp. milk
    d. ½ cup ice cream—¼ cup milk
  4. Major nutritional contribution
    a. Complete protein
    b. Calcium and phosphorus
    c. Vitamin A, vitamin D, thiamine, and riboflavin
B. Meat group—2 or more servings
  1. Includes
    a. Beef, veal, lamb, pork, variety meat
    b. Poultry and eggs
    c. Fish and shellfish
    d. Alternates—dry beans, dry peas, lentils, nuts, peanuts, peanut butter
  2. One serving includes
    a. 2 to 3 oz. lean cooked meat, poultry, or fish

    b. 2 eggs
    c. 1 cup cooked dry beans, dry peas, or lentils
    d. 4 tbsp. peanut butter
  3. Major nutritional contribution
    a. Complete protein
    b. Iron and phosphorus
    c. Vitamin B complex (especially pork and liver)
    d. Liver, excellent source of vitamin A, B complex, and iron
C. Vegetable-fruit group—4 or more servings
  1. Dark green or deep yellow, at least every other day
    a. Apricots, cantaloupe, mango, persimmon, pumpkin
    b. Broccoli, carrots, chard, collards, cress, kale, spinach, sweet potatoes, turnip greens, winter squash
  2. Vitamin C source—1 serving good source or 2 servings fair source every day
    a. Good source—grapefruit, orange, cantaloupe, guava, mango, papaya, strawberries, broccoli, Brussels sprouts, green pepper, sweet red pepper
    b. Fair source—honeydew melon, lemon, tangerine, watermelon, asparagus tips, raw cabbage, collards, garden cress, kale, kohlrabi, mustard greens, potatoes, sweet potatoes, spinach, tomatoes, turnip greens
  3. Major nutritional contribution
    a. Vitamins A and C
    b. Calcium, iron, thiamine, riboflavin
    c. Residue and bulk
D. Bread-cereal group—4 or more servings whole-grain, enriched, or restored
  1. Includes bread, cereal, flours, pastes, baked products containing these items
  2. Major nutritional contribution
    a. Thiamine, riboflavin, niacin (enriched)
    b. Iron (enriched), calcium (optional enrichment), phosphorus
    c. Carbohydrate, residue and bulk
E. Additional foods to meet recommended allowances for calories and all nutrients

NUTRITION AND PUBLIC HEALTH NURSING

1. **Objective of public health nutrition**
To promote, restore, and maintain health for all people through nutrition

---

*From Consumers All, The Yearbook of Agriculture 1965, U.S.D.A., Washington, D. C.

2. **Many organizations promoting public health nutrition through education, research, and service**

Following represents only small number of these organizations and their activities

A. International
  1. World Health Organization (WHO) interested in medical phases of nutrition
  2. Food and Agricultural Organization (FAO) provides technical assistance for agricultural problems in production, processing, and distribution of food products
  3. United Nations International Children's Fund (UNICEF) distributes food, equipment, and materials for child and maternal welfare
B. National
  1. Department of Health, Education and Welfare
    a. Public Health Service
      (1) Enrichment of food products
      (2) Sanitation of food
      (3) Research on food additives
      (4) Research, materials, and services for chronic diseases
      (5) Nutritional surveys
    b. Federal Food, Drug and Cosmetic Act provides for adequate and accurate labeling, safety, and wholesomeness of food
  2. Department of Agriculture engages in research, sanitation, education, distribution, analysis, inspection, and economy in food and nutrition through
    a. School lunch program
    b. Agriculture Marketing Service
    c. Federal Extension Service
    d. Agricultural Research Service
    e. Human Nutrition Service
  3. Academy of Sciences, National Research Council, Food and Nutrition Board promotes research and makes recommendations such as recommended dietary allowances
  4. Associations
    a. American Dietetic Association
    b. American Medical Association
    c. American Home Economics Association
    d. American Public Health Association
    e. American Heart Association
    f. American Red Cross
    g. American Diabetes Association
C. State and local efforts often patterned after national activities

3. **Public health nurse**

Works as member of health team to further community health; often works closely with individual or family; able to evaluate nutritional intake and to provide guidance, instruction, and assistance in meeting nutritional needs

4. **Situations involving nutrition frequently encountered by public health nurse**
A. Care of individuals during all phases of life cycle
B. Care of patients with chronic diseases such as diabetes, cardiac diseases, allergies, and arthritis
C. Inadequate nutritional intakes in all age groups as a result of
  1. Disease
  2. Lack of knowledge
  3. Food fads
  4. Idiosyncrasies
  5. Economic problems
  6. Cultural and social problems
D. Undernutrition and obesity

5. **Special nutritional considerations during life cycle**
A. Pregnancy and lactation
  1. Nutritional objectives
    a. To ensure good nutrition before, during, and after pregnancy and during lactation
    b. To provide adequate nutrition to meet mother's needs and additional needs for reproduction and lactation
  2. Observed nutritional influences
    a. Underweight women had higher incidence of prematurity and toxemia
    b. Teen-age pregnancies resulted in more premature births and toxemia
  3. Nutritional needs
    a. Calories to provide for approximately 25 pounds weight gain during pregnancy and to ensure adequate lactation
    b. Increased intake of all nutrients, especially protein, to provide for maintenance and repair, plus additional demands of growth and lactation
    c. Sources of vitamin D and iodine must be supplied
    d. Supplements of iron and folic acid recommended to prevent anemias
    e. Diet for pregnant teen-age girl must meet needs for her growth as well as those for pregnancy

4. Diet based on basic 4 food guide including 1 qt. milk daily during pregnancy and lactation plus additional serving of each of other groups to meet nutritional needs; additional fluids during lactation (see Guide for meeting nutritional adequacy—basic 4)
5. Complications of pregnancy and possible dietary modifications
   a. Underweight—carefully controlled intake to attain desirable weight gain and optimum nutrition
   b. Nausea and vomiting—limited fluids; small frequent feedings; restricted fat, high carbohydrate
   c. Constipation—increased fluids and roughage
   d. Toxemia—increased protein and calories

B. Infancy
1. Nutritional objectives
   a. To provide for adequate and consistent growth and development
   b. To establish good eating patterns
   c. To establish good relationship between mother and child
2. Emphasis on all nutrients to meet high energy requirements and demands of rapid growth and development of all tissues
3. Diet
   a. Breast-feeding
      (1) Has psychological value for both infant and mother
      (2) Is best suited to the needs of the infant
      (3) Reduces chance for infection and error
      (4) Provides an immunity factor
   b. Formula feeding must be sterile and nutritionally adequate
   c. Additions and changes introduced slowly and one at a time
      (1) From formula to orange juice, cereals, fruits, vegetables, meats, bread, eggs
      (2) From strained to chopped foods
      (3) From breast or formula to cup
   d. Supplementation of diet with vitamins A, C, and D
   e. Provision for variety
   f. Basic 4 food groups guide for diet from near end of first year through life (see Guide for meeting nutritional adequacy—basic 4)

4. Diseases and complications during infancy with possible dietary modifications
   a. Diarrhea—sterile feedings; decreased fat; decreased carbohydrate
   b. Constipation—increased fluids, added prune juice, change in type of carbohydrate
   c. Celiac disease—gluten-restricted diet
   d. Allergy—removal of offending food
   e. Inborn errors of metabolism
      (1) Phenylketonuria—restricted phenylalanine intake
      (2) Galactosemia—elimination of foods containing lactose or galactose

C. Childhood
1. Nutritional objectives
   a. To provide for adequate and consistent growth and development
   b. To establish good eating patterns
   c. To provide for increasing physical activity
2. Diet
   a. Change in consistency of food, from chopped to solid foods
   b. Change in method of feeding, finger food and self-feeding by spoon
   c. Provision for variety and attractiveness in menus
   d. Supplementation with vitamin D
   e. Provision of adequate diet with consideration for child's appetite, preferences, motor development
3. Nutritional problems
   a. Anemia and obesity
   b. Low intake of calcium, iron, vitamins A and C
   c. No breakfast

D. Adolescence
1. Nutritional objectives
   a. To provide adequate nutrition to meet demands of rapid growth and often tremendous energy expenditure
   b. To emphasize good eating patterns
      (1) Regular eating pattern
      (2) Proper kinds and amounts of snack foods
2. Nutritional needs high in all respects and adequate intakes of all nutrients should be stressed
3. Diet based on basic 4 food guide (see Guide for meeting nutritional adequacy—basic 4)

4. Nutritional problems
   a. Low intake of calcium, vitamins A and C; iron in girls
   b. Anemia and skin problems
   c. Underweight and overweight
   d. Inadequate intake resulting from
      (1) Psychological factors
      (2) Fear of overweight
      (3) Fad diets
      (4) Poor choice of snack foods
      (5) Elimination of breakfast
      (6) Irregular eating pattern
   e. Additional stress of pregnancy
5. Appeal for better nutrition made through its influence on physical appearance, figure control, complexion, physical fitness
E. Geriatrics
   1. Nutritional objective—to provide adequate nutrition to ensure and promote health
   2. Nutritional needs require
      a. Calories in relation to desired weight and activity
      b. Consistency of diet in relation to physical, physiologic, or mechanical capacity
      c. Adequate intake of all nutrients to meet adult needs
   3. Diet based on basic 4 food guide (see Guide for meeting nutritional adequacy—basic 4)
   4. Nutritional problems
      a. Low intake of calcium and vitamins A and C
      b. Obesity or overweight
      c. Faulty eating patterns resulting from
         (1) Lifelong eating habits
         (2) Psychological factors
         (3) Economic factors
         (4) Health status
         (5) Physical and physiologic capacity
         (6) Food fads
6. **Procedure for assisting family in meeting nutritional needs**
A. Establish rapport
B. Identify nutritional problem or problems
C. Note pertinent information that influences dietary patterns
   1. Age, weight, height, sex, and activity of family members
   2. General appearance and health status
   3. Cultural and religious customs
   4. Social and psychological meaning of food

   5. Financial status
   6. Physical and intelligence capacity
   7. Storage, preparation, and serving facilities
   8. Shopping and preparation methods—who, where, and what
   9. Family's knowledge of nutrition
   10. General interest and willingness to cooperate
D. Take nutrition history
   1. Kind and amounts of food in usual pattern on daily or weekly basis including between-meal snacks and differences of week-end pattern if any
   2. Distribution and time of meals and snacks
   3. Personal preferences
   4. Time and number of meals
   5. Where meals eaten
E. Evaluate nutritional intake based on basic 4 food guide and on recommended allowances of Food and Nutrition Board of National Research Council
F. Establish goals and suggest gradual changes and improvements in present pattern
G. Plan frequent follow-up visits for support, education, and encouragement
H. Utilize resource material
   1. Physician, dietitian, nutritionist
   2. Community agencies, associations, hospitals, clinics
   3. Textbooks, pamphlets, charts
7. **Planning, preparing, and serving menus**
A. Consider family preferences
B. Meet nutritional needs
C. Provide for attractiveness and variety through
   1. Color and shape
   2. Temperature
   3. Taste and flavor
   4. Arrangement
   5. Texture
   6. Preparation
8. **Economy planning**
A. Plan menus and market lists in advance
B. Select most economical shopping area
C. Take advantage of sales
D. Purchase foods in season
E. Purchase foods in sizes, amounts, and grades most suitable for use
F. Compare prices
   1. Fresh, dried, canned, frozen
   2. Edible portion vs. purchased price
   3. Homemade vs. precooked, mixes, ready-to-eat items

TABLE 6-2
DIET IN DISEASE

Disease	Possible modifications of normal diet	Purposes of dietary application	Remarks
Anemia	Adequate diet High protein, low fat, high iron	Provide adequate nutrition Correct nutritional deficiencies	Iron salts essential Vitamin C and vitamin C–containing foods aid iron absorption
Pernicious anemia	Soft, low fat	Facilitate swallowing	Low fat depresses secretion of HCl which is low in some cases; easily digested foods Therapy chiefly medical with administration of iron, liver concentrate, or B_{12}
Arthritis	Adequate diet	Maintain adequate nutrition	High caloric to increase weight; low caloric to decrease weight
Heart	Low calorie, easily available carbohydrate, moderate fat, moderate protein	Reduce strain on heart Improve efficiency of heart Supply adequate nutrition	Reduce calories for overweight individuals Small frequent feedings of easily manipulated and digested foods; foods nonirritating mechanically
	Karrell diet		Used in acute conditions; 800 ml. skim milk given in 4 feedings
	Restricted sodium	Reduce or prevent edema	May be as low as 200 mg. sodium with adequate protein; also used in hypertension
Coronary artery	Modified fat: high polyunsaturated, low saturated, low cholesterol		Reduce blood lipid levels
Hypertension	Restricted sodium	Reduce hypertension	
Diabetes mellitus	Diet designed to meet individual needs	Ensure adequate nutrition	Meet recommended amounts of all nutrients
	Reduced carbohydrate Reduced or modified fat Caloric	Ensure constant intake Maintain weight at slightly below desired weight	In-between and night feeding determined by medical therapy Weight reduction desirable for overweight diabetic
Diarrheas	Depending on etiology Low residue	Promote optimum assimilation Avoid irritation Provide adequate nutrition	No food during short acute cases Avoid chemical and mechanical stimulants Emphasis on supplying all nutrients lost in great quantities; adequate fluids and minerals to maintain electrolyte balance and water balance
Epilepsy	Ketogenic	Reduce number and severity of attacks	Produce state of ketosis High in fat; low in carbohydrate (10 to 30 gm.) adequate protein; used for children, diet likely to be deficient in minerals and vitamins
	Dry diet		Serve foods with little water content
	Normal diet		Drug therapy preferred
Fever	High calorie, high protein	Provide adequate nutrition Amounts to meet increased BMR	Modification in consistency as indicated; fluid maintenance important
Gallbladder	Low fat	Stimulate or depress flow of bile Relieve discomfort of patient	Cholecystitis: discomfort of patient indicates low-fat diet Avoid foods not readily tolerated
	Test diets		Fat-free meal and high-fat meal to determine functional capacity of gallbladder

Continued.

TABLE 6-2

DIET IN DISEASE—cont'd

Disease	Possible modifications of normal diet	Purposes of dietary application	Remarks
Gastro-intestinal surgery—			Diet depends on type of surgery
Preoperative	Restricted residue	Reduce residue in digestive tract	Highly seasoned foods limited; fiber minimal; consistency as indicated
	High calorie, high protein	Provide optimal nutrition Prevent shock Protect organs Promote recovery	Full diet with between meal nourishments
Postoperative	Liquid Low residue	Avoid discomfort of patient Stimulate peristalsis Restore electrolytes	Progressive diet: nothing by mouth, sips of water (no milk or fruit juice), liquid, soft (no milk or fruit juice), regular
	High calorie, high protein	Speed recovery Build and repair Provide optimal nutrition	
Dumping syndrome	High protein, high fat, low carbohydrate	Provide for slow and complete digestion and absorption	Small frequent feedings; fluids only between feedings
Gout	Low purine, low calorie, low fat	Provide adequate nutrition Reduce severity and number of attacks	Many patients overweight; limit meats; use easily digested foods; avoid highly seasoned foods, organ meats, anchovies, whole grain cereal products, alcohol
	Normal diet		Drug therapy preferred
Intestine, constipation	High or low roughage, high fluids, high fat	Stimulate peristalsis Provide adequacy	Spastic: foods low in mechanical stimulation, soft residue, high in chemical stimulants Atonic: high mechanical and chemical stimulation
Nontropical sprue	Gluten free		May be result of allergic response to protein in wheat, rye, oats, barley
Colitis, chronic, ulcerative	High protein, high calorie, low residue	Provide optimum nourishment Prevent irritation	Replace nutrient loss Avoid mechanical and chemical irritants Foods easily assimilated
Kidney Nephritis	Low and high protein, adequate calories	Supply adequate nutrition Spare damaged kidney Increase its efficiency Prevent complications	Protein may be specified as low, moderate, or high Low protein; acute stage Modified intakes of meat, milk, eggs, cheese Adequate calories for optimum protein utilization
Nephrosis	Restricted sodium High protein, low sodium	Reduce and prevent edema Replenish protein loss Reduce fluid retention	
Renal failure	Low protein, low potassium, low sodium, restricted fluids, adequate calories	Kidney unable to handle metabolic products	Butter balls: sweet butter, sugar
Stones		Prevent recurrence of stones	Diet depends on composition of stones
Liver	High protein (unless hepatic coma present or approaching), high carbohydrate Restricted sodium	Protect liver against stress Provide adequate nutrition Increase efficiency of liver Regenerate tissue Reduce ascites	Avoid highly seasoned foods and foods not readily tolerated

TABLE 6-2
DIET IN DISEASE—cont'd

Disease	Possible modifications of normal diet	Purposes of dietary application	Remarks
Coma	Low protein	Decrease metabolic production of ammonia	
Ulcers	High protein, high fat, bland	Provide adequate nutrition Decrease irritability Neutralize free acid Depress secretion of gastric juices	Avoid foods irritating chemically, mechanically (bland diet); small frequent feedings
	Sippy diet		Acute conditions: milk and cream every hour; gradual additions until patient on full diet
	Meulengracht	Neutralize gastric juice Shorten convalescence Favor blood regeneration Prevent digestion of clot	Hemorrhaging: advocates giving full ulcer diet first day in small frequent feedings
	Ewald fractional test meal	Determine free HCl	Composed of tea and dry toast

G. Compare nutritive return of foods in food group in relation to cost, e.g., non-fat milk solids most economical source of protein

MODIFICATION OF NORMAL DIET

1. **Purpose of nutrition in disease**
A. Supply adequate nutrition
B. Cure disease (nutritional deficiency)
C. Hasten recovery from disease
D. Improve function of injured or diseased tissue or system
E. Protect and provide materials for regeneration of diseased tissue
F. Reduce work of diseased or injured tissue or system
2. **Factors to consider in planning modifications of normal diet**
A. Underlying disease or pathologic situation that requires change in diet
B. Duration of disease
C. Modifications specified by physician
D. Patient's tolerance for food
E. Patient's dietary practices
F. Nutritional adequacy of modified diet
G. Patient's physical ability and home situation
3. **Modifications of normal diet in disease** (Table 6-2)
A. Consistency, bulk, residue
B. Nutrient distribution—increased or decreased content of
   1. Protein, fat, carbohydrate
   2. Minerals
   3. Vitamins—practical to increase only

vitamin A and vitamin C content by diet
C. Calories
D. Flavor or blandness
E. Selection of certain foods or food groups (allergy)
F. Number, time, and size of feedings
4. **Modifications in consistency, residue, and flavor**
A. Liquid
   1. Clear liquid includes foods in fluid state: broth, tea, gelatin dessert, coffee, tea, sugar, and occasionally clear fruit juices
   2. Includes foods that are fluid at room temperature; require no chewing
   3. Includes small particles of food in fluid medium; can pass through a tube or straw
   4. May be used for patients with acute infections, fevers, difficulty in swallowing or chewing, and for postoperative care
B. Soft
   1. Includes foods that are mechanically easy to eat; simply prepared and mildly seasoned
   2. Includes any food of soft consistency; used for patients without teeth
   3. May be used for patients with infections and inflammations, difficulty in swallowing and chewing, gastrointestinal diseases and disturbances, and for postoperative care
C. Residue restriction

TABLE 6-3
FOOD EXCHANGES*

---

1. One milk exchange—8 gm. protein, 10 gm. fat, 12 gm. carbohydrate, 170 calories

Whole milk, 1 cup	Skim milk, 1 cup (add 2 fat exchanges)
Evaporated milk, ½ cup	Buttermilk, 1 cup (add 2 fat exchanges)

---

2. One fruit exchange—10 gm. carbohydrate, 40 calories; all fruit prepared and served without sugar

Apple, 1 small	Dates, 2	Papaya, ⅓ medium
Applesauce, ½ cup	Figs, fresh, 2 large	Peach, 1 medium
Apricots, fresh, 2 medium	Figs, dried, 1 small	Pear, 1 small
Apricots, dried, 4 halves	†Grapefruit, ½ small	Pineapple, ½ cup
Banana, ½ small	†Grapefruit juice, ½ cup	Pineapple juice, ⅓ cup
Blackberries, ⅔ cup	Grapes, 12	Plums, 2 medium
Raspberries, 1 cup	Grape juice, ¼ cup	Prunes, dried, 2 medium
†Strawberries, 1 cup	Honeydew melon, ⅛	Raisins, 2 tbsp.
Blueberries, ⅔ cup	Mango, ½ small	†Tangerine, 1 large
†Cantaloupe, ¼	†Orange, 1 small	Watermelon, 1 cup
Cherries, 10 large	†Orange juice, ½ cup	

---

3. Vegetable exchange A—raw, as desired; cooked, 1 cup per meal

Asparagus	Cucumbers	‡Pepper
‡Broccoli	‡Escarole	Radishes
Brussels sprouts	Eggplant	Sauerkraut
Cabbage	‡Vegetable greens	String beans
Cauliflower	Lettuce	Summer squash
Celery	Mushrooms	‡Tomatoes
‡Chicory	Okra	‡Watercress

---

4. One vegetable exchange B—½ cup: 2 gm. protein, 7 gm. carbohydrate, 35 calories

Beets	Peas, green	‡Winter squash
‡Carrots	Pumpkin	Turnip
Onions	Rutabagas	

---

5. One meat exchange—7 gm. protein, 5 gm. fat, 75 calories

Meat and poultry (medium fat), 1 oz.	Fish
Beef, lamb, pork, liver, chicken	Haddock, 1 oz.
Cold cuts, 1 slice	Salmon, tuna, crab, lobster, ¼ cup
Salami, minced ham, bologna, liverwurst,	Shrimp, clams, oysters, 5 small
luncheon loaf	Sardines, 3 medium
Frankfurter, 1	Cheese
Egg, 1	Cheddar type, 1 oz.
Peanut butter, 2 tbsp.	Cottage, ¼ cup

---

6. One fat exchange—5 gm. fat, 45 calories

Butter or margarine, 1 tsp.	Cream cheese, 1 tbsp.	Oil or cooking fat, 1 tsp.
Bacon, crisp, 1 slice	Avocado, ⅛	Nuts, 6 small
Cream, light, 2 tbsp.	French dressing, 1 tbsp.	Olives, 5 small
Cream, heavy, 1 tbsp.	Mayonnaise, 1 tsp.	

---

7. One bread exchange—2 gm. protein, 15 gm. carbohydrate, 70 calories

Bread, 1 slice	Crackers
Biscuit, 1	Graham, 2
Muffin, 1	Oyster, 20
Cornbread, 1	Saltines, 5
Cereals	Soda, 3
Cooked, ½ cup	Round, thin, 6
Dry, ¾ cup	Vegetables
Rice, cooked, ½ cup	Beans, peas, dried, cooked, ½ cup
Spaghetti, cooked, ½ cup	Corn, ⅓ cup
Macaroni, cooked, ½ cup	Baked beans, ¼ cup

---

*Based on material in "Meal Planning With Exchange Lists" prepared by Committees of the American Diabetes Association, Inc., and The American Dietetic Association in cooperation with the Chronic Disease Program, Public Health Service, Department of Health, Education and Welfare.
†Sources of vitamin C.
‡Sources of vitamin A.

TABLE 6-3
FOOD EXCHANGES—cont'd

7. One bread exchange—cont'd

Flour, 2½ tbsp.
Sponge cake, plain, 1 to 1½″ cube
Ice cream, ½ cup (omit 2 fat exchanges)

Popcorn, 1 cup
Potatoes, white, 1 small
   White, mashed, ½ cup
Potatoes, sweet or yams, ¼ cup

8. Foods allowed as desired

Spices and herbs
Artificial sweeteners
Vinegar, onion, lemon, for seasoning
Coffee
Tea

Clear broth
Bouillon, without fat
Gelatin, unsweetened
Rennet tablets

Pickles, sour
Pickles, dill
Cranberries
Rhubarb

TABLE 6-4
SAMPLE MEAL PLAN, BASED ON FOOD EXCHANGE SYSTEM

Food	Exchange*	Protein (gm.)	Fat (gm.)	Carbohydrate (gm.)	Menu
Breakfast					
Fruit	1½			15	Orange juice, ¾ cup
Meat	2	14	10		Poached eggs, 2
Bread	2	4		30	Toast, 1 slice
					Cereal, cooked, ½ cup
Milk	1	8	10	12	Milk, whole, 1 cup
Fat	1		5		Butter for toast, 1 tsp.
Total		26	25	57	
Lunch					
Meat	2	14	10		Sliced chicken sandwich, 2 oz. cooked
Vegetable A					Lettuce
Bread	2	4		30	Bread, 2 slices
Fat	1		5		Mayonnaise, 1 tsp.
Milk	1	8	10	12	Milk, whole, 1 cup
Fruit	1½			15	Apple, 1 medium or 1½ small
Total		26	25	57	
Dinner					
Meat	3	21	15		Lean roast beef, 3 oz. cooked
Vegetable A					Sliced tomato, ½ raw on lettuce
Vegetable B	1	2		7	Frozen peas, ½ cup
Bread	2	4		30	Baked potato, 1 small
					Bread, 1 slice
Fat	2		10		Butter for potato, peas, and bread, 2 tsp.
Fruit	2			20	Sliced banana, 1 small
Total		27	25	57	
Bedtime or midafternoon snack					
Milk	1	8	10	12	Milk, whole, 1 cup
Meat	1	7	5		Cheese, cheddar, 1 oz.
Bread	1	2		15	Saltines, 5
Total		17	15	27	

Total for day: 95 gm. protein, 90 gm. fat, 200 gm. carbohydrate, 1990 calories

*See Table 6-3 for amounts of different foods per 1 exchange.

1. Includes foods that are almost completely digested and absorbed by body
2. May not meet recommended allowances for calcium and riboflavin
3. May be used for patients with diseases of lower gastrointestinal tract and in preparation for x-ray studies and surgery of lower gastrointestinal tract

D. Increased residue may be suggested for constipation, emphasizing foods high in fiber and increased fluid intake

E. Bland
1. Includes foods and quantities not irritating or stimulating mechanically or chemically
2. May be used for patients with ulcers and other gastrointestinal disturbances and diseases

5. **Meal plan modified in nutrient content**
A. Basic 4 food group as guide to meeting recommended allowances
B. Exchange system may be used to meet

specified contents of protein, fat, carbohydrate, and calories in diet (Table 6-3)
C. Sample meal plan using exchange system (Table 6-4)

6. **Meal pattern restricted in sodium**
A. Basic 4 food group as guide to meeting recommended allowances
B. General description
1. Foods should be processed, prepared, and served without addition of salt, baking soda, or baking powder
2. Labels must be checked on all canned, packaged, or frozen foods for added salt or sodium compounds
3. Salt substitutes, laxatives, medications must be taken on advice and knowledge of physician
4. Distilled water may have to be used for drinking and cooking purposes when sodium content of water supply is high
C. Selection of foods

TABLE 6-5
MODERATE RESTRICTION OF SODIUM

Food	Sodium (mg.)
Milk group*	
Whole milk, skim milk, 1 cup	122
Low-sodium cheese, 1 oz.	25
Meat group	
Fresh beef, lamb, veal, pork, poultry, fish (no shellfish), 1 oz.	21
Egg, 1	41
Fruit	
All fruit except candied fruit peel, currants, dried figs, and raisins, ½-cup serving	2.2
Cereal	
Shredded wheat, puffed wheat, puffed rice, cooked cereals without salt or sodium compounds, 1 serving	1
Vegetables	
Fresh or dietetic pack: asparagus, green beans, lima beans, navy beans, Brussels sprouts, cabbage, corn, cucumbers, endive, eggplant, lentils, lettuce, mushrooms, okra, onions, parsnips, peas, peppers, radishes, rutabagas, soybeans, squash, tomatoes, turnip greens, ½ cup	4.4
Bread,* regular, 1 slice	150
Fat*	
Butter or margarine, 1 tsp.	49
Cream, half-and-half, 1 tsp.	2.3
Oil	0
Miscellaneous	
Jelly, sugar, honey, tea, coffee, plain spices, herbs, vinegar	0

*For severe restriction in sodium content, low-sodium milk, low-sodium bread, and low-sodium butter indicated.

1. All items refer to fresh products or to processed foods without salt or sodium
2. Sodium content of foods must be calculated to meet physician's specifications (Table 6-5)

7. **Modifications with elimination or severe restriction of specific nutrients—inborn errors of metabolism**

A. Phenylketonuria
   1. Lack of enzyme necessary for converting phenylalanine to tyrosine in body
   2. Results in mental retardation if untreated or not treated in early stages
   3. Diet involves
      a. Restriction of phenylalanine to minimal requirement levels
      b. Restriction of protein—protein contains 4% to 6% phenylalanine
      c. Use of special proprietary foods that contain only minimal amounts of phenylalanine but supply other necessary amino acids (e.g., Lofenalac)
      d. Very careful calculation
      e. Supplementation with minerals and vitamins

B. Galactosemia
   1. Body unable to metabolize galactose
   2. Results in cataracts and in mental retardation if untreated
   3. Galactose (milk and milk products) eliminated from diet
   4. Use of special proprietary food that is lactose-free (e.g., Nutramigen)

REVIEW QUESTIONS FOR
NUTRITION AND DIET THERAPY

Questions are integrated in clinical chapters.

7

PHARMACOLOGY
AND
THERAPEUTICS

A.M.A. Drug evaluations, Chicago, 1971, American Medical Association.

American hospital formulary service, Washington, D. C., 1971, American Society of Hospital Pharmacists.

Bergersen, B. S., and Goth, A.: Pharmacology in nursing, ed. 12, St. Louis, 1973, The C. V. Mosby Co.

Di Palma, J. R.: Drill's pharmacology in medicine, ed. 4, New York, 1971, McGraw-Hill Book Co.

Falconer, M. W., Norman, M. R., Patterson, H. R., and Gustafson, E. A.: The drug, the nurse, and the patient, ed. 4, Philadelphia, 1970, W. B. Saunders Co.

Garb, S., and Crim, B. J.: Pharmacology and patient care, ed. 3, New York, 1970, Springer Publishing Co., Inc.

Goodman, L., and Gilman, A.: The pharmacological basis of therapeutics, ed. 4, New York, 1970, The Macmillan Co.

Hansten, P. D.: Drug interactions, Philadelphia, 1971, Lea & Febiger.

Modell, W., editor: Drugs of choice: 1972-1973, St. Louis, 1972, The C. V. Mosby Co.

Musser, R. D., and Schubkagel, B. L.: Pharmacology and therapeutics, ed. 4, New York, 1969, The Macmillan Co.

Rodman, M. J., and Smith, D. W.: Pharmacology and drug therapy in nursing, Philadelphia, 1968, J. B. Lippincott Co.

Sutherland, V. C.: A synopsis of pharmacology, ed. 2, Philadelphia, 1970, W. B. Saunders Co.

Periodicals

Nursing Outlook
American Journal of Nursing
Journal of the American Medical Association

It is suggested that a thorough review of pharmacology is best done with the help of several textbooks and the student's own notebook. It is emphasized that actions and manifestations of toxicity in addition to those listed in this review may occur.

INTRODUCTION TO PHARMACOLOGY

1. **Scope of pharmacology**
   A. Pharmacology—study of chemicals that have a biologic effect
   B. Drugs—chemical agents used to prevent, diagnose, treat, or cure disease
   C. Allied sciences that contribute to understanding and study of pharmacology
      1. Pharmacognosy—study of natural sources of drugs
      2. Pharmacy—techniques of preparing, compounding, and dispensing drugs
      3. Pharmacodynamics—study of actions and effects of drugs on living tissues
      4. Pharmacotherapeutics—use of drugs in preventing and treating disease
      5. Toxicology—study of adverse effects of drugs

2. **Drug standards**
   Established by means of assay and publications
   A. Assay—technique by which potency or purity of drug is determined
      1. Chemical—analysis of kind and amount of chemicals in drug

2. Biologic (bioassay)—determination of amount of drug needed to produce a particular effect on a living organism

B. Publications
1. *United States Pharmacopeia* (U.S.P.) —provides standards for identification and purity of drugs and for uniformity of strength; lists approved drugs used in modern medicine
2. The *National Formulary* (N.F.)—supplements the U.S.P.; lists drugs on basis of therapeutic value and usefulness; provides standards for older remedies
3. *Pharmacopoeia Internationalis* (Ph.I.) —published in several languages by the World Health Organization
4. *A.M.A. Drug Evaluations*—published annually under direction of the Council on Drugs, American Medical Association; not all drugs included have approval or official status
5. *The United States Dispensatory and Physicians' Pharmacology* — sponsored by the American Pharmaceutical Association; contains comprehensive information about drugs
6. *American Hospital Formulary Service* —published by the American Society of Hospital Pharmacists
7. Others

C. Drug legislation—provides for enforcement of drug standards; protects public from defraudment, adulteration, and unreliable or dangerous preparations
1. Federal Food, Drug and Cosmetic Act and its amendments—designed to enforce standards of U.S.P. and N.F.; protects against premature marketing; controls use of written and oral prescriptions, refilling of prescriptions, distribution and clinical study of drugs, labeling
2. Harrison Narcotic Act and its amendments—intended to regulate importation, manufacture, sale, and use of narcotics
3. State legislation

D. Enforcement agencies
1. Food and Drug Administration—empowered to enforce Federal Food, Drug and Cosmetic Act and its amendments
2. Division of Biologics Standards, National Institute of Health—establishes standards for the manufacture and licensure of biologic agents
3. Federal Trade Commission—controls advertising to the general public
4. Department of Justice, Bureau of Narcotics and Dangerous Drugs
5. Post Office Department, Fraud Section—controls use of mails to solicit customers or ship drugs for which fraudulent claims are made

3. **Names of drugs**
A. Official (generic, nonproprietary)—name under which drug is listed in official publications; does not change
B. Chemical — name describing chemical composition and placement of atoms
C. Trade (proprietary; brand)—name registered and legally owned by manufacturer

4. **Active constituents of plant drugs**
A. Alkaloids—bitter-tasting substances with alkaline properties; water-soluble salts are usually used in medicine; dosage is usually small; example: morphine
B. Glycosides—yield a carbohydrate grouping and another grouping when hydrolyzed; dosage is usually small; example: digitalis
C. Gums—exudates from plants, which swell to form gelatinous or mucilaginous materials when hydrolyzed; example: agar
D. Resins—complex organic substances that are insoluble in water; readily soluble in alcohol
E. Tannins—complex plant acids related to phenol; have astringent and precipitant properties; found in black tea and tannic acid
F. Oils—greasy liquids that are viscous and insoluble in water
1. Volatile—aromatic oils that evaporate readily when exposed to air; used as flavoring agents; example: oil of wintergreen
2. Fixed—feel greasy and do not evaporate readily; hydrolyze to form glycerin and fatty acids; example: olive oil
G. Waxes—chemically similar to oils but are solid at room temperature; example: beeswax

5. **Animal sources of drugs**
6. **Mineral sources of drugs**
7. **Chemical synthesis of drugs**
8. **Pharmaceutic preparations**
A. Solutions and suspensions

1. Aqueous solutions—contain one or more substances dissolved in water
   a. Waters—saturated solutions of aromatic substances dissolved in water; example: peppermint water
   b. True solutions—nonvolatile substances dissolved in water; example: epinephrine solution
   c. Syrups—aqueous solutions of sucrose, usually 85%, in which are dissolved flavoring or medicinal agents; used as demulcents, preservatives, and vehicles to disguise the taste of drugs; example: wild cherry syrup
2. Aqueous suspensions—finely divided drugs suspended, or intended to be suspended, in a liquid; drugs tend to settle out of solution; preparations need to be shaken before use
   a. Mixtures — aqueous preparations containing insoluble, nonfatty substances in suspension; example: cough mixtures
   b. Emulsions—suspensions of oil or fat in water; emulsifying agent is used; stabilizing agent sometimes used; example: cod-liver oil emulsion
   c. Magmas—white, bulky suspensions of insoluble preparations in water; may be referred to as milks; must be shaken before use; example: milk of magnesia
   d. Gels—aqueous suspensions of insoluble drugs in hydrated form; particles of drug are larger than those in magma; example: aluminum hydroxide gel
3. Spirits—concentrated alcoholic solutions of volatile substances; example: aromatic spirits of ammonia
4. Elixirs—aromatic, sweetened, alcoholic preparations often containing a flavoring agent; example: elixir of terpin hydrate
5. Tinctures—alcoholic or hydroalcoholic solutions of drugs; most tinctures are 10% solutions; exceptions are iodine, ferric chloride solutions; example: paregoric (camphorated tincture of opium)
6. Fluidextracts—concentrated fluid preparations of plant drugs; often 100% solution in alcohol; dose is usually quite small; example: cascara sagrada extract
7. Extracts—concentrated preparations of drugs obtained by removing active ingredients with solvents and then evaporating some or all of solvents; example: liver extract

B. Dosage forms—definite unit doses of drug, prepared by manufacturer in form for convenience of administration
   1. Capsule—gelatin container for drug, which prevents tasting the drug but dissolves readily when contacted by digestive juices
   2. Tablet—round, disc-shaped, oblong, triangular, and other forms prepared by molding and compression
   3. Timed-release tablet or capsule (sustained release, with prolonged, delayed, or repeat action)—used for slow continuous release, absorption, and effect of drug; achieved by coating parts or particles of the preparation with materials of varying solubility, absorbing the drug into a plastic matrix, or using particles of various sizes
   4. Enteric-coated tablet or capsule—coated with a substance that is unaffected by gastric juices but disintegrated by alkaline juices of intestinal tract
   5. Troche (lozenge)—flat, round, or rectangular preparation that is held in the mouth until dissolved, releasing the drug
   6. Pill—dosage form that is rarely manufactured; term is frequently used erroneously to describe oral dosage forms
   7. Powder—finely ground preparation of solid drug; usually enclosed in folded paper or gelatin capsule
   8. Ampule and vial—containers for powdered or liquid drug intended for injection; powder is dissolved with sterile diluent before use
      a. Ampule—sealed glass container; usually contains a single dose
      b. Vial—rubber-stoppered glass container; often contains multiple doses of drug
   9. Disposable syringe—syringe that may be prefilled with injectable drug; syringe or cartridge is discarded after use
   10. Repository suspension—suspension of drug in colloidal or fatty substance

from which it is released slowly, over an extended period of time

C. Other preparations
1. Liniments and lotions—liquid suspensions or dispersions for external application
   a. Liniment—usually contains anodyne and rubefacient; applied by rubbing
   b. Lotion—antiseptic or astringent drug in alcohol or water; patted onto skin
2. Creams—emulsions of oil in water or of water in oil
3. Ointments—semisolid preparations in fatty ointment base; applied externally by stroking
4. Pastes—heavy, ointmentlike preparations containing 50% powder; applied externally
5. Suppositories—molded preparations of drug; suitable for insertion into the rectum, vagina, or urethra

9. **Administration of medicines**
A. Major channels of administration
1. Local—action is confined to site of application; preparations are applied to the skin or mucous membranes and include ointments, lotions, creams, liniments, solutions, powders, and suppositories
2. Systemic—drug is absorbed into bloodstream and carried to tissues that respond to it
   a. Oral—safe, economic, convenient method; drug is swallowed with sufficient water to lubricate dosage form, dissolve, and dilute drug; not used if nausea or vomiting is present or when cooperation or swallowing reflex is absent
   b. Sublingual—dosage form is retained under tongue until dissolved and absorbed; example: nitroglycerin
   c. Buccal—dosage form is retained in buccal pouch (between teeth and cheek) until dissolved
   d. Rectal—suppository form releases drug slowly; retention enema gives less predictable effects
   e. Inhalation—breathing vapors of volatile drugs, gases, or aerosol (mist) obtained by nebulization of drug; provides almost instantaneous absorption
   f. Parenteral—includes all methods of injection; requires use of sterile materials and aseptic technique
      (1) Intradermal—injection into upper layers of skin
      (2) Subcutaneous (hypodermic)—injection into subcutaneous tissues; needle is inserted at angle of 45 to 60 degrees
      (3) Intramuscular—needle is inserted vertically into muscle tissues
      (4) Intravenous—drug is administered directly into vein by injection or infusion
      (5) Intraspinal—given by physician using technique of lumbar puncture
      (6) Intracardiac—given into muscle of heart by physician

B. Techniques of administration
1. Regulations related to administration of medicines are based on principles that protect patients and nurses
2. Nursing approach affects acceptance of medication
3. Skill in method of administration adds to comfort of patient

10. **Effects of drugs**
Drugs should be selected on *rational* basis of predictability of action, proved by scientific research, rather than on *empiric basis*
A. Sites of drug action
1. Local—acts at site of application
2. Systemic—acts only after absorption and distribution
B. Terms used to describe action or effect of drugs
1. Addiction—physiologic and psychic dependence on a drug such as morphine
2. Additive effect—simple addition or summation of effects in the body when drugs are given at the same time
3. Antagonism—opposite pharmacologic effects exerted by drugs in the body
4. Cumulation—effect produced when a drug is absorbed more quickly than it is excreted or destroyed
5. Depression—decrease in cellular functioning
6. Idiosyncrasy—abnormal response to a drug
7. Habituation—psychic craving for a drug

8. Hypersensitivity—allergic response to a drug
9. Irritation—some degree of tissue damage caused by drug
10. Physiologic—action on normal healthy tissues
11. Potentiation—intensified action of one drug by another
12. Therapeutic—action on diseased tissues or in the ill person
13. Tolerance—acquired reaction necessitating increased dosage to maintain therapeutic effects
14. Cross-tolerance—tolerance to chemically related drugs
15. Side effect—any effect other than one for which drug was administered
16. Stimulation—increased activity of cells
17. Synergism—exaggerated effect produced by two drugs working together
18. Untoward action—adverse side effect; may be harmful
C. Mechanisms of drug action
   1. Not understood for many drugs
   2. General concepts
      a. Alteration of some physicochemical process
      b. Modification of membrane's permeability to specific substances
      c. Interference with cell's chemical use of an essential substance
      d. Direct inhibition of an enzyme
      e. Influence on transportation of substances from surface to interior of cell
      f. Replacement of an essential biologic substance
D. Factors that influence or modify actions of drugs
   1. Dose—amount of drug needed for therapeutic effect; influenced by age, weight, sex, size, and condition of patient, response to therapy, sensitivity, tolerance, synergistic or antagonistic effects of concomitant medications, genetic and environmental factors, drug itself, time and method of administration
      a. Minimum—smallest dose that will produce therapeutic effect
      b. Maximum—largest dose that will produce therapeutic effect without producing toxic symptoms
      c. Toxic—dose that produces symptoms of poisoning
      d. Lethal—dose that results in death

2. Absorption—rate and amount are influenced by method of administration, dose, solubility of drug, nature of drug, particle size of drug, condition of absorbing surfaces, adequacy of circulation
3. Distribution—occurs by process of diffusion
4. Elimination—rapidity affects size of dose and frequency of administration; modified by hepatic and renal function

DRUGS AFFECTING THE CENTRAL NERVOUS SYSTEM (CNS)

1. **Central nervous system stimulants**
A. General stimulants—increase activity of central nervous system; principal site of action and toxicity vary with each drug
B. Selective stimulants
   1. Medullary stimulants
      a. Action—small doses combat respiratory and circulatory depression
      b. Toxicity—large doses may produce convulsions
      c. Preparations
         (1) Nikethamide (Coramine)
         (2) Pentylenetetrazol (Metrazol)
         (3) Picrotoxin (Cocculin)
         (4) Bemegride (Megimide)
   2. Reflex stimulants
      a. Action—stimulate medullary centers reflexly; stimulation arises from peripheral sites and carotid sinus
      b. Toxicity—some are extremely dangerous; effects are unreliable
      c. Preparation—aromatic spirits of ammonia
   3. Spinal cord stimulants (obsolete for medicinal purposes)
      a. Action—produce tonic convulsions
      b. Toxicity—important cause of accidental poisoning
      c. Preparation—strychnine
   4. Cerebral or psychic stimulants
      a. Action—stimulate cerebrum, producing increased alertness; used to improve mood
      b. Toxicity—symptoms include restlessness and insomnia
      c. Preparations
         (1) Xanthines
            (a) Action—induce wakefulness and alertness; unreliable as respiratory stimulants

  (b) Toxicity—restlessness, insomnia

  (c) Example—caffeine

 (2) Amphetamines and phenmetrazine

  (a) Action—used to induce wakefulness, treat narcolepsy and mild depression; questionable usefulness in treatment of barbiturate poisoning and obesity; psychic dependence and drug abuse may occur

  (b) Toxicity—insomnia, irritability, dizziness, cardiovascular effects, gastrointestinal symptoms, toxic psychoses; acute overdosage causes excitement, agitation, tachycardia, mydriasis, slurred speech, ataxia, hyperreflexia, rapid respiration; symptoms of chronic fatigue may occur during withdrawal of these drugs from abusers

  (c) Preparations
   (1) Amphetamine (Benzedrine)
   (2) Dextroamphetamine (Dexedrine)
   (3) Methamphetamine
   (4) Phenmetrazine hydrochloride (Preludin)

 (3) Diphenylmethane derivatives
  (a) Action—mild stimulation of mood, little effect on sleep
  (b) Toxicity — may produce hyperirritability, insomnia
  (c) Preparations
   (1) Pipradrol (Meratran)
   (2) Methylphenidate (Ritalin)

 (4) Monoamine oxidase inhibitors
  (a) Action—stimulate mood, appetite
  (b) Toxicity—may lower blood pressure; numerous serious side effects
  (c) Preparations
   (1) Nialamide (Niamid)
   (2) Others

 (5) Dibenzazepine group
  (a) Action — antidepressant; tranquilizer in normal persons
  (b) Toxicity — may produce toxic effects resembling those of atropine; sensitization; central nervous system effects may prove fatal
  (c) Preparations
   (1) Imipramine hydrochloride (Tofranil)
   (2) Amitriptyline (Elavil)
   (3) Others

2. Central nervous system depressants
 A. Nonselective depressants
  1. Narcotic analgesics
   a. Preparations containing whole opium
    (1) Used to relieve excessive peristalsis
    (2) Preparations
     (a) Tincture of opium (laudanum)
     (b) Camphorated opium tincture (paregoric)
     (c) Opium and belladonna suppositories
   b. Alkaloids of opium
    (1) Uses
     (a) Analgesic for severe pain
     (b) Preanesthetic medication
     (c) Relief of restlessness and apprehension in threatened abortion, pulmonary hemorrhage
     (d) Relief of cough (preparations containing codeine)
    (2) Preparations
     (a) Morphine sulfate
     (b) Codeine sulfate, phosphate
     (c) Others
    (3) Actions of morphine are representative; preparations differ in degree of action; act on cerebrum, producing these effects: relief of pain, depression of respiratory center, constriction of pupils, depression of cough center, diminished glandular activity of alimentary tract, increased tone of smooth muscles, decreased rhythmic contraction of smooth muscle
   c. Toxicity

(1) Tolerance is likely to lead to addiction
(2) Respiratory depression
(3) Dizziness, nausea, and vomiting
(4) Restlessness and insomnia
(5) Tremors, delirium
(6) Drowsiness, decreased level of concentration and thinking

2. Synthetic narcotic analgesics—resemble morphine in action, uses, and toxicity
   a. Meperidine hydrochloride (Demerol, Mepadin)
   b. Anileridine hydrochloride (Leritine)
   c. Methadone hydrochloride (Dolophine)
   d. Alphaprodine hydrochloride (Nisentil)
   e. Levorphanol tartrate (Levo-Dromoran)
   f. Piminodine esylate (Alvodine)
   g. Fentanyl citrate (Sublimaze)

3. Narcotic antagonists
   a. Action—antagonistic to excessive respiratory depression caused by narcotics; test for narcotic addiction
   b. Toxicity—depression of respiration if given in absence of narcotics
   c. Preparations
      (1) Levallorphan tartrate (Lorfan)
      (2) Nalorphine hydrochloride (Nalline)

4. Nonnarcotic analgesics
   a. Action—interrupt perception of pain
   b. Toxicity—nausea and vomiting
   c. Preparations
      (1) Propoxyphene hydrochloride (Darvon)
      (2) Darvon Compound
      (3) Ethoheptazine (Zactane)
      (4) Ethoheptazine with acetylsalicylic acid (Zactirin)
      (5) Pentazocine (Talwin)
      (6) Methotrimeprazine (Levoprome)
      (7) Acetaminophen (Tylenol)
      (8) Others

5. Analgesic antipyretics—important cause of poisoning in children
   a. Systemic actions
      (1) Antipyretic
      (2) Anti-inflammatory
      (3) Analgesic
   b. Toxicity
      (1) Gastrointestinal irritation
      (2) Tinnitus, headache, dizziness, confusion
      (3) Serious disturbances of acid-base balance
      (4) Allergic and anaphylactoid reactions
   c. Preparations exerting systemic actions
      (1) Acetylsalicylic acid (aspirin)
      (2) Sodium salicylate
      (3) Salicylamide
   d. Preparations exerting local actions
      (1) Salicylic acid—used as keratolytic agent
      (2) Methyl salicylate (oil of wintergreen)—flavoring agent, rubefacient
      (3) Sodium salicylate — sclerotic agent
   e. Other analgesic and antipyretic agents
      (1) Acetanilid
      (2) Phenacetin
   f. Drugs used to treat gout
      (1) Colchicine
         (a) Action—affects uric acid metabolism; specific for decrease of pain and inflammation of acute gouty arthritis
         (b) Toxicity—causes nausea, vomiting, abdominal pain, diarrhea; adverse effects due to cumulation are reduced by regulating dosage
      (2) Indomethacin (Indocin)
         (a) Action—anti-inflammatory, antipyretic, analgesic
         (b) Toxicity—vertigo, confusion, gastrointestinal disturbances, blood dyscrasia, jaundice
      (3) Probenecid (Benemid)
         (a) Action—inhibits reabsorption of urates; not useful for acute episodes
         (b) Toxicity—inhibits renal transport of some drugs; nausea, headache, rash, fever, CNS stimulation, gastrointestinal symptoms

(4) Phenylbutazone (Butazolidin)
  (a) Action—antipyretic, analgesic, and anti-inflammatory; useful for acute episodes
  (b) Toxicity—relatively high; symptoms include edema, nausea, vomiting, epigastric distress, gastrointestinal bleeding, rash, hepatitis, psychosis, and blood dyscrasias
(5) Allopurinol (Zyloprim)
  (a) Action—potent inhibitor of xanthine oxidase; used to treat chronic gout, especially if renal complications are present
  (b) Toxicity—skin eruptions, gastrointestinal disturbances, hypersensitivity reactions
(6) Sulfinpyrazone (Anturane)—increases urinary excretion of uric acid
(7) Salicylates
(8) Others
6. Hypnotics and sedatives—difference between hypnotic and sedative is in degree of central nervous system depression; usually can be related to dose
  a. Definitions
    (1) Hypnotic (somnifacient, soporific)—produces sleep soon after administration
    (2) Sedative—calms, relaxes, and quiets; does not produce sleep
  b. Barbiturates
    (1) Action—not well understood; depression of CNS
    (2) Toxicity
      (a) Marked symptoms of "hangover"
      (b) Rash, facial swelling, asthmatic attack
      (c) Nausea and vomiting
      (d) Nightmares, restlessness, delirium
      (e) Habituation
      (f) Restlessness, mental confusion, especially in presence of severe pain
      (g) Important cause of self-induced poisoning
    (3) Preparations
      (a) Phenobarbital (Luminal)
      (b) Mephobarbital (Mebaral)
      (c) Aprobarbital (Alurate)
      (d) Secobarbital (Seconal)
      (e) Pentobarbital (Nembutal)
      (f) Thiopental sodium (Pentothal)
      (g) Amobarbital sodium (Amytal)
      (h) Others
  c. Nonbarbiturate sedatives and hypnotics
    (1) Action—not understood; depression of CNS
    (2) Toxicity—relatively low; tolerance and habituation may occur
    (3) Preparations
      (a) Flurazepam (Dalmane)
      (b) Ethchlorvynol (Placidyl)
      (c) Ethinamate (Valmid)
      (d) Glutethimide (Doriden)
      (e) Methyprylon (Noludar)
      (f) Chloral betaine (Beta-Chlor)
      (g) Chloral hydrate
      (h) Methaqualone (Quaalude)
      (i) Paraldehyde
7. Anesthetics
  a. General anesthetics—drugs that produce loss of sensation and loss of consciousness
    (1) Action—cause irregular descending depression of central nervous system
    (2) Toxicity—varies with agent; influenced by
      (a) Skill of anesthetist
      (b) Use of preanesthetic agents
      (c) Combination of selected agents
      (d) Controlled use of analgesics during recovery
    (3) Groups
      (a) Volatile (gaseous) agents —administered by inhalation with oxygen; open, semiclosed, or closed method of administration
        (1) Ether (ethyl, diethyl)
        (2) Chloroform
        (3) Nitrous oxide
        (4) Ethylene
        (5) Cyclopropane
        (6) Ethyl chloride

(7) Halothane (Fluothane)

(8) Methoxyflurane (Penthrane)

(9) Fluroxene (Fluoromar)

(10) Trichloroethylene (Trilene)

(11) Vinyl ether (Vinethene)

(b) Nonvolatile—administered rectally or intravenously, producing hypnosis and unconsciousness; used as basal anesthetics; dose must be controlled very carefully

(1) Tribromoethanol (Avertin)

(2) Thiopental sodium (Pentothal)

(3) Hexobarbital sodium (Evipal sodium)

(4) Thiamylal sodium (Surital sodium)

(5) Methohexital sodium (Brevital)

(6) Ketamine hydrochloride (Ketalar)

b. Local anesthetics—drugs that produce analgesia without loss of consciousness

(1) Action—block nerve impulses along sensory and motor nerve fibers

(2) Toxicity—all are potentially toxic and may produce

(a) Central nervous system symptoms

(b) Cardiovascular symptoms

(c) Allergic manifestations

(3) Methods of administration

(a) Surface (topical)—drug is placed on surface of skin and mucous membranes

(b) Injection

(1) Infiltration—injection into skin and subcutaneous tissues

(2) Conduction (block)—injection near nerve trunk

(3) Spinal (subarachnoid)—injection into subarachnoid space

(4) Caudal—injection into sacral canal

(5) Saddle block

(4) Preparations

(a) Cocaine

(b) Procaine hydrochloride (Novocain)

(c) Chloroprocaine hydrochloride (Nesacaine)

(d) Lidocaine hydrochloride (Xylocaine)

(e) Piperocaine hydrochloride (Metycaine)

(f) Benoxinate hydrochloride (Dorsacaine)

(g) Benzocaine

(h) Butacaine (Butyn sulfate)

(i) Cyclomethycaine (Surfacaine)

(j) Dibucaine hydrochloride (Nupercaine)

(k) Dyclonine hydrochloride (Dyclone)

(l) Pramoxine hydrochloride (Tronothane)

(m) Tetracaine hydrochloride (Pontocaine)

(n) Others

8. Alcohols

a. Ethyl alcohol

(1) Local action—bacteriocidal, irritant, astringent

(2) Systemic actions

(a) Depresses central nervous system

(b) Dilates peripheral blood vessels

(c) Irritates gastrointestinal tract

(3) Toxicity

(a) Similar to anesthetic agents

(b) Cause of acute and chronic alcoholism

b. Methyl alcohol

(1) Action—depresses central nervous system; causes acidosis

(2) Toxicity—poisonous when ingested

c. Isopropyl alcohol

(1) Action—bacteriocidal

(2) Toxicity—ingestion produces severe poisoning and death

B. Selective depressants

1. Anticonvulsant drugs—prevent, mod-

ify, or reduce incidence of epileptic seizures

a. Barbituric acid derivatives
   (1) Action—appear to raise seizure threshold and lower excitability of cerebral cortex
   (2) Toxicity—sedation, skin rashes, fever, and others
   (3) Preparations
      (a) Phenobarbital
      (b) Mephobarbital (Mebaral)
      (c) Metharbital (Gemonil)
      (d) Primidone (Mysoline)
b. Hydantoins
   (1) Action—suppress grand mal, convulsions
   (2) Toxicity—varied; includes hyperplasia of gums, dermatitis, ataxia, nystagmus, diplopia, tremor, anemia, and lymphadenopathy
   (3) Preparations
      (a) Diphenylhydantoin sodium (Dilantin)
      (b) Mephenytoin (Mesantoin)
      (c) Ethotoin (Peganone)
c. Oxazolidones
   (1) Action—effective against petit mal, act as mild sedative and analgesic
   (2) Toxicity—photophobia, dermatitis, blood dyscrasias
   (3) Preparations
      (a) Trimethadione (Tridione)
      (b) Paramethadione (Paradione)
d. Succinimides
   (1) Ethosuximide (Zarontin)
      (a) Action—drug of choice for petit mal
      (b) Toxicity—gastrointestinal disturbances, headache, dizziness, rashes, ataxia, anemias, psychic disturbances
   (2) Methsuximide (Celontin)
      (a) Action—used to treat petit mal and minor motor seizures
      (b) Toxicity—high incidence of gastrointestinal and central nervous system disturbances
   (3) Phensuximide (Milontin)
      (a) Action—effective against petit mal

      (b) Toxicity—anorexia, diarrhea, drowsiness, ataxia, edema, liver damage, albuminuria
e. Other preparations
   (1) Phenacemide (Phenurone)
      (a) Action—effective against psychic and psychomotor equivalents of epilepsy
      (b) Toxicity—high incidence of liver damage, aplastic anemia, personality changes
2. Antipsychotic agents (major tranquilizers)—effect tranquil mental state without lessening mental faculties or consciousness; increase amenability to psychotherapy
a. Phenothiazine derivatives
   (1) Actions
      (a) Calm, without causing sleep or decreasing alertness and intellectual ability
      (b) Reduce emotions of hate, hostility, overactivity, anxiety, fear
      (c) Most preparations suppress nausea and vomiting
      (d) Potentiate drugs that act as central nervous system depressants, antihypertensive agents
   (2) Toxicity
      (a) Includes liver damage, blood dyscrasias, dermatitis, spasms of face and neck muscles, confusion, depression, atropine-like effects, orthostatic hypotension, and tachycardia
      (b) Use of epinephrine is contraindicated
   (3) Preparations
      (a) Chlorpromazine (Thorazine)
      (b) Acetophenazine maleate (Tindal)
      (c) Promazine hydrochloride (Sparine)
      (d) Promethazine (Phenergan)
      (e) Mepazine (Pacatal)
      (f) Trifluoperazine (Stelazine)
      (g) Prochlorperazine (Compazine)

(h) Thioridazine hydrochloride (Mellaril)
(i) Triflupromazine hydrochloride (Vesprin)
(j) Butaperazine maleate (Repoise)
(k) Carphenazine maleate (Proketazine)
(l) Fluphenazine (Prolixin)
(m) Mesoridazine (Serentil)
(n) Perphenazine (Trilafon)
(o) Piperacetazine (Quide)
(p) Thiopropazate hydrochloride (Dartal)
b. Thioxanthene derivatives
(1) Chlorprothixene (Taractan)
(2) Thiothixine (Navane)
c. Butyrophenone derivative—Haloperidol (Haldol)
d. Miscellaneous agents
(1) Flurothyl (Indoklon)
(a) Action — causes convulsions
(b) Toxicity—similar to electroconvulsive therapy
(2) Lithium carbonate
(a) Action—modifies mania of manic-depressive psychosis
(b) Toxicity—gastrointestinal and visual disturbances, muscle hyperirritability, sedation, and dizziness; severe reactions may occur
e. Rauwolfia group
(1) Action—tend to reduce overactivity and excitability
(2) Toxicity—depression; may produce or aggravate peptic ulcers; muscular rigidity, tremor, weight gain, diarrhea, nasal congestion
(3) Preparations
(a) Reserpine (Serpasil)
(b) Rescinnamine (Moderil)
(c) Deserpidine (Harmonyl)
(d) Others
3. Antianxiety agents (formerly called minor tranquilizers)
a. Uses—control mild to moderate anxiety and tension, often prescribed for persons with suicidal tendency
b. Action—depress central nervous system without clouding state of consciousness

c. Toxicity—may cause drowsiness, ataxia, decreased alertness and coordination; additive effect when combined with other central nervous system depressants; excessive doses cause coma, respiratory failure, vasomotor collapse
d. Group I
(1) Actions—acts on central nervous system, calms, relaxes smooth muscles
(2) Toxicity—similar to other antianxiety agents
(3) Preparations
(a) Chlordiazepoxide (Librium)
(b) Chlormezanone (Trancopal)
(c) Diazepam (Valium)
(d) Mephenoxalone (Trepidone)
(e) Meprobamate (Equanil, Miltown)
(f) Oxanamide (Quiactin)
(g) Oxazepam (Serax)
(h) Phenaglycodol (Ultran)
(i) Tybamate (Solacen, Tybatran)
e. Group II
(1) Action—calms; exerts antihistaminic, antiemetic, and anticholinergic effects
(2) Toxicity—similar to group I
(3) Preparations
(a) Hydroxyzine (Atarax, Vistaril)
(b) Buclizine (Softran)
f. Group III
(1) Actions—varies with preparation
(2) Toxicity—rashes, anticholinergic effects, anaphylaxis
(3) Preparations
(a) Benactyzine (Suavitil)
(b) Ectylurea (Levanil)
(c) Doxepin (Sinequan)
4. Antidepressants (p. 257)

AUTONOMIC DRUGS

1. **Adrenergic agents (sympathomimetic)**
A. Actions—degree of each action varies with preparation
1. Contract smooth muscle of blood vessels supplying the skin and mucous membranes
2. Relax smooth muscle of bronchi, ali-

mentary tract, and blood vessels supplying skeletal muscle

   3. Increase heart rate and cardiac output

   4. Stimulate central nervous system; stimulate respiration, increase wakefulness, decrease appetite

B. Toxicity—varied and complex; may include the following:

   1. Fear, anxiety, tremor, respiratory difficulty

   2. Blood pressure may be decreased (fainting) or be increased excessively, resulting in cerebral hemorrhage

   3. Cardiac arrhythmias, dilatation, palpitation

   4. Ventricular fibrillation (may be fatal)

   5. Pulmonary edema

   6. Sloughing and gangrene at site of injection; example: Levophed

C. Preparations

   1. Epinephrine (Adrenalin)

   2. Isoproterenol (Isuprel)

   3. Levarterenol bitartrate (norepinephrine, Levophed)

   4. Ephedrine

   5. Amphetamines

   6. Phenylephrine hydrochloride (Neo-Synephrine)

   7. Mephentermine (Wyamine)

   8. Metaraminol (Aramine)

   9. Angiotensinamide (Hypertensin)

   10. Methoxamine (Vasoxyl)

   11. Others

2. Adrenergic blocking agents (adrenolytic, sympatholytic)

A. Actions

   1. Inhibit response to adrenergic drugs, modifying body function

   2. Cause vasodilatation that lowers blood pressure; a transitory effect

   3. Increase muscle tone

   4. Increase activity of gastrointestinal tract

   5. Relieve vasospasm

B. Toxicity

   1. Postural hypotension, progressive if untreated

   2. Weakness, dizziness, blurred vision

   3. Numerous side effects

C. Preparations

   1. Azapetine phosphate (Ilidar)

   2. Phenoxybenzamine (Dibenzyline)

   3. Phentolamine (Regitine)

   4. Tolazoline (Priscoline)

   5. Others

3. Cholinergic drugs (parasympathomimetic)

A. Actions

   1. Slow the heart rate

   2. Increase gastrointestinal peristalsis and secretions

   3. Increase contractions of urinary bladder

   4. Cause sweating, peripheral vasodilatation

   5. Increase contraction of skeletal muscles and tone of bronchial muscle

   6. Produce miosis

B. Toxicity

   1. Nausea and vomiting, intestinal cramps

   2. Respiratory failure

   3. Atrioventricular block

   4. Others

C. Preparations

   1. Drugs that act similarly to acetylcholine

     a. Methacholine (Mecholyl)

     b. Carbachol

     c. Bethanechol (Urecholine)

     d. Pilocarpine

   2. Anticholinesterase drugs

     a. Physostigmine (Eserine)

     b. Neostigmine (Prostigmin)

     c. Pyridostigmine (Mestinon)

     d. Ambenonium (Mytelase)

     e. Echothiophate (Phospholine iodide)

     f. Isoflurophate (Floropryl)

     g. Edrophonium chloride (Tensilon)

     h. Benzpyrinium (Stigmonene)

4. Cholinergic blocking agents (parasympatholytic)

A. Actions

   1. Increase heart rate

   2. Relax smooth muscles

   3. Inhibit secretions of duct glands; decrease saliva and bronchial and gastric secretions

   4. Dilate pupils of eye; paralyze muscles of accommodation

   5. Reduce sweating

   6. Therapeutic doses increase rate and depth of respiration

B. Toxicity

   1. Photophobia; precipitate or worsen glaucoma

   2. Flushing, feeling of warmth; rapid, weak pulse

   3. Dryness of mouth, thirst, difficulty in swallowing and talking

   4. Stimulation of cerebrum; bizarre mental and neurologic symptoms

5. Rashes and other manifestations of allergic reactions

C. Preparations
  1. Belladonna and alkaloids
     a. Atropine
     b. Scopolamine (Hyoscine)
  2. Synthetic substitutes for atropine (mydriatics and cycloplegics)
     a. Homatropine hydrobromide
     b. Eucatropine hydrobromide
     c. Cyclopentolate hydrochloride (Cyclogyl)
  3. Synthetic substitutes for atropine (antispasmodics)
     a. Homatropine methylbromide (Novatrin)
     b. Methscopolamine bromide (Pamine)
     c. Methscopolamine nitrate (Skopolate)
     d. Propantheline bromide (Pro-Banthine)
     e. Others

5. Ganglion blocking agents
Some drugs stimulate and later depress activity at the autonomic ganglia. This is a complex group of drugs, since acetylcholine is the chemical mediator in the ganglia of both sympathetic and parasympathetic divisions. Nicotine is one of the blocking agents as well as tetraethylammonium chloride. A number of antihypertensive drugs belong to this group, mentioned under antihypertensive drugs.

DRUGS THAT AFFECT GASTROINTESTINAL ORGANS

1. Antacids
A. Action—lower gastric acidity and relieve pain by one of the following means:
  1. Chemical neutralization
  2. Physical adsorption
  3. Demulcent action
B. Toxicity—varies with each preparation
  1. Alkalosis with decreased renal function or milk-alkali syndrome
  2. Secondary increase of gastric acid
  3. Constipation or diarrhea
  4. Gastric distention, flatulence, and eructation due to release of carbon dioxide
C. Preparations
  1. Systemic antacids
     a. Sodium bicarbonate
     b. Sodium citrate
  2. Nonsystemic antacids
     a. Aluminum hydroxide gel (Amphojel)
     b. Aluminum phosphate (Phosphaljel)
     c. Magnesium trisilicate
     d. Calcium carbonate
     e. Magnesium oxide, magnesium hydroxide, milk of magnesia
     f. Polyamine-methylene resins (Exorbin, Resinat)
     g. Calcium phosphate, tribasic
     h. Dihydroxyaluminum aminoacetate (Robalate)
     i. Magnesium carbonate
     j. Magnesium phosphate, tribasic
     k. Magaldrate (Riopan)
  3. Mixtures
     a. Gelusil
     b. Maalox
     c. Mylanta
     d. Others

2. Digestants
Used to promote digestion; replacement therapy
A. Hydrochloric acid
  1. 10% preparation must be diluted
  2. Injures tooth enamel; to be given through a tube
B. Glutamic acid hydrochloride (Acidulin)
C. Pepsin
D. Pancreatin (Panteric, Viokase)
E. Pancrelipase (Cotazym)
F. Bile and bile salts
  1. Dehydrocholic acid (Decholin)
  2. Florantyrone (Zanchol)

3. Drugs used as diagnostic aids
A. To determine gastric acidity
  1. Histamine
     a. Action—stimulates secretion of hydrochloric acid
     b. Toxicity—headache, vertigo, flushing, hypotension
     c. Preparations
        (1) Histamine phosphate
        (2) Betazole hydrochloride (Histalog)
  2. Azuresin (Diagnex blue)
B. For roentgenographic studies
  1. Barium sulfate
  2. Organic iodide compounds for cholecystography
     a. Iodoalphionic acid (Priodax)
     b. Iopanic acid (Telepaque)
     c. Iophenoxic acid (Teridax)
  3. Others

4. Cathartics
Promote defecation, contraindicated as

long-term therapy or if impaction, ileus or undiagnosed abdominal pain is present; may cause electrolyte imbalance and multiple serious reactions

A. Bulk-forming cathartics
1. Action—stimulate peristalsis by increasing bulk
2. May cause fecal impaction and obstruction
3. Preparations
   a. Agar
   b. Plantago seed (psyllium seed, Metamucil, Konsyl)
   c. Methylcellulose (Cellothyl)
   d. Sodium carboxymethylcellulose (Carmethose)

B. Saline cathartics
1. Action—retain water in intestine, distending it and stimulating peristalsis
2. Toxicity—rare
3. Preparations
   a. Sodium sulfate (Glauber's salt)
   b. Magnesium sulfate (Epsom salt)
   c. Milk of magnesia (magnesium hydroxide)
   d. Magnesium citrate, oxide, or sulfate
   e. Sodium phosphate or sulfate
   f. Others

C. Emollient cathartics—liquid petrolatum (mineral oil) and others
1. Action—soften fecal mass; inhibit absorption of water
2. Undesirable effects—loss of fat-soluble vitamins, interference with healing in perineal and anal area

D. Fecal moistening agents
1. Dioctyl sodium sulfosuccinate (Colace, Doxinate)
2. Poloxalkol (Magcyl, Polykol)

E. Chemical irritants
1. Action—stimulate bowel, increasing peristalsis
2. Toxicity—may produce excessive purgation, abdominal cramping, exhaustion
3. Preparations
   a. Castor oil
   b. Cascara sagrada and other anthracene cathartics—aloe, rhubarb, and senna

F. Miscellaneous
1. Glycerin suppositories
2. Suppositories that bring about release of carbon dioxide (e.g., Pharmalax)
3. Bisacodyl (Dulcolax)

5. **Antidiarrheals**
A. Classification
1. Demulcents (e.g., bismuth salts)—soothe irritated mucous membranes
2. Adsorbents—adsorb gases and toxic substances
   a. Kaolin
   b. Kaolin mixture with pectin (Kaopectate)
   c. Activated charcoal
3. Hydrophilic agents (e.g., polycarbophil)
4. Anti-infectives—usually insoluble and not absorbed from gastrointestinal tract
   a. Sulfonamides
      (1) Sulfadiazine—used to treat bacillary dysentery, cholera
      (2) Salicylazosulfapyridine (Azulfidine)—used to treat infections secondary to colitis
   b. Antibiotics
5. Mixtures
   a. Cremomycin
   b. Cremosuxidine
   c. Diphenoxylate hydrochloride with atropine sulfate (Lomotil)
   d. Donnagel
   e. Furazolidone (Furoxone)
   f. Others
6. Sedatives and antispasmodics
   a. Opium tincture
   b. Camphorated opium tincture
   c. Belladonna and alkaloids (natural or synthetic)

DRUGS THAT AFFECT THE HEART, BLOOD VESSELS, AND BLOOD

1. **Drugs that affect the heart**
A. Cardiotonics
1. Cardiac glycosides
   a. Action—cumulative
      (1) Local action—marked irritation
      (2) Systemic actions
         (a) Alter mechanical and electrophysiologic action of heart muscle; increase force of contraction
         (b) Increase stroke volume and cardiac output, improve systolic emptying, and decrease heart size, blood volume, and central venous pressure
         (c) Stimulate vagus mechanism; slow heart rate

(d) Produce diuresis, a result of improved heart action and circulation
(e) May affect blood pressure
  b. Toxicity
    (1) Anorexia, salivation, nausea, vomiting, diarrhea, abdominal pain
    (2) Slow pulse (below 60), irregular rate or rhythm, tachyarrhythmias
    (3) Headache, malaise, hallucinations, visual disturbances
    (4) Lethargy, drowsiness, confusion
    (5) Electrocardiographic changes
    (6) Cardiac arrhythmias
  c. Preparations
    (1) Digitalis leaf
    (2) Digitoxin (Crystodigin, Purodigin)
    (3) Digoxin (Lanoxin)
    (4) Acetyldigitoxin (Acylanid)
    (5) Gitalin (Gitaligin)
    (6) Deslanoside (Cedilanid-D)
    (7) Lanatoside C (Cedilanid)
    (8) Ouabain
    (9) Others
B. Cardiac depressants (antiarrhythmic drugs)
  1. Digitalis glycosides—reduce automaticity of atria and decrease conduction through AV node; result in slower ventricular rate
  2. Quinidine preparations
    a. Action
      (1) Decrease cardiac excitability and rate of conduction across AV node
      (2) Increase refractory period
      (3) Slow the heart
      (4) Convert rapid, irregular pulse to slow, regular one
      (5) Relax smooth muscle
    b. Toxicity
      (1) Nausea, vomiting, abdominal cramps
      (2) Diarrhea, headache, vertigo, tinnitus, syncope, visual disturbances
      (3) Marked slowing of pulse, arrhythmias, severe hypotension, cardiac arrest
      (4) Hypersensitivity reactions
  3. Procainamide hydrochloride (Pronestyl)—similar to quinidine but action is more prolonged and toxicity is said to be lower
  4. Lidocaine hydrochloride (Xylocaine)
2. **Drugs that affect the blood vessels**
A. Drugs that produce vasoconstriction and increase rate and strength of heart's contraction; used to raise blood pressure, control superficial hemorrhage, relieve nasal congestion
  1. Epinephrine (Adrenalin)
    a. Actions
      (1) Constricts peripheral blood vessels
      (2) Large doses increase blood pressure briefly
      (3) Stimulates myocardium and increases cardiac output
    b. Toxicity
      (1) Excessive cardiac stimulation
      (2) Tissue anoxia may occur if used in presence of shock
      (3) Therapeutic doses may cause pallor, dizziness, headaches, anxiety, restlessness, palpitation, respiratory distress
      (4) Overdosage—convulsions, cerebral hemorrhage, arrhythmias
  2. Levarterenol bitartrate (Levophed, norepinephrine)
    a. Actions
      (1) Vasoconstrictor—raises and sustains blood pressure
      (2) Tends to slow pulse of patient in recumbent position; decreases cardiac output
    b. Toxicity
      (1) Dose must be adjusted to blood pressure to prevent excessive elevation of blood pressure
      (2) Necrosis and sloughing if extravasation of drug occurs
      (3) Anxiety, respiratory difficulty, headache, awareness of slow, forceful heartbeat
  3. Metaraminol bitartrate (Aramine)—similar to levarterenol; longer duration of action
  4. Mephentermine sulfate (Wyamine)
    a. Actions—produces prolonged vasoconstriction, increases cardiac output, dispels feelings of lethargy and fatigue
    b. Toxicity—nervousness, insomnia, headache
  5. Hydroxyamphetamine (Paredrine)—

similar to mephentermine; used to
treat orthostatic hypotension
6. Ephedrine—effects similar to those
of epinephrine but much more prolonged
7. Phenylephrine hydrochloride (Neo-
Synephrine)—has effects similar to
those of epinephrine; effect on blood
pressure is prolonged
8. Angiotensin amide (Hypertensin)
  a. Action—direct stimulation of
smooth blood vessels; powerful
vasoconstrictor; potency requires
continuous monitoring of blood
pressure, effectiveness decreases
with repeated use
  b. Toxicity—cumulative drug; symptoms of ergotism
9. Ergotamine tartrate
  a. Actions—stimulates smooth muscles of blood vessels and uterus;
used to treat migraine headaches
  b. Toxicity—dizziness, headache, urticaria, coronary insufficiency, renal constriction, bradycardia,
ventricular irregularities
10. Isoproterenol (Isuprel)
11. Drugs used to combat hypotension
related to anesthesia
  a. Methamphetamine hydrochloride
(Drinalfa)
  b. Methoxamine hydrochloride (Vasoxyl)
B. Drugs that produce vasodilatation—used
to treat hypertension, peripheral vascular
disease, and coronary disease
1. Nitrites and nitrates
  a. Actions—relax smooth muscles of
blood vessels, produce spasmolytic
effect on bronchi, urinary tract,
biliary tract, and gastrointestinal
tract; used to treat angina
  b. Toxicity
    (1) Headache until tolerance de-
velops (tolerance developed
and broken easily)
    (2) Dizziness and faintness
    (3) Nitrite reaction—flushing of
face and neck, throbbing headache, drop in blood pressure,
weak, rapid pulse, fainting
    (4) Hypoxia and/or circulatory
collapse
  c. Preparations
    (1) Amyl nitrite
    (2) Nitroglycerin

    (3) Pentaerythritol tetranitrate
(Peritrate)
    (4) Erythrityl tetranitrate (Cardi-
late)
    (5) Propranolol hydrochloride (In-
deral)
2. Papaverine
3. Aminophylline
4. Ethyl alcohol
5. Antihypertensive drugs
  a. Rauwolfia and derivatives
  b. Preparations of veratrum
  c. Hydralazine hydrochloride (Apre-
soline)
    (1) Action—reduces blood pressure
by acting on midbrain and by
antagonizing pressor substances
    (2) Toxicity—headache, palpita-
tion, anxiety, depression, dry
mouth, nausea, vomiting, cardiac pain, edema, chills, fever,
and manifestations of arthritic
and collagen diseases
  d. Ganglion blocking agents
    (1) Action—block impulses in sym-
pathetic and parasympathetic
ganglia; maximum effect occurs
in semisitting position
    (2) Toxicity—due to their potency,
dose must be determined by
blood pressure immediately
prior to administration of drug;
symptoms of toxicity include
hypotension, dry mouth, constipation, paralytic ileus, urinary
retention, and impotence
    (3) Preparations
      (a) Pentolinium tartrate (An-
solysen)
      (b) Chlorisondamine chloride
(Ecolid)
      (c) Mecamylamine hydrochlo-
ride (Inversine)
      (d) Trimethaphan camsylate
(Arfonad)
6. Thiazides and other diuretics used to
treat hypertension
  a. Chlorothiazide (Diuril)
  b. Hydrochlorothiazide (Esidrix)
  c. Furosemide (Lasix)
  d. Ethacrynic acid (Edecrin)
  e. Chlorthalidone (Hygroton)
  f. Quinethazone (Hydromox)
  g. Others
7. Guanethidine (Ismelin)
8. Methyldopa (Aldomet)

9. Pargyline hydrochloride (Eutonyl)

3. **Agents that affect the blood**

A. Antianemic (hemopoietic) drugs
1. Iron
a. Action
(1) Local—irritant and astringent
(2) Systemic—increases hemoglobin in iron-deficiency anemia, increases reserve supply of iron
b. Toxicity—nausea, vomiting, constipation or diarrhea, abdominal distress, headache; overdosage may cause death in children
c. Preparations
(1) Ferrous sulfate
(2) Ferrous gluconate (Fergon)
(3) Ferrocholinate (Chel-Iron, Ferrolip)
(4) Others
(5) Preparations for injection
(a) Iron-dextran injection (Imferon)
(b) Dextriferron (Astrafer)
(c) Iron sorbitex (Jectofer)
2. Cyanocobalamin (vitamin B_{12})—used in replacement therapy; treats pernicious anemia
3. Folic acid (Folvite)—useful therapy in selected cases of anemia
B. Blood, plasma, and plasma substitutes
1. Whole blood—used to restore blood passively and rapidly
2. Normal human serum albumin—used to restore blood volume, raise serum protein level, and decrease edema
3. Packed human blood cells—used to increase number of circulating red blood cells
4. Normal human plasma
5. Plasma protein fraction
6. Dextran used to expand plasma volume in selected cases
7. Polyvinylpyrrolidone (PVP)
C. Drugs that promote clotting
1. Vitamin K—essential to synthesis of prothrombin
a. Menadione
b. Menadione sodium bisulfite (Hykinone)
c. Menadiol sodium diphosphate (Synkayvite)
d. Phytonadione (vitamin K_1, Mephyton)
e. Vitamin K_5 (Synkamin)
2. Other systemic coagulants

a. Antihemophilic globulin (AHG)
b. Fibrinogen
c. Aminocaproic acid (Amicar)
3. Absorbable hemostatics—exert local action
a. Absorbable gelatin sponge (Gelfoam)
b. Oxidized cellulose (Oxycel)
c. Thrombin
d. Others
D. Anticoagulants
1. Actions—interfere with coagulation of blood, prevent formation of thrombi and emboli
2. Toxicity—overdosage causes bleeding; dosage controlled in relation to prothrombin time
3. Preparations
a. Sodium citrate
b. Heparin-antagonist: protamine sulfate
c. Coumarin derivatives
(1) Bishydroxycoumarin (Dicumarol)
(2) Ethyl biscoumacetate (Tromexan)
(3) Warfarin sodium (Coumadin, Panwarfin)
(4) Acenocoumarol (Sintrom)
(5) Phenprocoumon (Liquamar)
d. Indandione derivatives
(1) Phenindione (Danilone, Hedulin)
(2) Diphenadione (Dipaxin)
(3) Anisindione (Miradon)

HISTAMINE, ANTIHISTAMINES, AND DRUGS USED FOR MOTION SICKNESS

1. **Histamine**
A. Actions
1. Allergy causes release of abnormal amounts
2. Stimulates secretion of gastric acid
3. Diagnostic aid for pheochromocytoma
B. Toxicity—drop in blood pressure, headache, dyspnea, flushing, vomiting, diarrhea, shock, and collapse
2. **Betazole hydrochloride (Histalog)**—action similar to histamine; fewer adverse reactions
3. **Histamine-antagonizing agents**
A. Epinephrine
B. Antihistamines
1. Actions—probably prevent physiologic activity of histamine, suppress symptoms due to allergy

2. Toxicity—drowsiness, dizziness, dryness of mouth and throat, nausea, disturbed coordination, weakness, lassitude; additive effect with central nervous system depressants
3. Preparations
    a. Chlorpheniramine maleate (Chlor-Trimeton, Teldrin)
    b. Diphenhydramine hydrochloride (Benadryl)
    c. Tripelennamine hydrochloride (Pyribenzamine)
    d. Promethazine (Phenergan)
    e. Others
4. **Drugs used for motion sickness**
A. Action—unclear; appear to depress central nervous system and to decrease sensitivity of labyrinth
B. Toxicity—drowsiness, fatigue, blurred vision, dryness of mouth
C. Preparations
    1. Scopolamine
    2. Cyclizine (Marezine)
    3. Dimenhydrinate (Dramamine)
    4. Meclizine hydrochloride (Bonine)
    5. Trimethobenzamide hydrochloride (Tigan)
    6. Hydroxyzine (Vistaril, Atarax)
    7. Others

SKELETAL MUSCLE RELAXANTS

1. **Actions**
Inhibit nerve impulses at myoneural junction and inhibit certain reflexes in central nervous system
2. **Toxicity**
Respiratory paralysis, circulatory collapse, other central nervous system effects
3. **Preparations**
A. Curariform blocking agents (nondepolarizing agents)
    1. Tubocurarine chloride
    2. Dimethyltubocurarine iodide (Metubine)
    3. Gallamine triethiodide (Flaxedil)
B. Antagonists to curariform drugs (e.g., edrophonium chloride, Tensilon)
C. Drugs that prolong depolarization at the motor end plate
    1. Decamethonium bromide (Syncurine)
    2. Succinylcholine chloride (Anectine)—action prolonged by hexafluorenium bromide (Mylaxen)
D. Skeletal muscle relaxants that act centrally (in brain)

1. Mephenesin
2. Carisoprodol (Soma)
3. Diazepam (Valium)
4. Meprobamate (Equanil, Miltown)
5. Methocarbamol (Robaxin)
6. Orphenadrine citrate (Norflex)
7. Others

DRUGS THAT AFFECT ORGANS OF THE RESPIRATORY SYSTEM

1. **Drugs that stimulate respiratory center directly**
A. Carbon dioxide
B. Caffeine
C. Atropine
D. Nikethamide
E. Pentylenetetrazol (Metrazol)
2. **Antitussives—preparations to relieve cough**
A. Narcotic antitussives
    1. Action—suppress cough reflex
    2. Toxicity—depress respiration and ciliary, activity, may cause bronchial constriction, are habit-forming
    3. Preparations
        a. Codeine
        b. Hydrocodone bitartrate (Dicodid, Hycodan)
        c. Methadone hydrochloride (Dolophine)
        d. Others
B. Nonnarcotic antitussives
    1. Benzonatate (Tessalon)
    2. Carbetapentane citrate (Toclase)
    3. Noscapine (Nectadon)
    4. Dextromethorphan hydrobromide (Romilar)
    5. Glyceryl guaiacolate (Robitussin)
    6. Noscapine (Nectadon)
C. Demulcents—protect lining of upper respiratory tract
    1. Syrups
    2. Honey, hard candy, etc.
    3. Plain or medicated steam
D. Anti-infectives
    1. Antibiotics
    2. Sulfonamides
E. Expectorants
    1. Sedative expectorants—increase secretions by reflex stimulation of the gastric mucosa
        a. Ammonium chloride
        b. Ammonium carbonate
        c. Sodium and potassium iodide
        d. Glyceryl guaiacolate (Robitussin)
        e. Syrup of Ipecac

f. Enzymes (e.g., Mucomyst)
g. Detergents
(1) Tergemist
(2) Alevaire
2. Stimulating expectorants—decrease secretions
a. Terpin hydrate
b. Terpin hydrate and codeine elixir
3. **Drugs given to relax bronchial spasm**
A. Epinephrine (Adrenalin)
B. Ephedrine
C. Aminophylline
D. Belladonna
E. Isoproterenol hydrochloride (Isuprel)
F. Protokylol hydrochloride (Caytine)
G. Others
4. **Oxygen**

DRUGS THAT AFFECT THE SKIN AND MUCOUS MEMBRANES

1. **Anti-infective agents**
A. Antibiotics
B. Fungicides
1. Benzoic and salicylic acid (e.g., Whitfield's ointment)
2. Preparations containing cupric sulfate
3. Gentian violet
4. Nystatin (Mycostatin)
5. Propionate-caprylate compounds (e.g., Sopronol)
6. Propionate compound (Propion Gel)
7. Zinc undecylenate and zincundecate (Desenex)
8. Griseofulvin (Fulvicin, Grifulvin)
9. Salicylanilide (Ansadol)
10. Others
C. Miscellaneous local agents
1. Boric acid
2. Ammoniated mercury
3. Nitrofurazone (Furacin)
4. Selenium sulfide (Selsun)
5. Potassium permanganate
2. **Anti-inflammatory agents (e.g., topical corticosteroids)**
A. Hydrocortisone (Cortef, Cortone, Hydrocortone)
B. Triamcinolone (Aristocort, Kenalog)
C. Fluocinolone acetonide (Synalar, Syntex)
D. Others
3. **Antipruritics and local anesthetics—used to relieve itching and discomfort**
A. Dyclonine hydrochloride (Dyclone)
B. Menthol (e.g., Schamberg's lotion)
C. Phenol (e.g., phenolated calamine lotion)
D. Pramoxine hydrochloride (Tronothane)

E. Trimeprazine (Temaril) and other antihistaminic drugs
4. **Astringents**
A. Aluminum acetate (Burow's solution)
B. Silver nitrate
C. Tannic acid
5. **Cell stimulants and proliferants (e.g., vitamins A and D ointment)**
6. **Surface-active agents**
A. Benzalkonium chloride (Zephiran)
B. Benzethonium chloride (Phemerol)
C. Cetylpyridinium chloride (Ceepryn)
D. Methylbenzethonium chloride (Diaparene)
7. **Emollients, demulcents, and protectants**
A. Basic lotions and liniments
1. Hydrophilic lotion
2. Zinc oxide and talc lotions
B. Basic oils and other solvents
1. Collodion
2. Cottonseed oil
3. Glycerin (glycerol)
C. Basic ointments and protectants
1. Aluminum paste
2. Compound benzoin tincture
3. Petrolatum (Vaseline)
4. Rose water ointment (cold cream)
5. Silicone
6. Wool fat preparations (e.g., lanolin)
7. Zinc oxide (e.g., Lassar's paste)
D. Basic powders and demulcents
1. Oatmeal (e.g., Aveeno)
2. Collodial Soyaloid Soybean Complex
3. Cornstarch
4. Talc (talcum)
5. Zinc stearate
8. **Keratolytic agents—soften scales, loosen horny layers of skin**
A. Resorcinol
B. Salicylic acids
9. **Keratoplastic agents**
A. Preparations containing coal tar (e.g., pix carbonis, Zetar, liquid carbonis detergens—LCD)
B. Ichthammol (Ichthyol)
10. **Miscellaneous agents**
A. Arsenic preparations (e.g., Fowler's solution)
B. Chymotrypsin (Chymar)

DRUGS THAT AFFECT THE KIDNEY AND ORGANS OF THE URINARY TRACT

1. **Diuretics—increase flow of urine**
A. Water
B. Osmotic diuretics
1. Mannitol (Osmitrol)

2. Urea (Carbamide)
3. Sodium chloride
4. Potassium salts
5. Glucose and sucrose
C. Acid-forming salts (e.g., ammonium chloride)
D. Xanthine diuretics (e.g., aminophylline) —have limited use
E. Mercurial diuretics
 1. Action—interfere with absorption of sodium ion in tubules of kidney
 2. Toxicity—symptoms of mercurial poisoning, renal damage
 3. Preparations
  a. Meralluride (Mercuhydrin)
  b. Mercaptomerin (Thiomerin)
  c. Chlormerodrin (Neohydrin)
  d. Mercumatilin (Cumertilin)
  e. Others
F. Carbonic anhydrase inhibitors
 1. Action—interfere with reabsorption of sodium and bicarbonate ions in renal tubules; depress formation of aqueous humor
 2. Toxicity—multiple side effects may occur, including drowsiness, paresthesias of the face and extremities, and metabolic acidosis
 3. Preparations
  a. Acetazolamide sodium (Diamox)
  b. Ethoxzolamide (Cardrase)
  c. Methazolamide (Neptazane)
G. Thiazide diuretics
 1. Action—decrease reabsorption of sodium and chloride ions, may cause excretion of potassium
 2. Toxicity—allergic reactions, nausea, weakness, dizziness, paresthesias, muscle cramps; acidosis may occur
 3. Preparations
  a. Bendroflumethiazide (Naturetin)
  b. Chlorothiazide (Diuril)
  c. Hydrochlorothiazide (Esidrix, HydroDiuril)
  d. Methyclothiazide (Enduron)
  e. Others
H. Aldosterone antagonists—spironolactone (Aldactone), Triamterene (Dyrenium)
 1. Action—block effects of aldosterone, an adrenocortical hormone, causing retention of potassium and excretion of sodium and chloride ions
 2. Toxicity—low; electrolyte balance may be impaired
I. Cation exchange resins (e.g., carbacrylamine resins—Carbo-Resin)

J. Benzothiazides (e.g., ethacrynic acid—Edecrin)
K. Sulfonamide diuretics (e.g., furosemide —Lasix)
2. **Antidiuretics**
A. Posterior pituitary hormone—replacement therapy used in treatment of diabetes insipidus
3. **Drugs that affect the bladder**
A. Belladonna and derivatives—relax hypertonic bladder
B. Urinary antiseptics
 1. Sulfonamides
  a. Action—principally against gramnegative bacilli
  b. Toxicity—relatively low; includes nausea, vomiting, hypersensitivity reactions, renal disturbances, and blood dyscrasias
  c. Preparations
   (1) Sulfisoxazole (Gantrisin)
   (2) Sulfamethoxazole (Gantanol)
   (3) Sulfonamide mixtures
C. Antibiotics—choice of preparation depends on sensitivity of causative organism
D. Methenamine mandelate (Mandelamine)
E. Nitrofurantoin (Furadantin)
 1. Action—antibacterial effect on many organisms
 2. Toxicity—low; nausea and vomiting may occur
F. Nalidixic acid (NegGram)
G. Phenazopyridine (Pyridium)
 1. Action—produces analgesic effect on urinary mucosa
 2. Toxicity—may produce sensitivity
H. Others

DRUGS THAT ACT ON ORGANS
OF THE REPRODUCTIVE SYSTEM

1. **Oxytocics—drugs that promote uterine contractions**
A. Ergot and its derivatives
 1. Action—direct stimulation of uterus, constriction of blood vessels
 2. Toxicity
  a. Central nervous system stimulation —nausea, vomiting, tremor, weakness, excitement, convulsions, dilated pupils, rapid pulse
  b. Circulatory system—tingling, itching, coldness of skin; weak, rapid pulse
  c. Thirst, headache, dizziness, cramping and diarrhea

d. Chronic ergotism—gangrenous or convulsive
3. Preparations
   a. Ergonovine maleate (Ergotrate maleate)
   b. Methylergonovine (Methergine)
B. Posterior pituitary hormone
   1. Actions—stimulates uterine muscle, has antidiuretic effect, constricts peripheral blood vessels
   2. Toxicity—may cause uterine tetany
   3. Preparations
      a. Posterior pituitary injection
      b. Oxytocin injection (Pitocin, Syntocinon)
2. **Antispasmodics**
A. Relaxin (Releasin)
B. Lututrin (Lutrexin)
C. Magnesium sulfate
3. **Sex hormones**
A. Pituitary gonadotropic hormones
B. Placental gonadotropic hormones—chorionic gonadotropin
C. Ovarian hormones
   1. Action and uses—relieve some symptoms related to the menopause, suppress lactation, are used to relieve discomfort due to cancer of the prostate gland
   2. Toxicity—nausea, vomiting, diarrhea, rash
   3. Preparations
      a. Estrogens (natural)
         (1) Estrone (Theelin)
         (2) Estradiol
         (3) Others
      b. Conjugated estrogens
         (1) Estrogenic substances, conjugated (Premarin)
         (2) Piperazine estrone sulfate (Sulestrex)
      c. Synthetic estrogens
         (1) Diethylstilbestrol
         (2) Chlorotrianisene (Tace)
         (3) Others
      d. Luteal hormones
         (1) Actions—prepare uterus for implantation and nourishment of embryo, suppress ovulation during pregnancy, decrease irritability of uterine muscle
         (2) Toxicity—relatively low
         (3) Preparations
            (a) Progesterone
            (b) Medroxyprogesterone acetate (Provera)

            (c) Hydroxyprogesterone caproate (Delalutin)
            (d) Others
D. Ovulatory suppressants
   1. Norethynodrel with mestranol (Enovid)
   2. Norethindrone (Norlutin)
   3. Norethindrone with mestranol (Ortho-Novum)
   4. Ethynodiol diacetate with mestranol (Ovulen)
   5. Others
E. Ovulatory agents
   1. Action—stimulate ovulation
   2. Toxicity—ovarian enlargement, ovarian cysts
   3. Preparations—clomiphene citrate (Clomid), menotropines (Pergonal)
F. Androgens
   1. Testosterone preparations
   2. Norethandrolone (Nilevar)
   3. Others

ANTI-INFECTIVES—ANTIBIOTICS

1. **Antibiotics—chemical substances produced by microorganisms; inhibit or destroy other microorganisms**
2. **Sources of antibiotics**
A. Actinomycetes
B. Molds
C. Bacteria
D. Synthesis
3. **Action of antibiotics and problems resulting from action**
A. Bacteriostasis—inhibiting the growth of bacteria
B. Bacteriocidal effects—killing bacteria
C. Resistance—occurs when previously susceptible organisms develop ability to withstand action of an antibiotic
D. Allergic reactions—include anaphylaxis
E. Superinfection—infection that develops when normal protective flora of body is destroyed by action of antibiotic
4. **Antibiotics usually given for systemic effects**
A. Penicillins
   1. Action—bacteriostatic or bacteriocidal, depending on dosage; effective against many gram-positive bacteria, *Neisseria* and *Treponema* organisms
   2. Toxicity—relatively low; superinfections may occur, allergy, anaphylactic shock
   3. Preparations
      a. Semisynthetic penicillins

(1) Penicillin G
(2) Sodium methicillin (Staphcillin)
(3) Sodium oxacillin (Prostaphlin)
(4) Sodium nafcillin (Unipen)
(5) Ampicillin (Polycillin, Penbritin)
(6) Others
4. Penicillinase (Neutrapen)—enzyme capable of hydrolyzing penicillin; used to treat adverse reactions to penicillin
B. Streptomycins
1. Action—effective against causative organisms of tuberculosis, gram-negative organisms, *Pasteurella, Haemophilus,* and *Brucella* organisms
2. Toxicity—allergic reactions, contact dermatitis, toxic effects on liver and kidneys; dihydrostreptomycin seldom used, due to its damaging effect on eighth cranial nerve with resulting deafness and vertigo
C. Tetracyclines
1. Action—effective against wide range of bacteria, some large viruses, rickettsiae, and *Entamoeba histolytica;* among the few drugs that are effective against this group of organisms
2. Toxicity—nausea, vomiting, diarrhea; other reactions less frequent
3. Preparations
a. Chlortetracycline (Aureomycin)
b. Oxytetracycline (Terramycin)
c. Tetracycline (Achromycin)
d. Demecloycline (Declomycin)
e. Rolitetracycline (Syntetrin)
f. Tetracycline phosphate complex (Panmycin, Sumycin, Tetrex)
g. Others
D. Cephalosporins
1. Action—effective against wide range of gram-positive organisms including some penicillin-resistant organisms
2. Toxicity—local phlebitis and pain, blood dyscrasias, liver and kidney damage, allergic reactions
3. Preparations
a. Cephaloridine (Loridine)
b. Cephalothin (Keflin)
c. Cephalexin (Keflex)
E. Erythromycin
1. Action—range of antibacterial activity similar to penicillin
2. Toxicity—relatively low; gastrointestinal symptoms

F. Chloramphenicol (Chloromycetin)
1. Action—effective against wide range of organisms
2. Toxicity—depression of bone marrow, aplastic anemia, not used unless other antibiotics are ineffective or contraindicated
5. **Antibiotics used occasionally**
The following antibiotics are used occasionally and are beneficial in the treatment of certain infections; a few of the preparations listed are effective against organisms that have developed resistance to other antibiotics; the toxic nature of several preparations restricts their use
A. Amphotericin B (Fungizone)
B. Bacitracin
C. Colistin (Coly-Mycin)
D. Cycloserine (Seromycin)
E. Kanamycin (Kantrex)
F. Neomycin sulfate
G. Novobiocin
H. Oleandomycin
I. Vancomycin
J. Viomycin
K. Griseofulvin (Fulvicin)
L. Polymyxin B sulfate (Aerosporin)
M. Fumagillin
N. Nystatin (Mycostatin)
O. Tyrothricin
P. Gentamicin (Garamycin)
Q. Carbenicillin (Geopen, Pyopen)
R. Lincomycin (Lincocin)
S. Clindamycin (Cleocin)
T. Spectinomycin (Trobicin)

ANTI-INFECTIVES—SULFONAMIDES

1. **Conditions for which sulfonamides especially effective**
A. Meningococcic meningitis
B. Intestinal infections
C. Urinary tract infections
2. **Action—appear to inhibit growth of selected organisms, which permits body defenses to act more effectively; resistance known to occur**
3. **Toxicity—may produce nausea, vomiting, dizziness, headache, restlessness, irritability, drug fever, dermatitis, blood dyscrasias, renal damage**
4. **Preparations of sulfonamides**
A. Sulfadiazine
B. Sulfamerazine
C. Sulfacetamide (Urosulfon)
D. Sulfisoxazole (Gantrisin)
F. Salicylazosulfapyridine (Azulfidine)

G. Sulfamethoxazole (Gantanol)
H. Succinylsulfathiazole (Sulfasuxidine)
I. Sulfisomidine (Elkosin)
J. Others

ANTI-INFECTIVES—DRUGS USED IN TREATMENT OF TUBERCULOSIS, LEPROSY, MALARIA, AND CERTAIN OTHER PROTOZOAN DISEASES

1. Tuberculostatic drugs
A. Action—prevent multiplication of causative organism, *Mycobacterium tuberculosis*
B. Toxicity—relatively high in therapeutic doses
C. Primary drugs
   1. Streptomycin
   2. Para-aminosalicylic acid (PAS)
   3. Isoniazid
   4. Others
D. Secondary drugs
   1. Pyrazinamide
   2. Viomycin
   3. Cycloserine (Seromycin)
   4. Kanamycin (Kantrex)
   5. Ethionamide (Trecator)
   6. Ethambutol (Myambutol)
   7. Rifampin (Rifadin)
2. Drugs used in treatment of leprosy
A. Action—bacteriostatic for causative organism of leprosy
B. Toxicity—nausea, vomiting, hematologic reactions, dermatitis, hepatitis, and glandular enlargement; liver damage and psychosis occur infrequently
C. Sulfone preparations
   1. Dapsone (Avlosulfon)
   2. Sulfoxone (Diasone)
   3. Acetosulfone (Promacetin)
D. Others
3. Antimalarial drugs
A. Quinine
   1. Actions
      a. Effective against causative organism of malaria
      b. Antipyretic and analgesic
      c. Cause local irritation, unreliable stimulation of uterine muscle
   2. Toxicity—headache, nausea, dizziness, ringing in the ears, visual disturbances, renal damage, anemia, respiratory depression
B. Quinacrine hydrochloride (Atabrine)
   1. Action—similar to quinine but probably more effective
   2. Toxicity—nausea, vomiting, diarrhea, headache

C. Additional preparations
   1. Chloroquine phosphate (Aralen)
   2. Amodiaquin hydrochloride (Camoquin)
   3. 8-Aminoquinoline compound (Primaquine phosphate)
   4. Pyrimethamine (Daraprim)
   5. Others
4. Other antiprotozoan agents
Used in treatment of schistosomiasis, leishmaniasis, trypanosomiasis (African sleeping sickness), and some fungous infections; serious toxic effects may occur when these drugs are used
A. Suramin sodium
B. Nitrofurazone
C. Melarsonyl potassium
D. Tryparsamide
E. Melarsoprol
F. Pentaminidine isethionate
G. Nifurtimox

ANTI-INFECTIVES—ANTHELMINTHICS AND AMEBICIDES

1. Anthelminthics
A. Drugs used against cestodes and nematodes
   1. Quinacrine hydrochloride (Atabrine)—tapeworm
   2. Piperazine salts—whipworm, roundworm, pinworm
   3. Diethylcarbamazine (Hetrazan)—whipworm, roundworm
   4. Hexylresorcinol (Crystoids) — tapeworm, pinworm, hookworm
   5. Tetrachloroethylene—hookworm
   6. Thiabendazole (Mintezol) — threadworm, hookworm
   7. Ditheazanine iodide (Delvex)—whipworm, *Strongyloides stercoralis*
   8. Bephenium hydroxynaphthoate (Alcopara)—hookworm
   9. Niclosamide (Yomesan)—large tapeworms
   10. Pyrvinium pamoate (Povan)—pinworm
B. Drugs for schistosomiasis
   1. Antimony potassium tartrate (tartar emetic)
   2. Stibophen (Fuadin)
   3. Hycanthone mesylate
2. Amebicides
A. Drugs that act against extra intestinal amebiasis
   1. Emetine
   2. Chloroquine phosphate (Aralen)
B. Drugs used to treat intestinal amebiasis

1. Arsenicals
   a. Carbarsone
   b. Glycobiarsol (Milibis)
   c. Arsthinol (Balarsen)
2. Iodohydroxyquinoline compounds
   a. Diiodohydroxyquin (Diodoquin)
   b. Iodochlorhydroxyquin (Vioform)
3. Antibiotics
   a. Paromomycin (Humatin)
   b. Fumagillin (Fumidil)
   c. Others
C. Antitrichomonal agents
   1. Used to treat infections caused by *Trichomonas vaginalis*
   2. Toxicity—hypersensitivity reactions
   3. Preparations
      a. Metronidazole (Flagyl)
      b. Diiodohydroxyquin (Floraquin)
      c. Others
D. Scabicides and pediculicides—hygienic measures should accompany use of these agents
   1. Chlorophenothane (DDT)
   2. Crotamiton (Eurax)
   3. Gamma benzene hexachloride (Gexane, Kwell)
   4. Benzyl benzoate
   5. Others

MINERALS, VITAMINS, AND HORMONES

Used to replace or supplement natural components of diet and body secretions; excessive amounts may produce toxic effects
1. **Minerals**
A. Sodium and potassium
B. Calcium
   1. Calcium carbonate
   2. Calcium gluconate
   3. Calcium lactate
   4. Calcium gluceptate
   5. Calcium phosphate
2. **Vitamins**
A. Fat-soluble
   1. Vitamin A
   2. Vitamin D
   3. Vitamin E
   4. Vitamin K
B. Water-soluble
   1. Thiamin hydrochloride (B_1)
   2. Riboflavin (B_2)
   3. Niacin (nicotinic acid)
   4. Pyridoxine (B_6)
   5. Vitamin B_{12}
   6. Folic acid
   7. Ascorbic acid (vitamin C)
   8. Others

C. Multiple-vitamin preparations
3. **Hormones**
   Chemical substances secreted into the bloodstream by the ductless glands; exert specific physiologic effects on metabolism and regulate various body processes
A. Pituitary hormone
   1. Corticotropin injection (Acthar), ACTH—used as replacement therapy
   2. Antidiuretic hormone
      a. Action—increases absorption of water in renal tubules, treats diabetes insipidus
      b. Toxicity—excessive fluid retention, confusion, depression of central nervous system, vasoconstriction, hypersensitivity
      c. Preparations
         (1) Posterior pituitary, a powder
         (2) Posterior pituitary injection
         (3) Vasopressin (Pitressin)
         (4) Vasopressin tannate injection (Pitressin tannate)
B. Parathyroid hormone
   1. Use—relieves symptoms of tetany associated with parathyroid deficiency; calcium preparations are usually given also
   2. Toxicity—nausea, vomiting, weakness, confusion
C. Thyroid hormone
   1. Use—treatment of hypothyroid conditions
   2. Toxicity—rapid pulse, palpitation, pain over heart, insomnia, nervousness, sweating, tremor, weight loss
   3. Preparations
      a. Thyroid
      b. Thyroid extract (Proloid)
      c. Levothyroxine sodium (Synthroid)
      d. Sodium liothyronine (Cytomel)
D. Antithyroid drugs—interfere with formation, release, or action of thyroid hormones; lower the rate of basal metabolism
   1. Iodine and iodides
      a. Toxicity—gastrointestinal and respiratory symptoms, sore mouth, taste of iodine, edema of eyelids, headache, rash, drug fever, and others
      b. Preparations
         (1) Strong iodine solution (Lugol's solution)
         (2) Potassium iodide solution (SSKI)

(3) Sodium iodide solution
(4) Radioactive iodine (I^{131})—when dosage exceeds safety level of radioactivity, adequate precautions must be used to protect others; contamination with radioactive drug must be prevented

2. Propylthiouracil and related drugs
   a. Toxicity—symptoms of upper respiratory infection, rash, fever, loss of taste, enlarged salivary glands, enlarged lymph nodes in neck, edema of lower extremities, blood dyscrasias
   b. Preparations
     (1) Propylthiouracil
     (2) Methimazole (Tapazole)
     (3) Methylthiouracil

E. Hormones of adrenal gland (cortex)
1. Action
   a. Increase protein breakdown, increase excretion of uric and amino acids, produce negative nitrogen balance, cause cessation of tissue growth, modify inflammatory response
   b. Increase glucogenesis, increase blood sugar levels, cause glycosuria
   c. Alter distribution of fat and fat metabolism
   d. Cause retention of water and sodium; excretion of potassium
   e. Suppress secretion of ACTH; adrenal atrophy results
   f. Increase production of certain secretions—saliva, sweat, gastric juices
   g. Increase incidence of thrombosis and emboli formation
   h. May produce psychic manifestations

2. Toxicity
   a. Cushing's syndrome—moonface, striae, hirsutism, acne, hypothyroidism, osteoporosis, muscle wasting, retention of water and sodium, excretion of potassium, calcium, and phosphorus, hypertension
   b. Masking of symptoms of physical disease; aggravation of diabetes, tuberculosis, and peptic ulcers; delayed wound healing
   c. Mood swings and psychosis
   d. Others

3. Preparations

   a. Desoxycorticosterone acetate (DOCA)
   b. Aldosterone
   c. Cortisone and hydrocortisone
   d. Synthetic corticoids
     (1) Prednisone (Meticorten)
     (2) Prednisolone (Meticortelone, Hydreltrasol)
     (3) Triamcinolone (Aristocort, Kenacort, Kenalog)
     (4) Fludrocortisone (Florinef)
     (5) Methylprednisolone (Medrol)
     (6) Dexamethasone (Decadron)
     (7) Paramethasone (Haldrone)
     (8) Fluprednisolone (Alphadrol)
     (9) Betamethasone (Celestone)
   (10) Others

F. Insulin preparations
1. Action—lower blood sugar and promote storage of sugar in liver and muscle; used to control diabetes mellitus
2. Toxicity—symptoms of hypoglycemia; e.g., hunger, weakness, sweating, nervousness, anxiety, apprehension, pallor or flushing, aphasia, convulsions, coma, and death; treated with oral orange juice, sugar, or intravenous glucose
3. Preparations
   a. Insulin injection (regular insulin)
   b. Protamine zinc insulin suspension
   c. Globin zinc insulin injection (globin insulin with zinc)
   d. Isophane insulin suspension (NPH)
   e. Insulin zinc suspension, lente insulin
   f. Prompt insulin zinc suspension (semilente)
   g. Extended insulin zinc suspension (ultralente)

G. Oral hypoglycemic agents
1. Action—stimulate pancreas to secrete more insulin; lower the blood sugar
2. Toxicity—variable, by agent; fever, rashes, nausea, vomiting, blood disorders, neurologic and gastrointestinal symptoms, and hypoglycemia have been reported
3. Preparations
   a. Tolbutamide (Orinase)
   b. Chlorpropamide (Diabinese)
   c. Phenformin hydrochloride (DBI)
   d. Acetohexamide (Dymelor)
   e. Tolazamide (Tolinase)
   f. Others

H. Glucagon
   1. Action—pancreatic extract that opposes action of insulin and is useful in treatment of hypoglycemia
   2. Toxicity—nausea, vomiting, hypotension, hypersensitivity

ANTINEOPLASTIC (ANTIMALIGNANT, CARCINOSTATIC) DRUGS

Used with some success in controlling and eradicating malignancy that is not curable by irradiation or surgery
1. **Action**
   Not well understood
2. **Toxicity**
   In addition to other symptoms may include the following: sore mouth, abdominal pain, diarrhea, nausea, vomiting, paralysis, convulsions, alopecia, depression of bone marrow, thrombosis, and sloughing of tissue at site of injection if extravasation occurs
3. **Preparations**
A. Alkylating agents—nitrogen mustards and related compounds believed to react with essential molecules in cells of tumor to interfere with cell division; used to treat malignancy of breast, ovary, and reticuloendothelial system
   1. Mechlorethamine hydrochloride (Mustargen)
   2. Triethylenemelamine (TEM)
   3. Chlorambucil (Leukeran)
   4. Busulfan (Myleran)
   5. Thiotepa
   6. Cyclophosphamide (Cytoxan)
   7. Mephalan (Alkeran)
   8. Pipobroman (Vercyte)
   9. Uracil mustard
   10. Triethylenemelamine
B. Antimetabolites—drugs that interfere with use of some substance vital to growth and reproduction of cells of neoplasm (e.g., folic acid antagonists)
   1. Methotrexate
   2. Mercaptopurine (Purinethol)
   3. Fluorouracil (5-FU)
   4. Azathiopine (Imuran)
   5. Thioquanine
   6. Cytarabine (Cytosar)
C. Additional antineoplastic agents
   1. Dactinomycin (Cosmegen)
   2. Vincristine (Oncovin)
   3. Vinblastine (Velban)
   4. Others
D. Hormones—believed to slow growth of neoplasm by creating unfavorable environment for growth; androgens may be used to treat cancer of the breast; estrogens may be used to treat cancer of the prostate gland
E. Radioactive isotopes—agents that act like x rays and liberate cell-destroying radiation in vicinity of neoplasm
   1. Toxicity—nausea, vomiting, diarrhea, weakness, anemia, bone marrow depression, hemorrhage, infection
   2. Preparations
      a. Sodium radiophosphate (P^{32})
      b. Radiogold colloid (Au^{198})
      c. Sodium radioiodide (I^{131})
      d. Others

ENZYMES USED AS DRUGS
1. **Enzyme preparations**
A. Hyaluronidase (Alidase)
B. Streptokinase-streptodornase (Varidase)
C. Trypsin, crystallized (Tryptar)
D. Chymotrypsin

REVIEW QUESTIONS FOR PHARMACOLOGY AND THERAPEUTICS*
Multiple choice

Read each question carefully and consider all possible answers. When you have decided which answer is best, blacken in the corresponding space on the answer sheet. There is only one best answer for each question (or implied question).

Situation: Mrs. Hapler is admitted for a cholecystectomy. Preoperative orders include the following: secobarbital (Seconal) gr. 1½ at bedtime; meperidine (Demerol) 75 mg., promethazine (Phenergan) 25 mg., and atropine sulfate gr. 1/150 to be given ½ hour prior to surgical intervention. (See questions 1 to 8.)

1. The nurse should recognize which of the following amounts represent the approximate equivalent for the ordered dose of secobarbital?
   1. 50 mg.   3. 200 mg.
   2. 100 mg.   4. 125 mg.
2. Secobarbital is administered at 10 P.M. During which of the following time spans can the nurse expect this drug to exert its maximum effect?
   1. 10 P.M. to 10:15 P.M.
   2. 10:15 P.M. to 6:30 A.M.
   3. 11 P.M. to 5 A.M.
   4. 10:30 P.M. to 2 A.M.
3. Mrs. Hapler complains of pain when the nurse administers the secobarbital. If an analgesic is not given, the toxic effect that the nurse is most likely to observe is which of the following?
   1. Profound sleep with restlessness
   2. Respiratory depression with stertor

*Additional questions on pharmacology are integrated in clinical chapters.

3. Decrease in blood pressure
4. Mental confusion and restlessness

4. Drugs such as secobarbital which are used to produce sleep are called
   (a) Hypnotics   1. a and d
   (b) Sedatives   2. b and c
   (c) Tranquilizers   3. c and d
   (d) Narcotics   4. a and b

5. After administration of meperidine, Mrs. Hapler perspires profusely, becomes dizzy, and feels faint. Which of the following nursing actions should be carried out first?
   1. Take Mrs. Hapler's vital signs immediately
   2. Place Mrs. Hapler in a prone position
   3. Notify the nursing supervisor
   4. Instruct Mrs. Hapler to breathe deeply

6. Promethazine (Phenergan) will act primarily to
   1. Cause drowsiness and euphoria
   2. Counteract manifestations of allergy
   3. Prevent nausea and vomiting
   4. Potentiate the effects of meperidine

7. The atropine sulfate can be expected to
   (a) Increase ease of respiration 1. a and d
   (b) Decrease motility of gastrointestinal tract 2. b and c
      3. a, b, and d
   (c) Dilate pupils of the eyes 4. All the above
   (d) Decrease secretions and prevent laryngospasm

8. Which of the following characteristics of atropine sulfate explains why its use is preferred to the use of atropine?
   1. More soluble   3. More reactive
   2. More stable   4. Less toxic

Situation: A patient receives thiopental sodium (Pentothal sodium) as an anesthetic agent. (See questions 9 to 12.)

9. Thiopental sodium is used for
   1. Short nontraumatic surgical procedures
   2. Rapid and deep anesthesia
   3. Prolonging the effects of nitrous oxide
   4. Producing Stage II anesthesia

10. By which of the following methods is thiopental sodium administered?
    1. Inhalation   3. Intravenous
    2. Semiclosed   4. Rectal

11. If thiopental sodium is used as an anesthetic agent, the anesthesia will be known as which of the following types?
    1. Topical   3. Local
    2. General   4. Regional

12. During the course of anesthesia, the surgeon requests the anesthetist to increase muscular relaxation of the patient. Drugs that are specific for this purpose and likely to be used include which of the following?
    (a) Edrophonium chloride (Tensilon) 1. c only
    (b) Mephenesin (Tolserol) 2. b and c
       3. a and d
       4. c and d

(c) Tubocurarine chloride
(d) Succinylcholine (Anectine)

Situation: Mrs. Jones has had a bilateral radical mastectomy. The pathologist's report states that adenocarcinoma Grade IV was present in the tissue removed. (See question 13.)

13. A hormone that may be ordered as a part of Mrs. Jones' postoperative treatment as a palliative agent is
    (a) Diethylstilbestrol (Stilbestrol) 1. a and d
    (b) Dihydrotachysterol (Hytakerol) 2. b and c
       3. a, b, and c
    (c) Progesterone 4. All the above
    (d) Dromostanolone (Drolban)

Situation: Mr. Trum has a collagen disease. Drug therapy includes acetylsalicylic acid and one of the adrenal steroids. (See questions 14 to 18.)

14. Which of the following potential hazards may accompany steroid therapy?
    (a) Delay in wound healing 1. a and b
    (b) Impairment of blood circulation 2. c and d
       3. a, c, and d
    (c) Altered reaction of tissues 4. All the above
    (d) Hypokalemia and osteoporosis

15. Which of the following side effects may occur with overdosage from steroids?
    (a) Restlessness and euphoria 1. a and d
    (b) Edema and sodium retention 2. a and c
       3. b, c, and d
    (c) Hirsutism and striae 4. All the above
    (d) Rounded contour of the face

16. Which of the following conditions would contraindicate the use of steroid therapy?
    1. Recent administration of ACTH
    2. A healed tubercular lesion
    3. Orthostatic hypotension
    4. Ectodactylism

17. Mr. Trum, discouraged and believing that the steroid preparation is not helping his condition, discontinued use of "those little white tablets." Which of the following serious side effects may possibly occur as the result of abrupt discontinuance of corticosteroid therapy?
    1. Adrenal insufficiency
    2. Sodium retention
    3. Hypertension
    4. Cushing's syndrome

18. Prior to surgery on Mr. Trum, the physician is likely to order this change in steroid therapy:
    1. A gradual increase in dose
    2. A gradual decrease in dose
    3. Discontinuance of steroid therapy
    4. Several large doses of a steroid preparation

Situation: Mrs. Zicker is being prepared for thyroidectomy after discovery of some nodules in the thyroid gland. (See questions 19 to 21.)

19. Which of the following drugs might be used to inhibit thyroid production prior to surgery?
    (a) Thyroid extract   1. b only
    (b) Propylthiouracil   2. a and d
    (c) Strong iodine   3. b and c
        solution   4. a and c
    (d) Potassium triplex

20. Postoperatively Mrs. Zicker develops symptoms of tetany. Which of the following drugs is the physician most likely to prescribe in order to produce immediate relief of symptoms?
    1. Thyroid extract
    2. Calcium gluconate
    3. Parathyroid hormone
    4. Tetanus antitoxin

21. Mrs. Zicker receives decavitamin capsules each morning. Which of the following will be found on the label of this official preparation?
    1. N.F.   3. U.S.P.
    2. N.N.R.   4. ®

Situation: Mr. Spiker complains of epigastric distress that is unrelieved by antacids. (See questions 22 to 25.)

22. The antacid that Mr. Spiker has been taking is aluminum hydroxide gel (Amphojel). For which of the following purposes was this medication prescribed?
    (a) To systemically   1. b only
        neutralize gastric   2. a and c
        acidity   3. b and d
    (b) To chemically   4. All the above
        neutralize hydro-
        chloric acid of
        the stomach
    (c) To inhibit the
        secretion of
        hydrochloric
        acid

    (d) To exert a
        slower, prolonged
        antacid effect

23. Which of the following drugs may be used to stimulate the production of hydrochloric acid when a gastric analysis is done for the purpose of determining a diagnosis?
    1. Epinephrine
    2. Glutamic acid hydrochloride
    3. Histamine phosphate
    4. Polyamine-methylene resin

24. Mr. Spiker is told that he has achlorhydria and pernicious anemia. Which of the following is considered to be the most satisfactory medication for treatment of pernicious anemia?
    1. Folic acid   3. Ferrous sulfate
    2. Liver extract   4. Vitamin B_{12}

25. The nurse should teach which of the following principles related to the administration of hydrochloric acid to Mr. Spiker?
    (a) Hydrochloric acid   1. a and c
        should be diluted   2. b and d
        in ½ glass of   3. a, b, and c
        water before   4. All the above
        taking it
    (b) The prepared dose
        may be sipped
        with the meal
    (c) It should be
        taken through a
        tube in order
        to prevent injury
        to the teeth
    (d) Continual, regular
        use of hydrochloric
        acid over a period
        of several months
        will relieve
        symptoms of
        pernicious anemia

SCORES

NAME _____ DATE _____ DATE OF BIRTH _____ AGE _____ SEX _____ M OR F

LAST   FIRST   MIDDLE

SCHOOL _____ CITY _____ GRADE OR CLASS _____ INSTRUCTOR _____

NAME OF TEST _____ PART _____

DIRECTIONS: Read each question and its numbered answers. When you have decided which answer is correct, blacken the corresponding space on this sheet with the special pencil. Make your mark as long as the pair of lines, and move the pencil point up and down firmly to make a heavy black line. If you change your mind, erase your first mark completely. Make no stray marks; they may count against you.

SAMPLE:

1—1 a country
1—2 a mountain
1—3 an island
1—4 a city
1—5 a state

1. Chicago is

BE SURE YOUR MARKS ARE HEAVY AND BLACK.
ERASE COMPLETELY ANY ANSWER YOU WISH TO CHANGE.

Printed by the International Business Machines Corporation, Endicott, N. Y., U. S. A.   IBM FORM I. T. S. 1000 B 108

FOUR

BASIC NURSING

Fundamentals of nursing

complete physical,
mental & social
well being

CHAPTER

8

FUNDAMENTALS OF NURSING

The fundamentals of nursing discussed here are those aspects of nursing which are common to all clinical nursing areas. They are concepts and psychomotor skills that can be utilized in any and all nursing settings. Mastery of the basic concepts involves primarily the use of intellectual processes. In addition, no psychomotor skill can be employed safely unless it is thoroughly grounded both in knowledge and in how to use that knowledge in providing safe and effective nursing care for patients.

The concepts that follow are not unique to nursing. They are adapted from the social, biologic and physical sciences and they form the foundation upon which nursing is structured. Their value in nursing is centered mainly within the capacity of nurses to apply these concepts and their inherent theory to individualized patient care.

BASIC CONCEPTS

Health is an accepted value in society. One of the primary functions of the medical helping professions, including nursing, is to assist individuals, families, and groups to reach the highest level of wellness of which they are capable.
1. **Health defined**
A. A social value—Constitution of the World Health Organization sets forth the meaning of health as follows: "Health is a state of complete physical, mental and social well-being and not just the absence of disease or infirmity"

1. A fundamental right of man
2. Essential to local and worldwide peace and security
3. Requires full cooperation of individuals and agencies committed to its promotion and preservation
B. Concepts of health
1. As a continuum
a. Throughout life cycles of growth and development
b. Fluctuates in accord with biophysiologic function and energy expenditure
2. Halbert L. Dunn—levels of wellness
a. Health not merely the absence of illness or injury
b. Maximum vs. optimum levels
3. Stress
a. Hans Selye—the stress of life
b. Adaptation as the body's response to disease or injury
c. Degrees of adaptation
(1) Compensatory mechanisms
(2) Congenital and acquired disabilities
4. Adaptation
a. Rene Dubos—mirage of health
b. Environment and health
c. Social patterns of health and disease
5. George L. Engel—a unified concept of health and disease
a. Multiple causation of disease
2. **Factors influencing health**
A. Community—local, national, and international

285

1. Socioeconomic status
2. Geophysical environment
3. Agencies and resources available
4. Sociocultural deterrents to health

B. Individual in society
1. Cultural background
2. Socioeconomic class
3. Education
4. Environmental conditioning—susceptibility to mass-media advertising
5. Personal resources and values

3. **Delivery of health services**
A. Types of agencies
1. Official or public
2. Nonofficial or voluntary
3. Private and specialized

B. Classification of agencies
1. Geographic spheres
2. Support and control
3. Services available

C. Evolving patterns of services
1. Community health departments
2. Hospital centers—comprehensive care
facilities
3. Community health centers
4. Crisis intervention groups
   a. Suicide prevention
   b. Drug-addiction control
   c. Walk-in mental help
5. Changing role of hospital emergency
rooms
6. Shifting focus to communities rather
than agencies

D. Health services personnel—roles and
functions
1. Care today often given by health
teams
2. Professional health teams include the
following individuals
   a. Physician—colleague
   b. Registered professional nurse—colleague
   c. Physician's assistant
   d. Nurse's assistants
      (1) Licensed practical nurse
      (2) Nurse assistant
   e. Social worker
   f. Physical therapist
   g. Inhalation therapist
   h. Occupational therapist
   i. Others

The problem-solving process

In a world of exploding knowledge and
rapid social change, the most effective way
to function in the provision of nursing care,
presently and in the potential future, is
through use of the problem-solving process.

1. **Definition**
A. Problem-solving—the selection and utilization of relevant information in the
solution or alleviation of a felt difficulty

2. **Characteristics of the problem-solving
method**
A. Relies on validated facts
B. Encourages educated guesses that can be
tested
C. Sets a pattern of thinking that safeguards
against unwarranted assumptions
D. Provides reasonable alternate solutions
E. Rests on use of judgment

3. **Nursing and the problem-solving process**
A. Tentative identification of problems—
knowledge of deviations of health patterns in disease
B. Collection of data
   1. Sources of information
      a. Patient
      b. Chart
      c. Colleagues
      d. Family
      e. Literature
   2. Screening and retention of relevant
   facts
C. Delineation of specific problems—making
the nursing diagnosis
D. Formulation of the nursing care plan
E. Implementation of the care plan—making
adjustment to change in the patient's
condition or the acquisition of new
knowledge
F. Evaluation and revision—identifying additional resources, which were not immediately available but which can be available in subsequent situations

4. **Advantages of problem-solving process
in nursing**
A. Avoids stereotyped responses to problems
B. Makes allowance for individual patients'
responses to problems
C. Fosters flexibility and change in planning
and in giving nursing care

Man

Man responds to life as a total unit. All
aspects of his biologic being affect his
psychosocial being, and all aspects of his
psychosocial being affect his biologic function.

1. **Man is a unified being**
Man acts as a unit; therefore, his health

problems, actual or potential, are an expression of his life style

A. Biologic defects or deficiencies can lead to
1. Biologic limitations
2. Overcompensation—may be either adaptive or maladaptive

B. Psychosocial defects or deficiencies can result in
1. Limitations in performance
2. Overcompensation—may be adaptive or maladaptive
3. Somatic disease

C. Any health problem experienced by the individual grows out of
1. His genetic endowment
2. The kind of person he is
3. The pattern of life he lives
4. His total environment

2. **Physiologic health problems that may threaten unified man**

A. Impairment of vital capacity to function
1. Congenital or acquired defects can impair
   a. Absorption, transportation, and utilization of oxygen
   b. Ingestion and digestion of food; assimilation and utilization of essential nutrients
   c. Elimination of waste
   d. Equilibrium of regulatory function
   e. Perception, interpretation, and integration of total environment
   f. Coordination, mastery, and control of central nervous system motor activities
2. Successful adaptation or survival is dependent upon man's response to his health problem as it is affected by his individual total physiologic and psychosocial reserve

B. Adaptation and compensation
1. Some health problems are easily compensated
   a. Cause short-term discomfort or inconvenience
   b. Are reversible
2. Some health problems not easily compensated
   a. Require modifications in life style
   b. Not reversible
   c. Traumatize the psychosocial component (self-image, self-concept)
3. Some health problems a direct threat to life
   a. Occur in vital organs—heart, brain, etc.

   b. Generally (e.g., cancer) are perceived to have negative prognosis
   c. Are sources of high degrees of anxiety and fear in the individual and society

3. **Nursing responsibilities include**

A. Specific knowledge of the overt manifestations of common physiologic health problems

B. Awareness that no health problem evidences itself identically in all patients

C. Recognition and acceptance of the fact that emotional responses to health problems differ in individuals

D. Recognition and acceptance of variation in individual patients' responses to the impact of physiologic stress

E. Realistic support of patients through varying levels of adaptation in attempting to compensate for loss of vital capacity

F. Coping with the nurse's emotional response, and fulfilling the nursing role and function, when caring for patients whose health problems are irreversible

4. **Psychosocial health problems that may threaten unified man**

A. Basic to the ability to function effectively as a human being is a self-image that is reality oriented and permits satisfactory relationships with others
1. Sense of identity
2. Sense of purpose in life
3. Sense of belonging
4. Healthy balance of inner and outer motivation that permits the individual to function in the social setting without losing a sense of responsibility for his own behavior
5. Maintenance of a satisfactory social status
6. Accurate evaluation of feedback from others, which does not excessively inflate or deflate the ego

B. Cultural trends influence individual social behavior
1. Rapidly changing social values; old values not yet replaced with widely accepted new ones
2. Increasing interdependence of people, resulting from increased specialization of function in a technologic society
3. Increased social pressure for conformity to selected patterns of behavior
4. Decreased opportunity for fulfillment for the exceptional or dependent people in society

5. Existence of many subdivisions of value systems within the culture, especially in regard to health, often in conflict
C. Interplay between health and psychosocial adaptations
1. The capacity to accept health problems and their consequences is a fundamental tool in the process of successful adaptation
2. Health problems may interfere with established coping mechanisms that have been successful in the past
3. Health problems may lead to a change in self-perception: physical, psychological, social
4. Health problems may produce a change in family or community constellations that can place stress on individuals or groups
5. An individual may use health problems of many types as a means of solution to his own psychosocial problems
6. Psychosocial stress can lead to the development or accentuation of somatic pathology
7. Somatic pathology can lead to the development or accentuation of psychosocial pathology
8. Somatic pathology may damage the physiologic structure through which emotions are expressed
D. Reemphasis of interrelatedness—the inextricable interrelationships between all aspects of man are mediated by the central nervous system and the hormonal control system (pp. 22-36)
1. Partially under voluntary control
2. Partially not under voluntary control
3. Basic reason why knowledge and behavior are not always coordinated
5. Nursing responsibilities include
A. As much knowledge of the patient as a person as is possible
B. An acute awareness of the importance of value systems
C. An acute awareness of the significance of cultural differences
D. An acute sensitivity to the personal meaning of experiences to patients
E. Understanding that giving information may not result in a change in the patient's behavior
F. Full understanding that a patient will react to a nurse and a nurse will react to a patient, and that *this interaction is a nursing tool* to be directed in the patient's interest
G. A nurse must encourage and promote the patient's fullest participation in his care
H. A nurse must be able to give evidence of respect for the uniqueness and dignity of the individual
1. Listen, consider wishes when possible, explain, etc.
2. Avoid stereotyping, snap judgments, unjustified comparisons, etc.
3. Be nonjudgmental and nonpunitive in responses

Anxiety and stress

Anxiety, or a state of dis-ease, discomfort, or apprehension, is a universal human experience. Actual or potential health problems and their occurrence, or the setting in which they are treated, are often the source of stress that activates or heightens anxiety.
1. Anxiety is widespread and has a deep impact on the lives of people
A. Anxiety can range from mild to the extremes of panic or terror
B. Anxiety can be constructive when it motivates the individual to remove its source; this is usually a milder form of anxiety
C. Anxiety can be destructive when it results in varying degrees of personality disorganization
D. Anxiety can be expressed by any kind of behavior
E. Prolonged or severe anxiety is considered a primary causative influence in the development of some somatic health problems and by far the majority of personality maladjustments and mental health disorders
F. The patterns of situations that arouse anxiety and patterns of coping with it are the result of infant and childhood experiences; these can be modified by later life experiences
G. The response to and the expression of anxiety are always highly personal, being determined by the individual's past experience, by his selective perception of his environment, and by his existing repertory of coping behaviors
H. Cultural aspects of anxiety
1. A rapidly changing social order fosters the development of anxiety
2. Worldwide tensions, which affect everyone, are the results of

a. The continuing struggle for power
b. The rising expectations of the less-developed nations
c. The increased potential for destructiveness in military actions
3. Anxiety is contagious and can spread rapidly from person to person and especially among groups

2. Stress is a factor affecting the capacity to attain and maintain health

A. Definitions
1. General—intense strain
2. Technical—"Stress is the consequence of the rate of wear and tear on a biologic system." (Hans Selye)
   a. Produces the nonspecific response known as the general adaptation syndrome
      (1) Alarm reaction
      (2) Stage of resistance
      (3) Stage of exhaustion
B. Personal aspects of stress
1. Sources of stress for different people may vary widely
2. The ability to cope with stress also varies widely among people
3. Some people function better under a measure of stress, and some people have a low tolerance or threshold for any degree of stress
4. Prolonged severe stress tests to the utmost the individual's ability to maintain his equilibrium, biologically and psychosocially
5. Stress may arise from either internal or external sources

3. Patterns of coping behaviors in response to anxiety and stress
In general, it is difficult to determine personally, or in others, whether patterns of coping behaviors are operating on conscious or on unconscious mental levels

A. Patterns
1. Problem-solving
   a. Identification of the difficulty
   b. Collection of relevant background information
   c. Consideration of possible courses of action
   d. Selection of the best possible course
      (1) Attempt to remove the difficulty
      (2) Accept the difficulty as it is
      (3) Choose to seek another situation that would result in an improvement

e. Taking action
f. Evaluation of results and conclusions
2. Denial
   a. Of the past
   b. Of the present
3. Attack (directed hostility)
   a. Selective substitute attack for the real cause of anxiety—i.e., directing hostility toward persons or situations that are perceived as the cause of difficulties
   b. Holistic attack—i.e., generalized perception of all experiences as hostile
   c. Shifting attack to a theoretical or abstract basis—i.e., racism or political, social, or economic systems
4. Retreat from situation
   a. Actual physical removal from the situation or situations that produce stress
   b. Psychosocial distortion of reality to suit own need
5. Passive endurance—awareness of anxiety, accompanied by submission
6. Disorganization of personality—the individual loses, to various degrees, his ability to cope with actual life situations; disorganization can range from mild to severe
B. Factors affecting the ability to select and use patterns of coping behavior
1. The ability to cope with a variety of problems rests upon the individual's ego-strength resources
2. The wider the repertory of available coping behaviors, the better the individual's resources
3. The occurrence of a crisis, an event that requires new decisions and new directions, may precipitate the failure of previously successful coping behaviors and demand the development of new coping behaviors
4. Changing patterns of coping behaviors may require the use of support resources by the patient, family, health services, or the community

4. Nursing responsibilities in stress and anxiety include
A. Awareness of the very high stress-anxiety potential that exists in most health settings
1. In response to the health problem itself

2. Many treatments and procedures are threatening or painful
3. Common use of "medical jargon" isolates the patient

B. Constant anticipation of the presence of anxiety
C. Awareness of the contagion aspects of anxiety
   1. The nurse can arouse anxiety in a patient
   2. The patient can arouse anxiety in a nurse
D. Avoidance of either arousing or increasing anxiety in a patient is a positive nursing contribution
E. Knowing that anxiety cannot always be reduced or allayed
F. Providing patients with an opportunity to ventilate feelings
G. Using the art of listening—one of the most valuable nursing tools that exists
H. Explaining "what, how, when, where, and why" (at the patient's level), which may prevent or allay new anxiety and stress
I. Sometimes, using stress and anxiety to motivate the patient's participation in his health care regime
J. Searching for *patterns* of coping behavior rather than basing action on isolated instances of behavior
K. Realizing that adequate behavior patterns may become inadequate under stress
L. Remembering that much of behavior results from coping with stress and anxiety: the removal or changing of present behavior is possible only when the individual has replacement behaviors that enable him to maintain an equilibrium within himself and within his society
M. Recognizing the nurse's own anxiety and being able to cope with it

Communication

Productive communication is the mutually correct perception of messages exchanged between a receiver and a sender. Effective communication is a basic tool for the establishment of a therapeutic nurse-patient relationship. Clear, accurate communication among members of the health team, including the patient, is vital to support patient welfare.

1. **Importance of communication**
A. It is an extremely important factor in relationships with others

B. It is a way of conveying the meaning of experience
C. It is a two-way process that involves at least two people
D. It can improve the awareness of and sensitivity to others
E. Communication among members of the health team is basic to the coordination of their efforts

2. **Means of communication**
A. Verbal (words, tone of voice)
B. Nonverbal (facial expression, posture)
C. Written

3. **Factors affecting communication**
A. Perceptive fields of the message sender and receiver
B. Whether the motivation underlying communication is conscious or unconscious
C. Knowledge concerning human behavior
D. Command of language
E. Capacities of the individuals communicating
   1. Understanding of language, spoken or written
   2. Personal receptiveness
F. Promoting communication
   1. Focus on the patient
   2. Interest in the patient
   3. Listening
   4. Encouraging patient expression
   5. Availability
   6. Attention to detail
   7. Honesty
   8. Encouragement of patient participation in his health care plan
G. Inhibiting communication
   1. Superficial responses
   2. Stereotyped responses (to diagnosis, ethnic origin, etc.)
   3. Use of labels ("emotionally disturbed," "hostile," "sweet," etc.)
   4. Nonverbal conveyance of disapproval
   5. Use of criticism or ridicule
   6. Misinterpretation of communication
   7. Denying a patient expression
   8. Use of approval or disapproval to enforce conformity with "the good patient" role

4. **Nursing responsibilities in promotion of productive communication**
A. Awareness that effective communication requires skill in both sending and receiving messages
B. Awareness that communication is influenced by many factors other than what is said or how it is said

C. Keeping channels of communication open

D. Awareness that a positive approach to communication is more likely to be effective than a negative one

E. Understanding that productive communication is an effective means of promoting therapeutic changes in behavior

F. Full realization that patients can communicate only when someone is available to make this possible

G. Awareness that effectiveness of communication cannot be assumed but must be validated by feedback from the patient

H. Understanding that no stereotyped pattern of behavior will be effective in communicating with all patients

I. Knowing that the true meaning of communication is not always obvious

J. Awareness that the capacity of the patient (learning, language barriers, etc.) may require adaptations to the patient's abilities

K. Remembering that the establishment and use of channels of communication with relevant members of the health team is basic to patient welfare

Assessment

The ability to plan, implement, and evaluate nursing care effectively rests basically on exact and comprehensive assessment or appraisal of the biologic and the psychosocial status of the patient and on the interrelationship between the two.

1. **Importance of assessment**

A. Without adequate assessment, any plan for nursing action is inadequate—perhaps even destructive

B. Accurate assessment makes a very positive contribution to the quality of nursing care

2. **Biologic and physical areas of assessment**

A. Vital signs
   1. Temperature, pulse, and respiration
   2. Blood pressure

B. Color
   1. Specific for the individual patient (complexions, etc.)
   2. Deviations—general
      a. Pallor, cyanosis
      b. Ashen (gray)
      c. Flushing (rubor, redness)
   3. Local (nail beds, buccal mucosa, lips, sclera, skin surfaces)

C. Skin
   1. Turgor
   2. Lesions—rashes, abrasions
   3. Contusions
   4. Temperature
   5. Moistness or dryness

D. Sensory function
   1. Sight
   2. Hearing
   3. Touch (tactile sensations)
   4. Taste
   5. Smell

E. Motor function
   1. Locomotion (standing, sitting, walking)
   2. Body mechanics (reaching, lifting, grasping)
   3. Body posture

F. Rest and sleep
   1. Restlessness (tossing, turning, undue movement)
   2. Sleeplessness (insomnia)

G. Activity—exercise
   1. Inadequate capacity (lack of vigor)
   2. Overadequate capacity (excessive vigor)

H. Levels of consciousness and orientation
   1. Response to stimuli (when conscious, comatose, in coma, unconscious)
      a. Verbal
      b. Tactile
      c. Visual
      d. Painful
   2. Awareness (oriented, disoriented)
      a. Time
      b. Place
      c. Persons
      d. Circumstances

I. Nutrition
   1. Appetite (desire for or revulsion for food, anorexia, nausea)
   2. Ability to ingest, masticate, and swallow food (poor dental hygiene, dysphagia)
   3. Capacity to digest food (gastric distress, vomiting)
   4. Food preferences and/or fads (cultural, personal, social)
   5. Food allergies or sensitivities

J. Elimination
   1. Skin—water and sodium
      a. Excessive perspiration (diaphoresis)
      b. Excessive dryness (cracking, scaling)
   2. Respiratory tract—water and CO_2
      a. Labored respirations

ashen = gray

b. Irregular or depressed rate of breathing
c. Audible respirations (moistness, stertor, rales)
    3. Urinary and intestinal systems
    a. Characteristics of urine and fecal material (color, odor, consistency)
    b. Quantity (intake and output of fluid, solid food)
    c. Frequency
    d. Facility of disposal (pain, distress)
    e. Presence of abnormal constituents (gross or occult)
K. Critical signs and symptoms
    1. Essential—having knowledge of pathologic manifestations related to common health problems as they occur in patients
    2. Basic—recognizing significant findings in diagnostic tests
    3. Directly measurable by instruments and procedures—objective symptoms (blood pressure, TPR, fractional urinalysis, vomiting, hemorrhage, etc.)
    4. Subjective symptoms—patients' specific complaints (weakness, pain, nausea, vertigo, etc.)
3. Psychosocial areas of assessment
A. Socioeconomic background
B. Religion
C. Major aspects of value systems
D. Attitudes toward health
E. Level of education (formal or self-education)
F. Occupation
G. Behavior *patterns*
    1. Moods—emotional tone
    2. Response to stress
    3. Appropriateness (relative to individual and his situation)
    4. Family and the patient's place in the constellation
H. Resources within the individual
4. Assessment of interrelationships of biologic, physical, and psychosocial factors
A. Contribute to maintenance of homeostasis?
B. Lead to positive or to negative adaptation?
C. Affect the establishment of priorities in patient's nursing care?
5. Nursing responsibilities in assessment
A. Ability to observe, comprehensively and accurately
B. Ability to interpret observations
C. Ability to screen information from many

sources, including the patient, and select the valid and relevant information in planning nursing care
D. Ability to plan course of action based on knowledge of theory and on accurate interpretation of observations (use of judgment)

Rehabilitation

Nursing care plans for any patient must include appraisal of resources within the patient, the family, and the community for the maintenance or the restoration of biologic or psychosocial functions that have been impaired or are threatened with impairment.
1. Philosophy of rehabilitation
A. Health problems that cause disabilities are socially significant because of the number of people affected, the economic cost and loss, the distress of personal suffering, and the conditions in society that increase their incidence
B. Disabled persons need not necessarily be handicapped
C. Disabilities resulting from physiologic or psychosocial health problems may be compensated for or corrected (restored) to varying degrees
D. Attainable goals are determined by physiologic and psychosocial resources within individuals
E. Rehabilitation not only a field of specialization but also a point of view in all medicine
2. Constructs in rehabilitation practice
A. Major goals
    1. Prevent disability
    2. Restore capacity
    3. Retrain for usefulness
B. Immediate or potential rehabilitation problems present in all health problems
C. Accurate and comprehensive evaluation of each patient as an individual—all his physiologic and psychosocial irreversible limitations, optimal capacities, and useful resources
D. Realistic goal-setting
E. Clear-cut identification of short-term and long-range goals
F. Patient participation in and contribution to his own program
G. Promotion of independence
H. Importance of motivation and goal-directed activities
3. Nursing responsibilities in rehabilitation

A. Prevention of complications through a planned and consistently implemented program to combat the effects of prolonged bed rest and inactivity

B. Accurate assessment of the patient's condition, including his resources and potential capacity for restoration, essential if he is to achieve his optimal level of function

C. Institution of rehabilitation measures to maintain, to restore, and to retrain capacities for useful function as soon as possible

D. Encouragement and support for the patient to move from dependence to independence

E. Coordination of the patient's rehabilitation program as designed by the variety of health team members involved

F. Ability to use the complex of services available in the community to ensure continuity of care for the patient

G. Individualization of each nursing care plan, with respect for the patient as a person

Environment

The value system (often hidden) of a health care delivery system, as evidenced by governing policies, methods of operation, and power controls, has a marked effect upon the ability of all personnel, including nurses, to provide quality patient care.

1. Importance of a therapeutic environment

A. Physical environment has a definite impact, either positive or negative, on the people in it

B. Although organization is necessary, rigid policies and routines often conflict with the needs and interests of patients and personnel

C. The social value system of health care setting often place greater emphasis upon "getting things done" and "patient control" than upon patient needs

2. Physical aspects of the environment

A. Cleanliness, order, control of temperature, ventilation, and light are positive factors in the patient's environment

B. Control of noise, especially at night, can contribute to a therapeutic atmosphere

C. Environment should be safe for patients and personnel
   1. Cross-infection control
   2. All equipment in good working condition

3. Precautions against hazards (wet floors, collisions, falling from bed or chair, etc.)

4. Adequate and functioning signaling system

5. Fire prevention rules, enforced

3. Psychosocial aspects of environment

A. Interpersonal relationships and communications among team members have definite positive or negative effects on the quality of patient care

B. Increase in numbers of personnel groups involved in health care has in some cases resulted in overlapping of functions, lack of clear delineation of responsibilities, and, consequently, conflict among the groups (this has a negative impact on patient care)

C. In many situations the nurse has considerable power to control the patient situation; this power should be used in the patient's interest rather than to enforce conformity to the stereotyped "good patient" role

D. Frequently nurses are asked to assume responsibilities when they have no power or authority to control factors that affect their functioning; this may make it difficult to give the quality of nursing care they desire

E. Patient participation to the extent possible, in the process of decision-making concerning the patient, promotes or enhances health care plans

F. A prevailing attitude of impersonality, characteristic of many health care settings, denies the significance of the patient as a person; this can be combatted by
   1. Protection of privacy to the extent possible
   2. Use of names instead of diagnoses or room numbers as labels
   3. Explanations at the patient's level of understanding and tolerance
   4. Permitting personal possessions where practical
   5. Courtesy toward the patient, his family, and visitors

G. Diversional and recreational activities are a positive adjunct to the therapeutic atmosphere

H. A therapeutic environment is characterized by
   1. Permissiveness rather than authoritarianism

2. Valuing honesty in identifying and facing problems
3. Valuing the expression of feelings
4. Frankness and openness in discussion
5. Respect for other points of view

I. The patient population is increasingly knowledgeable about health and holds steadily rising expectations of health care services

4. Nursing responsibilities in promoting a therapeutic environment

A. Regulate and control, to the extent possible, the physical environment (temperature, ventilation, cleanliness, noise, etc.) in accord with patients' needs

B. Safeguard patients against danger and hazard in the environment, through application of scientific, mechanical, and practical knowledge: fire prevention, aseptic techniques, safe equipment, correct use of supportive and protective devices, etc.

C. Analyze the real goals of a social setting in which nursing care is given, as opposed to the usual verbalizing (e.g., is value placed on getting things done, "patient control," or on patient needs?)

D. Be an agent for change or support change
1. Identify the need for change
2. Propose alternative suggestions to bring about desired change
3. Obtain the commitment and involvement of those who must implement change
4. Bring the suggestions before those who have power to make change
   a. Persuasion
   b. Pressure
5. Support the implementation of change

E. Work effectively with health team colleagues
1. Bring conflicts out in the open
2. Maintain cooperative working relationships—not to be confused with submission

F. Support a social environment that sets priorities on patient needs

G. Retain flexibility in carrying out routines and policies

H. Encourage patient participation in decision-making that affects him, in so far as possible

I. Encourage expression of feelings, honesty in facing problems, and honesty in discussions

J. Approach patients not as "difficult" but as people with difficulties

K. Observe discretion in the use of power

L. Act as the patient's ombudsman in the provision of recreational and diversional activities

M. Have "the courage to change that which can be changed, the serenity to accept that which cannot be changed, and the wisdom to know the difference between the two"

Comfort

An assured state of physical, mental, and social ease or comfort is necessary to facilitate man's adaptation to stress and to provide essential support in any and all stages along the continuum of health.

1. **Components of comfort**

A. Physical
1. State of relative physiologic equilibrium (feeling of a returning level of wellness)
2. Absence of pain and distress

B. Psychosocial
1. A realistic self-identity and self-image
2. Constructive attitudes toward health and health problems
3. Satisfactory interpersonal relationships with all personnel within a health service: doctors, nurses, aides, therapists, technicians, orderlies, maids, etc.
4. Social security in relation to job, family and friends, as well as to other patients in the setting

2. **Causes of discomfort**

A. Physical factors
1. Symptoms produced by health problems (pain, fever, dyspnea, nausea, vomiting, etc.)
2. Prolonged inactivity and bed rest necessary in the treatment of health problems
3. Impairment of body mechanics, either caused by direct injury or resulting from disease
4. Ill-fitting or misused protective or supportive devices or appliances
5. Muscle fatigue due to weakness and debilitation
6. Local areas of pressure and decubiti resulting from prolonged retention of position—immobility
7. Inadequate provisions for physical hygiene needs (cleanliness, nutrition, elimination, etc.)

8. Rough, careless, insensitive, or incompetent physical manipulation by health team personnel

B. Psychosocial factors
   1. Anxiety induced by the health problem and/or the threat of death—real or anticipated
   2. Apprehension related to treatments or procedures necessitated by the health problem (injections, infusions, aspiration or decompression of body cavities, surgery, etc.)
   3. A nontherapeutic environment (for discussion of therapeutic environment see Chapter 12)

3. **Situations in which comfort has a high priority**
A. When the signs and symptoms of the health problem cause the patient undue physical distress (pain, fever, restlessness, sleeplessness, etc.)
B. When the patient's level of anxiety is high
C. When the patient is unable to communicate discomfort (aphasia, loss of mental faculties, language barrier, etc.)
D. When the patient is dying
   1. Stages of dying—Elisabeth Kübler-Ross
      a. Denial (not me) 1)
      b. Hostility (why me?) 2)
      c. Bargaining 3)
      d. Depression 4)
      e. Acceptance 5)
   2. Social attitudes toward death in the health care system
      a. Acceptance and honesty
      b. Evasion—avoidance
      c. Denial
      d. Indifference

4. **Nursing responsibilities in relation to comfort**
A. Accurate assessment and communication of the degree and extent of distress and discomfort, both physical and psychosocial
B. Awareness of the significance of discomfort or distress related to the health problem and the individual patient
C. Early and regular use of the specific measures designated to reduce or alleviate discomfort (medications, treatments, manipulation of environment, etc.)
D. Planning and carrying out nursing measures related to hygiene and comfort (bathing, back care, feeding, elimination,

care of appendages, etc.), with consideration for the individual patient's needs and wishes
E. Anticipating and, to the extent possible, providing for all the things the patient may need or desire but be unable to do for himself (adjusting pillows, making bedside equipment and personal belongings readily accessible, soothing an itch that the patient cannot reach, reducing glare of light, etc.)
F. Early institution of regular nursing measures to prevent or minimize the incidence of potential complications (turning and repositioning frequently, elevating the head of the bed, maintaining body alignment, supplying footboards, etc.)
G. Being acutely sensitive to the individual patient's response to touch
H. Recognizing the patient's behavior as expressions of the various stages of dying
I. Letting the patient talk about dying, if he wishes, or letting him be silent, if he wishes
J. Being aware that personal feelings are an important factor in the situation where the patient is dying
K. Being readily available to the patient who is dying
L. Creating to the extent possible an environment that is conducive to comfort

Nutrition

A balanced diet that provides the essential nutrients, caloric value, and types of food commensurate with the individual's need—relative to age, size, physical activity, physiologic function, and psychosocial satisfaction—is basic to an optimal degree of wellness.

1. **Basic aspects of nutrition**
A. Physiologic factors
   1. Correct balance of the essential nutrients required to maintain vital functions (proteins, carbohydrates, fats, vitamins, minerals, and water)
   2. Caloric value proportional to the energy needs of the body
   3. Ability to ingest, masticate, and swallow food
   4. Capacity to digest, absorb, transport, and assimilate the nutrients
B. Psychosocial factors
   1. There is a high degree of significance

associated with what, where, when, how, and with whom a person eats

2. Dietary patterns and habits of eating are determined by geographic location, economic status, and cultural orientation—within a nation, a family, and an individual

2. Factors that interfere with nutrition

A. Poverty—of society, community, family, and individual
   1. Unemployment, low income, high cost of living
   2. Ignorance, lack of knowledge related to nutrition (best sources of supply from the standpoint of availability and economy)
   3. Unavailability of certain foods in economically depressed areas

B. Affluence and culture in society
   1. Overabundance and ready availability of foods that are calorically rich but nutritionally poor
   2. A high-pressure system of advertising that results in compulsive buying and consumption of foodstuffs classified as having "empty calories"
   3. National dietary patterns that originated from religious and geographic conditions and tend to be unbalanced in regard to quality and quantity of nutrients as well as the use of seasonings or other agents in their preparation (Jewish, Oriental, French, Italian, German, South American, etc.)

C. Poor eating habits that primarily are rooted in psychosocial factors
   1. Nutritional deficiencies occur as a result of the deliberate exclusion of essential nutrients or calories from the diet ("food fads," indiscriminate dieting, lack of appetite, etc.)
   2. Nutritional excesses occur as a result of deliberately including in the diet unnecessary quantities of nutrients and caloric values (excessive consumption of certain types of food, intake of an excessive quantity of food)
   3. Malnutrition and obesity are two conditions prevalent in society, which predispose the individual to many other major health problems

D. Health problems that interfere with the ingestion, mastication, digestion, absorption, transportation, or assimilation of food not only impair nutrition but may be a threat to life

3. Dietary modifications and adaptations

A. The majority of health problems may require diet therapy or modification of nutritional intake in regard to quantity, quality, or consistency of food
   1. Quantity—low-caloric, high-caloric, supplementary feedings, etc.
   2. Quality—sodium-restricted, high-carbohydrate, low-cholesterol, etc.
   3. Consistency—fluid, puréed, soft, etc.

B. Many health problems require adaption in the manner of getting nutrients into the body
   1. Patient unable to feed himself
   2. Patient unable to ingest food
   3. Patient unable to digest, absorb, transport, or assimilate food

C. There are alternate methods used to supply and maintain the optimal level of nutrition possible in a variety of health problems
   1. Nasogastric or gastrostomy tube feedings of specially prepared fluid diets can be nutritionally adequate for a long period of time but may not satisfy the psychosocial aspect of eating
   2. Parenteral infusion of water, glucose, potassium, calcium, sodium, amino acids, and vitamins can sustain essentials of life for a certain length of time but do not provide total and adequate nutrition; prolonged use of infusion may lead to complicating health problems (e.g., malnutrition or fluid and electrolyte disturbances)

4. Nursing responsibilities include

A. Knowledge about the essential nutrients; sources and individual needs for quantity and quality of food throughout life cycles

B. Knowledge of modifications related to stress (growth and development, pregnancy, disease, injury)

C. Knowledge of the significance of the individual patient's specific dietary modification

D. Awareness of the psychosocial significance of food and eating habits to the individual patient

E. Making sure that the patient's dietary intake is adequate and satisfactory (feeding him or assisting him to eat)

F. Careful observation and communication of the actual nutritional intake—what is not eaten, as well as what is eaten

G. Providing for individual food preferences to the extent possible

H. Observation and communication of symptoms related to the nutritional status of the patient (appetite, weight gain or loss, skin tone and turgor, allergies, etc.)

I. Scheduling so that activities such as treatments do not coincide with mealtime except in emergency

J. Arranging so that the patient is as comfortable as possible when he is feeding himself (position, accessibility of food and utensils, ability to manage food, etc.)

K. Administering medications on time if the time of administration depends on when the patient eats (insulin, antacids, or any other a.c. or p.c. medication)

L. Teaching the patient what he needs to know about his diet and being sure he understands it

M. Including key family members in plans to help the patient carry out dietary modifications

Elimination of waste

Continuous or regular disposal of the waste products of metabolism in the individual person is necessary to maintain homeostasis that supports life. Physiologic dysfunction, physical limitation, dietary deficiencies, and psychosocial maladjustments commonly impair natural elimination and require supportive assistance to maintain or restore function.

1. Basic aspects involved

A. Physiologic factors
   1. The body requires an adequate intake of the essential nutritive elements to maintain this vital process
   2. The body must be able to effectively metabolize these elements
   3. The body must have the capacity to transport waste products to the organs of disposal (kidneys, colon, lungs, and skin)
   4. These organs must be able to excrete the toxic waste products from the body

B. Psychosocial factors
   1. Cultural dietary practices affect patterns of elimination
   2. Cultural values related to elimination produce both positive and negative feelings in patients toward the whole process of elimination
   3. A great majority of individuals are extremely sensitive about the total subject of elimination; it is a highly personal thing

2. Disturbances in the process of elimination

A. Deviations in patterns of elimination may be classified, by and large, in six categories
   1. Excesses or deficiencies in quantity (polyuria, oliguria, anuria, diaphoresis, etc.)
   2. Excesses or deficiencies in quality (consistency, appearance, or composition of the products, such as concentrated or dilute urine, loose stool)
   3. Presence of abnormal constituents that may be directly observable or determined through laboratory analysis (frank or occult blood in the stool, bile, clay-colored stool, mucus or pus in urine or feces, sugar or acetone in urine, "uremic frost" on skin, etc.)
   4. Difficulty or pain at any point along the body's waste transportation system—up to and including the point of disposal or excretion—possibly a sign of obstruction, inflammation, infection, in the major organs or their component parts
   5. Impairment of the ability to control excretion (incontinence)
   6. Inability of terminal organs to expel waste materials (urinary retention, constipation, obstipation)

B. Degree of deviation from usual patterns of elimination determines the extent of physiologic or psychosocial distress experienced by patients
   1. Alterations in patterns not due to pathologic changes in structure or function of the systems directly affect the level of wellness in patients and predispose them to complications (urinary retention postoperatively, incontinence following stroke, constipation resulting from dietary limitations or inactivity, fluid and electrolyte imbalance, and dehydration due to excessive perspiration, diarrhea, vomiting, or inadequate intake of food and fluid)
   2. Altered patterns of elimination resulting from pathologic changes in structure or function within the systems constitute serious health problems that may be a threat to life (renal failure, intestinal obstruction, respiratory acidosis or alkalosis, pulmonary edema, extensive burns of the body, heat exhaustion, etc.)

3. The psychosocial and cultural forces that prevail in society in general (dietary indiscretion, emotional tension and instability, injudicious use of drugs, etc.) have not been conducive to the development of sound health practices pertaining to elimination

4. Inadequate facilities in health as well as insufficient concern (on the part of health team personnel) for sound hygienic practices related to patients' elimination habits can compound elimination difficulties experienced by patients—whether they are directly or only indirectly due to a health problem (factors include failure to provide for needs promptly, failure to provide maximum privacy, failure to take measures to prevent disturbances, failure to keep accurate records of intake and output, etc.)

3. **Nursing responsibilities include**
A. Knowledge of the significance of deviations or changes in patterns of elimination
B. Critical observations related to the characteristics of the pattern of elimination (amount, color, odor, frequency, facility, etc.)
C. Ability to interpret observations in relation to the health problem and the patient
D. Knowledge of and the manual skill to carry out related procedures (fractional urinalysis, irrigation, catheterization, colostomy care, etc.)
E. Administration of medications accurately and at the appropriate time
F. Responsibility for the collection of necessary specimens, using correct procedural methods
G. Preparation of the patient for diagnostic and therapeutic procedures so that the patient knows what is expected and when it is expected
H. Promoting natural elimination (position, opportunity, privacy, skin cleanliness, promotion of pulmonary ventilation, etc.)
I. Maintaining accurate records on all aspects of elimination
J. Health teaching concerning elimination; measures of positive promotion, measures to alleviate transient difficulties, and external measures of intervention to maintain elimination (colostomy irrigations, catheter care, etc.)

K. Communicating to appropriate health personnel the patient's needs for assistance with elimination
L. A sensitivity to social, cultural, and individual values that affect attitudes toward elimination

Posture, activity, and rest

A relative degree of dynamic equilibrium between the total energy output of man and the reparative processes that occur through relaxation, rest, and sleep is required to sustain health as well as to restore an optimal level of wellness when injury or disease exists or threatens.

1. **Basic aspects involved**
A. Physiologic factors
1. All physical, mental, and mechanical functions of the body are directly affected by posture, activity, and rest
2. Correct body posture—standing, sitting, or lying—maintains alignment of articulating body parts and supports adequate function of vital organs (heart, lungs, intestines, etc.)
3. Routine activities of daily living (ADL)—bathing, eating, working, walking, writing, talking, reading, thinking—maintain mechanical efficiency in movable body parts and joints and promote an adequate level of physiologic function, both mental and physical
4. The human body requires regular periods of rest and sleep (times during which there is a reduction of all physical and mental activities) in order to restore the level of energy expended
B. Psychosocial factors
1. An adequate amount of sleep, regulated by individual need, is required to maintain a satisfactory level of mental hygiene and intellectual productivity
2. Periods of mental rest, relaxation, and diversion, regulated in accord with individual need and interest, are necessary to promote an optimal degree of mental and emotional stability
3. In a society that places a high value on "the body beautiful" correct body posture and efficient body mechanics are important to the emotional security of the individual
4. A wide variety of physical, mental,

and cultural activities provide emotional outlets for the individual

2. **Factors that impair posture, activity, and rest**

A. Disease and injury reduce the vital capacity of the body to maintain an adequate level of function related to posture, activity, and rest
  1. Debilitation resulting from acute and chronic illnesses (cardiac disease, chronic pulmonary disease, acute colitis, etc.) produces weakness, lethargy, apathy, and depression
  2. Enforced inactivity necessary in the treatment of disease (acute myocardial infarction, peripheral vascular disease, etc.) and injury inhibits physiologic and psychosocial function
  3. The physiologic and psychosocial stress (pain, fever, anxiety, fear, etc.) induced by illness and injury diminishes the capacity of the body to maintain a satisfactory level of rest, sleep, and diversional activity
  4. Diseases and injuries that disrupt motor function predispose to permanent deformity or loss of mechanical function and cause a high degree of emotional distress
  5. Congenital defects often inhibit physical growth and development and affect body mechanics, posture, and psychosocial activities; these require specific measures that will provide the individual optimal opportunity to substitute or compensate
  6. The extent to which disease or injury impairs the individual's correct posture, functional body mechanics, rest, and activity is determined largely by the degree of reversibility of the health problem and the quality of supportive, restorative, and prophylactic health care provided

B. Environmental factors in health agencies often are not generally conducive to promoting an optimal level of function related to posture, activity, rest and sleep
  1. Individuals who need to use the services of health agencies usually suffer a loss of independence, self-identity, and privacy
  2. The physical setting in many health agencies is not always comfortable (beds, chairs, space, sitting room, view of the outside world, etc.)
  3. Frequently there is a high level of physical, mental, and emotional stress due to environmental disturbances and distractions (noise, sense of alienation, unpleasant experiences related to self or to other patients with whom a patient may identify, etc.)
  4. In many health agencies facilities to provide for the physical and diversional activity needs of patients are inadequate, or patients are restricted in the use of them (walking inside or outside the hospital, going to the coffee shop or game rooms, sufficient personnel to plan and carry out individual physical and diversional activities, etc.)

C. The quality of health care provided by members of the health team, collectively and individually, influences the extent to which the patient's need to maintain or restore physical and mental function and activity is met; there are three conditions that can be directly responsible for the inadequate health care patients receive in this area
  1. Lack of knowledge and psychomotor skill
    a. Failure to institute specific measures to maintain body alignment regularly and consistently (positioning, repositioning, supporting dependent parts, etc.)
    b. Failure to use corrective and supportive devices appropriately to prevent further loss of function (footboards, splints, traction, etc.)
    c. Failure to use measures to reduce potential for complications (full range of motion exercises, promoting patient independence, physical hygiene, nutrition, etc.)
  2. Administrative limitations
    a. Hierarchic structures within health agencies may tend to limit the function of health teams and overlook the rights and needs of individual patients
    b. The high cost of health care services in society has resulted in a priority in many health agencies that allots more money for research and intensive care equipment and less for comfort and the activities of daily living

3. Lack of commitment on the part of health personnel
    a. There is an increasing tendency in our society to be more concerned about the condition of employment than the quality of services rendered to society
    b. In many situations the poor physical conditions and inadequate facilities available to provide health services result in feelings of apathy, hostility, indifference, and callousness toward striving for quality in patient care
3. **Nursing responsibilities include**
A. Critical observation of position or motion limitations or deviations
B. Consistent and regular alteration of position as an adjunct to minimal physical activity and for prevention of complications (bedsores, pneumonia, etc.)
C. Maintaining normal articulation of all body parts in any position
D. Providing for optimal level of correct body posture—lying, sitting, or walking
E. Institution of consistent and regular active and/or passive full range of motion exercises to prevent ankylosis
F. Employing appropriate methods and equipment to correct bizarre posture and to support weak and inert body parts, to reduce the hazard of permanent deformity and loss of function (shoulder, foot and wrist drop, pelvic tilt, lateral spine deviation, etc.)
G. Continuous critical evaluation of all corrective and supportive devices to determine their efficiency and be sure that
    1. They achieve the purpose for which they are being used
    2. Circulation to body parts involved is adequate
    3. They do not unnecessarily limit motion
    4. They do not cause the patient undue discomfort or pain
H. Providing an optimal level of hygienic care—cleanliness, nutrition, and elimination
I. Providing for optimal physical and diversional activity and promoting independence within the individual patient's limitation
J. Providing an optimal level of physical environmental and psychosocial comfort as prerequisite to rest and sleep
K. Communicating to other health team personnel significant information concerning the individual patient's needs, priorities, and wishes related to activity and rest
L. Ensuring continuity of care in the plans for activities necessary to maintain or restore sensory-motor function and to prevent or correct deformity
M. Consistently providing emotional support and realistic encouragement in accord with the needs, priorities, and wishes of the patient as a person

PSYCHOMOTOR SKILLS

In order to provide for the needs of patients related to health problems, a nurse not only requires knowledge but, in addition, must have ability to institute a variety of procedures effectively. Some of these the nurse carries out directly while others are carried out interdependently with the physician. Independent function requires nursing knowledge and judgment. Whereas interdependent function requires medical direction, it also implies that the nurse has specific responsibility involving judgment and decision in initiating, maintaining, or terminating many kinds of procedures.

Methods of procedure vary from one health agency to another, but there are certain basic elements that are universal. For arbitrary reasons, the procedures that are included here have been organized from the standpoint of the following: (1) their relatedness to basic nursing concepts, (2) their prevalence of use in a variety of health problems, and (3) their commonalities based on scientific knowledge and safe, effective practice.

1. **Measuring vital signs**
A. Important points
    1. Temperature
        a. Use appropriate thermometer (oral, rectal)
        b. Be certain it is clean and intact
    2. Pulse
        a. Evaluate quality of beat (weak, strong)
        b. Identify characteristics in rhythm (regularity, irregularities)
        c. Heart rate and rhythm are determined most accurately by stethoscope if function is impaired
        d. Apical and radial rates may be counted simultaneously by two nurses; when pulse rate is less than

apical rate, the numerical difference is the pulse deficit

3. Respiration
   a. Evaluate quality of ventilation (shallow, deep, adequate)
   b. Identify difficulties in breathing (dyspnea, orthopnea)
   c. Identify significant sounds (rales, stertor, wheezing)
   d. Identify irregularities in rhythm (periods of apnea, hyperpnea)
4. Blood pressure
   a. Use the same arm for consistency of readings
   b. Apply cuff efficiently
   c. Locate pulse digitally before inflating cuff
   d. Read manometer at eye level
   e. Calculate pulse pressure as the numerical difference between systolic and diastolic pressures

B. Common basic elements
   1. Accuracy of measurement
      a. Instruments used in good working order
      b. Reading and count precise
   2. Element of time
      a. Thermometer left in place sufficient length of time
      b. Pulse and respirations counted for full minute
      c. Blood pressure taken regularly as required (q. ½ h., b.i.d., q.i.d.)
   3. Physiologic factors
      a. Indicate vital capacity and function
      b. Variations in norms are related to individual physical constitution, as well as to health problems
      c. Deviations from normal limits in rate, rhythm, and characteristics of pulse and respiration are clinically significant
      d. Increase or decrease from normal limits in temperature and blood pressure levels is clinically significant

2. **Diagnostic procedures requiring special preparation**

A. Important points
   1. A wide variety of examinations require specific conditions to permit specific results
   2. The reliability of test results is directly proportional to the accuracy with which a procedure is carried out
B. Procedures frequently used

1. X-ray series (gallbladder, gastrointestinal, barium enema, pneumoencephalogram)
2. Obtaining specimens of body fluids or organs for laboratory examination (gastric analysis, lumbar puncture, liver biopsy, blood chemistries)
3. Measuring pressure within body chambers—vessels and cavities (cardiac catheterization, central venous, cerebrospinal)
4. Traces and scans of vital organs (thyroid, brain, liver)
5. Obtaining samples of bodily secretions for laboratory analysis (urine, stool, sputum)

C. Common basic elements
   1. Dietary modification
      a. Withholding food or fluid
      b. Giving special types of food or fluid
   2. Administration of medication
      a. Locally (anesthesia)
      b. Parenterally (intravenous dyes, narcotics)
   3. Administration of agents that permit visualization of organs (barium, radioactive isotopes)
   4. Elements of time
      a. When preparation begins
      b. When samples and specimens are collected
      c. When patient may resume usual activities of daily living of which he is capable (eating ambulation, etc.)
   5. Techniques in collecting and handling specimens
      a. Sterile or clean
      b. Correct storage and disposal
      c. Adequate sample for testing
   6. Physiologic factors
      a. Adequate cleansing of the intestinal tract (enemas, cathartics)
      b. Emptying the bladder (voiding, "clean catch," double-voided specimen, catheterization)

3. **Monitoring procedures**

A. Important points
   1. Fractional urinalysis
      a. Tests for the presence of sugar and acetone in the urine as a result of metabolic disorder
      b. Samples must be tested at specific times—at regular intervals related

to meals, sleep, and specific medicinal agents

   c. Positive reactions frequently require taking other measures to safeguard the patient (giving insulin, modifying diet)

2. Specific gravity of urine
   a. Indicates degree of concentration or dilution of urine (normal range 1.010 to 1.025)
   b. Reflects efficiency of renal function

3. Proteinuria
   a. Tests determine the absence or presence of albumin and plasma proteins, which are not normally present to any degree in urine (normal range 0 to trace in random samples)
   b. Positive reactions indicate degenerative or inflammatory processes within urinary system

4. Cardiac monitors
   a. Give visual indication of cardiac function
   b. Reflect irregularities in rate, rhythm, and force of contraction

B. Basic common elements
1. Laboratory procedures must be carried out correctly; each step taken is significant
2. Observations must be accurate (degree of reaction to specific reagents)
3. Interpretation of significance of reactions must be precise (e.g., 1+, 2+, 3+, 4+ sugar; positive or negative for acetone; specific gravity 1.040; deviate patterns in cardiac tracings)
4. Equipment used must be efficient to achieve the purpose (chemical reagents stable, hydrometer intact, cardiac monitor working and correctly attached to patient)
5. Severe deviations from norms can be crucial and require specific action

4. Procedures to support nutrition
A. Important points
1. Nasogastric feeding or gavage—introduction of a fluid (blender) diet through a syringe or funnel attached to a nasogastric tube
2. Gastrostomy feeding—introduction of a fluid diet through a syringe attached to a gastrostomy tube that has been surgically inserted into the stomach, through the abdominal wall
3. Parenteral and oral supplements—

nutritive elements in solution may be supplied by injection into the circulatory system or into body tissues
   a. Intravenous infusion—glucose, saline, potassium, calcium, vitamins, water, whole blood, plasma, etc.
   b. Intramuscular and subcutaneous injection—vitamins, hematinics, etc.
   c. Oral preparations—vitamins, antacids, iron, etc.

B. Basic common elements
1. Specific equipment required—tubes, syringes, needles
2. The patency and correct location (in site) of tubes and needles must be established
3. The factor of time
   a. Feedings and medications administered at appointed hours
   b. The rate of flow at which fluid is introduced by tube or intravenously controlled to avoid complications
     (1) Intravenous—drops per minute
     (2) Gastric tubes—slowly
4. Solutions and preparations used
   a. Correct type, concentration, and amount must be ensured
   b. Compatibility when given at room temperature
5. Aseptic factors
   a. Tube feedings and oral supplements
     (1) Utensils, equipment clean
     (2) Solutions and drugs free from contamination
   b. Parenteral infusions and injections
     (1) All equipment, solutions, and preparations sterile
     (2) Skin disinfection at the point of insertion
6. Inherent dangers
   a. Aspiration can occur
     (1) Tube not correctly in site
     (2) Regurgitation in patients who are comatose, dysphagic, paralyzed, etc.
   b. Thrombophlebitis
     (1) Needle not correctly in site (diffuse infiltration into tissues)
     (2) Response of vessels to trauma
7. Significance and use: an important aspect of nursing care in a wide variety of health problems
   a. Inability to ingest or metabolize any food or fluid

b. Excessive loss of essential nutrients by severe secretion and excretion

c. Excessive loss of essential nutrients abnormally, due to vomiting, diarrhea, hemorrhage, etc.

d. Dietary inadequacies due to anorexia or modifications required in treating health problems

5. Procedures to support elimination

A. Important points

1. Catheterization—insertion of a pliable tube or catheter into the urinary bladder

   a. Sterile technique used
      (1) Equipment sterile
      (2) Operator wears sterile gloves
      (3) Labia correctly disinfected

   b. Types of catheters
      (1) Plain (single or stat. catheterization)
      (2) Retention (continuous or intermittent drainage, Foley)

   c. Catheter drainage used to
      (1) Maintain elimination
      (2) Safeguard against cross-contamination
      (3) Keep record of urinary output

2. Enemas—introduction of solutions rectally

   a. Clean technique used

   b. Amount, type, and temperature of solution must be appropriate

   c. Employ a large volume (1,000 ml.) of water (tap, saline) or a smaller volume (150 ml.) of a hypertonic solution to stimulate evacuation

3. Irrigations and instillations

   a. Urinary bladder
      (1) Prophylactic or therapeutic
      (2) Continuous or intermittent

   b. Rectal
      (1) Colonic
      (2) Harris flush

   c. Colostomy
      (1) Single lumen
      (2) Double lumen
      (3) Temporary or permanent

B. Common basic elements

1. Purposes or objectives

   a. Assist the patient to eliminate retained waste (urine, stool, gas)

   b. Secure specimens for laboratory analysis (urine, stool)

   c. Relieve symptoms of inflammation and infection or prevent their occurrence (instillation of medications, irrigation with antiseptic solutions)

2. Physiologic factors

   a. Use appropriate equipment to ensure patient safety, comfort, and effective results

   b. Insert tubes safely and precisely into body cavities (lubrication, distance to insert, etc.)

   c. Position the patient anatomically and comfortably

   d. Ensure an adequate return flow of solution introduced into body cavities (bladder, intestines, colostomy stomas)

   e. Have temperature of solution conducive to physiologic function
      (1) Room temperature for bladder treatments and commercially prepared enemas
      (2) Other irrigations approximately 100° to 105° F.

3. Significant observations

   a. Undue distress the patient experiences

   b. Characteristics of return flow

6. Procedures to decompress body cavities

A. Important points

1. Gastrointestinal decompression—a tube may be inserted into the stomach or intestinal tract and suction be applied in order to aspirate food residue, fluid gas, or old blood

   a. Types of tubes
      (1) Nasogastric (Levin) for stomach
      (2) Cantor, Miller-Abbott for intestinal tract

   b. Negative pressure is created in a collection bottle attached simultaneously to an electrically powered machine (Gumco) and to the tube inserted into the cavity

   c. Procedures prophylactic or supportive
      (1) Following surgery, to prevent distention, vomiting
      (2) To relieve vomiting, distention

2. Abdominal paracentesis (tap)—fluid may be aspirated from the abdominal cavity by surgical insertion of a trocar attached to tubing that provides gravity drainage

   a. Patient's bladder must be empty to avoid inadvertent puncture

---

b. Usually a large volume of fluid is removed

3. Thoracentesis (chest tap)—removal of fluid from the thoracic cavity by inserting a needle into the pleural space and aspirating into an attached syringe

4. Lumbar puncture (spinal tap)—removal of fluid from the spinal canal by inserting a needle into the space and aspirating into a syringe or allowing gravity drainage

B. Basic common elements
1. Purposes or objectives
   a. To reduce within cavities pressure that impairs vital function
      (1) Cerebral
      (2) Respiratory
      (3) Circulatory
      (4) Digestive
   b. To secure specimens for laboratory analysis
2. Specialized equipment and techniques required
   a. Instruments and equipment necessary to implement procedures must be adaptable and functioning
   b. Aseptic measures indicated
      (1) Shaving skin areas through which instruments will be inserted
      (2) Disinfection of skin surfaces
      (3) Sterile equipment and techniques when body surface is punctured
      (4) Meticulous oral hygiene for patients who have decompression tubes in site
3. Physiologic factors
   a. Rapid reduction of internal pressure can result in serious circulatory shifts that produce shock
   b. Any negative pressure exerted on body cavities must be controlled to avoid injury to internal organs or tissues
4. Significant assessment
   a. Ensuring patency of drainage tubes
   b. Noting characteristics of fluid aspirated
   c. Checking vital signs and symptoms during institution of procedures and, following termination of them, until the patient's general condition is stable

7. **Procedures to promote safety in patient's environment**
A. Important points
1. Biologic
   a. Prevention of cross-infection
      (1) Use medical aseptic techniques
      (2) Use surgical aseptic techniques
   b. Avoid direct patient contact when you have a local or systemic infection
2. Physical
   a. Use correct body mechanics in moving, lifting, or turning patient and thus prevent injury to the patient and nurse
   b. Check mechanical equipment and furniture for safety before use
   c. Use or operate equipment correctly
B. Basic common elements
1. Medical aseptic techniques
   a. Hand washing before and after patient contact
   b. Gowns, gloves, and masks protect personnel in contact with patients who have infectious diseases
   c. Utensils and equipment free from contamination before use for patient service
   d. Concurrent and terminal disinfection of contaminated articles to be reused
   e. Immediate safe disposal of contaminated materials (excreta, dressings, sputum, etc.)
2. Surgical aseptic techniques
   a. Gloves, masks, and gowns protect patients against cross-infection by health personnel
   b. Skin disinfection before injections reduces hazard of infection
   c. Sterile equipment used when body areas are susceptible to initial or superimposed infection
      (1) Care of all wounds—simple or complex (dressing, irrigating)
      (2) Any procedure that requires intrusion of instruments or devices into body cavities or areas that are normally sterile or clean (bladder, tissue, stomach)
3. Physical factors
   a. Precautions to prevent accidents to patients and personnel (side-rails, strap supports, dry floors, safe electrical equipment, etc.)

b. Being sure of identity of patient before nursing services (administration of medications, serving meals, transporting to diagnostic or therapy departments, etc.)

c. Using necessary physical assistance in moving or lifting helpless patients

d. Using available service resources to replace or restore defective equipment or furniture (wheelchairs, mechanical lifts, stretchers, etc.)

8. **Procedures to support oxygen need**
A. Important points
  1. Administration of oxygen
    a. Methods of delivery
      (1) Mask, catheter, cannula
      (2) Oxygen tent
      (3) IPPB apparatus
        (a) Delivers O_2 under pressure on inspiration
        (b) Combined with bronchodilating and mucolytic agents—nebulizers
    b. Regulation of supply
      (1) Flow of liters per minute as required
        (a) 4 to 8 per minute via catheter, mask
        (b) 8 to 10 per minute via tent
        (c) Pressure of IPPB prescribed for the individual, usually 15 to 20 cm. H_2O
      (2) Regulated by a special gauge attached to source (central piping, cylinder)
      (3) Humidification
    c. Safety precautions against fire must be used in the presence of free oxygen
  2. Tracheostomy—in certain respiratory health problems a hollow metal tube is surgically introduced into the trachea to facilitate oxygen intake and permit drainage or aspiration of mucus
    a. Tracheostomy care
      (1) Size of tube varies in relation to size of patient
      (2) Outer cannula remains in site
      (3) Inner cannula removed and cleaned as often as necessary
      (4) Suction as often as necessary (soft catheter attached to suction machine)

b. Other procedures used in conjunction
  (1) Oxygen
  (2) Respirator
B. Basic common elements
  1. Devices used to facilitate respiration must be applied and secured correctly
    a. Nasal catheter not visible in the throat and affixed in site
    b. Mask must be snug around nose and/or mouth
    c. Tent secured against excessive leakage
    d. Tracheostomy tube (outer cannula) firmly tied around neck to prevent expulsion due to coughing
  2. All devices used to deliver a supply of oxygen must remain patent
  3. Delivery of an adequate supply of oxygen must be ensured
  4. Critical assessment of signs and symptoms of respiratory distress (dyspnea, cyanosis, etc.)
  5. Meticulous oral and nasal hygiene is basic nursing care in all respiratory health problems

9. **Procedures in administration of medications**
A. Important points
  1. Oral preparations
    a. Forms available—tablet, capsule, pill, liquid, powder
    b. Unpalatable tastes may be disguised
    c. Patients may have difficulty in swallowing tablets, but these can be crushed
  2. Parenteral injections
    a. Sites commonly used
      (1) Hypodermic—subcutaneous tissue in the deltoid area
      (2) Intramuscular—ventrogluteal muscle
    b. Angle of insertion of needle
      (1) Hypodermic—approximately 45° angle
      (2) Intramuscular—90° angle
    c. Certain chemical agents alter, lose effect, and may be injurious if mixed with other agents for injection
    d. Forms of preparations available
      (1) Ampules, vials of usually prescribed dosage in solution (e.g., 1 ml. = 100 mg. of drug)
      (2) Vials with powdered drugs to

which sterile water or saline may be added to make a required dose

B. Basic common elements
1. Accuracy must be ensured
   a. Skill in preparation (pouring, drawing up, etc.)
   b. Knowledge of pharmacologic preparations—names, physiologic effects, uses, toxic signs, untoward effects
   c. Knowledge of symbols and equivalent measures in the metric and apothecary systems
   d. Skill in calculation of prescribed dosage that is greater than or less than the available supply

   Example: give 75 mg. of Demerol I.M. stat. when ampule available reads 1 ml. = 100 mg.
   Solution: Drug as Solution: Drug
   $$x : 75 \text{ mg.} :: 1 \text{ ml.} : 100 \text{ mg.}$$
   $$100x = 75$$
   $$x = \frac{75}{100} = \frac{3}{4} \text{ ml.}$$
   16 minims = 1 ml.
   12 minims = ¾ ml.
   ∴ 12 minims of solution = 75 mg. Demerol

   e. Skill in reading orders and labels
2. Skills and techniques in administration
   a. Identification of patient required
   b. Ability of patient to ingest and swallow oral preparations established
   c. Skillful insertion of needle in the correct anatomic site is necessary
   d. Clean and sterile techniques employed as indicated
3. Clarity and accuracy in recording and reporting the administration of medications and responses of patients to them
10. Summary
All psychomotor skills in nursing require both the use of underlying physiologic knowledge, knowing "how to do it," and the use of psychosocial skills in administration

REVIEW QUESTIONS FOR FUNDAMENTALS OF NURSING

Read each question carefully and select the single best answer proposed. Indicate your response by blocking out the corresponding number on the answer sheet following this chapter.

Situation: Mr. Davis is a 55-year-old man who is admitted to the hospital following a stroke. He is paralyzed on the right side and is experiencing dysphagia and dysphasia. His nursing care includes taking vital signs frequently. Questions 1 through 15 apply to Mr. Davis.

1. Temperature should be taken by
   1. Mouth   3. Rectum
   2. Groin   4. Axilla
2. Mr. Davis' temperature is 102.2° F. The equivalent of this in centigrade measurement is
   1. 39°   3. 40°
   2. 37°   4. 38°
3. Systolic pressure is the point on the manometer scale where the pulse beat is heard
   1. Loudest   3. Muted
   2. First   4. Last
4. Pulse pressure is the
   1. Deficit in apical-radial rate
   2. Force exerted against an arterial wall
   3. Degree of ventricular contraction
   4. Difference between systolic and diastolic readings
5. Mr. Davis is experiencing difficulty in
   1. Swallowing   3. Hearing
   2. Focusing   4. Understanding
6. Blood pressure should not be taken on his right arm because circulatory impairment may
   1. Produce inaccurate readings
   2. Result in unnecessary pain
   3. Hinder restoration of function
   4. Precipitate emboli formation
7. The patient's dysphasia requires that the nursing care plan initially must provide for
   1. Effective communication
   2. Routine hygiene needs
   3. Prevention of aspiration
   4. Withholding solid foods

Three days after admission, Mr. Davis has a nasogastric tube inserted and is to receive a prescribed liquid formula diet six times daily.

8. The amount of liquid administered at one time should not exceed
   1. 150 ml.   3. 450 ml.
   2. 350 ml.   4. 250 ml.
9. Location of the tube in the stomach is best established by
   1. Slowly inserting 20 ml. of water
   2. Observing the patient's color
   3. Asking the patient if he feels the fluid
   4. Aspirating a small amount of gastric content
10. The formula temperature most compatible for administration is
    1. Chilled   3. Room
    2. Body   4. 108° F.
11. During feedings the position of choice for Mr. Davis is
    1. Semi-Fowler's (sitting)
    2. Lateral prone
    3. Trendelenburg
    4. Dorsal

12. Tube-feeding diets are administered slowly to reduce the hazard of
   1. Indigestion
   2. Regurgitation
   3. Flatulence
   4. Distention
13. Mr. Davis' body alignment must be maintained in order to prevent
   1. Pneumonia
   2. Decubiti
   3. Contractures
   4. Regurgitation
14. Meticulous cleanliness, skin care, and frequent repositioning are positive nursing measures because they
   1. Induce a sense of well-being
   2. Are common cultural values
   3. Insure a fuller recovery
   4. Reduce incidence of complications
15. Full range of motion exercises may be instituted for Mr. Davis
   1. Immediately
   2. In 48 to 72 hours
   3. When he wishes
   4. In 2 weeks

Situation: Mrs. Evans, a 60-year-old homemaker, is admitted because of possible intestinal obstruction. A Cantor tube has been inserted and attached to suction. Questions 16 through 25 apply to Mrs. Evans.

16. A serious danger to which Mrs. Evans is exposed because of intestinal suction is excessive loss of
   1. Protein enzymes
   2. Energy carbohydrates
   3. Water and electrolytes
   4. Vitamins and minerals
17. Critical assessment of Mrs. Evans includes observation for
   1. Dehydration
   2. Nausea
   3. Edema
   4. Belching
18. The solution of choice used to maintain patency of the Cantor tube is
   1. Hypertonic glucose
   2. Isotonic saline
   3. Hypotonic saline
   4. Sterile water
19. A strong priority in Mrs. Evans' hygiene care is
   1. Skin and back
   2. Genital areas
   3. Nails and extremities
   4. Oral and nasal regions
20. A significant nursing responsibility related to Mrs. Evans and the decompression therapy is
   1. Ensuring that the tube is in site
   2. Irrigating the tube at regular intervals
   3. Noting the character of materials aspirated
   4. Aspirating with a 50 ml. syringe if tube is occluded

Mrs. Evans is scheduled for a colostomy after diagnostic work-up. Her anxiety is overt and realistic

21. The most effective way to help Mrs. Evans at this point is to
   1. Encourage her to express her feelings
   2. Reassure her that many people cope with this problem
   3. Explain the procedure and postoperative course
   4. Administer a sedative and tell her to rest
22. A significant aspect of nursing related to Mrs. Evans' preoperative care is helping her to identify the
   1. Necessary dietary adaptations involved
   2. Specific cause of her anxiety
   3. Activity limitations required after surgery
   4. Community resources available after discharge
23. During the preoperative shaving preparation, Mrs. Evans starts to cry and says, "I'm sorry you have to do this messy thing for me." The choice response for a nurse at this time is
   1. I don't mind it
   2. Nurses get used to this
   3. This is part of my job
   4. You are upset

Following satisfactory surgery, Mrs. Evans is to have a colostomy irrigation

24. The basic knowledge necessary before a nurse can institute the procedure correctly for Mrs. Evans is the
   1. Capacity of the patient to participate
   2. Kind of tumor excised during surgery
   3. Type of surgical procedure that was done
   4. Presence of pathogenic organisms
25. The primary step toward long-range goals in Mrs. Evans' rehabilitation is her
   1. Mastering techniques of colostomy care
   2. Readiness to accept her altered body function
   3. Knowledge of the dietary modifications necessary
   4. Awareness of community resources available to her

Situation: Mr. Jasper, a 40-year-old obese gourmet chef, hospitalized for medical work-up, was recently found to have diabetes mellitus. He is now ambulatory. He is receiving Dymelor once a day and requires fractional urinalysis q.i.d. Questions 26 through 36 refer to Mr. Jasper.

26. Mr. Jasper will probably experience difficulty in adjusting to his
   1. Dietary restrictions
   2. Hygienic regimen
   3. Urinary testing
   4. Medical surveillance
27. In addition to his carbohydrate regulation, Mr. Jasper would probably be required to reduce his intake of
   1. Water
   2. Protein
   3. Calories
   4. Vitamins
28. Fractional urinalysis is a test to determine the amount of
   1. Albumin
   2. Urea nitrogen
   3. Specific gravity
   4. Sugar and acetone
29. A major priority in Mr. Jasper's nursing care plan is providing him with specific knowledge about
   1. Community resources
   2. The specific health problem
   3. Medical supervision
   4. Activity limitations
30. In maintaining physical hygiene, Mr. Jasper would be especially attentive to
   1. Foot and toenail care
   2. Dental and oral care
   3. Elimination
   4. Water intake
31. Meticulous hygiene is significant for Mr. Jasper because people who have diabetes generally tend to be more

1. Careless about health practices
2. Inclined to deny the health problem
3. Restrictive of physical activity
4. Prone to local infections

32. A major point in the nursing plan to teach Mr. Jasper how to test his urine is that he must
    1. Understand the reagents used
    2. Know the normal blood sugar level
    3. Demonstrate what he has learned
    4. Correctly dispose of the specimen
33. The nursing care plan for Mr. Jasper must make sure he understands that he
    1. May have to change his job
    2. Must adhere to his diet
    3. Should modify all activity
    4. Cannot take alcohol in any form
34. The teaching plan related to Mr. Jasper's health problem ought to include a
    1. Member of his family
    2. Social service worker
    3. Representative from community service
    4. Physical therapist
35. Concerning diabetes mellitus, it is of primary importance that Mr. Jasper know
    1. Factors pertaining to heredity
    2. Associated health problems resulting from it
    3. Its prevalence as a disease in society
    4. Symptoms of incipient shock or coma
36. Teaching related to Mr. Jasper's medication must place emphasis on the significance of
    1. Manifestations of toxicity
    2. Untoward reactions
    3. Taking it regularly on time
    4. Increasing dosage when necessary

Situation: Mr. Vincent, a 65-year-old self-employed grocer was admitted to the hospital with congestive heart failure and ascites. His treatment includes oxygen by mask, retention catheter for drainage (irrigated with normal saline t.i.d.), digoxin, Diuril, and low-sodium diet. He is dyspneic, apprehensive, and restless. Questions 37 through 51 refer to Mr. Vincent.

37. The number of liters of oxygen per minute comfortable for Mr. Vincent most probably is
    1. 12 to 14   3. 2 to 4
    2. 6 to 8   4. 16 to 18
38. Safety precautions are especially important in Mr. Vincent's room because oxygen
    1. Is flammable
    2. Has unstable properties
    3. Increases apprehension
    4. Supports combustion
39. Mr. Vincent's safety can be best ensured through rigid enforcement of regulations pertaining to
    1. Restriction of visitors
    2. Hospital routines
    3. Housekeeping activities
    4. Disaster prevention
40. Mr. Vincent's restlessness is dangerous because it
    1. Decreases the amount of oxygen available
    2. Interferes with normal respiration
    3. Increases the cardiac work load
    4. Produces elevation in temperature
41. Mr. Vincent's apprehension may be critical because it reduces his capacity to

1. Rest and sleep   3. Talk and relate
2. Move and turn   4. Eat and drink

42. In planning nursing care for Mr. Vincent, major emphasis ought to be placed on supporting physiologic and psychosocial factors in relation to
    1. Nutrition   3. Elimination
    2. Comfort   4. Rehabilitation
43. After receiving a sedative, Mr. Vincent says to the nurse, "I guess you're too busy to stay with me." The best choice of response in this circumstance is
    1. "I have to see other patients."
    2. "The medication will help you rest soon."
    3. "I have to go now but I will come back in 10 minutes."
    4. "You will feel better; I'll adjust your oxygen mask."
44. Before giving Mr. Vincent digoxin, it is necessary to measure his
    1. Pulse   3. Blood pressure
    2. Apical beat   4. Respirations
45. Nursing care of Mr. Vincent includes observation for symptoms of electrolyte depletion due to
    1. Sodium restriction
    2. Inadequate intake
    3. Continuous bladder drainage
    4. Diuretic therapy
46. Mr. Vincent's catheter is irrigated regularly, primarily to
    1. Dilute the urine
    2. Prevent infection
    3. Maintain patency
    4. Alter pH of urine
47. When irrigating Mr. Vincent's catheter a safety precaution to be taken is
    1. Warm the solution to 105°
    2. Aspirate to initiate return flow
    3. Be sure that equipment is clean
    4. Avoid undue force in instilling
48. Mr. Vincent's lunch includes 6 ounces of soup and 4 ounces of milk. His fluid intake for this meal is
    1. 300 ml.   3. 400 ml.
    2. 240 ml.   4. 150 ml.
49. Mr. Vincent requires a paracentesis. This procedure involves the removal of fluid from the
    1. Spinal canal
    2. Abdominal cavity
    3. Pleural space
    4. Myocardial space
50. Mr. Vincent's ascites is critical because it
    1. Interferes with digestion
    2. Contributes to constipation
    3. Impairs local circulation
    4. Burdens cardiopulmonary function
51. Prior to the paracentesis, a major nursing responsibility supporting Mr. Vincent's safety is
    1. Procuring correct equipment
    2. Local skin preparation
    3. Making sure of legal consent
    4. Explaining the procedure

Situation: Miss Carlow, a 35-year-old executive secretary, is hospitalized for treatment of hypertension. She requires bed rest with bathroom privileges, low-sodium diet, Serpasil, Hygroton, and phenobarbital. She is a person who is used to a fully active business and social life, who smoked an average of a pack of cigarettes daily, and who usually had two alcoholic cocktails before dinner. She is required to stop smoking. Questions 52 through 60 refer to Miss Carlow.

52. Miss Carlow is angry and expresses disgust with her regimen and dissatisfaction with the nursing care. Such behavior is probably a manifestation of her
 1. Ill manners
 2. Disdain for nurses
 3. Reaction to medications
 4. Fear of her health problem
53. Phenobarbital is probably indicated for Miss Carlow because it will
 1. Promote rest
 2. Induce sleep
 3. Alleviate headache
 4. Reduce hostility
54. Miss Carlow is receiving Hygroton because it is an effective
 1. Antihypertensive   3. Diuretic
 2. Tranquilizer   4. Analgesic
55. You discover a pack of cigarettes in Miss Carlow's bathrobe. The best course of action to take at this time is to
 1. Report the situation to the head nurse
 2. Let the patient know you found them
 3. Discard them and say nothing
 4. Call the physician for advice
56. When Miss Carlow is being overtly verbally hostile, the most appropriate nursing response is
 1. Reasonable explanation of situations
 2. Complete withdrawal from the setting
 3. Silent acceptance of her behavior
 4. Verbal defense of your position
57. Since Miss Carlow requires bed rest, related nursing care includes
 1. Planning diversional activities
 2. Ensuring safety with bedrails
 3. Maintaining a semi-Fowler position
 4. Changing linen frequently
58. Miss Carlow refuses to eat her dinner. Angrily, she says, "I will not eat food without seasoning." The response of choice in this situation is
 1. Salt is bad for high blood pressure
 2. The doctor ordered this diet
 3. I wish I could change it
 4. Your diet upsets you
59. The nurse may help Miss Carlow to accept diet restriction by teaching her about
 1. Sodium content in foods
 2. Palatable nonsalt seasonings
 3. Available salt substitutes
 4. Fluid and electrolyte balance
60. In discussing rehabilitation plans, the nurse must be sure Miss Carlow understands that a major realistic goal for her is
 1. Altering her personality
 2. Retraining for employment
 3. Modifying her life style
 4. Controlling her environment

Situation: Mr. Soloman, a 54-year-old Hebrew insurance broker, is terminally ill with metastatic cancer of the lung. He and his 44-year-old wife have a 20-year-old daughter who is a college student and a 16-year-old son in high school. His plan of care includes a soft diet with between-meal nourishment, meperidine, 100 mg. p.r.n. for pain, and intermittent positive pressure breathing treatments twice a day. Mr. Soloman is weak, emaciated, and apathetic. Questions 61 through 75 refer to Mr. Soloman.

61. Nursing care plans for Mr. Soloman ought to give priority to
 1. Diet and nutrition
 2. Hygiene and comfort
 3. Intake and output
 4. Body mechanics and posture
62. Mr. Soloman expresses aversion for his meals and eats only small amounts each time. Nursing care that may alleviate this situation is to provide him with
 1. Only foods that he likes
 2. Supplementary vitamins
 3. Extra nourishment between meals
 4. Small portions at frequent intervals
63. The term used to describe Mr. Soloman's response to food most accurately is
 1. Anorexia   3. Apathy
 2. Anoxia   4. Anosmia
64. In preparing Mr. Soloman's medication the nurse should know that meperidine is commonly available for dispensation as
 1. Darvon   3. Demerol
 2. Doriden   4. Donatal
65. As directed, Mr. Soloman may be given his medication
 1. As he desires
 2. After meals
 3. Whenever necessary
 4. Before meals
66. Mr. Soloman receives his medication subcutaneously. The supply is labeled 1 ml. = 150 mg. The number of minims you would administer is
 1. 12½   3. 7½
 2. 10   4. 5
67. The IPPB treatment may be more helpful to Mr. Soloman if given before mealtime since this can temporarily
 1. Facilitate expectoration
 2. Stimulate appetite
 3. Reduce apathy
 4. Alleviate fatigue
68. In view of Mr. Soloman's state of extreme weakness, nursing care plans ought to include
 1. Limiting family visiting hours
 2. Encouraging family to feed and assist him
 3. Giving all care at once to allow longer rest time
 4. Promoting self-activity to preserve muscle tone
69. On one occasion Mr. Soloman says to you, "If I could just get something to take away my pain for a few days I might be able to eat more and get some strength back." In reference to the "stages of dying" identified by Dr. Kübler-Ross, the patient indicates the stage of
 1. Anger   3. Bargaining
 2. Acceptance   4. Depression
70. While Mr. Soloman is sleeping after dinner,

his wife approaches you. She is overtly anxious and states, "My husband has been ill so long, the hospital and doctor bills keep mounting, I don't know where it will lead us." Your best choice of response is
1. You are concerned for family security
2. I know how costly health care is
3. Is your husband heavily insured
4. Now, don't upset yourself, Mrs. Soloman

71. Some time later, while you are caring for Mr. Soloman, he says, "I don't really mind dying, but I worry about my boy, he is so young." This statement may be indicative of the stage of
   1. Acceptance   3. Denial
   2. Bargaining   4. Depression

72. Your response of choice to Mr. Soloman's statement in question 71 is
   1. You must get more rest
   2. He will be all right
   3. You feel your son needs you
   4. What about your wife and daughter

73. When Mr. Soloman reaches the point of acceptance in the stages of dying, it may be manifested in his behavior by his psychological state of
   1. Euphoria   3. Apathy
   2. Detachment   4. Emotionalism

74. For the duration of Mr. Soloman's acceptance of his dying and death, nursing care plans ought to place emphasis on
   1. Support of all family members
   2. Increased diversional activity
   3. Nutritional adequacy
   4. Control of emotional lability

75. When Mr. Soloman dies, his son becomes angry and cries as he says to you, "Doctors are dumb, hospitals are dumb, they did not help my father, they killed him." Your best choice of response is
   1. Your father was a very sick man
   2. You must buck up and be strong
   3. You loved your father very much
   4. Your mother and sister need you now

Situation: Mrs. Lopez, a 21-year-old mother, has been discharged 5 days following delivery of her second child. Her first child is 15 months old. She had no prenatal care during either pregnancy and was admitted while in labor in both instances. Mrs. Lopez was referred for home care follow-up and you are assigned to make the visit. Questions 76 through 85 refer to the Lopez family.

76. In planning for this visit it may be vital to identify any limitations relative to
   1. Psychosocial factors
   2. Effective communication
   3. Cultural influences
   4. Economic security

77. The initial visit to Mrs. Lopez will be more productive if scheduled when
   1. You have more time to expend
   2. She is feeding the children
   3. Her husband is at work
   4. It is convenient for the family

78. The role most likely to foster sound interpersonal relationships during the first visit to the Lopez home is that of

1. Stranger   3. Counselor
2. Teacher   4. Surrogate

79. When you first talk with Mrs. Lopez, the type of interview that is likely to be most productive is
   1. Information-giving   3. Exploratory
   2. Problem-solving   4. Directive

On arrival for the first visit at 10 A.M., you find Mr. Lopez is home. He is temporarily collecting unemployment benefits and the family is on welfare. Mrs. Lopez is worried and ill at ease in the situation. The infant is due for bottle feeding, the toddler is playing on the floor.

80. At this time your best action would be to ask Mr. Lopez if he would mind
   1. Giving the baby a bottle
   2. Taking the toddler for a walk
   3. Leaving you and Mrs. Lopez alone
   4. Participating in the discussion

81. Mrs. Lopez's uneasiness in your presence may be a significant clue to the existence of conflict between her and her husband about
   1. Finances   3. Job stability
   2. Health care   4. Birth control

82. Mrs. Lopez tells you that she did not have prenatal care because she "is ashamed to go to the clinic." An effective response to this may be to
   1. Explain health services as a contribution to society
   2. Tell her about the dangers of pregnancy
   3. Assure her that poverty is nothing to be ashamed of
   4. Make her aware of the incidence of congenital defects

83. The 15-month-old child has had no inoculations. Mr. Lopez says he does not believe in them. Your best choice of response to his statement may be
   1. Scientific evidence proves you wrong
   2. Have you discussed this with a doctor?
   3. How can you risk the life of your child?
   4. You feel they may be harmful

84. Action directed toward resolving the problem resulting from Mr. Lopez's skepticism ought to include
   1. Reporting him to the child care bureau
   2. Providing him with suitable and related literature
   3. Arguing the merits of prophylactic health care
   4. Scheduling him for a tour of the local health center

85. When Mr. Lopez leaves for a job interview, Mrs. Lopez confides that she would have the children inoculated but her husband has forbidden it. You may best assist her in this dilemma by advising her to
   1. Avoid family conflict and let the matter go
   2. Take the children to clinic and not tell him
   3. Try to get him to go with her for family counseling
   4. Force the issue and argue it despite consequences

Situation: Mr. Farrentino, a 20-year-old college senior, is admitted for ulcerative colitis. He is the youngest of three sons and the first member of his family to attend college. He works part time. His major support comes from his parents and his brothers. He is grossly underweight, pale, and dehydrated. His care plan includes intravenous infusion, a low-residue, bland, high-protein diet, vitamins B, C, and K and electrolytes parenterally, and stool examination daily. Questions 86 through 102 refer to this situation.

86. Mr. Farrentino is receiving vitamins and electrolytes parenterally because
   1. Intestinal absorption may be inadequate
   2. More rapid action can be attained
   3. They are ineffective when taken orally
   4. Colon irritability is increased by their presence

87. Mr. Farrentino is to receive 2,000 ml. of fluid intravenously in about 12 hours. Nursing responsibility includes maintaining the rate of flow so that the number of drops per minute is approximately (drop factor is 10 gtts. = 1 ml.)
   1. 48 to 50   3. 27 to 29
   2. 30 to 32   4. 40 to 42

88. Another specific nursing responsibility related to Mr. Farrentino's infusion includes
   1. Securing parental consent for the treatment
   2. Continuous observation for tissue infiltration
   3. Immobilizing the patient's arm to reduce trauma
   4. Making sure the procedure is instituted on time

89. Mr. Farrentino's diet will reduce
   1. Gastric acidity
   2. Intestinal malabsorption
   3. Colon irritation
   4. Electrolyte depletion

90. The high protein content of his diet is necessary to
   1. Correct anemia
   2. Improve muscle tone
   3. Decrease colon spasms
   4. Repair tissues

91. Mr. Farrentino is receiving electrolytes parenterally because colitis can result in
   1. Potassium depletion
   2. Inability to metabolize
   3. Sodium retention
   4. Impaired absorption

92. Stool examinations in this situation are done commonly to determine
   1. Culture and sensitivity
   2. Occult blood and organisms
   3. Ova and parasites
   4. Fat and undigested food

Mr. Farrentino's medical evaluation includes internal examination and fluoroscopic and x-ray visualization.

93. Mr. Farrentino most probably will be scheduled for
   1. Proctoscopy   3. Cystoscopy
   2. Anoscopy   4. Sigmoidoscopy

94. The procedure of value in diagnosing Mr. Farrentino's condition is
   1. Gastrointestinal series
   2. Barium enema
   3. Flat plate of the abdomen
   4. Cholecystography

95. Specific nursing responsibility in preparing Mr. Farrentino for these procedures includes
   1. Withholding food and fluid for 8 hours beforehand
   2. Giving soapsuds enemas until clear
   3. Maintaining him on complete bed rest
   4. Making sure that he understands what is to happen

96. During the acute phase of Mr. Farrentino's illness, nursing care includes critical observation for symptoms of
   1. Dysentery   3. Perforation
   2. Constipation   4. Diverticulosis

Mr. Farrentino is unhappy with his diet. He is depressed because he feels he won't feel stronger without food.

97. During dinner he pushes his tray aside and says, "I hate to be a pest and bellyache about it, but I can't eat the stuff; it's like nothing." Your best choice of response to him is
   1. This diet will help you gain strength
   2. Have you discussed it with the doctor
   3. What kind of food do you usually eat
   4. You have every right to complain

98. On one occasion you find Mrs. Farrentino about to give her son a bowl of homemade minestrone soup. Nursing action indicated here is to
   1. Take away the soup and discard it
   2. Tell them that hospital rules forbid this
   3. Explain how such food will affect the patient
   4. Strain the soup and let him have the liquid

99. Later you learn from Mrs. Farrentino that her son asked her to bring the soup. Such behavior may be indicating
   1. Denial of the health problem
   2. Marked egocentricity
   3. Maternal dependency
   4. Rejection of medical care

100. Mr. Farrentino is anxious about prolonged hospitalization. He asks you directly, "Do you think the doctor will discharge me in time to take my exams?" Your best choice of response is
   1. You must not worry; it is bad for you
   2. Your are concerned about your schoolwork
   3. You won't be discharged until you are well
   4. Unless you eat your diet, you won't be strong enough

101. A major goal in nursing care plans for Mr. Farrentino is helping him to
   1. Understand nutrition and disease
   2. Establish a pattern of bowel hygiene
   3. Accept and live with chronic disease
   4. Avoid all stressful life situations

102. Nursing care plans for Mr. Farrentino must place emphasis on maintaining his regime. This probably may be achieved most effectively through
   1. Peer relationships
   2. Strict authoritarianism
   3. Maternal gentleness
   4. Psychological support

Situation: Nancy Hand, a 5-year-old only child, is admitted to the hospital with rheumatic fever. She requires bed rest, full soft diet, liberal fluid intake, and Ampicillin, 250 mg. p.o., q.i.d. Nancy is restless and fretful and tells you that her "legs hurt." Questions 103 through 112 refer to Nancy.

103. Nancy's medication is classified as an
   1. Analgesic   3. Anti-infective
   2. Antibiotic   4. Antipyretic
104. The medication label reads "1 dram equals 200 mg." You would give Nancy
   1. 5 ml.   3. 4 ml.
   2. 8 ml.   4. 3 ml.
105. Nancy may be more comfortable if her
   1. Position is changed frequently
   2. Bed is elevated at the head
   3. Legs are supported on a pillow
   4. Body alignment is maintained
106. The immediate priority in Nancy's nursing care is
   1. Nutrition   3. Exercise
   2. Rest   4. Elimination
107. Nursing care likely to be most effective in alleviating Nancy's fretfulness is
   1. Giving her a jig-saw puzzle
   2. Putting her in a room by herself
   3. Letting her play with a doll
   4. Reading a story to her
108. The best choice of between-meal nourishment for Nancy is
   1. Fresh fruit   3. Fruit gelatin
   2. Hard candy   4. Creamed soup
109. The most serious complication that may threaten Nancy is
   1. Endocarditis
   2. Pneumonitis
   3. Tenosynovitis
   4. Rheumatoid arthritis
110. When you bring Nancy her dinner tray she says, "I'm too sick to feed myself." Nursing action indicated is to tell her to
   1. Try to eat as much as she can
   2. Be a big girl and not to act like a baby
   3. Let it go until she feels better
   4. Wait 5 minutes and you will help her
111. Nancy's statement is most likely indicative of
   1. Immaturity   3. Regression
   2. Lonesomeness   4. Temper tantrum
112. Nancy is apathetic about eating. Nursing care directed toward supporting her nutrition ought to include
   1. Providing diversional activity at mealtime
   2. Eliminating all between-meal nourishment
   3. Asking her parents to visit at mealtime
   4. Giving her only the foods she likes best

Situation: Mrs. O'Hanlon, a childless widow, was born in Ireland. She has been an outpatient in medical clinic for 6 months, under treatment for diabetes and hypertension. Her regimen includes Orinase, a low-sodium, diabetic diet, and Serpasil b.i.d. On the occasion of a regular visit her urine sample shows sugar, 3+ and acetone, a trace. She is employed as cook in the sandwich shop of the local department store. Questions 113 through 118 refer to Mrs. O'Hanlon.

113. As the nurse interviewing Mrs. O'Hanlon, you would first be most concerned to find out about any changes in her
   1. Eating habits   3. Weight range
   2. Blood pressure   4. Serum glucose

114. Mrs. O'Hanlon tells you that sometimes she forgets to take the Serpasil when she is in a hurry. Your best choice of response to her is
   1. You cannot forget something so important
   2. Can't you find someone to remind you?
   3. Try leaving it at your place at table
   4. If you neglect it, you can have a stroke
115. In discussing the patient's present metabolic state, a factor that ought to be dealt with is that people taking oral antidiabetic agents
   1. Should not work where food is readily accessible
   2. Consciously or unconsciously may tend to relax dietary rules
   3. Are not as threatened by their disease as those on insulin
   4. Need not be concerned about serious complications
116. Mrs. O'Hanlon tells you she can't "eat big meals." She prefers to "snack" throughout the day. You would carefully explain to her that in her condition
   1. Small, frequent meals are better for digestion
   2. Large meals can contribute to a weight problem
   3. Salt and sugar restriction is her main concern
   4. Regulated food intake is basic to her control
117. Mrs. O'Hanlon is scheduled to have a serum glucose test the following morning. To ensure accuracy in the result, you would instruct her to
   1. Take her regular dose of Orinase
   2. Abstain from food and fluid
   3. Have clear fluids for breakfast
   4. Eat her usual diet
118. The patient complains that she finds the low-salt foods "very tasteless." Your best choice of response may be
   1. Salt can be very harmful to your health
   2. I know how difficult it is for you
   3. You miss your ham and cabbage
   4. Ask the doctor if you can splurge occasionally

Situation: Mrs. Lobinski, a 75-year-old Polish woman, is admitted for diagnostic evaluation for arteriosclerotic heart disease. In the year since her husband's death, she has lived with her son and daughter-in-law. Presently, she is not physically distressed, but is apprehensive and alienated. Questions 119 through 125 refer to Mrs. Lobinski

119. Nursing care that may help Mrs. Lobinski to feel more at ease includes
   1. Telling her that everything will be all right
   2. Giving her a copy of hospital regulations
   3. Reassuring her that there is nothing to fear
   4. Orienting her to the environment and personnel
120. In your initial approach to creating a therapeutic environment you would give priority to
   1. Identifying individuality
   2. Promoting independence
   3. Maintaining safety

4. Explaining procedures

121. Mrs. Lobinski's apprehension is most probably related to
    1. Invasion of privacy
    2. Dependent tendencies
    3. Fear of death
    4. Loss of self-direction

122. In providing emotional support for Mrs. Lobinski, a nurse ought to remember that
    1. Senile behavioral changes are irreversible
    2. The aging can have useful inner resources
    3. Polish mothers respond to overt affection
    4. A firm direct approach is most effective

123. On one occasion after her family has been visiting, the patient is angry and says to you, "My daughter-in-law says they can't take me home until the doctor let's me go. She doesn't understand; she isn't Polish." Your best choice of response would be

1. Oh, what nationality is she?
2. You wish she were Polish
3. The doctor is the authority
4. You feel she doesn't want you home

124. In discussing the future resumption of previous activities with Mrs. Lobinski, nursing care plans should focus on
    1. Avoiding stress in living
    2. Establishing realistic goals
    3. Resolving all family problems
    4. Supporting dependent behavior

125. In discussing Mrs. Lobinski's rehabilitation with the family, you would emphasize their role in helping her to feel
    1. Important   3. Useful
    2. Dependent   4. Secure

SCORES

NAME ______________________ (LAST) (FIRST) (MIDDLE) DATE __________ 1 ______ 5 ______ DATE OF BIRTH ______________ AGE ______ SEX ______ (M OR F)

SCHOOL ______________ CITY ______________ 2 ______ 6 ______ GRADE OR CLASS ______ INSTRUCTOR ______________

3 ______ 7 ______

1 ______________ 2 ______________ 4 ______ 8 ______ NAME OF TEST ______________ PART ______

DIRECTIONS: Read each question and its numbered answers. When you have decided which answer is correct, blacken the corresponding space on this sheet with the special pencil. Make your mark as long as the pair of lines, and move the pencil point up and down firmly to make a heavy black line. If you change your mind, erase your first mark completely. Make no stray marks; they may count against you.

SAMPLE:

1. Chicago is
1—1 a country
1—2 a mountain
1—3 an island
1—4 a city
1—5 a state

1 ▯1 ▯2 ▯3 ▮4 ▯5

1	31	61	91	121
2	32	62	92	122
3	33	63	93	123
4	34	64	94	124
5	35	65	95	125
6	36	66	96	126
7	37	67	97	127
8	38	68	98	128
9	39	69	99	129
10	40	70	100	130
11	41	71	101	131
12	42	72	102	132
13	43	73	103	133
14	44	74	104	134
15	45	75	105	135

BE SURE YOUR MARKS ARE HEAVY AND BLACK.
ERASE COMPLETELY ANY ANSWER YOU WISH TO CHANGE.

16	46	76	106	136
17	47	77	107	137
18	48	78	108	138
19	49	79	109	139
20	50	80	110	140
21	51	81	111	141
22	52	82	112	142
23	53	83	113	143
24	54	84	114	144
25	55	85	115	145
26	56	86	116	146
27	57	87	117	147
28	58	88	118	148
29	59	89	119	149
30	60	90	120	150

Printed by the International Business Machines Corporation, Endicott, N. Y., U. S. A.

IBM FORM I. T. S. 1000 B 108

FIVE

CLINICAL NURSING

Medical-surgical nursing

Obstetric and gynecologic nursing

Pediatric nursing

Psychiatric nursing

Rehabilitation nursing

CHAPTER

9

MEDICAL-SURGICAL NURSING

Adams, J. C.: Outline of fractures, ed. 4, Baltimore, 1964, The Williams & Wilkins Co.

Adams, J. P., editor: Current practice in orthopaedic surgery, vol. 4, St. Louis, 1969, The C. V. Mosby Co.

Anderson, G., Arnstein, M. G., and Lester, M. R.: Communicable disease control, ed. 4, New York, 1962, The Macmillan Co.

Anderson, H. C.: Newton's geriatric nursing, ed. 5, St. Louis, 1971, The C. V. Mosby Co.

Anderson, O. W.: Syphilis and society—problems of control in the United States 1812-1964, Research Series no. 22, Chicago, 1965, University of Chicago Press.

Andrews, G. C., and Domonkos, A. N.: Diseases of the skin, ed. 10, Philadelphia, 1971, W. B. Saunders Co.

Beeson, P. B., and McDermott, W., editors: Cecil-Loeb textbook of medicine, ed. 13, Philadelphia, 1971, W. B. Saunders Co.

Beland, I.: Clinical nursing, ed. 2, New York, 1970, The Macmillan Co.

Benenson, A. S., editor: Control of communicable diseases in man, ed. 11, Washington, D. C., 1970, American Public Health Association.

Bergersen, B. S.: Pharmacology in nursing, ed. 12, St. Louis, 1973, The C. V. Mosby Co.

Blumberg, J., and Drummond, E.: Nursing care of the long-term patient, ed. 2, New York, 1971, Springer Publishing Co., Inc.

Brunner, L. S., Emerson, C. P., Ferguson, L. K., and Suddarth, D.: Textbook of medical-surgical nursing, ed. 2, Philadelphia, 1970, J. B. Lippincott Co.

Carini, E., and Owens, G.: Neurological and neurosurgical nursing, ed. 5, St. Louis, 1970, The C. V. Mosby Co.

Crenshaw, A. H.: Campbell's operative orthopaedics, ed. 5, vols. 1 and 2, St. Louis, 1971, The C. V. Mosby Co.

Diagnostic standards and classification of tuberculosis, New York, 1969, Committee on Revision of Diagnostic Standards, National Tuberculosis Association.

Dubos, R. J., and Hirsch, J. G., editors: Bacterial and mycotic infections of man, ed. 4, Philadelphia, 1965, J. B. Lippincott Co.

Duff, R. S., and Hollingshead, A. B.: Sickness and society, New York, 1968, Harper & Row, Publishers.

Engle, D. J., editor: Life and disease, New York, 1963, Basic Books, Inc.

Ferguson, A.: Orthopedic surgery in infancy and childhood, ed. 3, Baltimore, 1968, The Williams & Wilkins Co.

Field, M.: Patients are people, ed. 3, New York, 1967, Columbia University Press.

Finnegan, J., and LeMaitre, G.: The patient in surgery, Philadelphia, 1966, W. B. Saunders Co.

Freeman, R. B.: Community health nursing practice, Philadelphia, 1970, W. B. Saunders Co.

The future of tuberculosis control: a report to the Surgeon General by a Task Force on Tuberculosis Control, U. S. Public Health Service, Public Health Service Pub. no. 1119, Washington, D. C., 1966.

Garb, S.: Laboratory tests in common use, ed. 5, New York, 1971, Springer Publishing Co., Inc.

Gartland, J. J.: Fundamentals of orthopaedics, Philadelphia, 1965, W. B. Saunders Co.

Gunther, J.: Death be not proud, New York, 1949, Harper & Brothers.

Harrison, T. R., et al.: Principles of internal medicine, ed. 5, New York, 1966, McGraw-Hill Book Co.

Health information for international travel, 1967-1968, Public Health Service Pub. no. HE 20-2302 T-69, Washington, D. C., April, 1970.

Hinman, E. H.: World eradication of infectious diseases, Springfield, Ill., 1966, Charles C Thomas, Publisher.

Hollander, J. L., editor: Arthritis and allied conditions: a textbook of rheumatology, ed. 7, Philadelphia, 1966, Lea & Febiger.

319

Horsfall, F. L., Jr., and Tamm, I., editors: Viral and rickettsial infections of man, ed. 4, Philadelphia, 1965, J. B. Lippincott Co.

Huckstep, R. L.: Typhoid fever and other *Salmonella* infections, Edinburgh, 1962, E. & S. Livingstone, Ltd.

Johnston, D. F.: Essentials of communicable disease: with nursing principles, St. Louis, 1968, The C. V. Mosby Co.

Kallins, E. L.: Textbook of public health nursing, St. Louis, 1967, The C. V. Mosby Co.

Krusen, F. H., Kottke, F. J., and Ellwood, P. M.: Handbook of physical medicine and rehabilitation, ed. 2, Philadelphia, 1971, W. B. Saunders Co.

Larson, C. B., and Gould, M. L.: Orthopaedic nursing, ed. 7, St. Louis, 1970, The C. V. Mosby Co.

Lawton, E. B.: Activities of daily living for physical rehabilitation, New York, 1963, McGraw-Hill Book Co.

Lichtenstein, L.: Bone tumors, ed. 4, St. Louis, 1972, The C. V. Mosby Co.

MacBryde, C. M., and Blacklow, R. S.: Signs and symptoms, ed. 5, Philadelphia, 1970, J. B. Lippincott Co.

Matheney, R. V., and Topalis, M.: Psychiatric nursing, ed. 5, St. Louis, 1970, The C. V. Mosby Co.

Metheny, N. M., and Snively, W. D.: Nurses' handbook of fluid balance, Philadelphia, 1967, J. B. Lippincott Co.

Miller, B. F., and Blackman, C. B.: Encyclopedia and dictionary of medicine and nursing, Philadelphia, 1972, W. B. Saunders Co.

Modell, W., Schwartz, D. R., Hazeltine, L. S., and Kirkland, F. F.: Handbook of cardiology for nurses, ed. 5, New York, 1966, Springer Publishing Co., Inc.

Pack, G., and Irving, A., editors: Tumors of the soft somatic tissues and bone, vol. 8, ed. 2, New York, 1964, Paul B. Hoeber, Inc.

Paul, H.: The control of diseases (social and communicable), ed. 2, Baltimore, 1964, The Williams & Wilkins Co.

Pitorak, E. F., Hudak, C., O'Gureck, J., and Hanusz, P. P.: Nurse's guide to cardiac surgery and nursing care, New York, 1969, McGraw-Hill Book Co.

Podair, S.: Venereal disease: man against a plague, Palo Alto, Calif., 1966, Fearon Publishers, Lear Siegler, Inc.

Raney, R. B., Sr., and Brashear, H. R., Jr.: Shands' handbook of orthopaedic surgery, ed. 8, St. Louis, 1971, The C. V. Mosby Co.

Rehabilitative aspects of nursing—a program instruction series: Part I. Physical therapeutic nursing measures. Unit 1. Concepts and goals, 1966; Unit 2. Range of joint motion, 1967. Available at National League for Nursing, 10 Columbus Circle, New York, N. Y. 10019.

Reported tuberculosis data, Public Health Service Pub. no. HE-20-28 13, p. 971, Washington, D. C., 1971.

Robinson, J. O.: Surgery, Boston, 1965, Little, Brown & Co.

Rusk, H. A.: Rehabilitation medicine, ed. 3, St. Louis, 1971, The C. V. Mosby Co.

Safer ways in nursing, New York, 1962, National Advisory Service, National Tuberculosis Association and National League for Nursing.

Saunders, W. H., Havener, W. H., Fair, C. J., and Hickey, J. T.: Nursing care in eye, ear, nose, and throat disorders, ed. 2, St. Louis, 1968, The C. V. Mosby Co.

Schmeisser, G.: A clinical manual of orthopedic traction techniques, Philadelphia, 1963, W. B. Saunders Co.

Schwartz, D.: The elderly ambulatory patient: nursing and psychosocial needs, New York, 1964, The Macmillan Co.

Secor, J.: Patient studies in medical-surgical nursing, Philadelphia, 1967, J. B. Lippincott Co.

Secor, J.: Patient care in respiratory problems, Philadelphia, 1969, W. B. Saunders Co.

Shafer, K. N., Sawyer, J. R., McCluskey, A. M., Beck, E. L., and Phipps, W. J.: Medical-surgical nursing, ed. 5, St. Louis, 1971, The C. V. Mosby Co.

South, J.: Tuberculosis handbook for public health nurses, ed. 4, New York, 1965, National Tuberculosis Association.

Stewart, H. C. H.: Influenza and other virus infections of the respiratory tract, Baltimore, 1965, The Williams & Wilkins Co.

Top, F. H., Sr., and Wehrle, P. F.: Communicable and infectious diseases, ed. 7, St. Louis, 1972, The C. V. Mosby Co.

Turek, S. L.: Orthopaedics: principles and their application, Philadelphia, 1967, J. B. Lippincott Co.

Watson, J. E.: Medical-surgical nursing and related physiology, Philadelphia, 1972, W. B. Saunders Co.

Williams, R. H., editor: Textbook of endocrinology, ed. 4, Philadelphia, 1968, W. B. Saunders Co.

Williams, S. R.: Nutrition and diet therapy, St. Louis, 1969, The C. V. Mosby Co.

Winter, C. C., and Roehm, M. M.: Nursing care of patients with urologic diseases, ed. 3, St. Louis, 1972, The C. V. Mosby Co.

Periodicals

American Heart Journal
American Journal of Nursing
Cancer, a journal of the American Cancer Society
Journal of American Physical Therapy Association
Nursing Clinics of North America
Journal of Geriatrics
Medical Clinics of North America
Morbidity and Mortality Weekly Reports
Nursing Outlook
Nursing Research
Surgical Clinics of North America
The Journal of Social Casework
World Health

BASIC NURSING PRECEPTS

1. Definitions

A. Comprehensive nursing care—includes functions associated with nursing diagnosis, nursing therapy, maintenance and promotion of health, and rehabilitation for patient and/or his family
   1. Knowledge of and ability to apply

principles from following areas essential
- a. Biophysical sciences
- b. Psychosocial sciences
- c. Psychiatric nursing
- d. Pathology
- e. Fundamentals of nursing
- f. Rehabilitation

2. Inherent in medical-surgical nursing, since varying levels of adaptation may occur on different levels of organization within the individual
- a. Biochemical
- b. Cellular
- c. Organic
- d. Psychological
- e. Interpersonal or social

3. Includes primary, secondary, and tertiary prevention

B. Medical-surgical nursing—includes
1. Therapy specifically aimed at
- a. Curing sick individual
- b. Modifying course of disease so that progress is slowed and disability limited
- c. Modifying effects of disease so that person is maintained in as active and comfortable state as possible for as long as he lives

2. Primary, secondary, and tertiary prevention

2. Concepts of adaptation

A. Ranges on a spectrum from positive to negative
1. Maintenance of homeostasis without undue effort
2. Maintenance of homeostasis, with effort required
3. Damage or loss at any level of organization that requires development of compensatory adaptive mechanisms
4. Compensatory adaptive mechanisms as a problem
5. Total decompensation

B. Varying levels in same individual—age, heredity, environment

C. Interrelatedness of categories of all levels —entire organism, time, flexibility, economy of energy

D. Dynamic mobility from one level to another

E. Affected by problems of living
1. Genetic
2. Evolutionary history
3. Social innovation
4. Cultural innovation

5. Environment—external, internal
6. Technologic changes
7. Aging
8. Disease (chronic) and disability

F. Levels of comprehensive nursing care in medical-surgical nursing (each level includes previous nursing care)
1. Maintenance of homeostasis without undue effort
- a. Promotion of health
  - (1) Teaching
  - (2) Role model
  - (3) Therapeutic environment
- b. Prevention of disease
  - (1) Immunizations
  - (2) Identifying potential stress areas and planning approaches to prevent stress

2. Maintenance of homeostasis under stress, with effort required
- a. Observation
  - (1) Signs and symptoms
  - (2) Adaptive capacity of individual
- b. Therapy
  - (1) Maintenance at positive adaptive level—content of environment
  - (2) Restoration to stage of homeostasis without undue effort

3. Damage or loss at any level of organization, requiring adaptive mechanisms
- a. Support the positive adaptive mechanism to prevent further stress
- b. Intervene when adaptive mechanism is stressful
- c. Identify and meet dependent needs
- d. Assist in moving toward independence

4. Adaptive mechanism as a stressor
- a. Prevent additional stress
- b. Assist patient to recognize that adaptive mechanism is the stressor and help to cope with the negative adaptation, changing to a more positive adaptation

5. Adaptation is impossible
- a. Nursing evaluation of how long an individual can be maintained in a reasonably comfortable and useful state
- b. Support of family
- c. Recognize own negative adaptive mechanism toward death

3. **Etiologic factors or stressors**
A. Factors that cause stress by virtue of their physical and/or chemical properties
   1. External—physical or chemical factors that may impinge on man from the external environment; examples: mechanical forces, poisons, heat, cold, radiation, electricity, etc.
   2. Internal—substances formed or forces developed within the body that alter or injure by virtue of change in quantity or location; examples: excess insulin, action of gastric juice on esophagus, increased intracranial pressure, excess or increase in hormones, growth change, etc.
B. Factors that cause stress by being insufficient or unavailable
   1. Deficiency state—an interference with the essential elements the organism must obtain from the environment
      a. Oxygen
      b. Water
      c. Electrolytes
      d. Nutrients
      e. Vitamins
      f. Others
   2. Insufficiency state—an interference with the production or utilization of essential substances formed in the body
      a. Hormones
      b. Enzymes
      c. Others
C. Factors that cause stress by stimulating the body's rejection mechanism; examples: microorganisms, parasites, foreign proteins, etc.
D. Psychological factors
   1. Actual or threatened, real or imaginary loss of psychic objects
      a. Relationships with significant adults
      b. Role alterations
      c. Short- or long-term goals
      d. Valued possessions
      e. Self-image
      f. Ideals—self, religious, social-cultural
   2. Actual or threatened, real or imaginary injury to the body
      a. Infliction of pain
      b. Mutilation
      c. Alteration in body functioning
   3. Actual or threatened, real or imaginary interference with adaptive behavior by which the individual attempts to satisfy either a primary or a secondary drive—results in some degree of stress
      a. Primary drives—inborn needs, mainly physiologic in nature, and largely concerned with vital bodily functions
      b. Secondary drives—acquired needs derived from, and by association with, primary drives; account for emotional responses and formation of attitudes

4. **Understanding individuals with**
A. Inadequate emotional development; see also Chapter 12
   1. Psychoneurotic disorders—anxiety, dissociative, conversion, phobic, obsessive, compulsive reactions, etc.
   2. Psychophysiologic disorders—psychogenic rheumatism, pruritus, hyperventilation syndromes, peptic ulcer, hypertension, migraine, etc.
   3. Personality disorders
      a. Personality pattern disturbances (e.g., schizoid, paranoid)
      b. Personality trait disturbance (e.g., emotionally unstable, passive-aggressive, compulsive personalities)
      c. Sociopathic personality disturbances (e.g., sexual deviate, addict)

5. **Principles of psychiatric nursing essential to care of all patients; see Chapter 12**

6. **Knowledge of deviate patterns of behavior and related nursing care essential; see Chapter 12**

7. **Nursing the aging patient**
A. Special considerations of developmental tasks of the life cycle and implications for nursing essential
B. Individual does not age at the same rate in all areas
   1. Chronologic age—related to length of time individual has lived; may differ with how individual has actually aged —physically, psychologically, and/or socially
   2. Biologic age—considers the deterioration of a mature organism as the result of irreversible changes that occur with time and are intrinsic to all members of the species
   3. Psychological age—considers the adaptive capacity of the individual and his reactions to, and concepts of, himself as an individual; result of behavior patterns and attitudes that have developed over a lifetime

4. Social age—considers the role and social habits of the individual as they relate to the expectations of his peers and society

C. Aging patient
  1. Normal changes
    a. Physiologic patterns
      (1) Decrease in number of cells in the body, with some decrease in efficiency of organs
      (2) Gradual decline in activity and acuity of the senses
      (3) Delay in speed of reactions
      (4) Decrease in the basal metabolic rate
      (5) Loss of elasticity of skin and blood vessels
      (6) Skin drier and thinner
    b. Psychological developments
      (1) Major developmental tasks—coping with grief and bereavement and also adapting to changes in family constellation
      (2) Learning takes place at a slower rate
    c. Sociologic patterns
      (1) Retirement with reduction in income
      (2) Reduction in social activities
  2. Problems resulting from normal aging
    a. Greater susceptibility to accidents
    b. Decrease in ability to recover from acute illness
    c. Difficulty in accepting failures in achieving life's goals
    d. Difficulty in accepting changes that occur with age; greater chance of economic dependency
  3. Common complicating factors
    a. Existence of several chronic diseases that may have developed gradually
    b. Chronic brain deterioration
  4. Understanding nursing care especially required for
    a. Basic needs of elderly
      (1) Include security, sense of belonging, some occupation, and someone to love
      (2) Never to be treated as children; helped to maintain sense of dignity and respect
      (3) To be encouraged to maintain independence
    b. Personal and hygienic needs
      (1) Fewer baths but special skin care
      (2) Diet adjusted to patient's ability to chew and/or digest certain foods
      (3) Special devices and care for certain senses usually needed
      (4) Sedation for sleep frequently undesirable (increases cerebral anoxia); warm drink or quiet conversation may be more effective
      (5) Light exercise essential, since inactivity produces atrophy and contractures
    5. Nurse should know financial aid available for needy: Social Security, old age assistance funds, aid for totally disabled, aid for blind
    6. She should be aware of, and help patient to use, community agencies and other services

8. **Infection of some type (bacteria, viruses, protozoa, helminths, and fungi) basic in pathology of many diseases**
  A. Infection—invasion of organ by pathogenic microorganism; to prevent serious infection, microorganism must be prevented from invading organ or from flourishing in sufficient quantities to produce disease; staphylococci responsible for most human skin infections (see B through K)
  B. Etiology—several phase types of *Staphylococcus aureus*
  C. Transmission—method unknown; believed to be direct contact with infected patient, environmental transmission undetermined; asymptomatic carriers considered possible; newborn, surgical, maternity, and elderly debilitated patients at high risk
  D. Incubation period—indefinite; from 24 hours to several weeks
  E. Manifestations—range from cutaneous lesions to fatal bacteremia; typical finding, a purulent lesion; hospital-acquired infection a major problem
  F. Diagnosis—bacteriologic examination of exudate from lesion; smears, cultures, and slide tests
  G. Systemic care of infections
    1. Constitutional rest—heart, lungs, and alimentary tract (soft, easily digested foods)
    2. Mental and emotional rest
    3. Adequate elimination
      a. Encourage fluids, but watch output, since kidneys may be damaged

b. Mild cathartics only if necessary
4. Relief of pain
5. Antibiotics when indicated
H. Local care of infections
   1. Rest part
   2. Elevate part, if possible
   3. Apply moist heat
   4. Antibiotics and chemotherapy to relieve infections
I. Systemic infections exist when pathogenic microorganism, its toxins, or products of tissue destruction are absorbed into bloodstream in sufficient quantities to produce generalized reaction
   1. Symptoms include
      a. Markedly elevated temperature
      b. Anorexia
      c. Chills
      d. Delirium
      e. Rapid pulse
      f. Increased white blood count
      g. Increased sedimentation rate
   2. Care of systemic infections
      a. Includes systemic care
      b. May also include local care
J. Nursing—strict isolation and medical asepsis (gown, mask, gloves to change dressings, thorough hand washing); care depends on specific diagnosis; release from isolation based on bacteriologic examination
K. Prevention—no immunization; hazard increases with extensive surgical procedures and prolonged anesthesia
   1. Surveillance and supervision by infection control committee
   2. Increased emphasis on hand washing
   3. Bacteriologic study of hand lotions for contamination by gram-negative bacteria
   4. When 2 or more cases occur at the same time, considered to be a serious problem; all cases reportable to the Public Health Department
L. Brucellosis (undulant fever), Bang's disease in animals—a disease of animals transmitted to humans; 188 cases in 1972 in the United States
   1. Etiology—a coccobacillus
   2. All forms pathogenic for man—include *Brucella melitensis, Brucella abortus, Brucella suis*
   3. Transmission—inoculation by handling infected animals, carcasses, or excreta, or by ingestion of infected milk and milk products

4. Incubation period—days to months
5. Symptoms—fever 101° to 105° F., aching, splenomegaly, enlarged liver, anorexia, nausea, vomiting, abdominal pain, malaise, intestinal bleeding, neurologic symptoms; (disease marked by remissions and exacerbations)
6. Diagnosis—agglutination tests; cultures of blood, feces, urine, sputum; biopsy of lymph nodes and bone marrow
7. Treatment—bed rest, broad-spectrum antibiotics, analgesics, corticosteroids
8. Nursing—isolation; disinfection of vomitus, stools, urine; emotional support
9. Prevention—testing of dairy cattle, immunization of calves, pasteurization of milk, interstate and international control of domestic animals and feed materials

9. **Wounds and healing process**
A. Classification according to
   1. Presence or absence of microorganisms—clean, contaminated, or infected
   2. Presence or absence of break in the surface tissue—closed or open
   3. Cause of wounds
      a. Mechanical
      b. Chemical
      c. Heat
      d. Cold
      e. Pathogenic organisms
   4. Manner of occurrence
      a. Abraded
      b. Contused
      c. Incised
      d. Lacerated
      e. Penetrating
      f. Puncture or stab
B. Inflammation—nature's response to injury, characterized by
   1. Redness
   2. Heat
   3. Pain
   4. Limitation of function
   5. Swelling
C. Suppuration—occurs when pus formed
   1. Abscess—pus contained in membrane or "wall"
   2. Cellulitis—infection spreads through lymph channels to other cells; distinguished by "red streaks"
D. Healing—closure of wound
   1. By primary intention—occurs when

"clean" wound heals by direct union, with minimal scar tissue

2. By secondary intention—healing by granulation or indirect union; often follows infection

3. By third intention—two opposing granulation surfaces are brought together; occurs when a deep wound either has not been sutured early or breaks down and then is resutured later

E. Factors that promote healing
1. Relief of physical and mental discomfort
2. Rest for part affected
3. Adequate nutrition, especially protein, and vitamins K and C
4. Absence of infection
5. Adequate blood supply to area
6. Normal blood-clotting time
7. Careful asepsis

F. Factors that retard healing
1. Anemia
2. Debris of any kind in wound
3. Lowered body resistance—malnutrition, disease, etc.
4. Lack of electrolyte balance
5. Abnormal blood conditions
6. Movement of part
7. Age
8. Edema
9. Hormones
10. Irradiation

10. Shock
A. Definition—condition of collapse or prostration accompanied by depression of vital functions, especially those of circulation

B. Characteristics
1. May be part of many diseases or functional disorder syndromes
2. Produced by any set of circumstances that affects force of heartbeat, size of vascular bed, or blood volume
   a. Primary—neurogenic or fainting
   b. Secondary or hypovolemic—oligemic, hemorrhagic, traumatic, or surgical
   c. Normovolemic—cardiogenic and septic
3. Must be treated before further treatment of diseases can be undertaken

C. Symptoms
1. Premonitory signs—restlessness, apprehension, and thirst
2. Listlessness and apathy

3. Depression of reflex responses
4. Cool, moist, pale skin
5. Low blood pressure—arterial and venous
6. Weak, thready, rapid pulse
7. Body temperature usually subnormal
8. Change in respiration rate
9. Decreased urinary output
10. Loss of consciousness

D. Treatment and nursing care—depend to some extent on cause
1. Keep patient quiet, head lowered, and body heat maintained
2. Control pain
3. Give fluids unless contraindicated
4. Give oxygen if indicated
5. Restore blood volume; blood transfusion, plasma or plasma expander such as dextran
6. Use drugs with caution; Levophed, Aramine, deoxycorticosterone acetate, Pituitrin, ephedrine, and caffeine–sodium benzoate
7. Position as ordered—head low (Trendelenburg), elevation of lower extremities at 45° angle from hip, or flat
8. Monitor vital signs frequently
9. Keep accurate records of intake and output

11. Hemorrhage
A. Definition—condition in which blood escapes from vascular system—arterial, venous, or capillary
B. May be primary or secondary
C. May be internal or external
D. Treatment
1. Stop loss of blood
2. Restore fluid loss
E. Severe hemorrhage will produce shock, but restlessness, air hunger, and thirst may precede definite shock
1. Control external hemorrhage by pressure, elevation, and cold
2. Nurse's role in control of internal hemorrhage
   a. Chiefly in recognizing symptoms
   b. Keeping patient quiet
   c. Helping to decrease anxiety and fear
F. Blood transfusions may be given; nurse should
1. Be sure correct blood given right patient; check name, type, Rh factor, etc.
2. Keep blood in refrigerator before giving

3. Allow blood to drip slowly
4. Stop blood immediately if these re-actions occur
  a. Restlessness
  b. Pain in back or substernally
  c. Nausea
  d. Generalized pain
  e. Dyspnea
  f. Cyanosis
  g. Rapid pulse or low blood pressure
5. Watch for delayed reactions that may occur a few days later
  a. Jaundice
  b. Hematuria
  c. Urticaria
  d. Fever
  e. Later, nephrosis
6. Inspect first urine specimen after transfusion for gross hemoglobinuria
7. Be responsible for
  a. Recording
    (1) Time begun and ended
    (2) Amount given
  b. Keeping solution running
  c. Observing for reactions
  d. Care of equipment

12. Requirements of patients treated surgically

A. In planning nursing care, the nurse should be aware of the
1. Patient as an individual person
2. Risks to which patient is exposed during this period
3. Relationship between route of approach to the organ or tissue and nursing needs of the patient
4. The involved organ or region of the body
5. Disorder under treatment and the effects of therapy
6. Patient's perception of the nature of this disorder, the therapy, and his prognosis

13. Preoperative nursing care

A. Principles
1. Maintain nutritional adequacy (oral route best)
2. Maintain adequate elimination
3. Help patient accept surgery with as little trauma as possible
4. Maintain cleanliness
5. Safeguard patient's property
6. Prepare patient physically and psychologically as much as feasible for eventual rehabilitation
7. Prepare patient for postsurgical environment and treatments; practice special activities

B. Nutrition and fluids important
1. Lack of adequate nutrition may cause
  a. Lag in healing
  b. Increased tendency to wound dehiscence
  c. Increased tendency to develop
    (1) Decubiti
    (2) Shock
    (3) Infections
    (4) Lack of intestinal motility
2. Protein increased to avoid depletion of body protein and reduction in hemoglobin level (normal 16 gm. per 100 ml.) essential for oxygen transport
3. Vitamins essential
  a. Ascorbic acid
  b. Riboflavin
  c. Thiamin
  d. Nicotinic acid
  e. Vitamin K for prothrombin
4. Dehydration and chemical imbalance cause compensatory shifts in extracellular fluid and disturbance of electrolyte balance; may be accompanied by acidosis

C. Care of patient on operative day
1. Give all emotional support possible
2. Carry out and chart orders meticulously
3. Do not forget that relatives also may need support
4. Make provisions for patient's belongings, including dentures and any other prosthesis
5. Report any change in patient's condition, including mental or emotional distress
6. Be sure that operative permit is signed and attached to patient's chart
7. Accompany patient to operating room and remain until member of the surgical unit receives him

14. Postoperative nursing care

A. Principles
1. Safeguard patient
2. Restore him to maximum health
3. Rehabilitate him to maximum usefulness

B. Immediate postoperative nursing care
1. Place patient in position ordered, always keeping respiratory tree in natural unrestricted position
2. Check vital signs frequently
3. Note all tubes, dressings, and other

devices; be sure to understand their purpose before proceeding

4. Carry out "stat." and standing orders
5. Attach tubes that require attaching
6. Keep intake and output records
7. Change patient's position at least every 2 hours; encourage deep coughing and breathing unless contraindicated
8. Stay with or near patient until full reaction is seen
9. Note and report any signs of complications
10. Reassure relatives

C. Frequent postoperative discomforts
1. Pain in wound
2. Vomiting—nurse should take measures to prevent aspiration
3. Inability to void; patient should be watched for return of urinary function and for retention with overflow
4. "Gas pains" may cause much discomfort and some abdominal distention; this should be differentiated from ileus

15. **Postoperative complications**
A. Wound complications
1. Hemorrhage—inspect dressing at intervals for external bleeding and observe for symptoms of internal hemorrhage
2. Dehiscence—separation of wound, or evisceration—protrusion of viscera
   a. Characteristics
      (1) Pain in wound
      (2) Pinkish, watery discharge
      (3) Perhaps shock
   b. Maintain aseptic technique until surgeon can repair wound
3. Infection—occurs 3 to 4 days after surgery
B. Respiratory complications—many can be prevented by turning patient frequently and by having patient practice deep breathing and coughing
1. Atelectasis—bronchus or bronchiole plugged with mucus or aspirated material
   a. Symptoms
      (1) Dyspnea
      (2) Rise in temperature
      (3) Profuse perspiration
      (4) Restlessness
      (5) Pallor
   b. If obstruction not dislodged by

changing position and coughing, bronchoscopy may be indicated

2. Pneumonia (pneumococcal)—either lobar or bronchial—condition of lungs characterized by exudate in interstitial and cellular portions of lungs; sporadic occurrence, increased incidence during influenza epidemics
   a. Etiology—any of cocci bacteria, Friedländer bacillus, *Haemophilus influenzae;* may be primary or secondary infection
      (1) About 75 immunologic groups; 8 groups cause three fourths of infections
   b. Transmission—direct or indirect contact with droplet infection; carrier transmission possible
   c. Incubation period—24 hours to 3 days
   d. Symptoms include
      (1) Fever
      (2) Pain in chest
      (3) Increased pulse and respirations
      (4) Dyspnea
      (5) Cough
      (6) Cyanosis
   e. Treatment and nursing care
      (1) Mental and physical rest
      (2) Appropriate antibiotic or sulfonamide agents
         (a) Isolate until 24 hours after beginning antibiotic therapy; use concurrent disinfection
      (3) Oxygen
      (4) Fluids
      (5) Relief of pain
      (6) Relief of distention and constipation
      (7) Close observation for complications
      (8) Other medications may include
         (a) Codeine or Hycodan for relief of cough and pain
         (b) Prostigmin for relief of distention
         (c) Chloral hydrate or barbiturates for rest
         (d) Antipyretics if indicated
   f. Complications
      (1) May be serious in any type pneumonia, since it is debilitating disease

(2) Include
  (a) Phlebitis
  (b) Decubitus ulcers
  (c) Urinary tract infections
  (d) Empyema
  (e) Septicemia
  (f) Atelectasis
  (g) Unresolved pneumonia
3. Viral pneumonia (atypical pneumonia)
  a. Etiology—strains of several groups of viruses
    (1) *Mycoplasma pneumonia* causes Eaton pneumonia, a primary atypical pneumonia not of viral origin
  b. Transmission—direct contact with droplet infection
  c. Incubation period—variable; depends on specific virus; may be days to weeks; for Eaton pneumonia, 3 weeks
  d. Symptoms—mild upper respiratory tract infection followed by chills, malaise, headache, anorexia, fever, and cough
  e. Complications—rare
  f. Diagnosis—clinical signs, x-ray film of chest; laboratory examinations of little diagnostic value
  g. Treatment—no specific therapy; hydration, bed rest, oxygen for cyanosis, sedative cough mixture
  h. Nursing—same as for bacterial pneumonia, isolation unnecessary
4. Lung infarct—area of necrosis in lung due to obstruction of circulation to area
  a. Symptoms
    (1) Acute, progressive cyanosis
    (2) Dyspnea
    (3) Weak pulse
    (4) Agitation
    (5) Apprehension
  b. Treatment and nursing care include
    (1) Oxygen
    (2) Change of position
    (3) Endotracheal suction
    (4) Chemotherapy
    (5) Aminophylline, I.V.
C. Cardiovascular complications
  1. Pulmonary embolism—obstruction of pulmonary artery; may be rapidly fatal
    a. Symptoms
      (1) Sudden, severe, crushing chest pain

      (2) Severe dyspnea
      (3) Rapid pulse
      (4) Cyanosis
      (5) Apprehension
      (6) Loss of consciousness
    b. Treatment and nursing care
      (1) Immediate administration of oxygen
      (2) Morphine
      (3) Rest
      (4) Anticoagulants
      (5) Reassurance
      (6) Later, diagnosis by electrocardiogram
  2. Circulatory depression—shock (p. 325)
  3. Coronary occlusion—occlusion of coronary vessel
    a. Symptoms
      (1) Crushing pain in chest that may radiate to abdomen and arms
      (2) Cyanosis
      (3) Dyspnea
      (4) Low blood pressure
    b. Treatment and nursing care
      (1) Oxygen
      (2) Morphine
      (3) Mental and physical rest
D. Abdominal complications
  1. Mechanical intestinal obstruction—obstruction that does not permit flow of intestinal contents
    a. Possible causes
      (1) Adhesions
      (2) Tumors
      (3) Volvulus
      (4) Intussusception that usually occurs 1 to 3 weeks postoperatively
    b. Symptoms
      (1) Severe, cramping pains with each peristaltic wave
      (2) Abdominal distention above obstruction
      (3) Projectile vomiting containing bile
    c. Treatment and nursing care
      (1) Gastric suction
      (2) Nothing by mouth
      (3) May require surgery to remove obstruction
      (4) Electrolyte balance needs to be maintained
  2. Paralytic ileus—marked lessening or loss of peristalsis due to overactivity of sympathetic nerves

a. Symptoms
   (1) Acute abdominal distention
   (2) No peristalsis
   (3) General discomfort due to pressure
   (4) Emesis
b. Immediate care
   (1) Abdominal suction
   (2) Measures (including drugs) to stimulate peristalsis
   (3) Parenteral fluids
   (4) Intake and output records important

E. Other complications
   1. Central respiratory depression
      a. Symptoms
         (1) Slow, shallow, or gasping respiration
         (2) Cyanosis or pallor
         (3) Restlessness
         (4) Apprehension
      b. Treatment and nursing care directed toward stimulating respiratory center
         (1) Characteristic procedures
            (a) Oxygen
            (b) Position to promote easy respiration
            (c) No sedation
   2. Laryngeal spasm—spasm of muscles of larynx; in severe cases may entirely obstruct respirations
      a. Symptoms
         (1) Characteristically labored or "crowing" respiration
         (2) Cyanosis
         (3) Rapid pulse
         (4) Restlessness
      b. Treatment
         (1) Oxygen under pressure, given by physician or anesthetist
         (2) Artificial respiration may be given until oxygen obtained

NURSING PATIENTS WITH NEOPLASTIC CONDITIONS

1. **Basic principles of nursing**
A. Objective threefold
   1. To assist in primary and secondary prevention
   2. To achieve complete recovery and return patient to useful life
   3. To make life more endurable when recovery impossible
B. Remember that prevention depends on early recognition and treatment; continuously interpret these concepts
C. Keep patient as active as possible
D. Encourage patient to be independent, especially in regard to personal and distasteful tasks
E. Reactivate pride and self-respect; hope will follow
F. Provide religious activities when desired; "Man shall not live by bread alone"
G. Provide occupational and recreational therapy
H. Ensure that relatives and friends are not afraid of patient's disease
I. Know community resources and help patient and family to use these resources
J. Give relatives special consideration, especially in inoperable cases
K. Rehabilitation vital, especially when mutilating surgery has controlled disease

2. **Neoplasms**
A. Definition—new formations that tend to grow and to persist; that fulfill no function and appear without apparent cause
B. Benign tumors—not dangerous, unless exerting pressure on vital organ and interfering with its function; characteristics
   1. Encapsulation
   2. Localization
   3. Slow growth
   4. Nonrecurrence after removal
   5. Adult type of cells
   6. Closely resemble parent tissue
C. Precancerous tumors
   1. Require observation and treatment if changes occur
      a. In size
      b. In color
      c. In consistency
      d. Ulceration that will not heal
   2. Extremely important to recognize such tumors and alarming changes
D. Malignant tumors—second cause of death in United States today; main examples are cancers of lung, breast, colon and rectum, prostate, stomach, kidney and bladder, uterus
   1. Characteristics
      a. Infiltration
      b. Metastasis
      c. Rapidly multiplying embryonic cells
      d. Progression of symptoms
      e. Local recurrence after removal
      f. Invasive growth

g. Tend to be anaplastic—less differentiated than the normal cells from which they are derived
h. Cause loss of weight and strength, anemia, cachexia, and eventually death
2. Cause or causes of cancer unknown; many theories have considerable substantiative evidence
   a. Embryonal theory
   b. Cell autonomy
   c. Chemical or metabolic
   d. Trauma or chronic irritation
   e. Inherited tendency
   f. Infection—filtrable agent
   g. Glandular imbalance
3. Carcinoma or epithelioma (from entoderm and ectoderm) most common malignant tumor; metastasizes through lymphatic system
4. Sarcoma (from mesoderm) metastasizes very rapidly through bloodstream

3. **Prevention and control**
A. Primary prevention
   1. Eliminating or protecting from carcinogenic agents
   2. Identifying and removing precancerous lesions
   3. Avoiding sources of chronic irritation
B. Nurse can assist by
   1. Supporting research projects
   2. Supporting community efforts to improve environmental conditions
   3. Practicing self-protection in situations where exposure to carcinogens is possible
   4. Observing and reporting precancerous lesions in herself and others; encouraging others to do likewise
   5. Educating the public
   6. Having knowledge of facilities for education and care
C. Secondary prevention—based on identification of a cancer while it is still localized
   1. Warning signals of cancer
      a. Any sore that does not heal
      b. Any lump or thickening in breast or elsewhere
      c. Unexplained bleeding or discharge
      d. Persistent indigestion or difficulty in swallowing
      e. Change in a wart or mole
      f. Persistent hoarseness or cough
      g. Change in normal bowel habits

2. Cancer detection examinations
3. Microscopic and x-ray examinations, endoscopic and tissue examinations
4. Isotopes
   a. Isotope dilution tests—to determine plasma volume or cardiac output
   b. Selective localization (due to increased vascularity)—used in diagnosing brain tumors
   c. Selective uptake—used in helping diagnose thyroid, liver, or renal function
   d. Intestinal absorption—useful in diagnosing various blood dyscrasias
   e. Metabolism of iron—useful in diagnosing various blood dyscrasias
   f. Colloid measurements—help determine regional blood supply

4. **Nursing patients with malignancies**
A. Hygienic care
   1. Special mouth care
   2. Protection of skin with massage and oil
   3. Use of deodorants when indicated
   4. Prevention of infections of lesions
B. Dietetic care
   1. Prevention of malnutrition
   2. Intake and output record
   3. Extreme diligence with patients who have cancer of mouth, neck, esophagus, or stomach
C. Palliative care
   1. Positioning for comfort
   2. Helping prevent complications
   3. Placing patient near someone who will give moral support
   4. Providing light and air
   5. Giving medications as ordered
   6. Keeping dressings clean and odorless
   7. Relieving physical and mental distress as much as possible
D. Guard against complications
   1. Pneumonia and other respiratory conditions due to aspiration
   2. Decubitus ulcers
   3. Malnutrition, cachexia
   4. Hemorrhage
   5. Secondary infection, toxicity
E. Psychological care of utmost importance

5. **Treatment and nursing care**
A. Surgery—used if cancer can be removed or as palliative measure
   1. Operations lengthy and radical; often disfiguring and mutilating
   2. Postoperative care much as for any other major, radical surgery

a. Danger of aspiration great
b. Sepsis and malnutrition often problem
c. Psychological care most important; nurse must
  (1) Have calm, reassuring attitude
  (2) Inspire hope but must never lie to patient
  (3) Divert patient's attention by encouraging visitors, radio, television, books, etc., as condition permits
3. After mutilating surgery such as colostomy or radical mastectomy, rehabilitation important

B. Radiotherapy—used for larger areas that cannot be removed surgically, as palliative measure for inoperable cancers, and sometimes before or after surgery (p. 149)
1. Never speak of "x-ray burns"; tissues given all of therapy advisable and become red, followed by tanning
2. Blistering and peeling (radiodermatitis) or even necrosis may occur if too much given
3. Infections in irradiated areas heal very slowly because of diminished blood supply
4. Many patients develop radiation sickness characterized by
  a. Nausea and/or vomiting
  b. Diarrhea
  c. Headache
  d. Fever
  e. Loss of appetite
  f. Feeling of malaise
  g. Symptoms may be only temporary, lasting from a few days to a week or more
5. X-ray therapy removes hair—usually will grow again
6. Full effects of treatment not evident for about 6 months

C. Radon seeds used for small localized tumors, especially posterior tongue
1. Radon seeds—small tubes filled with radioactive emanations from radium
2. After radiotherapy or radon seed implantation in oral cavity, patient needs special mouth care; secretions greatly diminished
  a. Patient should not smoke
  b. Good oral hygiene and mouthwash at bedside most desirable
  c. Food may have metallic flavor that affects appetite adversely

d. Precautions should be taken to prevent swallowing tubes if tissue sloughs

D. Radium implantations used for local tumors, especially cervix
1. Radium enclosed in metal tubes inserted in affected tissue area
2. Patient needs support, since usually necessary to remain in one position
3. Often causes extremely unpleasant odor
4. Use rubber gloves and long forceps when handling radium; place it in special lead container and return to radiotherapy department
5. Note time for removal carefully
6. May also cause radiation sickness
7. Patient should be instructed in how to care for self after radium therapy to cervix
  a. Report immediately any bladder or bowel dysfunction
  b. Usually advised to take douches at body temperature and report any adverse symptoms
8. Nurse should spend as little time near patient as possible while radium in place

E. Radioactive isotopes—isotopes of elements rendered radioactive combined with substances having same body chemistry; used in diagnosis and treatment of certain types of malignancies
1. Radioactive iodine (I^{131}) given orally; eliminated largely in urine and in small amounts in other body discharges
2. Radioactive gold (Au^{198}) injected into pleural cavity; unless it escapes, requires minimal precautions; rubber gloves worn when applying dressings and isolation precautions observed
3. Radioactive phosphorus (P^{32}) used in treatment of bone cancer; eliminated chiefly in feces
4. Each hospital using radioactive isotopes has definite routines for safety of patient and nurse; nurse should be familiar with these routines before caring for patients receiving these substances
5. Types of radioisotope therapy include teletherapy, external molds, intracavitary, interstitial and internal irradiation

F. Alkylating agents (mechlorethamine [nitrogen mustard], triethylene melamine [TEM], chlorambucil [Leukeran], busulfan [Myleran], dimethanesulfonoxybutane)—given intravenously to selected patients with Hodgkin's disease, lymphosarcoma, and other types of generalized carcinoma

1. Nitrogen mustard—tissue irritant; characteristically produces nausea, vomiting, extreme malaise that can be helped by sedatives and Thorazine.
2. Complications can be serious; patient should be observed for bone marrow depression, local thrombophlebitis, and toxicity; less toxic drugs being developed for future use

G. Antimetabolites (folic acid and purine antagonists—methotrexate, aminopterin, 6-mercaptopurine) may be used to depress growth of rapidly reproducing cells; toxic symptoms must be watched for
1. Nausea
2. Anorexia
3. Abdominal cramps
4. Ulceration of buccal mucosa

H. Steroid compounds, ACTH, oophorectomy, adrenalectomy, and pituitarectomy —alteration of endocrine environments for tumors arising in organs usually under hormonal control (e.g., prostate [castration] and breast [androgens and estrogens]); toxic signs are
1. Fluid retention
2. Increased libido
3. Hirsutism
4. Nausea
5. Vomiting

I. Miscellaneous drugs—antibiotics (actinomycin D, mitomycin C and streptonigrin); plant alkaloids (vinblastine [Velban] and vincristine [Oncovin]); toxic effects are
1. Nausea, vomiting, leukopenia, skin changes, and epilation (vinblastine, used in Hodgkin's disease)

J. Extracorporeal perfusion—administration of anticancer drug to particular area of body which has been isolated from general systemic circulation
1. Cobalt 60 in special chamber—for operating room; systemic blood occluded from area; oxygenated blood containing drug is introduced into artery, passes through area, and passes out through cannulated vein; systemic circulation then restored

2. Preprocedure care consists of many tests, including bone marrow aspiration, cardiac and renal function, and complete blood studies
3. Postprocedure care is that given any postoperative patient; includes observation for
   a. Hemorrhage at site—anticoagulants used predispose to bleeding
   b. Circulatory disturbances in area— phlebitis, edema, embolism, etc.
   c. Evidence that drug has leaked into general circulatory system— erythema, toxicity, urinary suppression, diarrhea, and reduced leukocytes and thrombocytes
4. Nurse should know nature and purpose of drug used and be aware of complications that might occur
5. Patient needs encouragement throughout process
6. Patient may need protective isolation because of reduced leukocytes and lymphocytes

K. Arterial perfusion with antimetabolic chemotherapy—usually used in conditions that have not responded to other therapy
1. Usually given to patients with malignancies of cranial, nasopharyngeal, or oral regions; catheter inserted into external carotid artery
2. Rate of flow and patency of catheter noted carefully
3. Patient watched closely for symptoms of respiratory difficulty (tracheotomy may be necessary) and toxicity due to the drug
4. Complications often unpleasant and/ or serious
   a. Oral ulceration
   b. Renal dysfunction
   c. Reduced leukocytes and lymphocytes
   d. Emotional distress
   e. Epistaxis

L. Total body irradiation—experimental procedure
1. Cobalt 60 in special chamber—for leukemia when other treatment has failed
2. Followed by bone marrow replacement
3. Pretreatment preparation
   a. Antibiotics
   b. Crew cut, shampoo, hexachlorophene bath

c. Antinauseants
4. Posttreatment nursing care
   a. Strict isolation, sterile clothing, linens, etc.
   b. Careful handling, good personal hygiene
   c. Bone marrow intravenously
   d. Understanding and support
5. Complications
   a. If bone marrow does not function, no production of erythrocytes, leukocytes, platelets; patient's blood incapable of destroying bacteria
   b. Emaciation, stomatitis, purpura, petechiae, nervous system involvement, diarrhea, bleeding, death

NURSING PATIENTS WITH RESPIRATORY PROBLEMS

1. Basic principles of nursing

A. Ensure adequate rest; may be disturbed by
   1. Coughing
   2. Pain
   3. Dyspnea
   4. Apprehension
   5. Worry
B. Promote ease in respiration; dyspnea may be found in
   1. Pulmonary conditions
   2. Abnormalities in circulation
   3. Acidosis
   4. Disturbance in mental apparatus—fear, anxiety
C. Provide good ventilation; cool, moist, medicated air may be desirable
D. Maintain adequate nutrition; coughing, expectoration, nausea, and/or a vile taste in mouth may prevent proper intake
E. Maintain adequate oxygen; proper positioning, clearing of air passages, and/or concentrated oxygen may be required
F. Prevent spread of infectious conditions
G. Help patient maintain calm emotional attitude; maintain quiet, cheerful environment
H. Help prevent complications, including secondary infections
I. Help patient understand disease and precautions desirable
J. Help patients with disabling conditions make adjustments necessary to useful life with minimal disability
K. Emphasis on health education, prevention, control, and community concern important

2. Changes seen with respiratory involvement—signs, symptoms, complications

A. Changes in breathing
   1. Dyspnea, apnea, Cheyne-Stokes respirations
   2. Unusual sounds
B. Cough
C. Chest pain
D. Changes in sputum
E. Increased body temperature if infection is present
F. Hypoxia—oxygen deficiency at the cellular level
   1. Causes
      a. Breathing a low-oxygen mixture of gases
      b. Obstructive airway disease and asphyxia
      c. Structural irregularities of the intrathoracic space
      d. Decreased function of respiratory muscles
      e. Respiratory-depressant drugs
      f. Loss of functional pulmonary tissue
      g. Intracranial trauma and infections
   2. Symptoms
      a. Air hunger, dyspnea
      b. Anorexia
      c. Tachycardia with increased cardiac output
      d. Increased systolic blood pressure
      e. Increased renal output
      f. Increased temperature
      g. Nausea, vomiting
      h. Headache
      i. Disorientation
      j. Cyanosis
   3. Treatment aimed at
      a. Alleviating cause
      b. Treating symptoms
      c. Administering oxygen-rich gas mixture
G. Hypercapnia—retention of excessive amounts of carbon dioxide
   1. Causes—same as hypoxia; in addition
      a. Hypothermia and cardiopulmonary bypass procedure
      b. Excessive carbon dioxide inhalation
   2. Symptoms
      a. Confusion
      b. Lessened sensory acuity
      c. Severe respiratory acidosis
      d. Coma
      e. Death
   3. Treatment aimed at
      a. Treating underlying pathology

(handwritten margin notes: "↑ pulse", "↑ CO_2", "hypoxia ↓ O_2", "hypercapnia ↑ CO_2")

b. Improving ventilation
c. Correcting acidosis

H. Hypocapnia—excessive loss of carbon dioxide, due to overventilation
  1. Causes
    a. Hypermetabolism
    b. Excessive stimulation of respiratory center
    c. Salicylate overdosage
    d. Improper use of mechanical respirators
    e. "Voluntary"
  2. Symptoms
    a. Respiratory alkalosis
    b. Marked vasoconstriction, causing cerebral ischemia, skin pallor, and increased cardiac output
  3. Treatment aimed at
    a. Correcting predisposing pathology
    b. Treating the alkalosis
    c. Supplying carbon dioxide by inhalation

I. Acid-base irregularities
  1. Respiratory acidosis—produced by high serum carbonic acid from increased retention of carbon dioxide by the lungs
    a. Can be caused by any of conditions producing hypercapnia
    b. Symptoms—many and varied
    c. Treatment
      (1) Acute—improve ventilation
        (a) Intermittent positive pressure breathing
        (b) Mucolytic, detergent, and bronchodilating agents
        (c) Suction
        (d) Tracheostomy
        (e) Mechanical breathing devices in paralysis of respiratory muscles
        (f) Antibiotics
        (g) I.V. chemical buffers such as Ringer's lactate solution, THAM
      (2) Less severe—breathing exercises to increase pulmonary depth and volume
      (3) If uncorrected, can cause serious derangement of body functions
  2. Respiratory alkalosis—caused by carbonic acid deficit in plasma attributed to increased excretion of carbon dioxide through the lungs
    a. Primary cause—overventilation plus those conditions that cause hypocapnia
    b. Symptoms
      (1) Neuromuscular
      (2) Palpitations
      (3) Vertigo, lightheadedness
      (4) Blurred vision
      (5) Diaphoresis
      (6) Low carbon dioxide tension
      (7) Elevated pH
    c. Treatment aimed at
      (1) Alleviating cause
      (2) Rebreathing expired air
      (3) I.V. administration of Ringer's solution, with added potassium if necessary
      (4) Carbon dioxide inhalation—rarely used—may produce hyperventilation

J. Cyanosis—caused by increase of reduced hemoglobin in superficial capillaries
  1. Causes
    a. Most frequent—cardiovascular disorders
    b. Inadequate ventilation from
      (1) Airway obstruction
      (2) Paralysis of respiratory muscles
      (3) Depression of respiratory center
    c. Emphysema, asthma, pulmonary edema
      (1) Pulmonary fibrosis
      (2) Obesity and severe kyphoscoliosis
      (3) Anxiety and exposure to low environmental temperatures
  2. Mild—may be masked by natural skin pigments or presence of abnormal amounts of bilirubin
  3. Nursing responsibilities include
    a. Identification of physical or emotional influences that induce or increase cyanosis
    b. Minimization of activities that produce or increase cyanosis
    c. Maintaining patent airway
    d. Providing sufficient amounts of oxygen when oxygen therapy is being used
    e. Exercise and positioning as necessary

K. Cor pulmonale—serious condition of right heart failure associated with pulmonary disease due to increased pressure within the pulmonary artery; may be
  1. Acute—result of pulmonary embolism

2. Chronic—result of chronic lung disorder such as emphysema, silicosis, and fibrosis of lung after an infection

3. Signs and symptoms similar to those of congestive heart failure from other causes

4. Treatment aimed at
   a. Relief of lung disorder causing condition
   b. Relieving pulmonary insufficiency
   c. Treating heart failure
   d. Phlebotomy may be indicated

L. Pulmonary edema (p. 339)

3. Causes of irregularities in pulmonary ventilation and pulmonary diffusion

A. Loss of optimal integrity of respiratory muscles
   1. Bulbar poliomyelitis
   2. Myasthenia gravis
   3. Amyotrophic lateral siderosis
   4. Syringomyelia
   5. Tetanus
   6. Electric shock
   7. Drug intoxication
   8. Viruses, infectious diseases of central nervous system
   9. Traumatic injuries
   10. Metastatic lesions

B. Alterations in airway compliance and patency
   1. Chronic obstructive emphysema
   2. Bronchial asthma
   3. Bronchiectasis
   4. Chronic bronchitis
   5. Acute obstructive laryngitis
   6. Foreign bodies, neoplasms, polyps, rhinitis, colds, laryngitis, drowning, food lodged in esophagus

C. Alterations in the length of the upper airway
   1. Tracheostomy

D. Alterations in intrapleural pressure
   1. Spontaneous pneumothorax
   2. Hydrothorax
   3. Hemothorax
   4. Pleurisy
      a. Pleural effusion
      b. Empyema
      c. Fibrinous pleurisy

E. Loss of functioning pulmonary tissue
   1. Pulmonary infarction
   2. Lung abscess
   3. Bronchogenic carcinoma
   4. Pulmonary fibrosis
   5. Pneumoconiosis
   6. Pneumonia

7. Pulmonary tuberculosis
8. Pulmonary edema

F. Alterations in pulmonary capillary pressure
   1. Pulmonary hypertension

G. Alterations in composition of ambient air
   1. Pollution of inhaled air from heavy atmosphere contamination and from cigarette smoking causes serious irritation of respiratory tissues
   2. Preexisting airway disease
   3. Tracheostomy

4. Procedures and diagnostic tests commonly used in respiratory pathology

A. Pulmonary function tests—done with a spirometer and designed to determine ventilation capacity of the lung (vital capacity, residual volume, maximum breathing capacity, etc.)
   1. Special preparation not usually required
   2. Inform patient that he is to have test

B. Roentgenograms

C. Bronchogram—x-ray examination of bronchial tree after a radiopaque dye is instilled
   1. Sedative and atropine given prior to procedure
   2. Meal usually withheld to prevent aspiration from regurgitation
   3. Use of local anesthetic such as cocaine or pontocaine to prevent gagging and coughing when tube is passed nasally
   4. Food and fluids withheld until the effects of local anesthetic worn off
   5. Regimen of postural drainage may be instituted
   6. Surgery may be postponed for 2 months

D. Peroral techniques—examination of the respiratory tract by means of illuminated instrument introduced through mouth
   1. Laryngoscopy
   2. Bronchoscopy
   3. Esophagoscopy
   4. Procedures usually done in semidarkened room under local anesthesia
   5. Preprocedure care concerned with getting patient quiet, very relaxed; given nothing by mouth for 6 to 8 hours previously
   6. Postprocedure care includes observation for laryngeal edema, emphysema, and difficulty in swallowing

E. Thoracentesis—aspiration of fluid from pleural cavity

1. May be therapeutic or diagnostic procedure
2. Done under aseptic conditions
3. May be disagreeable procedure for patient
4. Antibiotics or other medication may be injected

F. Routine examinations of nose and throat require good illumination—natural light best
1. Patient placed in sitting position if possible
2. Babies wrapped in "mummy" sheet

G. Sputum studies—for infection, neoplasm
1. Necessity to be familiar with proper means of collection of specimen
2. Patient should be informed and instructed how to aid in collection

H. Arterial blood analyses—specimens for analysis drawn through an indwelling catheter, usually in radial or femoral artery
1. Oxygen tension (P_{O_2}), if being done to test ventilatory efficiency, should be performed before oxygen therapy is started
2. pH—slight alteration beyond normal limits (7.35 to 7.45) produces serious consequences
3. Carbon dioxide tension (P_{CO_2})

I. Venous blood analysis
1. Carbon dioxide tension
2. Carbon dioxide combining power
3. Carbon dioxide content (carbon dioxide capacity)
4. White blood cell count
5. Red blood cell count
6. Erythrocyte sedimentation rate
7. Lactic dehydrogenase (LDH, SLDH)
8. C-reactive protein test (CRPA)

J. Tuberculin test (Mantoux, tine, Heaf tests)

K. Histoplasmin test

L. Serum electrolytes

M. Nose and throat cultures

N. Isotope lung scanning—for emboli, tumors, or ischemia

O. Biopsies—malignancies
1. Pleural
2. Prescaline and mediastinal
3. Lung

P. Angiography—alterations in vascularity in emphysema, massive embolization, pulmonary infarct
1. Major danger—development of car-

diac arrhythmias as catheter is passed through heart chambers
2. Requires continuous ECG monitoring until catheter is removed

5. **Nursing patients with upper respiratory tract infections**
A. General principles
1. Bed rest if temperature elevated
2. Fluids freely
3. Well-balanced diet
4. Irrigations for pharyngitis or tonsillitis
5. Nose drops used sparingly for relief of discomfort
6. Mild sedatives
7. In some instances, chemotherapy—antibiotics or antihistaminics
8. All irrigations and sprays given with steady, gentle pressure

6. **Diseases of upper respiratory tract**
A. Common cold, or coryza—most prevalent and most infectious of all communicable diseases
1. Symptoms
a. Malaise
b. Aching
c. Sneezing
d. Watery discharge from nose
e. All degrees of severity
2. Complications may be serious
a. Sinusitis
b. Tonsillitis
c. Pharyngitis
d. Laryngitis
e. Tracheitis
f. Bronchitis
g. Pneumonia
h. Rheumatic fever
i. Glomerulonephritis
j. Otitis media
k. Mastoiditis

B. Acute respiratory disease or grippe—severe coryza with elevated temperature

C. Deformities of nose
1. Absence of nose
2. Flattened
3. Bifid
4. Humped
5. Long
6. Crooked
7. Saddle
8. Deviated nasal septum

D. Injuries of nose include various types of fractures and perforation of septum

E. Epistaxis, or nosebleed
1. Requires reassurance

2. Patient kept quiet and in sitting position
3. Application of pressure and/or ice
4. Adrenalin packs or electrocoagulation may be required in severe cases

F. Rhinitis—inflammation of mucous membranes of nostrils; may be acute, chronic, hypertrophic, atrophic, or diphtheric
   1. Complications may be serious; chronic rhinitis frequently continues for life
   2. Various sprays or irrigations may give symptomatic relief

G. Carcinoma of nasal sinuses
   1. Symptoms
      a. Begins insidiously
      b. Resembles cold
      c. Later some bleeding
      d. Much later protrusion of eyeballs or loosening of teeth may occur
      e. No pain until antrum filled with growth
      f. Metastasis to pterygoid region may follow
   2. Treatment
      a. Resection only treatment
      b. X rays or radium may be used as palliative measure

7. **Nursing patients with surgery of upper respiratory tract**

A. Nursing care after submucous resection and/or sinus operations
   1. Patient placed in sitting position and observed closely for edema
   2. Ice compresses placed over nose, and sedative given as needed
   3. Packing usually removed second day, and nostrils gently washed out with warm saline solution
   4. Patient should not blow his nose for few days; then very gently, one side at a time

B. Care of patient with fracture of nose
   1. Symptoms of internal or external hemorrhage should be noted, including spitting or swallowing blood
   2. Nostrils may be packed and ice applied to control hemorrhage
   3. Usually patient kept in sitting position and given sedatives for pain
   4. Nurse should determine that tetanus antitoxin has been given

8. **Pathology of throat**

A. Acute tonsillitis
   1. Symptoms
      a. Pain
      b. Fullness in throat
      c. Difficulty in swallowing
      d. Marked temperature elevation
      e. Generalized aching
      f. Swollen pharynx, tonsils, palate, and uvula
   2. Often forerunner of other diseases
      a. Acute rheumatic fever
      b. Scarlet fever
   3. Conservative treatment
      a. Warm irrigation
      b. Ice collar
      c. Antibiotics
      d. Fluids
      e. Sedatives
   4. Indications for tonsillectomy
      a. Repeated attacks
      b. Earache
      c. Cervical adenitis
      d. Rheumatic heart due to infected tonsils
      e. Tonsils from which pus can be expressed
      f. Mechanical obstructions

B. Injuries to larynx—death may occur from asphyxiation—should be kept with face down to prevent blood from entering trachea

C. Obstruction of larynx in addition to tumors and injuries
   1. Foreign bodies—removed with bronchoscope
   2. Paralysis of recurrent laryngeal nerve due to trauma, surgery, injury; tracheotomy may be necessary for severe dyspnea
   3. Laryngeal spasm or laryngismus stridulus in children after tetanus or head injuries
   4. Chronic stenosis of larynx due to narrowing by scar tissue

D. Stridor—important symptom in laryngeal pathology
   1. Inspiratory stridor—characterized by hoarse or windlike blowing and incoordination of muscles of glottis; "crowing" sound
   2. Expiratory stridor—breath expelled with "grunt," neck often looks swollen

E. Carcinoma of larynx manifested by hoarseness that becomes progressively worse; cough, discomfort, and dyspnea much later; pain very late
   1. Types
      a. Intrinsic—on vocal cords; cords become infiltrated and fixed; finally

grows beyond cord region to fill larynx and blocks airway; low-grade type malignancy

b. Extrinsic—arises from epiglottis; spreads rapidly and metastasizes to regional lymph glands, airway, esophagus, and deep structures of neck to form one indurated, ulcerating mass

2. Treatment

a. In surgical cases

(1) Laryngectomy done with permanent tracheostomy

(2) Trachea sutured to surrounding skin

(3) Nursing care

(a) Tracheostomy care (see next column)

(b) Teaching patient to manage own tracheostomy and to accept disability

(c) Assisting patient in learning esophageal speech

b. In inoperable cases

(1) Patient may be given repeated doses of x rays as palliative measure

(2) Nursing care includes all principles of caring for patient with malignancy (p. 329)

9. **Nursing patients with surgery of throat**

A. Nursing care of patient with tonsillectomy

1. Careful observation for symptoms of internal or external hemorrhage principal nursing responsibility

2. Patient placed in position to facilitate drainage: children on abdomen or right side; conscious adults in Fowler's position

3. Adults may be given ice collar, may chew Aspergum

4. Discourage coughing and clearing of throat; liquid or nonirritating diet given; any elevation of temperature noted

5. Some patients will have earache for few days

6. Follow-up examination should be done about 1 week later

B. Nursing tracheotomized patient (always remember that patient under great mental and emotional strain)

1. Preoperative care

a. Complete explanation to patient

b. Preparation of room for patient's return

(1) Suction apparatus

(2) Sterile tracheotomy set

(3) Pad

(4) Pencil

(5) Materials for cleansing inner cannula

2. Postoperative care

a. Positioning in dorsal recumbent, semi-Fowler's position with sandbags to hold head steady

b. Observation

(1) For respiratory embarrassment

(a) Increased respiratory rate

(b) Change in sound—crowing or wheezing

(c) Restlessness and apprehension

(d) Indrawing respirations—first noticed at suprasternal fossae, in soft tissues around clavicles, and in intercostal spaces

(2) For color changes—pallor to cyanosis

(3) For excessive edema

(4) For persistent hemorrhage

(5) For aspiration

c. Suction inner cannula every 10 to 15 minutes and p.r.n. and remove and clean inner cannula p.r.n.; give continuous emotional support, meticulous oral hygiene

d. Humidification of respiratory tract necessary—by atomizer, nebulizer, or steam

e. Do not encourage patient to talk first few days

f. Gradually close opening with cork or stopper to decannulize

g. For permanent tracheostomy, patient taught how to adjust to tube and how to care for it; warned not to go swimming or take showers, to avoid infections, and to carry dilator at all times

h. When larynx removed, patient needs speech therapy

10. **Diseases of bronchi and lungs**

A. Bronchitis—acute or chronic inflammation of bronchial tree

1. Symptoms of acute bronchitis

a. Headache

b. Malaise

c. Chilliness

d. Hoarseness

e. Elevated temperature

f. Muscular aches
g. Cough
2. Treatment
   a. Same as for cold, and symptomatically
   b. Antibiotics may be used
3. Chronic bronchitis may result from repeated attacks of acute infections
   a. Symptoms
      (1) Irritating morning cough
      (2) Production of sputum
      (3) Later, dyspnea
   b. Pneumonia most frequent complication of bronchitis; usually some degree of bronchiectasis develops
   c. Protection from extremes in weather and excessive fatigue essential

B. Bronchiectasis—dilatation of walls of bronchi
   1. Symptoms
      a. Cough
      b. Expectoration
      c. Foul breath
      d. Hemoptysis
      e. In severe cases, elevated temperature
   2. Surgical treatment—removal of portion of lung
   3. Conservative treatment
      a. Postural drainage twice daily
      b. Antibiotics
      c. Rarely, bronchoscopy to remove mucus plugs
      d. Nurse should remain with patient during severe coughing spells

C. Pleurisy—inflammation of pleural serous membrane; pain characteristic symptom and should be combated because it causes shallow breathing and sets stage for lung pathology

D. Pleural effusion—collection of fluid in pleural cavity; reduces negative pressure (normally 14 pounds on inspiration and 81 pounds on expiration)
   1. Primary pleural effusion may be first sign of disease; secondary pleural effusion is a complication of disease
   2. General care similar to that given patients with respiratory conditions
      a. Antibiotics may be effective
      b. Thoracentesis may be necessary

E. Pneumothorax—air in pleural cavity—may be induced (therapeutic), traumatic, or spontaneous
   1. Tension pneumothorax occurs when opening into pleural cavity will admit air, but will not let it out; air rapidly accumulates in cavity with high positive pressure
      a. Air must be prevented from entering pleural cavity, by any means available, or patient may die
      b. Results in cardiac displacement, pressure on vena cava, downward displacement of diaphragm
   2. Spontaneous pneumothorax may be due to pulmonary disease or may occur in apparently healthy persons
      a. Symptoms include sudden chest pain, dyspnea, sometimes sensation of rubbing without pain
      b. Limited activity for few weeks usually sufficient treatment

F. Hemothorax—presence of blood in pleural cavity

G. Empyema—presence of pus in pleural cavity
   1. Symptoms—those of primary disease; also
      a. Chest discomfort
      b. Dyspnea
      c. Malaise
      d. Cough
      e. Elevated temperature
      f. Elevated leukocyte count
   2. Treatment—elimination of infective organism; may be accomplished by
      a. Chemotherapy
      b. Thoracentesis—aspiration
      c. Closed or open drainage
      d. Thoracoplasty
   3. Exercises to prevent deformities should be instituted

H. Pneumonia (see Postoperative complications, p. 327)

I. Pulmonary edema—sudden or gradual escape of serous fluid from capillaries into lung tissue, alveoli, bronchioles, often bronchi
   1. Causes
      a. Mechanical forces
      b. Infections
      c. Toxins
      d. Diseases of central nervous system
      e. Pregnancy
      f. Shock
      g. Others
   2. Symptoms appear gradually or suddenly
      a. Feeling of apprehension
      b. Pain in chest

c. Rapid breathing with dyspnea or orthopnea

d. Short cough with copious frothy or bloody fluid

e. Feeble pulse

f. Bubbling rales

g. Eventually, falling temperature and blood pressure

3. Treatment varies with cause, but fluid must be removed from respiratory tree or patient cannot survive

4. Nursing measures

a. Intratracheal suctioning

b. Administration of oxygen

c. Positioning to facilitate drainage

d. Measures to relieve apprehension

e. Special mouth care

J. Pulmonary emphysema—alveoli of lungs become overdistended and rupture or become filled with air or fluid

1. Caused by any condition that causes loss of elasticity of pulmonary alveoli and eventually interferes more with expiration than inspiration

2. Symptoms begin insidiously and progress

a. Shortness of breath

b. Puffiness

c. Moderate cyanosis

d. Dyspnea

e. Edema of extremities

3. Treatment—oxygen, chemotherapy, bronchodilators, and intermittent positive pressure breathing; tracheobronchial drainage; no cure

4. Nursing care

a. Teaching patient importance of prevention of infections

b. Limitation of exertion

c. Abdominal support

d. Exercises to promote force of exhalations

K. Atelectasis—pressure on alveoli of lungs causing collapse; many causes; complication of variety of medical conditions and procedures

1. Degree of severity of symptoms varies widely; ranges from no symptoms, if only small portion of lung involved to severe symptoms if large area involved

2. Symptoms of massive involvement

a. Diminished or absent respirations

b. Chest wall flat

c. Intercostal spaces narrowed

d. Heart, mediastinum, and diaphragm moved toward affected side

e. Sudden dyspnea

f. Prostration

g. Pain in lower part of chest

h. Anxiety

i. Temperature elevated

j. Pulse rate increased

k. Respiration increased

l. Elevated leukocyte count

3. Nursing duties

a. Moving patient from side to side

b. Encouraging deep breathing

c. Reassuring patient

d. Assisting doctor

L. Pneumoconiosis—pathology of lungs due to inhalation of injurious dusts

1. Degree of symptoms varies greatly in relation to both severity and time of appearance

2. More common harmful dusts

a. Silica—inhalation causes silicosis; nodules may encroach on vital lung tissue; serious complications include emphysema, cor pulmonale, congestive heart failure

b. Coal dust—accumulation around pulmonary blood vessels results in serious complications, including emphysema, cor pulmonale, massive consolidation

c. Asbestos or fibrous particles—produce interstitial fibrosis of lungs resulting in dyspnea, cor pulmonale, cardiac failure

M. Tumors of lungs—carcinoma most important malignancy

1. Symptoms insidious—72% develop between ages of 40 and 72 years; only early symptom, persistent cough with ordinary mucoid or mucopurulent sputum

2. Treatment—surgical: lobectomy or pneumonectomy

3. Benign growths cause little damage

N. Tuberculosis

1. Infectious disease caused by one of several closely related mycobacteria, including *M. tuberculosis, M. bovis,* and *M. avium;* usually involves lungs but also involves, and sometimes produces gross lesions in, other organs and tissues; distribution worldwide; one of most important communicable diseases: 33,635 new active cases reported in the United States in 1972

2. Atypical mycobacteria—produce pul-

monary disease that is undistinguish-able from tuberculosis (Runyon's classification)

a. Found in various geographic locations

  (1) Group I, *M. kansasii* (photochromogens), widely distributed

  (2) Group II, scotochromogens, found in soil and water

  (3) Group III, Battey bacillus, southeastern United States, mainly Georgia

  (4) Group IV, *M. fortuitum* (rapid growers)

b. Respond poorly to antituberculosis drugs; often require surgery

c. Not believed to be airborne; isolation not required

d. Occur most commonly in persons in high socioeconomic areas

e. More common in men than women; more in middle-aged or older

f. Patients usually on chemotherapy for at least 2 years; careful medical follow-up required

g. May have infection with both typical and atypical bacteria at same time

3. Transmission—inhalation of tubercle bacilli into lungs: droplet nuclei from air; droplet infection questionable, dust-borne transmission uncertain

4. Predisposing factors—environmental, socioeconomic, familial (habits, attitudes, defense mechanisms, and immunologic factors)

a. Urban environment—increased incidence, serious problem in large cities

b. High incidence in slums, ghettos, reduced financial resources

c. Occupational groups at special risk: doctors, nurses, health workers, and workers in occupations with dust, coal, asbestos, silicone

d. Family disease—family members 3 to 4 times more likely to have disease if contact with case in family

e. Attitudes—social stigma of tuberculosis causes delay in examination; developing habits of preventive measures often difficult

f. Lowered resistance to infection—poor food habits, loss of sleep, respiratory infections, overwork, fa-tigue, teen-age pregnancy, frequent pregnancies, debilitating diseases, mental stress and illness

g. Evidence of immunity—not conclusive

5. Pulmonary tuberculosis

a. Primary infection

  (1) Tubercle bacilli may be deposited in any part of lung parenchyma; nearly always in hilum and mediastinal lymph nodes

  (2) May heal with no recognized symptoms—resolution, calcification

  (3) May be progressive with bronchogenic spread to other lung areas

  (4) May spread by lymph or blood vessels, causing generalized infection

  (5) Miliary tuberculosis, tuberculous meningitis, or death may occur

  (6) Estimated that 5% of persons with healed primary lesions will develop active tuberculosis sometime in their lives

b. Postprimary tuberculosis

  (1) May be exogenous—new infection from without

  (2) May be endogenous—breakdown of primary infection

    (a) Rupture of lymph node into bronchus

    (b) Lymphatic or bloodstream spread from lung node

    (c) May occur months or years after initial lesion

  (3) Lesions in apex of lung or other areas of parenchyma; rarely in mediastinal nodes

  (4) Fibrosis and cavity formation

  (5) Productivity and contiguous spread

  (6) Healing by fibrosis partly or completely fills cavity, or cavity is filled with caseous material; some cavities remain open and clean

c. Extrapulmonary tuberculosis—decreasing due to animal control and chemotherapy

  (1) Generalized hematogenous spread may involve every organ and tissue in body

(2) Miliary tuberculosis may involve lungs, spleen, kidneys, bones, other organs; more common in children

(3) Tuberculosis of bones, joints—a result of hematogenous spread or *Mycobacterium bovis*

    (a) Rapid destruction of bone with abscess formation; spine, hip, knee frequent sites (p. 424)

6. Complications—usually result of active progressive pulmonary tuberculosis

a. Hemoptysis — varies from blood-streaked sputum to massive hemorrhage; always a medical emergency

b. Spontaneous pneumothorax—tuberculosis empyema may result

c. Pleurisy with effusion

d. Tuberculosis laryngitis

e. Chronic lung disease may coexist with pulmonary tuberculosis

7. Classification of tuberculosis — may vary throughout course of disease

a. Extent of disease

(1) Minimal—no cavitation

(2) Moderately advanced—one or both lungs; no cavitation, or cavity less than 4 cm.

(3) Far advanced—lesions with cavitation progressed beyond moderately advanced stage

b. Activity of disease—evidenced by roentgenographic examination

(1) Active—new lesions and extension of cavitation

(2) Quiescent—lesions and cavities present; no indication of extension

(3) Inactive—lesions healing and bacteriologic findings negative

8. Symptoms

a. Primary tuberculosis—usually none, unless progressive; only a slight cold

b. Postprimary, uncomplicated

(1) Onset insidious: weight loss, malaise, fatigue, night sweats, low-grade fever, cough becoming productive, anorexia, nausea, amenorrhea in women, anemia

(2) Symptoms vary with extent and activity of disease

9. Diagnosis—personal and family history, physical examination, bacterio-logic and roentgenologic examinations, tuberculin testing (Mantoux, Sterneedle; tine test and jet injector)

a. Specific diagnosis must be based on identification of tubercle bacillus; repeated examination may be necessary

(1) Examination of sputum, gastric washings; may include spinal fluid, urine, pleural fluid, and biopsy examinations

(2) Positive when organisms are found; negative—failure to isolate organism after adequate examination

(3) Roentgenologic procedures

    (a) Standard x-ray film of lungs

    (b) Planigram of lungs

    (c) Fluoroscopic examination

    (d) Bronchogram

10. Treatment of tuberculosis—chemotherapy; all patients do not respond to the same drugs or drug combinations

a. Drug sensitivity tests prior to beginning of therapy essential to ensure the most effective treatment

(1) Primary drugs—streptomycin, para-aminosalicylic acid (PAS), isonicotinic acid hydrazide (isoniazid)

(2) Secondary drugs—pyrazinamide, viomycin, cycloserine, kanamycin, ethionamide, ethambutol

b. A typical tuberculosis responds poorly to primary drugs

c. Chemotherapy initiated when diagnosis is made and is continued for 2 years

d. Advantages of chemotherapy

(1) Renders sputum negative and prevents spread of infection

(2) Provides greater success for resectional surgery

(3) Decreases need for prolonged hospitalization

(4) May allow patient to return to employment

(5) Reduces socioeconomic and emotional factors related to prolonged confinement in institution

e. Surgical treatment may be indicated in event medical treatment does not check disease

(1) Pneumonectomy
(2) Segmental lobe resection
(3) Wedge resection
(4) Thoracoplasty
(5) Decortication of lung—surgical removal of fibrinous deposition in pleura
  f. Collapse therapy rarely used today
11. Immunity—present evidence cannot confirm an active immunity resulting from primary infection or from other contact with organism
  a. Artificially acquired active immunity—Bacilli Calmette-Guérin (BCG) vaccine—prepared from viable strains of attenuated tubercle bacillus
    (1) Administered only to persons with negative tuberculin test
    (2) National Tuberculosis Association recommends vaccine be given to specific high-risk groups
      (a) Children in high endemic areas
      (b) Hospital personnel who are at risk
      (c) Tuberculin-negative persons in homes where exposure is possible
      (d) Persons in prisons, mental hospitals where incidence is high
    (3) U. S. Public Health Service does not recommend use of BCG in the United States
12. Nursing care in pulmonary tuberculosis
  a. Special hospital—techniques prescribed by the institution
  b. General hospital—may have communicable disease unit or room; isolation of patients with positive sputum or coughing; medical asepsis, concurrent and terminal disinfection
    (1) Patient to cover nose and mouth when coughing
    (2) Careful collection, handling, and disposal of sputum; sputum cups not recommended
    (3) Disinfection of urine, feces, and vomitus unless public sewerage system available
    (4) Most important factor is good ventilation to disperse droplet

nuclei so they may be carried where they can be killed by sunlight
    (5) Prompt handwashing after patient care or handling sputum, contaminated dressings, or excretions
    (6) Diet high-caloric and well-balanced
    (7) Rest and emotional support
    (8) Terminal cleaning—routine cleaning of room; expose pillows and mattress to sunlight 6 to 8 hours and air room thoroughly
  c. Collection of sputum specimens
    (1) Use container designed for purpose
    (2) Take first sputum raised in morning—prior to patient's brushing teeth, rinsing mouth, or food
    (3) Mark container "contaminated"
    (4) Place container in clean paper bag and send to laboratory
13. Prevention and control
  a. Case finding
  b. Long-term follow-up
  c. Surveillance of high-risk groups
  d. Recommended procedures
    (1) Tuberculin testing of all preschool children, including infants between 6 and 12 months of age; some advise testing all schoolchildren
    (2) Examination of all contacts in new cases of tuberculosis
    (3) Routine chest x-ray film on all hospital admissions
    (4) Tuberculin test, x-ray film if indicated, and prophylactic therapy for all school personnel
      (a) Teachers
      (b) Custodians
      (c) Bus drivers
      (d) Practice teachers
      (e) Nursery school personnel
      (f) Workers in Head Start programs
      (g) Baby-sitters
      (h) All others who have contact with infants and young children
    (5) Administration of prophylactic isoniazid

(a) All tuberculin reactors under 3 years of age
(b) All adolescents with recent infections
(c) Persons of any age whose tuberculin tests have converted from negative to positive
(d) All persons with healed lesions where reactivation is possible
(e) Family contacts in active cases
(f) Individuals with conditions that place them at risk: persons with positive tuberculin test results who are receiving steroid therapy; patients in inactive cases who have diabetes or are pregnant
(6) Medical and nursing students with negative tuberculin tests, retest every 3 months; if conversion occurs have x-ray film and in the absence of disease, isoniazid therapy
(7) Tuberculosis in all forms is reportable to the Public Health Department

11. Nursing patients with chest injuries
A. Intercostal block to control pain often done for fractured ribs, other painful conditions that affect respiration
B. Observe for
1. Hemorrhage and/or shock
2. Infection of pleural cavity
3. Cyanosis, dyspnea
4. Sudden, sharp pain which could indicate bronchopleural fistula
C. Maintain high-caloric, high-protein intake with added vitamins
D. Plasma or blood may be given for fluid volume, protein, or to correct low hemoglobin
E. Oxygen may be given as symptomatic, supportive measure

12. Nursing patients with chest surgery
A. Preoperative care (patients characteristically apprehensive; need assurance and support)
1. Provide pleasant environment with plenty of sunshine and fresh air
2. Provide high-caloric diet with added vitamins
3. Vaccines and antibiotics given as indicated

4. Teach necessity of deep breathing and coughing after surgery; demonstrate correct method
B. Postoperative care
1. Patient usually placed in Fowler's position and turned from back to affected side; position must be changed frequently
2. Observation of vital signs; oxygen given for cyanosis
3. Encourage patient to breathe deeply, cough, splint chest with hands for more comfort when coughing
4. Chart accurately all secretions and drainage, including amount and description
5. Control pulmonary secretions with suction
6. Start exercises early to prevent deformity
C. Closed or underwater drainage—used to promote and maintain negative pressure within pleural cavity
1. Drainage bottle should always be kept below level of patient's body
2. Outside air (atmospheric pressure) must never be permitted to enter circuit—sudden inrush of air could cause death
3. Maintain sterile conditions at all times
4. If pleural pump used, amount of pressure should be carefully regulated (20 cm. pressure)
5. Drainage bottle should be emptied and contents measured, charted at same time of day
D. Common late complications of chest surgery
1. Atelectasis
2. Sepsis
3. Pericarditis
4. Cerebral abscess
5. Deformities, especially scoliosis in thoracotomy patient

NURSING PATIENTS WITH CARDIOVASCULAR PATHOLOGY

1. Basic principles of nursing
A. Maintenance or promotion of adequate supply of oxygenated blood to all parts of body
B. Decreasing burden on heart; increasing efficiency of heart; removal of edema
C. Promotion of a calm, accepting attitude and reduction of fear
D. Teaching patient and/or family how to live with disability

E. Planning with individual for rehabilitation and assisting with implementation of these plans
F. Emphasizing dangers of infection in predisposing to various cardiovascular disorders; important preventive factor
G. Preventing those diseases and conditions likely to cause heart disease
H. Understanding of and help with psychological, social, and economic problems

2. **Nursing patients with cardiac pathology**
A. Essential to gain cooperation of patient
B. Activities regulated according to amount of cardiac damage; absolute bed rest—no physical, mental, or emotional activity
C. Relief of dyspnea important
D. Relief of anxiety—anxiety may produce symptoms of early cardiac failure
E. Drug therapy
   1. Digitalization—one of most common drug therapies used
   2. Diuretics—to increase elimination of intracellular fluids
   3. Nitrates—nitroglycerin, amyl nitrate—to dilate coronary vessels and relieve coronary pain
   4. Morphine—for cardiac distress and to promote rest
   5. Anticoagulants—for prevention of thrombi
F. Acutely ill cardiac patient—requires complete mental and physical rest
   1. Positioned for ease in respiration—usually Fowler's or orthopneic position
   2. Care of skin important, since edema conducive to formation of decubitus ulcers
   3. Light, easily assimilated diet (often sodium-poor) should be given; if patient on complete bed rest, must be fed
   4. Oxygen given for dyspnea; may be given under pressure for pulmonary edema
   5. Sedative, usually morphine, for relief of discomfort and for rest
   6. Complete passive range of motion exercises should be instituted
   7. Severe attacks of paroxysmal cardiac dyspnea demand prompt, energetic treatment
      a. Positioned in upright or orthopneic position
      b. Sedatives given
      c. Atropine or other medication may be ordered for pulmonary edema
      d. Oxygen given immediately
   8. Only very mild laxatives used; straining at stool to be avoided
G. Chronic or compensated cardiac patient needs to observe certain precautions in daily life
   1. Activities regulated, some exercise
   2. Easily digested diet, frequently low-sodium
   3. Cheerful surroundings with minimum stress
   4. Patient and some member of family instructed in what to do in emergency or pain
   5. Patient must understand illness and purposes of health regimen he must follow

3. **Symptoms of cardiac pathology**
A. Dyspnea—breathlessness or shortness of breath; present when one becomes conscious of his breathing—normal on unusual exertion
   1. Different from rapid breathing (tachypnea) in which no feeling of distress and the deep breathing (hyperpnea) of acidosis
   2. As vital capacity decreases, dyspnea increases; dyspnea at rest more indicative of pathology than dyspnea on movement
B. Paroxysmal dyspnea—sudden attacks of dyspnea, often while patient asleep
   1. Occur frequently in cardiac pathology from hypertension, coronary artery disease; aortic insufficiency and aortic stenosis; all diseases that cause strain in left ventricle
   2. Attacks accompanied by tachycardia
C. Orthopnea—more advanced stage of dyspnea, in which patient has great difficulty in breathing in horizontal position
D. Cheyne-Stokes respiration or periodic breathing—due to incoordination of neural and chemical factors that control respirations; results from inability of heart to supply adequate nourishment to brain
E. Edema—retention of water and salt in intracellular spaces; patient may retain 10 to 20 pounds fluid before any objective signs
F. Cough and expectoration—frequent in cardiac patients; cough produced by reflex from congested lungs and bronchi, or, in some cases, may result from

pressure of aneurysm or enlarged left ventricle
G. Hemoptysis—bleeding from lungs or bronchial mucosa frequent in heart failure; in severe pulmonary edema, bloody froth may pour from mouth
H. Anorexia, nausea, and vomiting—especially common in congestive failure; hiccoughs present in myocardial infarction indicate serious prognosis
I. Abdominal pain—in upper right quadrant common symptom of congestive failure, result of enlarged, tender liver
J. Cerebral anoxia—common with symptoms of cerebral dysfunction, but usually does not appear until patient reaches stage of dyspnea at rest
   1. Characterized by
      a. Irritability
      b. Restlessness
      c. Difficulty in fixing attention
   2. Presenting symptoms in myocardial infarction
      a. Changes in personality
      b. Mild delirium
      c. Mental depression
K. Anxiety state—present when person knows he has heart disease
   1. Degree and manner in which anxiety expressed depends on individual
   2. Anxiety may produce symptoms of early heart failure
L. Cardiac pain—appears when metabolism of heart muscle exceeds available blood supply and metabolites increase
   1. Inadequate coronary circulation may occur due to
      a. Narrowing or obstruction of coronary vessels
      b. Cardiac hypertrophy without increase in number of capillaries
      c. Interference with coronary circulation because of aortic insufficiency, aortic stenosis, or advanced mitral stenosis
   2. Cardiac pain typically substernal; radiates down ulnar aspects of one or both arms
   3. A dull precordial ache, tenderness on palpation, may occur in pericarditis or myocarditis
M. Pulse irregularities—the rate usually not affected until it increases in course of complete failure
   1. Collapsing, water-hammer, or Corrigan's pulse; "jerky" pulse with dull

expansion and sudden collapse; frequently found in aortic regurgitation
   2. Extrasystole—premature contraction of one of chambers of heart, independent of normal rhythm; if it originates in ventricles, there may be compensatory pause
   3. Paroxysmal tachycardia—sudden onset and cessation of rapid, regular heartbeats; feeling of faintness, shortness of breath, and apprehension
   4. Fibrillation—irregular and rapid contractions of groups of muscle fibers in auricles, working independently of ventricles
      a. Pulse completely irregular in time sequence and in strength of beat
      b. Pulse deficit
      c. Apical-radial pulse should be taken; indicative of serious cardiac damage
      d. Often controlled with digitalis
N. Pulmonary edema (p. 359)
O. Heart block—occurs when stimuli arising in sinus node or auricles delayed or obstructed in passage; may be due to structural damage, toxic effects of drugs, nutritional changes, or vagal disturbances
   1. First- and second-degree heart block usually not serious
   2. Third-degree heart block causes decrease in cardiac output; function of heart cannot be increased on demand
      a. Symptoms
         (1) Slow, forceful pulse (35 per minute)
         (2) Dyspnea and dizziness on exertion
         (3) Headache
         (4) Weakness
         (5) Fatigue
         (6) Sometimes, syncope
      b. Heart failure may result
P. Murmurs—may or may not be important symptom; when valves become hardened, scarred, or rough, they form obstacles that produce sound as blood passes through
Q. Ventricular fibrillation—rapid, ineffective twitching of the ventricles, resulting from insufficient blood supply to the heart; may occur in coronary disease, during the administration of general anesthesia, or from electric shock
   1. Characteristics

a. Pulse and blood pressure unobtainable
b. Unconsciousness
c. Convulsions
d. Results in death if ventricles cannot be made to contract
e. Important cause of cardiac arrest

R. Cardiac arrest—occurs as result of cardiac standstill (ventricular asystole) or ventricular fibrillation
1. Characteristics
   a. Absence of respirations, peripheral pulse, blood pressure, and heart sounds
   b. Dilatation of pupils
   c. ECG reading incompatible with effective cardiac action
2. Treatment—within 3 to 5 minutes, to avoid fatality or irreversible damage to the brain from anoxia
   a. Maintenance or restoration of respiration by means of artificial respiration and the administration of oxygen
   b. Prompt use of mouth-to-mouth resuscitation at first, followed by insertion of an endotracheal tube and the administration of oxygen intratracheally
   c. External cardiac resuscitation by properly trained individuals
   d. Drug therapy as indicated
   e. Defibrillation

4. **Procedures and diagnostic tests commonly used in cardiac pathology**
A. Cardiac catheterization—small catheter passed through vein in forearm, through superior vena cava, into right auricle, ventricle, and into pulmonary artery for diagnosis of anatomic and functional disorders
   1. Painless procedure, but patient may be apprehensive
   2. Solid food withheld before procedure, and sedatives may be ordered
   3. After procedure, pulse taken frequently for first few hours and patient closely observed for any untoward symptoms
B. Electrocardiogram—record of electric activity of heart muscles, used to determine types of heart damage and amount of myocardial damage
   1. Painless procedure but may be frightening to patient

2. Patient should be relaxed before procedure; no special aftercare
C. Central venous pressure—used as diagnostic procedure or for evaluation of patient's condition after heart surgery
   1. Measured by attaching a pressure-sensitive device to end of small catheter inserted in one of the large veins
   2. Zero point on instrument should be on level with right atrium of heart
   3. Minimum for postsurgical patient 5 to 10 cm. of pressure (saline); may go safely as high as 20 to 25 cm. immediately after surgery
D. Angiocardiogram
E. Arteriogram
F. Ballistocardiogram
G. Laboratory tests
   1. Blood counts
   2. Urinalysis
   3. Sedimentation rate
   4. Blood urea nitrogen
   5. Prothrombin time
   6. Transaminase test
   7. Venous clotting time
H. Pulmonary circulation time—cardiac function test in which speed with which blood circulates through lungs is determined by injecting Decholin in antecubital vein and noting when recipient is first aware of bitter taste
I. Arterial oxygen saturation—cardiac test in which percentage of oxygen in blood specimen is compared with that of aliquot sample fully saturated with air; normal, approximately 95%
J. Vital capacity—maximum volume of air person can exhale; expirogram—graphic recording of expiration, indicating both amount of air and time

5. **Specific cardiac conditions**
A. Developmental heart pathology
   1. Interventricular septal defect—most common congenital cardiac anomaly; defect in interventricular septum may be small or large; no symptoms unless defect large; rarely affects life expectancy
   2. Patent ductus arteriosus—ductus arteriosus between pulmonary artery and aorta remains open
      a. Symptoms
         (1) Murmur
         (2) Retardation of development
         (3) General ill health

(4) Shorter life expectancy (25 years)

(5) Tendency to subacute bacterial endocarditis and heart failure

b. Early surgery only known treatment

3. Coarctation of aorta—narrowing of aorta, which causes increased pressure in left ventricle

a. Symptoms

(1) Higher blood pressure in upper extremities than in lower

(2) Resultant hypertension in upper part of body

b. Unless defect repaired surgically, patient usually succumbs to cerebral vascular accident or to rupture of aorta

c. Inoperable patients should avoid infections and physical exertion and strain

d. Nursing after surgery

(1) General postoperative care

(2) Blood pressure taken in both upper and lower extremities

(3) Careful observation for thrombus formation

(4) Measures to prevent pulmonary infections

4. Tetralogy of Fallot (blue babies)—condition with four defects that result in large proportion of blood not oxygenated

a. Defects

(1) Pulmonary stenosis

(2) Hypertrophy of right ventricle

(3) Interventricular septal defect

(4) Dextroposition of aorta

b. Symptoms

(1) Weakness

(2) Pallor

(3) Increased red blood count

(4) Clubbed fingers

(5) Decreased growth

(6) Susceptibility to infections

c. Surgery (Blalock-Taussig operation) only treatment, but gives dramatic results

d. Child and parents need emotional support

e. Postoperative care especially concerned with maintaining fluid intake; pulse on side of operation not palpable

f. Complications

(1) Hemorrhage

(2) Atelectasis

(3) Failure of heart

5. Transposition of the great vessels—pulmonary artery arises from left ventricle and carries oxygenated blood back to lungs; aorta arises from right ventricle and carries unoxygenated blood into systemic circulation

a. Symptoms

(1) Cyanosis

(2) Clubbing of fingers and toes in older children and adults

b. Surgery (palliative or corrective)

6. Septal defects—arterial or ventricular

a. Surgery only treatment

B. Rheumatic heart disease—defect of valves after rheumatic fever; scarring of mitral valve most common defect

1. Rheumatic fever—produced by products of hemolytic streptococci; particularly common between ages of 4 and 30 years

a. Symptoms

(1) Migrating pains

(2) Tenderness

(3) Swelling of joints

(4) Chorea

(5) Inflammation of heart

(6) Increased sedimentation rate

b. Nursing care

(1) Bed rest

(2) Salicylates

(3) Antibiotics

(4) Care of complications

(5) Prevention of infection

(6) Child kept quiet during acute period

2. Mitral stenosis most common sequela of rheumatic fever

a. Left auricle becomes hypertrophied and congestive heart failure may ensue

b. Mitral commissurotomy may be performed

3. Other complications of rheumatic heart disease

a. Auricular fibrillation

b. Subacute endocarditis

c. Thrombi formation

d. Congestive heart failure

4. Nursing care and treatment of rheumatic heart disease

a. All principles of cardiac care

b. All excessive activity, infections, and emotional stress should be avoided

C. Hypertensive heart disease found in conjunction with vascular hypertension
   1. Characteristics
      a. Hypertrophy of the heart muscle
      b. Ischemia of heart muscle
      c. Finally, heart failure
   2. Nursing care and treatment
      a. Principles of cardiac care
      b. Principles of vascular hypertension care
D. Acute cardiac failure
   1. Failure of left ventricle
      a. Characterized by congestion in pulmonary circuit
      b. Symptoms
         (1) Dyspnea
         (2) Cough
         (3) Moist rales
         (4) Asthmatic breathing or paroxysmal dyspnea followed by blood-streaked sputum and prostration
   2. Failure of right ventricle
      a. Characterized by congestion in systemic circulation
      b. Symptoms
         (1) Engorgement and visible pulsation in neck veins
         (2) Edema of feet and legs
         (3) Engorgement of liver
         (4) Albuminuria
         (5) Cyanosis
   3. Nursing care and treatment
      a. Principles of cardiac care
      b. Absolute physical and mental rest
      c. Head elevated
      d. Cool room
      e. Chemotherapy
      f. Oxygen
      g. Apical and radial pulse (note deficit)
      h. Record fluid intake and output
      i. Record daily weight of patient
E. Syphilitic heart disease—usually involves aorta: aortitis, aortic insufficiency, or aortic aneurysm
   1. Penicillin may arrest disease, but will not reverse damage
   2. Treatment and nursing care symptomatic; patient must learn to live in manner that will not overburden damaged heart
F. Coronary heart disease—greatest single health problem in the United States
   1. Angina pectoris—probably due to temporary inadequacy of blood supply to cardiac muscles
      a. Characterized by paroxysmal attacks of severe pain that radiate down arm; may be triggered by exertion
      b. Patient must learn to live within his capacity, since any attack can produce more serious complications
         (1) Avoid stress and emotional episodes; any emotional upset may cause attack
         (2) Reduce if overweight
         (3) Periodic rest cures beneficial
      c. Nitroglycerin or amyl nitrate specifics for condition; aminophylline I.V. may be necessary in severe attacks
   2. Myocardial infarction—due to blocking of coronary artery; severity depends on amount of interference in cardiac function
      a. Characteristics
         (1) Severe, viselike, substernal pain
         (2) Restlessness
         (3) Apprehension
         (4) Dyspnea
         (5) Cyanosis
         (6) In severe cases, shock
         (7) Ventricular aneurysm may form first few weeks postinfarct
      b. Treatment and nursing care
         (1) Absolute mental and physical rest
         (2) Sedatives
         (3) Oxygen
         (4) Anticoagulants
         (5) Continuing nursing care
         (6) Surgery for ventricular aneurysm
      c. After recovery from attack, patient should be evaluated for cardiac reserve and classified for work and physical activity as indicated
   3. Surgery (grafts, Vineberg operation) sometimes indicated
      a. Incisional pain postoperatively may be similar to that of anginal pain
      b. Patient will need considerable reassurance and emotional support
6. Complications of cardiac diseases
A. Pericarditis—inflammation of pericardium; may be fibrinous (dry) or serofibrinous (wet)
   1. Symptoms
      a. Pain

b. Dyspnea
c. Pericardial friction rub
2. Pericardial effusion—complication of pericarditis
    a. Characteristics
        (1) Dull pain
        (2) Dyspnea or orthopnea
        (3) Cough
    b. Treatment
        (1) Aspiration of pericardial sac and/or
        (2) Injection of medication
3. Chronic constrictive pericarditis—fibrous adhesions between epicardium and pericardium may follow pericarditis
B. Subacute bacterial endocarditis—condition in which pathogenic microorganisms carried by bloodstream invade heart
    1. Symptoms
        a. Recurring attacks of fever
        b. Petechiae
        c. Rapid progression if not treated
    2. Treatment and nursing care
        a. Massive doses of antibiotics
        b. Bed rest
        c. General cardiac nursing
C. Chronic myocardial diseases
    1. Fibrosis of myocardium
    2. Fatty degeneration
    3. Chronic myocarditis
D. Congestive heart failure (myocardial insufficiency, cardiac decompensation)—resulting from some preexisting heart disease, functional or organic
    1. Clinical course variable; pulmonary edema (p. 339) may cause death in few hours
    2. Often patient has successive attacks, increasing in severity and duration
    3. Treatment and nursing care directed toward
        a. Decreasing burden on heart
        b. Increasing efficiency of heart
        c. Removing edema
7. **Cardiac surgery**
May be closed or open; an open-heart procedure employs extracorporeal circulation (cardiopulmonary bypass) to maintain functions of the cardiac and respiratory systems during the operation
A. Preoperative care—same as for any major surgery
    1. Meeting with patient and family for discussion
    2. Complete explanation of postsurgical condition, including type and care of oxygen therapy, tubes, drainage, central venous pressure
    3. Practice in postsurgical procedures such as coughing with manual splinting of diaphragm, deep breathing, use of respirator, and any other special activity
B. Postsurgical care
    1. Postoperative room should contain
        a. Oxygen equipment
        b. Cardiac monitor
        c. Sterile cardiac arrest kit
        d. Suction apparatus
        e. Intravenous trays
        f. Underwater drainage
        g. Thoracentesis set
        h. Tracheotomy set
        i. Any other special equipment requested, such as hypothermia mattress
    2. Treatment same as that for major surgery and cardiac patient; patient usually very uncomfortable and restless; may be emotionally disturbed or disoriented
    3. Chest catheter and suction tubing attached
    4. If cardiac monitor used, it is attached; patient checked continuously for cardiac distress, arrhythmias, and irregular cardiac rate
    5. Vital signs including both apical and pedal pulse noted frequently
    6. Position changed at least every 2 hours; deep breathing and coughing practiced
    7. Administration of fluids, intake and output computation, and exercise of extremities important
    8. Observation for symptoms of pneumothorax and for hemorrhage
    9. Complications include hemorrhage, cardiac arrest, pulmonary edema, pneumothorax, cardiac distress, emboli
    10. Rehabilitation started before surgery and continued until maximum results obtained; conducted by health team
C. Special techniques
    1. Hyperbaric oxygenation—in certain forms of congenital heart disease
    2. Hypothermia—used less frequently now
    3. Extracorporeal circulation (pump oxygenator or heart-lung machine)
    4. Grafts

5. Artificial heart or heart-assist devices
D. Heart transplantation
1. Major problem—immunologic rejection
2. Ethic, moral, and economic problems also of great significance
3. Observation and psychological support of prime importance
E. Surgery for congenital heart disease (see developmental heart pathology)
F. Artificial pacemaker—used in selected cases involving trauma to or disease of atrioventricular conduction system
1. Type of electrical stimulation selected dependent on anticipated duration of treatment
   a. Emergency
   b. Temporary (few days to weeks)
   c. Permanent (months to years)
2. Three basic types of pacing
   a. Fixed rate, asynchronous—stimulate ventricles at constant rhythm
   b. Standby or demand—used in persons who develop episodes of spontaneous or drug-induced bradycardia or asystole
   c. Synchronous (variable rate)—responsive, within preset limits, to normal physiologic variations of sinus mechanism; best used in younger, more active patient
3. Problems after pacemaker insertion include infection, wire breakage, pacemaker failure, and battery failure
4. Implanted in subcutaneous tissue; platinum electrodes implanted directly into myocardium to stimulate ventricle; regulated to about 70 beats per minute
5. Nursing care as for open heart surgery, with special emphasis on reducing fear
6. Narcotics given sparingly; arm and leg exercises, passive and active, practiced consistently
7. Normal activities resumed when wound healed
8. Rehabilitation ideally should include work-health evaluation team consisting of physician, nurse, social worker, occupational therapist, and any other specialist indicated
9. Pacemaker will stimulate contractions for about 5 years; present cost over $600
G. Insertion of prosthetic heart valve—for aortic or mitral valve insufficiency

1. Usual preoperative care plus selective electrocardiograms, cardiac catheterization, phonocardiograms, and usually digitalization, low-salt diet, and diuretic regimen
2. Usual cardiac postoperative care after commissurotomy—patent airway, central venous pressure, underwater drainage, oxygen, fluids, and exercise
3. Nurse must be alert for changes in valve sound, widening pulse pressure, arrhythmias and tachycardia—may lead to cardiac arrest
4. Possible postsurgical complications—electrolyte disturbance, hemorrhage, pneumonia, thrombotic problems, and failure of suture to hold

8. **Nursing patients with vascular pathology**
A. Purpose of nursing care—to limit disease and prevent complications
B. Adequate supply of blood must be kept flowing through vessels
1. Warmth, cleanliness, and avoidance of infection and trauma help prevent complications
2. Rest, exercise, correct posture, and avoidance of constriction help to maintain free circulation
3. Smoking generally believed to be contraindicated in patients with vascular diseases
4. Emotional stress should be avoided, since it affects sympathetic nerves

9. **Diagnostic procedures**
A. Sympathetic block—injection of procaine into ganglion of sympathetic nerves supplying area; done to determine probable value of sympathectomy or to control pain
B. Oscillometer readings—measuring pulsations of arteries by means of oscillometer to determine relative effectiveness of arteries in certain area
C. Angiography—x-ray studies of arteries after injection of radiopaque material to determine anomalies and patency of arteries

10. **Specific vascular pathology**
A. Structural abnormalities
1. Aneurysm—local, arterial dilatation due to weakened condition of vessel wall and/or pressure of blood forms sac of clotted blood
   a. Dissecting aneurysm of aorta most serious; may rupture into pericardial sac or left bronchus or may

cause serious complications due to pressure

  b. Treatment surgical if it can be done without loss of blood supply to distal areas; heparin or Dicumarol usually given as anticoagulant

2. Thrombosis and embolism—clot of blood or other material, circulating in bloodstream, lodges in artery and obstructs blood supply to area

  a. All degrees of severity

  b. Treatment and nursing care

    (1) Keeping patient quiet

    (2) Anticoagulants (e.g., Dicumarol and heparin) delay clotting time

    (3) Embolectomy

    (4) Sometimes, vasodilators

    (5) If patient receiving anticoagulants, must be observed closely for hemorrhage

3. Arteriovenous fistula—communication between artery and vein; may be acquired or congenital

  a. Symptoms

    (1) Swelling

    (2) Elevated skin temperature over area

    (3) In severe cases may cause cardiac embarrassment

  b. Treatment—surgical: excision of fistula, or ligation

4. Tumors of arteries usually benign, but pressure may cause difficulty or, as in case of hemangioma, may hemorrhage

B. Peripheral vascular diseases—diseases in which blood flow through extremities disturbed by functional or structural abnormalities of blood vessels

1. Arteriosclerosis—degenerative condition with inflammatory changes in which artery loses elasticity, thickens, hardens; there are two main types

  a. Arteriosclerosis proper—hardening as result of fibrous and mineral deposits in middle layer of artery wall

  b. Atherosclerosis—fatty and other substances collect in inner lining of arteries

  a. Symptoms

    (1) Elevated blood pressure

    (2) Pain

    (3) Tingling

    (4) Numbness

    (5) Ischemia

    (6) Lack or lessening of function

    (7) In severe cases part may atrophy or become gangrenous

  b. No specific treatment—good hygiene, protection of part, and postural exercise may help

2. Raynaud's disease—disturbance of vasomotor mechanism, resulting in arterial spasms

  a. Symptoms

    (1) Paroxysmal, bilateral blanching or cyanosis of extremities (usually upper)

    (2) Numbness

    (3) Attacks often precipitated by emotion or cold

    (4) Gradual onset

  b. Treatment

    (1) Psychotherapy

    (2) Protection from cold

    (3) Regional sympathectomy for progressive type

    (4) Vasodilator drugs for attacks

    (5) Cessation of smoking

3. Thromboangiitis obliterans (Buerger's disease)—inflammatory type of obliterative vascular disease affecting chiefly arteries and veins; more common in young adult males

  a. Symptoms

    (1) Periods of progression and quiescence

    (2) Coldness of extremity

    (3) Severe pain, especially after exercise

    (4) Cyanosis of part, especially when dependent

    (5) Intermittent claudication

    (6) If unrelieved, edema, ulceration, and gangrene

  b. Treatment and nursing care

    (1) General care for diseases of vascular system

    (2) Suction and pressure therapy

    (3) Oscillating bed

    (4) Bilateral sympathectomy

    (5) In rapidly progressive cases, amputation may be indicated

4. Varicose veins—dilatation of veins due to deficiency of valves, producing venous stasis

  a. Symptoms

    (1) Dilated, tortuous veins

    (2) Local edema

    (3) Indolent ulceration

    (4) Pigmentation

    (5) Stabbing or aching pain

  b. Treatment and nursing care con-

cerned with emptying veins; methods used
(1) Elevation
(2) Removal of all constricting and hydrostatic pressure
(3) Elastic bandage or stocking
(4) Unna's paste boot or Dome-Paste bandage
(5) Stripping vein
(6) Injection with sclerosing substance

5. Thrombophlebitis—venous obstruction by thrombus, secondary to infection and accompanied by inflammatory reaction in walls of affected vein
   a. Phlebothrombosis — noninflammatory thrombus of vein; frequently can be prevented by proper exercise and positioning
   b. Symptoms
      (1) Usually appear suddenly
      (2) May be mild or severe depending on size of thrombus
      (3) Pain, local tenderness, edema, and mottled cyanosis may or may not be present
      (4) Ulcers may result
   c. Treatment
      (1) Prevention much better than treatment
      (2) Drug therapy with anticoagulants
      (3) Rest and elevation of part
      (4) Heat
      (5) If pain severe, sympathetic block

C. Hypertension—condition characterized by higher blood pressure than normal
   1. Factors that affect blood pressure
      a. Strength of heart contractions
      b. Volume of vascular fluid
      c. Viscosity of vascular fluid
      d. Peripheral resistance
   2. Arteriosclerotic hypertension—arteries become inelastic
      a. Characteristics
         (1) High systolic and normal or low diastolic pressure
         (2) Usually found in persons over 50 years of age
      b. Treatment—chiefly palliative
         (1) Rest
         (2) Sedation
         (3) Drugs to reduce blood pressure
   3. Spastic hypertension—elevation of both systolic and diastolic pressure

a. Kidney type—found in conjunction with renal pathology
b. Adrenal type—found in conjunction with conditions that result in increased adrenaline production
c. Essential hypertension—cause unknown—most common type of serious hypertension
d. Symptoms of spastic hypertension
   (1) Rising blood pressure
   (2) Dizziness
   (3) Headache
   (4) Tinnitus
   (5) Precardial pain
e. Complications dangerous and sudden
   (1) Heart failure
   (2) Myocardial infarction
   (3) Renal failure
   (4) Cerebral vascular accidents
   (5) Arteriosclerosis of coronary vessels
   (6) Hypertensive encephalopathy
f. Treatment and nursing care
   (1) Lower blood pressure
   (2) Prevent complications
   (3) Mental and physical rest
   (4) Sedation
   (5) Hypotensive drugs
   (6) Weight reduction in overweight persons
   (7) In some cases, sympathectomy
g. Hypotensive drugs (p. 267)
   (1) Have been greatly improved
   (2) Many have toxic side effects
   (3) Require close observation
   (4) Commonly used drugs
      (a) Reserpine (Serpasil)
      (b) Chlorothiazide (Diuril)
      (c) Chlorthalidone (Hygroton)
      (d) Hydralazine (Apresoline)
      (e) Pentolinium tartrate (Ansolysen)
      (f) Guanethidine sulfate (Ismelin)

D. Hypotension—condition manifested by blood pressure lower than normal; seldom serious; not disease; many times not even manifestation of disease

11. Lymphatic diseases
A. Lymphedema
   1. Cause
      a. Any obstruction of lymph flow, in lymphatic vessels or nodes
      b. After surgery in which lymph vessels removed

2. Treatment—chiefly palliative
   a. Elevation of area
   b. Care to prevent trauma
   c. Antibiotics
   d. In applicable cases, surgery may help
   e. In specific instances, elastic bandages and exercise
B. Lymphomas—tumors of lymphoid tissue

12. **Surgical procedures frequently used in treatment of vascular conditions**
A. Lumbar sympathectomy—surgical procedure in which spinal ganglion or preganglionic fibers removed to facilitate dilation of the vessels in area affected
B. Bilateral thoracic or thoracolumbar sympathectomy—surgical procedure used for selected patients to relieve essential hypertension; shock and hypotension principal complications; may be relieved only temporarily
C. Amputation—surgical procedure in which part or all of extremity removed (p. 425)
   1. Preoperative care
      a. General preoperative care
      b. Additional testing for adequate circulation (oscillometer readings)
      c. Attention to mental and emotional preparation
   2. Postoperative care
      a. General postoperative care
      b. Measures to avoid retraction of soft parts
         (1) Good alignment
         (2) No pillows under stump
      c. Tourniquet available at all times
      d. Attitude of empathy and hopefulness
   3. Postoperative complications to guard against
      a. Shock
      b. Hemorrhage
      c. Infection
      d. Phantom pain
      e. Deformity
   4. Rehabilitation must be psychological as well as physical

NURSING PATIENTS WITH DISEASES OF THE BLOOD AND BLOOD-FORMING ORGANS

1. **Basic principles of nursing**
A. Correction of cause if possible
B. Emotional support and help in accepting knowledge that he has chronic disease
C. Maintenance of hopeful, cheerful attitude and environment
D. Maintenance of adequate nutritional intake high in vitamins, protein, and iron
E. Protection from trauma and infections
F. Observation for hemorrhage—internal and external

2. **Nursing patients with blood dyscrasias**
A. Good mouth care; mouth and tongue often sore; may be bleeding
B. Frequent short periods of rest and adequate diet may help in reducing fatigue frequently present
C. Bland diet advisable because of tendency to bleed and anorexia
D. Care of patient receiving nitrogen mustard intravenously
   1. Avoidance of contact with skin; usually injected from vial into infusion that has already started
   2. Care of nausea and vomiting occurring 1 to 3 hours after injection; barbiturates help to control discomfort
E. Care of patient receiving sodium radiophosphate (P^{32})
   1. Includes isolation precautions
      a. P^{32} emits beta rays; half-life of 14.3 days
      b. Nurse should know hospital or clinic regulations concerning management of patients receiving P^{32}
   2. Patient experiences no discomfort
F. Care of patient with sternal bone marrow biopsy
   1. Procedure performed under local anesthetic, and specimen saved in sodium oxylate specimen container
   2. Procedure mildly uncomfortable for patient, but often very frightening; may be local tenderness for few days

3. **Diseases of blood and blood-forming organs**
A. Anemia—any deficiency in quantity or quality of blood as manifested by reduction in number of red corpuscles or in amount of hemoglobin or both
   1. Anemias due to blood loss characterized by
      a. Reduced blood volume
      b. Low hemoglobin
      c. Reduced red blood cell count
      d. Hypochromia
   2. Anemias due to defective formation of blood

a. Causes
   (1) Nutritional deficiency
   (2) Depression of bone marrow
   (3) Unknown causes
b. Symptoms
   (1) Harshness of skin and hair
   (2) Excessive menstrual flow in women
   (3) Brittle, ridged nails
   (4) Small red blood cells with low volume index
c. Iron especially needed during growth, pregnancy, and menstruation

3. Pernicious anemia due to lack of intrinsic factor normally found in gastric secretions
  a. Characteristic symptoms
    (1) Lack of hydrochloric acid
    (2) Macrocytic red blood cells
    (3) Low red and white blood cell counts
    (4) Digestive symptoms
    (5) Low blood pressure
    (6) Weakness
    (7) Characteristic smooth, shiny, atrophic tongue
    (8) Irregular, low-grade fever
  b. Later, neural symptoms
    (1) Disorders of sensation
    (2) Persistent numbness and tingling of hands and feet
    (3) Defects of special senses
    (4) Cardiac and nephritic symptoms
  c. Treatment and nursing care
    (1) Administration of B_{12}
    (2) Physical therapy for neural symptoms
    (3) Special mouth care
    (4) Teaching importance of continuing medications
    (5) Maintaining good nutrition
    (6) Emotional support

4. Anemias due to increased destruction of blood—may vary from slight to severe; due to destruction of erythrocytes
  a. Extrinsic causes include chemicals and infections
  b. Intrinsic hemolytic anemias
    (1) Sickle cell anemia
    (2) Hemolytic spherocytic anemia associated with splenomegaly
    (3) Erythroblastosis (incompatible Rh factor)

B. Polycythemia vera—chronic, slowly progressive disease of unknown origin, in which spleen enlarged and red blood cell count greatly increased
  1. Symptoms
    a. Reddish purple appearance of skin
    b. Increased viscosity of blood
    c. Increased volume of blood
    d. Enlarged spleen
    e. Lassitude
    f. Increased sweating
    g. Headache
    h. Vertigo
    i. Dyspnea
    j. Increased tendency to hemorrhage
    k. Digestive disturbances
  2. Treatment and nursing care
    a. Avoidance of mental and physical strain
    b. Venesection
    c. Irradiation of long bones
    d. Triethylene melamine (radioactive phosphorus)
    e. Diet low in iron
    f. Avoidance of trauma or anything conducive to hemorrhage

C. Leukemia—malignant condition—shows increase in white blood cells; loosely classified as cancer of white blood cells; two major types—myelogenous; lymphatic
  1. Acute leukemia of either type
    a. Symptoms
      (1) Develops abruptly with symptoms of "cold"
      (2) Elevated temperature
      (3) Rapidly developing anemia
      (4) Spontaneous hemorrhages (due to low platelet count)
      (5) Prostration
      (6) Usually rapidly fatal
    b. Treatment
      (1) Whole blood transfusions, packed red blood cells, and platelets
      (2) Folic acid antagonists (mercaptopurine, aminopterin)
      (3) Supportive care
  2. Chronic myelogenous leukemia
    a. Symptoms
      (1) Slow, insidious onset
      (2) Anemia
      (3) Enlarged spleen and bone marrow
      (4) Tendency to bleed
      (5) Infiltration of white blood cells into various structures of body

(6) Dyspnea
(7) Secondary infections
b. Treatment may bring about remissions, but life-span usually less than 5 years after diagnosis
  (1) Blood transfusions
  (2) Folic acid antagonists
  (3) Radioactive sodium radiophosphate (P^{32})
  (4) Spray x-ray
  (5) Antibiotics
  (6) Corticosteroids
  (7) Nitrogen mustard I.V.
3. Chronic lymphatic leukemia has most hopeful prognosis
a. Symptoms
  (1) Enlarged lymph nodes and bone marrow
  (2) Fatigue
  (3) Weakness
  (4) May have dyspnea due to pressure of lymph nodes
b. Treatment and nursing care
  (1) Directed toward relief of symptoms
  (2) Any of above-mentioned procedures may be used
  (3) High-protein diet is important
D. Hodgkin's disease—characterized by marked enlargement of lymph nodes
1. Symptoms
a. Anemia, including pallor, fatigue
b. Interference with breathing and swallowing develops
2. Remissions and exacerbations of symptoms with elevation of temperature rule; usually fatal within few years
3. Treatment and nursing care
a. Nitrogen mustard intravenously
b. X-ray therapy
c. Surgical removal of enlarged nodes
d. Blood transfusions
e. Local care of pruritus
f. Avoidance of infections
g. Rest
h. Psychological encouragement and support
E. Lymphosarcoma—rapidly growing malignant tumor of lymph nodes; enlarged nodes commonly seen in neck
1. Treatment
a. Node may be removed to prevent pressure on vital point or for biopsy
b. Radiation therapy
c. Nitrogen mustard and related drugs

2. Nursing care includes principles of cancer nursing
F. Purpura—group of diseases characterized by extravasations of blood into skin and mucous membranes; areas of discoloration range from petechiae to large ecchymoses
1. Thrombocytopenic purpura—number of platelets in the blood greatly decreased; many causes
2. Idiopathic thrombopenic purpura (purpura hemorrhagica)—acute or chronic purpura characterized by marked, unaccountable diminution in number of blood platelets and by spontaneous hemorrhages from mucous membranes
a. Symptoms
  (1) Spontaneous capillary bleeding
  (2) Fever in acute episodes
  (3) Spleen enlarged in chronic types
  (4) Low platelet count
  (5) Increased bleeding time
  (6) Normal white count
  (7) Usually no pronounced feeling of discomfort or malaise
b. Treatment and nursing care
  (1) Iron for anemia
  (2) Good hygiene
  (3) Blood transfusions
  (4) ACTH or cortisone
  (5) Removal of spleen that has been destroying blood platelets prematurely
  (6) Splenectomy gives symptomatic relief in about 70% of chronic types of purpura
G. Hemophilia—hereditary disease in which coagulation time of blood greatly prolonged; occurs only in male, but transmitted through female
1. Symptoms
a. Excessive bleeding after injury
b. Bleeding in and around joints that eventually leads to hypertrophy
c. Frequent hemorrhage into other structures
d. Usually proves fatal before or in early adult life
2. Prevention—problem of eugenics
3. Treatment and nursing care
a. Absolute quiet
b. Morphine
c. Local application of thromboplastic substance
d. ACTH or cortisone

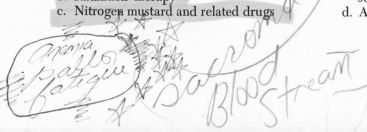

e. Blood transfusions

f. Special dental care

g. Utmost care to prevent trauma

H. Agranulocytosis—blood dyscrasia in which granulocytes not formed, due to maturation arrest of bone marrow; characterized by extreme leukopenia and destructive, ulcerative lesions of throat, skin, or gastrointestinal tract

1. Symptoms appear rapidly
   a. High fever
   b. Headache
   c. Chills
   d. Malaise
   e. Sore throat
   f. Enlarged cervical lymph nodes
   g. Progressive infection
   h. Disease fatal unless controlled

2. Treatment and nursing care
   a. Discontinuance of drugs that may be cause
   b. Control of infections
   c. Blood transfusions

I. Malaria
   Worldwide distribution; in 1972, 810 cases in the United States

1. Etiology—protozoan parasite of genus *Plasmodium*
   a. Species of *Plasmodium*
      (1) *Plasmodium vivax*, most common
      (2) *Plasmodium falciparum*, most serious
      (3) *Plasmodium malariae*
      (4) *Plasmodium ovale*, rare

2. Transmission—carried from man to man by mosquito and from man to mosquito; may be transmitted by blood transfusions, contaminated syringes and needles

3. Incubation period—varies with specific species of *Plasmodium*; *P. vivax* 12 to 14 days, but may be 8 to 10 months; period shorter if from blood transfusion

4. Symptoms—similar for all species: three stages
   a. Severe shaking chill, 10 to 15 minutes' duration
   b. Fever 103° to 106° F., skin hot, dry, and flushed, headache, nausea, vomiting, aching, abdominal pain, duration 4 to 6 hours
   c. Profuse sweating and weakness

5. Diagnosis—laboratory examination of blood smears

6. Treatment—quinine sulfate; new synthetic agents being used: chloroquine phosphate, chloroguanide, amodiaquin, pyrimethamine, primaquine

7. Nursing—give external heat, hot drinks psychological support; analgesics, ice cap to head, tepid sponges for fever; keep dry during sweating stage; no isolation

8. Prevention—eliminate vectors' breeding places, screen homes and public buildings, use repellents, spray homes; global eradication necessary

4. **Pathology of spleen**

A. Splenomegaly—enlargement of spleen
   1. Causes
      a. Chronic malaria
      b. Infections
      c. Certain types of cysts
      d. Tumors
      e. Banti's syndrome
      f. Hodgkin's disease

B. Anomalies of spleen
   1. Absence of spleen
   2. Subdivided spleen
   3. One or more accessory spleen
   4. Variations in size
   5. Movable or floating spleen found in any part of abdomen

C. Tumors and cysts of spleen
   1. Benign tumors frequent but of no clinical importance
   2. Carcinomas always secondary; one of terminal manifestations
   3. Lymphosarcoma a primary splenic tumor; rapidly fatal, since diagnosis almost always too late for splenectomy
      a. Symptoms
         (1) Pain
         (2) Tenderness
         (3) Fever
         (4) Pressure
         (5) Mass
         (6) Anemia
         (7) Emaciation
   4. Cysts
      a. Congenital or acquired
      b. Simple, parasitic (*Echinococcus*)
      c. Neoplastic (dermoid)

D. Thrombosis—may be partial or complete
   1. Spleen becomes congested or enlarged and gastric hemorrhage may result
   2. Chronic thrombosis may be accompanied by ascites, anemia, and leukopenia
   3. Diagnosis is rarely made before death

E. Abscess of spleen—relatively rare condition; abscesses usually multiple; rarely noticed before rupture

F. Rupture of spleen—may be due to trauma or disease
1. Symptoms
   a. Shock
   b. Low blood pressure
   c. Sudden local pain and tenderness
   d. Fullness in both flanks
   e. Only treatment—surgery

G. Splenectomy—removal of spleen—relatively simple surgical procedure, but reason for removal usually quite serious
1. Preoperative care depends to some extent on purpose of splenectomy; patient usually given
   a. Blood transfusions
   b. Antibiotics
   c. X-ray therapy to reduce large spleen in blood dyscrasias
   d. General preoperative care
2. Postoperative care
   a. Hemorrhage chief complication; symptoms of external or internal bleeding should be noted carefully
   b. ACTH or cortisone may be given
   c. Temperature may remain elevated for few days
   d. Abdominal suction, Prostigmin, or Pitressin may be given for abdominal distention
   e. Evisceration sometimes late complication

NURSING PATIENTS WITH RENAL AND GENITOURINARY PROBLEMS

1. Basic principles of nursing

A. Emphasis on prevention; health education

B. Tact and professional attitude essential in caring for patients with urologic conditions

C. Avoiding unnecessary exposure of patient

D. Patient, sympathetic explanations and education essential

E. Occupational and diversional therapy necessary, especially for patient who has led active life

F. Helping patient adjust to condition important; often difficult responsibility of nurse

G. Cleanliness mandatory; urine irritating to wounds and to normal skin

H. Correct collection of specimens important, since disturbance of urinary function often discovered by urinalysis, amount, and microscopic examination of urine
1. All specimens must be clean; specimens for culture must be sterile
2. Time of urine collection to be indicated clearly on label
3. Specimens kept cool if not examined immediately; in some instances, preservative can be used

I. Understand psychologic approach, since condition often frightening, painful, and embarrassing

J. Teach self-care to patient and/or his family and how to prevent complications

K. Help with plans for future care of patient; prolonged convalescence and/or continued ill health may create economic and social problems

L. Renal dysfunction integral part of many diseases, especially those that affect circulatory system; influences prognosis

M. Large amounts of fluids indicated in most instances of renal pathology; often patient needs instruction in importance of adequate fluid intake

N. Free drainage maintained at all times; plugged catheter more dangerous than no catheter

O. Diet important part of treatment; may require much teaching and help on part of nurse; diets commonly used (p. 246)
1. Salt-poor
2. Nephritic
3. High-vitamin
4. Alkaline ash or acid ash

2. Nursing patient with renal system disease; in addition to above

A. Continuous secretion of urine

B. Drugs (p. 271)
1. Diuretics
2. Antidiuretics
3. Urinary antiseptics
4. Antibiotics
5. Acidifying or alkalizing drugs

C. Management of urinary drainage integral part of nursing patient with urinary pathology
1. Prevent tube from becoming kinked or blocked—roll tube between fingers to determine presence of sediment
2. Force fluids and keep intake and output records
3. Fasten tube securely so that patient may move about freely

4. Keep apparatus clean; do not allow urine to remain on skin
5. Instruct patient discharged with drainage apparatus
   a. How to manage it
   b. What complications to watch for
D. Tidal drainage—procedure in which bladder is filled to predetermined intervesicular pressure and emptied by suction and gravity; often used when patient has neurogenic or "cord" bladder
   1. Nursing care
      a. Check working condition of apparatus at least every 4 hours
      b. Keep bottles filled with sterile solution
      c. Keep equipment clean
      d. Keep accurate intake and output record
      e. Fluid intake must be maintained
E. Peritoneal dialysis—sterile solutions introduced into peritoneal cavity, left for specified time, and then drained from cavity
   1. Purpose—to reduce abnormal electrolyte concentration in body fluids by allowing equilibrium to be established by dialysis, between infused solutions and body fluids
   2. Usually 2,000 ml. of prepared solution introduced into peritoneal cavity, left 60 to 90 minutes, then allowed to drain out
   3. Keep exact measurement of fluid introduced and fluid returned; report immediately any major imbalance
   4. Check vital signs
   5. Observe patients for complications—peritonitis, abdominal pain, restlessness, bleeding, abdominal distention and/or ileus
F. Artificial kidney—external mechanism through which arterial blood can be shunted in order to rest patient's kidney
   1. Nursing care during this procedure usually done by specially trained personnel; patient must be observed closely for hemorrhage and shock
   2. Unless damaged kidneys begin to function in relatively short time, procedure becomes impracticable
3. **Nursing patient with genitourinary problems; in addition to basic principles**
A. Usually duty of nurse to keep urologic instruments in good working order and ready for use

4. **Procedures in urinary pathology**
A. Pathologic conditions of urine and voiding
   1. Glycosuria—excessive amount of sugar in urine; usually does not indicate kidney damage
   2. Hematuria—red blood cells in urine; may give reddish or smoky color; very important symptom, since rarely normal
   3. Pyuria—pus in urine; usually indicates nephritis or infection in urinary tract
   4. Bacteriuria—bacteria in urine
   5. Dysuria—painful urination; tenesmus —painful, ineffectual straining
   6. Polyuria—daily output over 3,000 ml.
   7. Oliguria—daily output between 50 and 500 ml.
   8. Anuria—daily output less than 50 ml.
   9. Suppression of urine—no urine secreted by kidneys
   10. Retention of urine—urine retained in bladder
   11. Residual urine—urine retained in bladder immediately following urination
   12. Nocturia or nycturia—excessive urge to void at night
   13. Albuminuria—albumin in urine; usually due to nephritis, but may be temporary following strenuous exercise or during acute fevers
   14. Casts in urine—many kinds; often found with albuminuria
   15. Bence Jones protein in urine—indicates malignancy in urinary tract
B. Renal function tests
   1. Concentration test—done in order to ascertain power of kidney tubules to concentrate or dilute urine; if kidney unable to concentrate or dilute urine, specific gravity said to be "fixed"
   2. Blood urea nitrogen (BUN)—blood test to estimate relative amount of urea nitrogen in blood; normal kidney function will clear blood to 8 to 20 mg.%
   3. Nonprotein nitrogen (NPN)—blood test to ascertain amount of nonprotein nitrogen in blood; normal in fasting blood 20 to 35 mg.%
   4. Urea clearance test—measures amount of plasma cleared of urea in 1 minute and represents glomerular filtration rate; when rate falls to 50% of normal (130 ml. per minute), blood urea elevated

5. Phenolsulfonphthalein (PSP)—indicates amount of excretion of dye by kidney tubules
6. Intravenous urography—x-ray examination of urinary structures after intravenous injection of radiopaque dye (Diodrast, Neo-Iopax, Urokon)
7. Cystoscopy—procedure in which hollow, lighted instrument inserted into bladder; affords direct vision of bladder; ureters may be catheterized at this time if indicated
   a. Patient often quite uncomfortable following procedure; heat usually gives some relief
   b. Often some blood in urine, but large amounts of bleeding should be investigated
8. Retrograde pyelograms—radiopaque dye inserted directly through ureteral catheters into kidney and x-ray studies made
9. Renal arteriography—radiopaque dye injected into aorta and x-ray films taken of dye as it travels through renal arteries and veins; complications may include thrombosis, fibrillation, cardiac arrest
10. Radioisotope renogram—radioactive substance (Hippuran) injected intravenously; vascular, secretory, and excretory ability of renal vessels determined by measuring radioactivity over renal areas

5. Pathology of renal system
A. Malformations of renal structures—may be almost any type; anomalies in number, size, form, location, fusion, rotation, and/or omission
   1. Kidney malformations
      a. Horseshoe kidney
      b. Lack of or nonfunctioning kidney
      c. Failure of kidney to fuse
   2. Anomalies of ureters
      a. Strictures
      b. Diverticuli
      c. Spiral twist or torsion
      d. Double ureter
      e. Anomalies of insertion or termination
      f. Ureterocele
      g. Extra valves or folds in ureteral lumen
   3. Anomalies of bladder
      a. Absence of or aplasia
      b. Double bladder
      c. Hourglass bladder
      d. Exstrophy (absence of lower abdominal wall and anterior wall of bladder)
      e. Hypertrophy of bladder neck
   4. Urethral anomalies
      a. Narrowing of meatus
      b. Double urethra
      c. Diverticuli of male urethra
      d. Epispadias or hypospadias of male urethra
B. Tumors
   1. Classification
      a. Primary or metastatic
      b. Benign
      c. Malignant
      d. Embryonic
   2. Carcinoma of kidney (hypernephroma) most common malignancy of adult; metastasizes rapidly; characterized by hematuria; later, fever and anemia
   3. Congenital polycystic kidney and Wilms' tumor (adenocarcinoma) chief malignancies of kidney in children
   4. Carcinoma of renal pelvis and bladder metastasizes more slowly; characterized by symptoms of cystitis
   5. Treatment—surgery or irradiation
C. Uremic syndrome—clinical pattern characterized by renal insufficiency and nitrogen retention; may be due to kidney damage or to extrarenal causes
   1. Symptoms include
      a. Acidosis
      b. Dehydration
      c. Muscular irritation
      d. Urea retention
      e. Toxic manifestations
   2. Treatment—palliative and symptomatic, unless cause can be removed; effort made to maintain fluid and electrolyte balance; peritoneal dialysis or artificial kidney routines sometimes employed
   3. Nursing care
      a. Exacting
      b. Special mouth and skin care (pruritus may be severe)
      c. Observation for and care of mental symptoms
      d. Frequent change of position
      e. Maintenance of adequate fluid intake and output
      f. Special diet
      g. Understanding and kindness
D. Nephritis—inflammatory and degenerative condition of kidney; acute, subacute,

chronic glomerulonephritis and nephrosclerosis included in general category
1. Characteristic symptoms
   a. Hematuria
   b. Edema
   c. Headache
   d. Malaise
   e. Increasing blood pressure
   f. Anemia
   g. Low specific gravity of urine
2. Terminal symptoms may be
   a. Anuria and uremia
   b. Heart failure
   c. Cerebral vascular accident due to high blood pressure
3. Treatment and nursing care in acute stages
   a. Concerned with mental and physical rest
   b. Usually salt-poor, low-protein diet
   c. Fluid intake as ordered
   d. Daily weight
   e. Intake and output records
   f. Special skin and mouth care
   g. Observation for and treatment of complications
   h. ACTH or cortisone may be given
   i. Mercurial diuretics contraindicated
4. In chronic or subacute nephritis
   a. Motto is "moderation in all things"
   b. High-protein, low-sodium diet
   c. Treatment for hypertension if present
   d. Avoidance of colds and infections usually advocated
   e. Diuretics may be indicated
E. Infections of urinary tract—may be caused by bacteria, viruses, or parasites
   1. Urethritis—female urethra quite vulnerable to bacterial invasion, unless strict personal hygiene; predisposes to other infections of urinary tract
   2. Cystitis—acute or chronic infection of bladder
      a. Symptoms
         (1) More or less pain on urination
         (2) Frequency
         (3) Pyuria
         (4) Sometimes hematuria and elevated temperature if kidneys involved
      b. Treatment and nursing care
         (1) Specific drugs for infecting organism
         (2) Large amounts of fluids
         (3) Antispasmodics

         (4) Heat for pain
         (5) Sedatives
         (6) Rest
         (7) Special diets
         (8) Bladder irrigations if indicated
   3. Pyelonephritis—acute or chronic infection of kidney; pyelitis may be included in this category
      a. Symptoms
         (1) Attacks of chills and fever
         (2) Pain
         (3) Backache
         (4) Sometimes bladder irritation or infection
      b. Treatment and nursing care
         (1) Antibiotic therapy
         (2) Fluids
         (3) Adequate rest
         (4) Relief of obstruction when present
F. Urinary calculi (nephrolithiasis)—painful; may cause hematuria, infection, or hydronephrosis due to obstruction
   1. Bed rest encourages formation of stones; hence all patients kept as active as possible
   2. Large amounts of fluids and exercise encourage stones to pass spontaneously; all urine should be strained; may be necessary to remove larger stones by cystoscopy and very large ones by surgery
   3. To prevent recurrence of stones patient should
      a. Avoid infections
      b. Take large amounts of fluids
      c. Omit certain types of foods, depending on chemistry of stones
      d. If etiologic factor ascertained, measures should be taken to correct it
G. Hydronephrosis—condition of fluid being retained in kidney pelvis due to obstruction of ureter from any cause
   1. Symptoms
      a. May be "silent" or quite severe
      b. Include pain, nausea, vomiting
      c. If not relieved, eventual infection of kidney
   2. Treatment and nursing care concerned with
      a. Reestablishing drainage
      b. Preventing as much damage to kidney as possible
H. Lipoid nephrosis—childhood disease characterized by depletion of plasma protein

1. Characteristics
   a. Massive edema
   b. Albuminuria
   c. Changes in blood serum
2. Treatment and nursing care
   a. Much the same as for chronic nephritis
   b. High-protein diet usually considered essential

6. **Common urologic disorders**
A. Infections of male genital tract
   1. Balanitis—inflammation of glans penis
   2. Cellulitis of penis—may be due to acute gonorrhea, severe balanitis, periurethral infections, or ulcerative chancre
   3. Seminal vesiculitis—infection of seminal vesicles—may be due to tuberculous gonorrhea, *Staphylococcus,* or *Escherichia coli;* may be acute, subacute, or chronic
      a. Symptoms range from mild to severe and include frequent, painful nocturnal ejections with blood and pus in semen; pain, urgency, frequency, and nocturia—urinary symptoms; backache; suprapubic and lower abdominal pain; fever
      b. Treatment and nursing care
         (1) Antibiotics
         (2) Local heat
         (3) Sedatives
         (4) Persistent massage for chronic infection
         (5) Vasectomy may become necessary for chronic type
   4. Vasitis (deferentitis)—infection of vas deferens; usually follows epididymitis
   5. Epididymitis—inflammation of epididymis; most common inflammatory condition of scrotum; usually secondary to seminal vesiculitis or may be complication of prostatic surgery
      a. Symptoms may be slight or severe and include local tenderness, pain; may produce local abscess
      b. Treatment and nursing care
         (1) Antibiotics
         (2) Local heat
         (3) Rest
         (4) In some cases, epididymectomy or orchiectomy
   6. Orchitis—infection of testes; may be complication of mumps
      a. Symptoms
         (1) Pain
         (2) Swelling
         (3) Marked rise in temperature
      b. Treatment
         (1) Usual treatment for infection
         (2) Early incision and drainage of associated hydrocele
   7. Prostatitis—acute or chronic infection of prostate gland
      a. Symptoms
         (1) Gland swells and becomes painful
         (2) Severe swelling causes obstruction
         (3) Produces urinary symptoms and hematuria
      b. Treatment
         (1) Antibiotics
         (2) Heat
         (3) Rest
         (4) Fluids
B. Benign prostatic hypertrophy—occurs in about one third of male population over 60 years of age; cause unknown but may be hormonal
   1. Symptoms characteristically those of urinary obstruction
      a. Difficulty in starting urination
      b. Small stream
      c. Dribbling
      d. Later, complete obstruction
   2. Treatment—prostatectomy
C. Congenital malformations may occur in any part of male reproductive tract; most common
   1. Cryptorchism—failure of one or both testicles to descend into scrotum
      a. Treatment
         (1) With hormones
         (2) If unsuccessful, operation indicated
   2. Hypospadias—urethral opening on ventral wall of penis
   3. Epispadias—urethral opening on upper surface of penis; plastic surgery usually required
   4. Phimosis—foreskin so narrow cannot be retracted over glans; circumcision done to remove foreskin
D. Tumors of male reproductive system
   1. Carcinoma of skin of penis rare; treated as skin cancer
   2. Malignant tumors of testicle usually occur during years of greatest sexual activity
      a. Symptoms
         (1) Early metastasis

(2) Gradual swelling of testicle
(3) Backache
(4) Pain in abdomen
(5) Loss of weight
(6) Weakness
  b. Treatment
    (1) Irradiation
    (2) Orchiectomy
    (3) Further irradiation
3. Sarcoma of prostate relatively rare but occurs 50% of time in children
  a. Often infiltrates bladder wall, seminal vesicles, and rectum, causing urinary infection and obstruction
  b. Treatment
    (1) Surgery preferred but few cases diagnosed early enough
    (2) Palliative
      (a) Radiotherapy
      (b) Urinary drainage
      (c) General care for patient with inoperable malignancy
4. Carcinoma of prostate—occurs chiefly in middle-aged or older men; 3 distinct types recognized
  a. Small and causes no symptoms but may metastasize widely
  b. Mixed with benign hypertrophy
  c. Unmixed, grows more rapidly; infiltrates gland and capsule
    (1) Characteristics
      (a) Local increase in size
      (b) Hard lump in prostate
      (c) Low back pain
      (d) Metastasis to bones
      (e) Increased blood phosphatase
      (f) No pain until urinary obstruction occurs
  d. Treatment and nursing care
    (1) Depends on stage of tumor—4 commonly performed surgical procedures
    (2) Radical prostatectomy done in operable cases
    (3) Palliative treatment
      (a) Relief of obstruction if present
      (b) Transurethral resection or permanent suprapubic cystotomy
      (c) Hormonal therapy—estrogens or orchiectomy
      (d) Sometimes cortisone
    (4) Nursing care—similar to that

given to patients with inoperable malignancies
7. **Nursing patients with renal and urologic surgery**
A. Preoperative preparation
  1. Psychological support
  2. Large amounts of fluids
  3. Adequate nutrition
  4. Free drainage
  5. Number of tests will be performed
  6. Extensive study to determine amount of invasion if malignancy involved
  7. Any infections controlled
  8. General preoperative care
B. Commonly performed surgical procedures
  1. Nephrectomy—removal of kidney
  2. Pyelotomy—opening of renal pelvis
  3. Nephrolithotomy—opening into kidney for removal of calculi
  4. Nephrostomy—formation of artificial fistula into renal pelvis
  5. Nephropexy—surgical attachment of floating kidney
  6. Ureterolithotomy—incision into ureter for removal of calculi
  7. Ureteral transplant—for diversion of urine from bladder
  8. Cystectomy—removal of bladder, may be total or subtotal
  9. Suprapubic cystotomy—opening into bladder above pubis
  10. Kidney transplants (limited at this time)
  11. Vesiculectomy—removal of seminal vesicles; rare procedure performed through perineal incision; may result in impotency
  12. Prostatotomy—usually done for drainage of prostatic abscess; since advent of antibiotics, procedure rarely necessary
  13. Vasectomy—removal of all or part of vas deferens to sterilize patient or to prevent epididymitis following prostatectomy
  14. Epididymectomy—removal of epididymis; used in malignancy of epididymis
  15. Orchiectomy—removal of body of testes, epididymis, and scrotal portion of vas deferens
  16. Orchiopexy—surgery to correct faulty descent of testes
  17. Transurethral prostatectomy—excision

Balanitis — inflam. glans penis.

of part or all of prostate gland through urethra

18. Suprapubic prostatectomy—removal of prostate through incision of abdominal wall and urinary bladder; may be 1- or 2-stage operation

19. Perineal prostatectomy—removal of prostate gland through perineal incision

20. Retropubic prostatectomy—excision of prostate gland through abdominal incision, but without entering bladder

C. Postoperative care
    1. Nursing care—general care for major surgery
    2. Drainage tubes may be initiated in surgery and must be connected with sterile tubing with patent lumen
    3. Dressings contaminated with urine should be changed frequently, and deodorants used if indicated
    4. Observation for hemorrhage, abdominal distention, pain, and mental distress needed
    5. Painful epididymitis (scrotal swelling) may require scrotal support
    6. Usually fluids urged; accurate intake and output record kept
    7. Strict asepsis desirable, since infection a serious complication and in younger men may cause sterility
    8. Patients with surgery on reproductive system need understanding and help
    9. If postoperative incontinence or "dribbles" or residual urine, measures to correct conditions or methods to manage secretions instituted; patient given necessary help and instruction

D. Postoperative care following nephrectomy
    1. Patient positioned on side of operation and on back
    2. Passive and active exercise to prevent peripheral vascular complications
    3. Observation for hemorrhage and toxicity
    4. Following hospitalization, patient should be warned not to do any heavy lifting for at least a year

E. Postoperative care following bladder surgery
    1. Urine may empty through catheter inserted through pelvis, urethra, or may drain into rectum; cleanliness special problem
    2. Psychological care especially impor-

tant following radical bladder surgery

3. Complications include shock, pulmonary difficulties, decubitus ulcers, excoriation of skin, and later infection of urinary tract
4. Preparation for future health care very vital

8. **Venereal disease**
   Worldwide problem
   A. Syphilis
      1. Etiology—*Treponema pallidum;* organism very fragile
      2. Transmission—direct contact through sexual intercourse; infection of fetus in utero
      3. Incubation period—10 to 90 days
      4. Classification of syphilis
         a. Primary
         b. Secondary
         c. Early syphilis
         d. Late syphilis—of 4 years' duration
         e. 25,719 cases of primary and secondary types in 1972 in the United States
      5. Symptoms
         a. Primary syphilis—chancre about anogenital area; lesion at point of inoculation by organism; painless; serology usually negative during early stage; highly infectious
         b. Secondary syphilis—6 weeks to 3 months following primary lesion; slight fever, sore throat, malaise, lesions may appear on skin and mucous membranes—skin rash with macules, papules, pustules; lesions on palms of hands and soles of feet, moist lesions in mouth (mucous patches), elevated flat lesions (condylomata lata) about genitalia; alopecia, lymphadenopathy, serology reactive; highly infectious
         c. Early syphilis—only symptom, reactive serology
         d. Late syphilis—15 to 20 years after onset, serology reactive; small number develop complications
      6. Diagnosis—bacteriologic and serologic
         a. Dark-field examination of serous exudate from primary lesions for *Treponema pallidum;* skill needed to obtain specimen
         b. Serologic examination—if negative but dark-field is positive, patient is treated; if both are negative, serol-

ogy is repeated at intervals for 3 months

c. Spinal fluid examination—lumbar puncture for central nervous system involvement; *Treponema* antibody present in 30% with secondary syphilis

7. Serologic tests—many developed, only a few in use
    a. Nontreponemal (reagin)
        (1) Complement-fixation technique —example, Kolmer
        (2) Flocculation, lipoidal antigen tests—example, Kahn; cardio-lipin tests—example, VDRL— the most widely used test today
    b. Treponemal antigen tests
        (1) Whole viable organism—example, *Treponema pallidum* im-mobilization test (TPI)
        (2) Whole nonviable organism— examples, fluorescent trepo-nemal antibody modification (FTA-200) and fluorescent treponemal antibody absorbed (FTA-ABS)
        (3) Chemical fraction of *Trepo-nema*—example, Reiter pro-tein complement-fixation test (RPCF)

8. Treatment
    a. Infectious syphilis—primary and secondary
        (1) Benzathine penicillin (Bicillin or Permapen) 2.4 million units I.M. in 1 divided dose with 4 ml. in each gluteal muscle; al-ternate treatment: procaine penicillin G in oil with alumi-num monostearate (PAM) 1.2 million units biweekly until total of 4.8 million units has been given
    b. Early syphilis
        (1) Benzathine penicillin same as in infectious syphilis; or pro-caine penicillin G 600,000 units daily for 10 days
    c. Late syphilis
        (1) Procaine penicillin G biweekly for a total of 7.2 million units or 400,000 units of benzathine penicillin weekly for 3 weeks

9. Nursing
    a. Isolation unnecessary
    b. Thorough hand washing after care

of patients with infectious syphilis

c. Gloves for enemas if anogenital lesions present
d. Gloves when changing dressings
e. Care to avoid puncture wounds if doing procedures such as starting intravenous infusions

B. Gonorrhea—worldwide, and incidence ex-tensive: 755,615 cases in 1972 in the United States

1. Etiology—*Neisseria gonorrhoeae* (gon-ococcus); organism fragile
2. Transmission—sexual contact, includ-ing homosexual relationships; ophthal-mia neonatorum may result from in-fected birth canal
3. Incubation period—variable, average 3 to 5 days
4. Symptoms
    a. Male—burning sensation on urina-tion, redness and edema of urinary meatus, mucopurulent discharge
    b. Female—vaginal discharge; symp-toms may be lacking
5. Complications
    a. Male—prostatitis, epididymitis, stricture; seminal vesicles and vas deferens may be involved; gonor-rheal arthritis, sterility
    b. Female—abscess of Bartholin's glands and Skene's ducts, salpin-gitis, endocervicitis, pelvic inflam-matory disease, gonorrheal arthritis, sterility
6. Diagnosis—bacteriologic smear and culture techniques; fluorescent anti-body (FA) cytochrome oxidase test, a paper test with color reaction; sero-logic test for syphilis always done
7. Treatment
    a. Male—2,400,000 units aqueous pen-icillin G or PAM in 1 injection; methacycline—1,200 mg. orally
    b. Female—4,800,000 units of peni-cillin G in 1 divided dose
    c. Complicated gonorrhea—crystalline penicillin G 4 to 10 million units with administration at 2- to 4-hour intervals
    d. Ophthalmia neonatorum—aqueous penicillin G 150,000 to 300,000 units daily for 7 days
8. Nursing—isolation unnecessary; care as in syphilis
9. Prevention of syphilis and gonorrhea

a. Case finding through interviewing of contacts
b. Early sex education in home and school
c. Public education
d. Control of prostitution
e. Uniform legislation for premarital and prenatal serologic examinations
f. Need to deal with social, economic, cultural, and personality problems
g. Prophylactic penicillin questioned by some; if given, serology follow-up for several months

NURSING PATIENTS WITH PROBLEMS IN CELLULAR NUTRITION

1. **Basic principles of nursing**
A. Health education in nutrition, elimination, and normal functioning of gastrointestinal tract
B. Nutrition of very young and of aged present special problems; if neglected, may be responsible for many disorders
C. None of essential dietary factors can be formed in body; therefore, must be obtained in diet
D. Maintenance of patency of entire gastrointestinal tract
E. Maintenance of electrolyte balance of system
F. Control of emotions for satisfactory digestion
G. Maintenance of nutritional and fluid needs of patient
H. Rehabilitation of patients with gastrointestinal disorders
I. Observation and accurate recording of all alimentary tract discharge
J. Allowance for individuality of eating patterns when possible
K. Provision for patient's cultural and religious preferences for foods
L. Observation and reporting subjective and objective symptoms
M. Maintenance of cleanliness and avoidance of infection
N. Emotional support of utmost importance
2. **Causes of problems in cellular nutrition**
A. Alteration in fluid and electrolyte balance
1. Changes in sodium
2. Changes in potassium
3. Changes in calcium
4. Mixed depletions
5. Changes in body fluid volume
6. Changes in hydrogen ion concentration

B. Imbalance in supply of essential factors
1. Nutritive
2. Quantitative
C. Inadequate ingestion
1. Interference with mastication
2. Interference with swallowing
D. Inadequate digestion
1. Abnormal motility
2. Abnormality of enzymes or digestive juices
3. Inadequate digestive area
E. Inadequate absorption
1. Inadequate absorption
2. Biochemical abnormalities
3. Inadequate absorptive surface
4. Lymphatic obstruction
5. Altered bacterial flow
F. Inadequate transportation
G. Inadequate utilization by cells
H. Abnormal excretion of waste products
3. **Nursing patients with gastrointestinal pathology**
A. Accurate intake and output records especially important
B. Usually additional vitamins and/or special diets required to maintain nutrition
C. Patients with various types of tubes for ingestion of nutrients or disposal of waste products need special instructions concerning care of equipment
D. Emotional support needed, since distressing to be unable to enjoy food
E. Education concerning foods for adequate nutrition and importance of mental tranquility for proper digestion
F. Important observations
1. For blood in stool, sputum, and other discharges—amount, time, duration, and any distinctive characteristics should be noted
2. For pain—emotional distress, food intolerances, food fads, anorexia, dysphagia, nausea, and other symptoms of dysfunction of nutritional process
4. **Diagnostic and therapeutic procedures in gastrointestinal pathology**
A. Gastric analysis—fasting specimen of gastric contents examined for components and amount (p. 301)
1. Procedure
a. Specimen obtained through gastric tube
b. Histamine given✓
c. Desired number of specimens (usually 3) taken every 15 minutes
d. Important to label specimen bottles clearly, noting exact time obtained

2. Adrenalin should be available for use in event patient reacts to histamine
3. Amount of hydrochloric acid in gastric contents important finding

B. Cholecystogram—to determine adequacy of gallbladder
1. Radiopaque substance, Priodax, given orally; stored in gallbladder in same manner as bile
2. Roentgenogram taken 12 to 24 hours later; if gallbladder patent, patient may be given "fat" meal and another roentgenogram taken in 2 or 3 hours

C. Percutaneous transhepatic cholangiogram—aid to distinguish between stones and neoplasms in gallbladder
1. Bile aspirated from liver, and dye (75% diatrizoate sodium with diatrizoate methylglucamine) injected
2. Outlines and filling of ducts observed with television monitor

D. Complete gastrointestinal series—barium swallowed and/or administered by enema
1. Order for n.p.o. for 6 to 8 hours prior to test
2. Cathartics may be ordered after barium swallow
3. Enemas usually after a barium enema

E. "Oscopy" examinations
1. Gastroscopy—n.p.o. for 8 hours prior to test and several hours afterward
2. Sigmoidoscopy and proctoscopy
   a. Laxatives administered evening before test
   b. Enemas until clear on morning of test

F. Decompression—commonly referred to as intubation—suction siphonage and nasogastric suction
1. Therapeutic uses
   a. Removal of gas and fluids in prevention and treatment of distention following abdominal operations
   b. Study with x-ray films the response of alimentary tract to opaque liquids introduced through the tube
   c. Removal of contents from alimentary tract
   d. Removal of stomach contents as preparation for and during anesthesia
2. If irrigation is required, important to use physiologic solution so that electrolytes are not washed out

5. Common nutritional disorders
A. Undernutrition or starvation—may be due to inadequate intake or absorption, impaired utilization, or increased metabolism
1. Many diets in America deficient in thiamin, nicotinic acid, riboflavin, ascorbic acid, or calcium, because of poor selection of food
2. Starvation manifested in four successive stages
   a. Tissue depletion, characterized by
      (1) Weight loss
      (2) Headache
      (3) Fatigue
      (4) Irritability
      (5) Insomnia
      (6) Depression
   b. Biochemical disturbance, characterized by
      (1) Hypoproteinemia
      (2) Lack of vitamins K and C
   c. Functional disturbances, characterized by
      (1) Emaciation
      (2) Weakness
      (3) Edema
      (4) Muscle atrophy
      (5) Premature aging
      (6) Poor teeth
      (7) Evidence of pituitary, thyroid, and gonadal failure
   d. Anatomic lesions
      (1) Pathologic fractures
      (2) Bleeding gums
      (3) Hemorrhaging into skin
      (4) Dermatitis
      (5) Glossitis
      (6) Edema
      (7) Infections or ulcers that heal slowly if at all; may affect any structure
3. Treatment and nursing care
   a. Supplying adequate nutrition, including "protective foods"
   b. Treatment of concurrent diseases

B. Obesity—refers to physical state in which amount of fat stored in body is excessive; occurs when caloric intake exceeds expenditure of energy
1. May arise from intake greater than normal, energy expenditure less than normal, or both
2. Probably majority of cases due to combination of physical and psychological factors
3. Symptoms
   a. In addition to overweight
      (1) Dyspnea

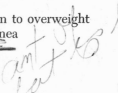

(2) Fatigue on exertion
(3) Lower back pain
(4) Flat feet
b. Predisposes to
(1) Arthritis
(2) Diabetes
(3) Arterial hypertension
c. Increases probability of heart failure in heart disease and exaggerates symptoms due to impaired circulation
4. Treatment
a. Prevention easier than remedy
b. Psychological and/or physical causes should receive first consideration
c. Eventually, decrease in caloric intake only cure

C. Gout—disturbance of purine metabolism characterized by deposition of urates in tissues of joints, particularly in cartilages
1. Symptoms
a. Attacks appear
(1) Joint becomes
(a) Painful
(b) Tender
(c) Swollen
(d) Deep red or purplish
(e) With distended veins
b. Attacks subside
(1) Cuticle peels
(2) Local itching
c. May eventually lead to podagra, ulcerations, and/or amputation
2. Treatment and nursing care
a. Purine-free diet (low in fats, rich in carbohydrates and proteins) (p. 246)
b. No alcohol
c. Colchicine tablets, probenecid, and phenylbutazone
d. Rest of affected parts
e. Hot compresses during exacerbations
f. Alkalies
g. Excision of tophi
h. Adrenal steroids used with some success

D. Sprue—chronic afebrile disease with exacerbations and remissions
1. Characteristics
a. Glossitis
b. Gastrointestinal disturbances
c. Diarrhea with frothy stools
2. Treatment
a. Parenteral liver therapy

b. Folic acid
c. Fat-restricted diet
d. Brewer's yeast
e. Calcium lactate and phosphate
f. Can be cured if treated in time

E. Acidosis—term referring to decrease of alkaline reserve of blood
1. True acidosis when there is increase in hydrogen ion concentration of blood; e.g., diabetic coma
2. Treatment
a. Restoring alkaline reserve with sodium chloride, Hartmann's solution, or other solution containing required electrolytes

F. Alkalosis—excess of alkalies in body fluids
1. Treatment
a. Supplying chlorides lost because of persistent vomiting or gastric suction
b. Discontinuing sodium bicarbonate (sometimes taken for gastric distress)

6. Vitamin deficiency diseases
Extreme deficiencies rare in United States at present
A. Vitamin A deficiency
1. Characteristics
a. Atrophy and keratinization of epithelial tissue
b. Infections of eye
c. Infections of respiratory organs
d. Infections of genitourinary tract
e. Infections of mouth
f. In severe cases, night blindness and xerophthalmia
2. Treatment
a. Obtaining vitamin A
(1) Naturally, from
(a) Liver
(b) Kidney
(c) Lungs
(d) Animal fats
(e) Green and yellow vegetables and fruits
(f) Fish oils and milk
(2) Medically, from
(a) Concentrated fish-liver oils
(b) Carotene
(c) Synthetic vitamin A
b. Continuing treatment for 3 to 4 months until beneficial results observed

B. Vitamin B₁ deficiency (beriberi)
1. Characteristics

a. Peripheral neuritis
b. Edema
c. Muscular atrophy
d. Cardiovascular changes
e. Extremities may be atrophied
2. Treatment
a. Obtaining sufficient amounts of thiamin
(1) Naturally, from
(a) Whole grains
(b) Lean meat
(c) Eggs
(d) Vegetables
(e) Milk
(2) Medically
(a) Dried brewer's yeast
(b) Crystalline vitamin B
(c) Thiamin hydrochloride may be given intravenously, intramuscularly, or orally
C. Pellagra (vitamin B complex deficiency)
1. Characteristics
a. Fatigue
b. Insomnia
c. Loss of teeth
d. Infections
e. Food idiosyncrasies
f. Glossitis
g. Stomatitis
h. Tremors
i. Labile emotional states
j. Sometimes, dermatitis
2. Prevention
a. Well-balanced diet
b. Brewer's yeast
c. Wheat germ
d. Proteins
3. Treatment and nursing care
a. High-protein, high-caloric diet
b. Adequate rest
c. Crude liver extract
d. Vitamin B complex (niacin, nicotinic acid, riboflavin, pyridoxine)
e. Thiamin hydrochloride
D. Riboflavin deficiency—may be the most prevalent deficiency disease today
1. Characteristics
a. Stomatitis
b. Fissures of corners of mouth
c. Glossitis
d. Corneal vascular irritation
e. Failing vision
2. Prevention—proper diet
a. Milk
b. Liver

c. Whole grains
3. Treatment—synthetic riboflavin will correct symptoms in few days
E. Vitamin C deficiency (scurvy)
1. Characteristics
a. Apathy
b. Anorexia
c. Fatigue
d. Loss of strength
e. Edema
f. Accumulation of fluid in body cavities
g. Increased tendency to infection
h. Hemorrhage
i. Mental depression
2. Prevention depends on diet adequate in ascorbic acid, found in
a. Citrus fruits
b. Green vegetables
c. Tubers
3. Treatment—ascorbic acid may be given orally
F. Vitamin D deficiency (rickets)
1. Characteristics
a. Inability to metabolize calcium and phosphorus
b. Deficient deposits of lime in bones and cartilage, leading to soft, deformed bones
2. Prevention includes sunlight and vitamin D
3. Treatment—vitamin D found in cod-liver oil, viosterol (irradiated ergosterol), and irradiated milk
G. Vitamin K deficiency—causes lowered blood prothrombin
1. Characterized by hemorrhagic manifestations
2. Treatment consists of giving vitamin K (Synkayvite, menadiol sodium diphosphate) unless deficiency is due to inability of liver to utilize vitamin K
7. Diseases of upper gastrointestinal tract
A. Oral mucosa often reflects general condition
1. Koplik's spots before measles
2. Bleeding from gums in jaundice
3. Atrophy in pernicious anemia
4. Many others
B. Stomatitis—infection of oral cavity
1. Symptoms
a. Swelling
b. Redness
c. Tenderness of gums
2. Types
a. Catarrhal

b. Ulcerative

c. Gangrenous

C. Herpes simplex (fever blisters)—group of vesicles on erythematous base, due to latent filtrable virus that may be activated by infection, digestive disturbances, and menses (p. 392)

D. Vincent's angina (trench mouth)—acute infection of oral mucosa with fusiform bacillus and spirochete described by Vincent

1. Symptoms
   a. Fever
   b. Anorexia
   c. Pain
   d. Foul breath
   e. Enlarged cervical and submental glands
   f. Purplish red gums covered by gray membrane
2. Treatment
   a. Antibiotics
   b. Mouthwashes
   c. Sometimes, dental care

E. Parasitic stomatitis (thrush)—fungous infection of oral mucosa characterized by dry mucous membrane covered with adherent white patches resembling milk curd

F. Ludwig's angina—streptococcal infection of floor of mouth and submaxillary glands

1. Symptoms
   a. Severe infection
   b. Malaise
   c. Elevation of temperature
   d. Swelling under jaw, extending to neck
   e. Pain
   f. Salivation
   g. Toxemia
   h. Edema of glottis
   i. Difficulty in swallowing and talking
2. Treatment and nursing care
   a. Antibiotics
   b. Warm saline irrigations
   c. High fluid intake
   d. In severe cases, incision and drainage and/or tracheotomy

G. Leukoplakia—white, smooth patches on mucous membranes or tongue; may be precancerous lesions

1. Causes
   a. Tobacco
   b. Infected teeth
   c. Electrogalvanic charge between dissimilar dental appliances

d. Highly spiced foods

e. Any chronic irritation

2. Treatment
   a. Elimination of cause or causes
   b. If persistent, radical removal of lesions

H. Tumors of mouth create difficult medical and nursing problem; nurse should miss no opportunity to inspect mouth and gums for symptoms of beginning malignancy

1. Epithelioma of lip, tongue, or cheek most common cancer of mouth
   a. Symptoms
      (1) Metastasis to lymph nodes of neck
      (2) Later, pain and soreness
      (3) Excessive salivation
      (4) Complications due to aspiration
2. Only effective treatment—radical surgery or radiotherapy

I. Salivation—excess salivation to 10 liters daily (normal, 3 to 4 liters); may be a symptom or an idiopathic condition

1. Causes
   a. Drugs
   b. Poisons
   c. Local inflammation or irritation
   d. Infectious diseases
   e. Reflex stimulation of stomach
   f. Diseases of nervous system
   g. Idiopathic
2. Symptoms
   a. Excess salivation
   b. Indigestion
   c. Vomiting
   d. Disordered taste
   e. Thickened speech
3. Cause should be treated and measures taken to prevent swallowing large amounts of saliva

J. Inflammation of salivary gland—sometimes called surgical parotitis (differentiate from mumps caused by virus); usually due to *Staphylococcus aureus*

1. Symptoms
   a. Pain
   b. Tenderness
   c. Rise in temperature
   d. Marked swelling
   e. Dysphagia
   f. Redness
   g. Shininess
   h. Fluctuation of overlying skin
2. Precautionary measures
   a. Scrupulous cleansing of mouth

b. Chewing gum for lubrication

c. Adequate fluids

3. Treatment and nursing care

a. Antibiotics

b. Warm packs

c. Fluids

d. Sometimes, incision and drainage

K. Salivary calculi or tumors—if they cause symptoms, excision may be indicated

L. Acute pharyngitis—acute inflammation of mucous membranes of pharynx

1. Symptoms

a. Slight cold

b. Dry, painful throat

c. Painful or difficult swallowing

d. Granular, chronic, hypertrophic, or atrophic pharyngitis may result

M. Retropharyngeal abscess—accumulation of pus in submucous connective tissue of pharynx, usually due to streptococcal infection

1. Symptoms

a. Malaise

b. Fever

c. Chills

d. Difficulty in swallowing

2. Treatment and nursing care

a. Antibiotics

b. Fluids

c. If severe, incision and drainage

d. Head held in lowered position to facilitate drainage and prevent choking if abscess ruptures or incision is made

8. Surgical procedures of upper alimentary tract

A. Radical surgery of mouth or tongue

1. Preoperative care

a. Careful oral hygiene that may require large, frequent irrigations

b. Oil to mouth if dry

c. Use of dental floss

d. Antibiotics

e. Nutritional therapy

f. Fluids given

g. Emotional support, since surgery often mutilating

2. Postoperative care

a. Usual postoperative care

b. Head kept to one side to help prevent aspiration

c. Suction p.r.n.

d. Close observation for hemorrhage, edema, and complications due to aspiration

e. Patient's nutrition and electrolyte balance maintained

B. Radiation therapy, radium, or radon seeds—usually used when lesion on posterior part of tongue

1. Radon seeds may not need removing

2. Radium needles have strings attached; may cause difficulty in talking or swallowing

3. Radiation therapy applied directly

4. Any of these procedures may cause systemic reaction

a. Loss of appetite

b. Nausea

c. Vomiting

d. Headache

e. Malaise

5. Smoking should be prohibited; mouthwash should be available at all times, since mouth will be very dry and have bad odor

9. Diseases of esophagus

Rare but very serious, since life without normally functioning esophagus very difficult

A. Congenital abnormalities—part may be missing, or either end may connect with trachea and require surgery; portion may be too narrow and require dilatation

B. Diverticulum of esophagus—sac or pouch protruding from wall of esophagus

1. Symptoms—range from none to inability to swallow or to regurgitation of food eaten days before

2. Treatment and nursing care

a. May be dilatation if small or surgery if large

b. Surgery of esophagus usually involves

(1) Temporary gastrostomy

(2) Thoracic surgery

(3) Maintaining nutrition and fluid balance

C. Inflammation of esophagus—may occur during course of infections or may be due to chemical irritants

1. Chemical irritants cause strictures and may eventually require gastrostomy

2. Treatment and nursing care of patients who have swallowed chemical irritants

a. Combat pain and shock

b. Antidotes

c. Fluids

d. Later, pass silk thread and bougie to prevent strictures

D. Spasms of esophagus—result of imbalance between sympathetic and parasympathetic stimulation when lower portion of esophagus is affected, known as cardiospasm

1. Symptoms may begin gradually or suddenly
   a. Gastric pain
   b. Varying degrees of dysphagia
   c. Regurgitation
2. Treatment and nursing care
   a. Dilatation (passage of French sound followed by hydrostatic dilator)
   b. Maintenance of nutritional and fluid balance
   c. Emotional support

E. Esophageal varices—bleeding varicose veins of esophagus, usually found with portal hypertension; unless bleeding can be controlled, patient will not live
   1. Due to inaccessibility of veins in esophagus, controlling hemorrhage can be very difficult; several methods used to control bleeding
      a. Esophageal tamponade—Sengstaken-Blakemore tube
      b. Pitressin or Pituitrin and vitamin K
      c. Portacaval or splenorenal shunt to reduce pressure
   2. Nursing care very exacting
      a. Observation for hemorrhage
      b. Maintenance of nutritional and fluid balance
      c. Reassurance; care of tube
      d. Meticulous oral hygiene given frequently because blood leaves foul taste in mouth

F. Tumors of esophagus—benign tumors and sarcomas rare, but carcinoma probably most important disease of esophagus
   1. Symptoms begin insidiously with dysphagia; poor nutrition much later
   2. Surgery only treatment, but usually discovered too late; gastrostomy necessary in either case

10. **Surgical procedures for esophageal pathology**

A. Preoperative care for surgery on esophagus
   1. Normal nutrition and fluid balances need to be restored
   2. Patient needs explanations and reassurance
   3. Usually many laboratory tests required
   4. General preoperative care given

B. Postoperative care
   1. General postoperative care

2. Oxygen
3. Care of thoracic surgery and of gastrostomy

C. Nursing patient with gastrostomy—gastric fistula through abdominal wall
   1. Area around opening kept covered with heavy bland ointment, since gastric juices digest protein
   2. Accurate intake and output record kept; fluid intake maintained at high level
   3. Feedings at room temperature, given slowly; water given at end of each feeding
   4. Good mental hygiene for both patient and nurse important
   5. Excellent mouth care important; chewing gum may help keep secretions normal

11. **Diseases of stomach**

A. Acute gastritis—inflammation of stomach wall due to exogenous or endogenous causes; chronic gastritis may be atrophic or hypertrophic due to previous acute gastritis or to other irritants or neuroses

B. Hypertrophic stenosis of pylorus—congenital obstructive narrowing of pylorus with hypertrophy of pyloric muscles
   1. Usually noted in infants
   2. Characteristics
      a. Projectile vomiting
      b. Loss of weight
      c. Decreased fecal and urinary output
   3. Treatment
      a. Medical—sedatives and small, frequent feedings
      b. Surgical—Ramstedt operation

C. Foreign bodies in stomach may penetrate wall and cause abscess or peritonitis
   1. Bezoars—conglomeration of swallowed material such as hair balls
   2. No treatment except laparotomy for sharp, penetrating articles; roentgenogram usually taken

D. Diaphragmatic hernia—protrusion of stomach through diaphragm into pleural cavity; repaired through chest wall; care same as for thoracic surgery (p. 344)

E. Peptic ulcer—loss of mucosa of area of stomach or duodenum
   1. Symptoms
      a. Gnawing pain
      b. Definite food intolerances
      c. Tenderness of epigastrium
      d. Weight loss
      e. Relief with certain foods and alkalies

f. Remissions and exacerbations of symptoms
g. If severe, vomiting and/or bleeding

2. Treatment and nursing care
   a. Purpose
      (1) To promote healing of ulcer
      (2) To prevent recurrence
   b. In mild cases
      (1) Rest—mental, physical, and emotional
      (2) Psychotherapy
      (3) Sedation
      (4) Bland diet
      (5) Neutralization of hydrochloric acid by antacids such as Amphojel, aluminum hydroxide, calcium carbonate
      (6) Observe for alkalosis, indicated by
         (a) Loss of appetite
         (b) Lassitude
         (c) Vomiting
   c. In severe cases
      (1) Surgery may be necessary in severe cases and for complications such as severe hemorrhage, perforation, or intractable pain
      (2) Surgical procedures performed
         (a) Subtotal gastrectomy
         (b) Gastrojejunostomy
         (c) Gastroenterostomy
         (d) Vagotomy

F. Cancer of stomach—"silent neoplasm"
   1. Types
      a. Polypoid
      b. Infiltrating
      c. Ulcerating
      d. Diffuse infiltrating
   2. Symptoms
      a. Vague and atypical
      b. Absent or diminished hydrochloric acid in gastric contents
      c. Slight digestive symptoms
      d. Gastric fullness and dyspepsia
      e. Later, pain induced by eating and relieved by vomiting
      f. Much later, anemia, metastasis, hemorrhage, and obstruction
   3. More than half metastasize before diagnosis; carcinoma of stomach metastasizes to lymph nodes and liver; spreads by direct extension and infiltration, and by transplantation to ovaries
   4. After 50 years of age, any gastric distress should be investigated; x-ray most valuable means of diagnosis
   5. Only treatment for gastric malignancy—radical surgical removal; only contraindication to surgery—unresectability
   6. Palliative procedures
      a. Radiation therapy to delay growth of cancer cells; may increase nausea and vomiting
      b. Gastroenterostomy—surgical anastomosis of stomach and small bowel; may give 6 to 18 months of fairly comfortable life

12. Nursing patient with gastric surgery
A. Preoperative care
   1. General condition as nearly normal as possible; if necessary, blood, vitamins, proteins, and electrolytes given
   2. Patient should have adequate explanations and should feel as secure as possible
   3. In addition to usual preoperative tests, blood chemistry and gastric acidity tests done (normal acidity after histamine, 25% to 50%); stomach gavaged and tube left in place during surgery
   4. Other immediate preoperative care much the same as for any major surgery

B. Postoperative care
   1. Usually placed in shock position at first, then in Fowler's position
   2. Gastric tube connected to suction apparatus
   3. Deep breathing, coughing, and frequent changes in position desirable
   4. Sedatives and medications for distention (Prostigmin) given as needed
   5. Accurate intake and output record
   6. Good mouth care in order to avoid aspiration and parotitis
   7. Supplemental vitamins (B_{12}) may be necessary to supply intrinsic maturation factor, especially when large portion of stomach removed
   8. Diet based on smaller, more frequent feedings, with elimination of (p. 246)
      a. Concentrated sweets
      b. Acids
      c. Raw vegetables or fruits
      d. Condiments
      e. Most meat stocks

C. More usual postoperative complications
   1. Shock and/or hemorrhage
   2. Complications involving lungs

a. Atelectasis
b. Pulmonary infarct
c. Pneumonia
3. Complications involving stomach
  a. Ileus
  b. Mechanical obstruction
  c. Acute dilatation, especially after vagotomy
  d. Dumping syndrome
  e. Diarrhea
4. Peritonitis
5. Thrombosis and embolism
6. Wound evisceration

13. Diseases of small intestine

A. Visceroptosis—prolapse or falling of viscera; not disease, but manifestation of lean, lank body with loss of abdominal muscle tone; important only when kidney or spleen becomes strangulated in pelvis

B. Diverticulitis—infection of diverticuli in intestine
1. Symptoms
  a. Signs of peritoneal irritation
  b. Elevated temperature
  c. Elevated leukocyte count
  d. Loss of weight
  e. Discomfort
2. Treatment and nursing care
  a. Rest in bed
  b. Antibiotics
  c. Heat to abdomen
  d. Symptomatic care of complications
  e. With complications—radiation therapy, resection, or colostomy may be required
3. More usual complications
  a. Perforation
  b. Fistula
  c. Obstruction

C. Meckel's diverticulum—remnant of mesenteric duct that normally disappears within a few weeks after birth, persists as fibrous cord
1. May cause
  a. Volvulus
  b. Strangulation
  c. Intussusception
  d. Inflammation similar to appendicitis
2. Treatment—surgery

D. Regional ileitis—nonspecific inflammation of distal loops of small intestine with "cobblestone" ulceration
1. Symptoms
  a. Those of low-grade infection
  b. Diarrhea
  c. Abdominal pain

d. Loss of weight
e. May progress to exhaustion or to formation of fistula to abdominal wall or to other hollow organs
f. Rarely fatal
2. Treatment and nursing care
  a. Supportive
  b. Bland diet with vitamins
  c. Sunlight
  d. Transfusions
  e. Emotional tranquility
  f. Antibiotics

E. Neoplasms of small intestine—benign tumors more common than malignant tumors
1. Adenoma the usual benign tumor found; causes trouble only if complicated by
  a. Hemorrhage
  b. Perforation
  c. Obstruction
2. Carcinoma and sarcoma sometimes found
  a. Symptoms
    (1) Early
      (a) Indefinite until lesions far advanced
      (b) Indigestion
    (2) Much later
      (a) Nausea
      (b) Vomiting
      (c) Loss of weight
      (d) Hematemesis or melena
      (e) Cachexia
      (f) Pain
      (g) Symptoms of obstruction
3. As for all malignancies, treatment surgical or palliative

F. Trichinosis—first stage of infestation with parasite *Trichinella spiralis;* enters body through ingestion of insufficiently cooked pork containing encysted larvae
1. Symptoms
  a. Early—when larvae enter mucosa of intestine and mesenteric lymphatics
    (1) Nausea
    (2) Vomiting
    (3) Diarrhea
    (4) Sometimes, eruptions of skin
  b. Later
    (1) Myositis
    (2) Remittent fever
    (3) Edema
    (4) Dehydration
    (5) Hallucinations

also called Crohn's disease

Crohn's disease

2. Treatment and nursing care
   a. Purging
   b. High fluid intake
   c. Sedation
3. Preventive measures important
   a. Thorough cooking of all pork
   b. No feeding of raw garbage to hogs
   c. Extermination of rats and mice

G. Appendicitis—inflammation of vermiform appendix; most common major surgical condition—over 20,000 in United States yearly
   1. Symptoms
      a. Acute appendicitis
         (1) Abdominal pain that localizes in lower right quadrant
         (2) Tenderness and rigidity
         (3) Nausea and vomiting
         (4) Increased leukocyte count
         (5) Constipation
         (6) Low-grade fever
      b. Chronic appendicitis
         (1) Exacerbations and remissions
         (2) Symptoms of acute appendicitis in milder form
   2. Palliative treatment and nursing care
      a. Fowler's position
      b. Nothing by mouth
      c. Ice bag to lower right quadrant
      d. No cathartics
      e. Close observation of T.P.R. and leukocyte count
   3. Surgical treatment—appendectomy
   4. Complications of appendicitis
      a. If not controlled
         (1) Perforation
         (2) Formation of abscess
         (3) Spontaneous subsidence
         (4) Production of intestinal obstruction
      b. Most serious complication—ruptured appendix with peritonitis
         (1) Symptoms
            (a) Sudden sharp pain followed by comparative comfort
            (b) Rapid rise in temperature and leukocyte count
            (c) Few hours later
               (1) Shallow thoracic breathing
               (2) Anxiety
               (3) Dehydration
               (4) Increasing shock
         (2) Treatment
            (a) Immediate appendectomy, usually with drainage

            (b) Local and systemic antibiotics
            (c) Semi-Fowler's position
            (d) Fluids
            (e) Blood transfusions

H. Bowel obstructions—mechanical obstruction; ileus

14. Pathology of large intestine
A. Diarrhea—infection of large bowel, characterized by evacuation of watery or unformed stool
   1. Diarrhea—symptom of many disorders; symptoms vary greatly in severity and duration; when persistent, should receive careful investigation
   2. Symptoms
      a. Frequent, watery stools—no blood
      b. Nausea and vomiting
      c. Abdominal cramps
   3. Treatment of simple diarrhea
      a. Rest in bed
      b. No food for 24 hours
      c. Fluids and no enemas or rectal irrigations

B. Ulcerative colitis—inflammatory disease of unknown etiology; theories involve infection and/or emotional problems; no bacteria found
   1. Symptoms progressive; may lead to chronic invalidism
      a. Diarrhea
      b. Passage of blood and mucus
      c. Loss of appetite
      d. Nausea and vomiting
      e. Fever in severe cases
      f. Death possible from exhaustion, perforation, or peritonitis
      g. Possible remissions and exacerbations
   2. Treatment and nursing care
      a. No known specific treatment
      b. Rest in bed
      c. Heat to abdomen
      d. Bland nourishing diet
      e. Vitamin K for bleeding
      f. Mental and emotional tranquility
      g. Sedatives

C. Constipation—passage of unduly hard and dry fecal material; probably most mismanaged health problem in United States
   1. Consistency of stool more important than frequency or quantity expelled
   2. Atonic constipation—constipation with no abdominal distress; often follows years of "laxative habit"
      a. Treatment

(1) Establishment of "habit time"
(2) Diet adequate in laxative foods
    (a) Oatmeal
    (b) Spinach
    (c) Prunes
    (d) Vegetables
    (e) Fruit juices
    (f) Whole wheat bread
    (g) Others
(3) Ability to relax should be cultivated

D. Irritable colon or functional bowel distress
1. Possible causes
    a. Excessive irritation by cathartics
    b. Foods
    c. Enemas
    d. Emotional disturbances
    e. Any combination of these
2. Symptoms
    a. Feeling of fullness and distress
    b. Usually constipation
    c. Frequently nausea
    d. Sometimes large amounts of mucus expelled
3. Treatment and nursing care
    a. Relief of anxiety and worry concerning condition
    b. Establishment of "habit time"
    c. Dietary control
    d. Antispasmodics such as tincture of belladonna, atropine, or phenobarbital
    e. Glycerin suppositories
    f. Small enemas
    g. Opiates, cathartics, and smoking contraindicated

E. Acute dilatation of colon—usually complication of other pathology; three principal types
1. Gaseous—may follow functional bowel distress, abdominal surgery, or febrile illness such as pneumonia
2. Obstructive—usually due to new growths; requires surgery
3. Megacolon or Hirschsprung's disease —congenital condition of extreme dilatation of colon; child's growth stunted, abdomen enlarged, and bowel movements very infrequent (may be weeks apart)

F. Cancer of colon—principal pathologic condition of colon, especially common in sigmoid and rectum; rectal examinations should be integral part of all physical examinations

1. Symptoms
    a. Vague and slow to develop
    b. Progressive over long period of time
    c. Distention
    d. Increasing constipation, sometimes alternating with diarrhea, cramps, vague soreness in lower abdomen
    e. Blood in stools
    f. "Pencil" stools
    g. Anemia
    h. Weight loss
2. Treatment—surgical removal and permanent colostomy
3. Polyps often pathogenic of carcinoma; may need to be removed
4. Diverticuli seldom become malignant; usually treated conservatively with antibiotics

15. **Nursing patients with intestinal surgery**
A. Preoperative care
1. Care given all major surgical patients
2. Low-residue diet high in proteins; liquid diet at prescribed interval before surgery
3. Antibiotics for lower intestinal tract, such as Sulfasuxidine or neomycin
4. Complete intestinal tract may be intubated
5. Give laxatives as directed to cleanse bowel by catharsis
6. Administer enemas and colonic irrigations to rid bowel of feces and gas

B. Postoperative care
1. All principles of major surgical care
2. Retention of urine and flatus and lack of peristalsis may require special nursing procedures
3. Oral intake started cautiously; laxatives may be contraindicated
4. Ensure function of the suction tube for as long as needed
5. Complications
    a. Intra-abdominal disease
    b. Intracolonic infections
    c. Wound infections
6. Encourage patient to have follow-up examinations

C. Nursing patient with cecostomy or with temporary colostomy
1. Since both conditions temporary, emotional distress of patient not great; may be very distasteful, however; nurse should never let patient see signs of revulsion in her attitude

2. Bowel near opening usually irrigated, done gently
3. Patient kept clean; odors controlled as much as possible; skin around opening coated with protective ointment

D. Nursing care of patient with permanent colostomy likely to be difficult for both patient and nurse
1. Helping patient accept colostomy emotionally, an important nursing duty
2. Protective ointment kept around opening to protect skin
3. As soon as possible, patient should begin to practice caring for his own colostomy
4. Irrigations should be done at same time every day to establish "habit time"
5. Diet should be selected to produce soft, formed stools
6. Cathartics contraindicated
7. Colostomy bag may be desired by patient; but usually more satisfactory to control expulsion of feces so that few pieces of gauze give all protection needed after daily morning evacuation

16. Pathology of rectum and anus
A. Fissure in ano—crack or fissure in anal skin caused by infection or trauma
1. Characterized by excruciating pain with each bowel movement and inability to heal, since it becomes reinfected
2. Treatment may be palliative or surgical
B. Fistula in ano—tiny tubular tract between anal canal and skin near anus, characterized by continuous drainage of pus
1. Treatment surgical; requires complete exposure of tract from primary to secondary opening
2. One of two methods of aftercare used
   a. Constipating—no bowel movement for 4 days
   b. Stool kept at liquid or very soft consistency
3. Sedatives, sitz baths, and observation for hemorrhage necessary
C. Hemorrhoids—varicose veins in rectum; may be internal (above internal sphincter) or external; embarrassing; many wait too long before seeking medical help
1. Preventive measures
   a. Sufficient roughage in diet
   b. Daily exercise
   c. Adequate fluids
   d. Regular bowel habits
   e. Early treatment of anal conditions
   f. Early help for symptoms
2. Treatment
   a. Palliative
      (1) Avoidance of heavy labor
      (2) Application of warm wet packs after defecation
      (3) Sitz baths
      (4) Prevention of constipation
   b. Nonsurgical
      (1) Injection of sclerosing substances into varicosities
      (2) Application of electric energy in one of its various forms
   c. Surgical—hemorrhoidectomy, excision of varicosities
   d. Nursing care
      (1) Cleanliness of area
      (2) Comfort of patient (bowel movements very painful following hemorrhoidectomy until wound healed)
      (3) Teaching patient proper bowel habits
      (4) Heat and sedatives for comfort
D. Ischiorectal abscess—abscess located in fatty tissue near anus
1. Usually requires large incision and drainage
2. Feces kept liquid or soft during postoperative period
E. Carcinoma of rectum—most serious of rectal diseases; adenocarcinoma that metastasizes through inguinal lymph nodes most common type
1. Symptoms
   a. Vary
   b. Change in bowel habit
   c. Bleeding, sometimes pain
   d. Much later, loss of weight
2. Treatment—surgical
   a. Abdominoperineal resection with permanent colostomy
   b. Patients in inoperable cases may benefit from local cauterization
3. Preoperative preparation
   a. Routine care given in major surgical cases
   b. Decompression of large bowel
   c. Both abdominal and rectal surgical preparation
4. Postoperative care
   a. General postoperative care

b. Care of colostomy
c. Care of Foley catheter
d. Care of rectal wound
e. Care of abdominal incision
f. Usually sitz baths given for perineal wound after few days
g. Help with emotional adjustment
h. Help and teaching to prepare patient and/or his family to care for colostomy and to be on alert for further symptoms or complications

17. **Pathology of mesentery and abdominal wall**

A. Mesenteric thrombosis—occlusion of mesenteric vessels by thrombus or embolism that usually leads to death of some part of abdominal wall
  1. Symptoms
    a. Sudden, severe, generalized pain
    b. Vomiting
    c. Sometimes, bloody diarrhea
    d. Condition frequently fatal
  2. Surgical treatment—affected area brought to outside and resected to line of demarcation
B. Wounds and contusions of abdominal wall—serious in proportion to amount of visceral damage
  1. Difficult to judge amount of injury
  2. Time of utmost importance
  3. Severe abdominal injuries should be investigated immediately
  4. Urine should be examined for blood
C. Abdominal hernia—congenital or acquired condition characterized by protrusion of viscus through abdominal wall; hernias may be classified anatomically or according to degree of severity
  1. Most common abdominal hernias
    a. Inguinal
    b. Femoral
    c. Umbilical
  2. Degree of severity more important than location
    a. Reducible hernias—those whose contents will return to abdominal cavity with patient in supine position
    b. Incarcerated hernias—those in which intestinal flow is completely arrested
    c. Strangulated hernias—those in which both intestinal flow and blood supply to area are obstructed
  3. Usual treatment of hernia—surgery; trusses or injections of sclerosing material sometimes used

4. Nursing care of herniorrhaphy
  a. Usual preoperative care
  b. Postoperative care
    (1) Observation
    (2) Relief of pain
    (3) Prevention of urinary retention
    (4) Patient usually may return to work in about 60 days
5. Postoperative complications rare, but may include
  a. Pneumonia
  b. Collapse of lung
  c. Epididymitis
  d. Phlebothrombosis
  e. Wound infection
  f. Scrotal hernia
  g. Pulmonary embolus
  h. Hydrocele

18. **Pathology of biliary tract**

A. Jaundice—due to accumulation of bile pigments in bloodstream
  1. Possible causes
    a. Too rapid breakdown of red blood cells
    b. Disease of liver
    c. Obstruction in posthepatic system
  2. Characteristics
    a. Yellow pigmentation
    b. Dark urine
    c. Clay-colored stools
    d. Pruritus
B. Diseases of liver
  1. Cirrhosis—fibrous replacement of normal liver cells, due primarily to dietary deficiency
    a. Symptoms
      (1) Weight loss
      (2) Increased susceptibility to hepatitis
      (3) Ascites
      (4) Chills and fever
      (5) May predispose to portal hypertension
    b. Serious complication—portal hypertension (Banti's syndrome) characterized by
      (1) Congested spleen
      (2) Ascites
      (3) Esophageal varices
      (4) Hemorrhoids
      (5) Jaundice
      (6) Edema
      (7) Telangiectasis
      (8) Patient may have complete liver failure
    c. Treatment and nursing care

(1) High-protein, low-fat, salt-poor diet
(2) Vitamin B complex
(3) Special skin care because of subcutaneous edema
(4) Diuretics
(5) Care of complications
(6) Ascites may require frequent paracentesis
(7) Intake and output records kept
(8) Esophageal varices discussed on p. 372

2. Hepatitis—may be due to infection, to serum, or to toxic causes
    a. Infection or serum the cause
        (1) Virus A—epidemic jaundice; infectious hepatitis (IH): 54,-340 cases in 1972 in the United States
        (2) Virus B—homologous serum hepatitis (SH): 8,817 cases in 1972 in the United States
    b. Toxic—due to chemicals such as arsenine, carbon tetrachloride, phosphorus, and gold compounds
        (1) Symptoms—mild cases resemble those of epidemic hepatitis
        (2) Treatment—supportive
    c. Transmission—anal-oral route and blood
        (1) Virus A—anal-oral route and blood
        (2) Virus B—blood and blood products
        (3) Food, water, contaminated shellfish, contaminated syringes
        (4) Asymptomatic carriers possible
    d. Incubation period
        (1) Hepatitis A, 15 to 50 days
        (2) Hepatitis B, 50 to 160 days
    e. Symptoms—three phases; virus A and virus B indistinguishable
        (1) Preicteric phase
            (a) Abrupt onset
            (b) Anorexia
            (c) Chill
            (d) Nausea and vomiting
            (e) Abdominal discomfort
            (f) Diarrhea
            (g) Fever 100° to 104° F.
            (h) Cervical adenopathy, splenomegaly
            (i) Duration 24 hours to 3 weeks

        (2) Icteric phase—duration about 4 weeks
            (a) Jaundice and pruritus
            (b) Enlargement of liver
            (c) Weight loss
            (d) Irritability
            (e) Central nervous system symptoms
            (f) Return of preicteric symptoms
            (g) Urticaria
        (3) Posticteric phase—jaundice fades; convalescence
    f. Diagnosis—no immunologic tests; a number of liver function tests usually done
    g. Treatment—symptomatic only
    h. Nursing—isolation for IH for 7 days; no isolation for SH
        (1) Wear gloves for enemas, rectal temperatures, venipunctures, and dressings
        (2) Use disposable syringes and needles
        (3) Autoclave or boil for 30 minutes; hepatitis virus resistant to chemical disinfection
        (4) Encourage 3,000 to 4,000 ml. of fluid daily
        (5) Take measures to relieve pruritus
        (6) Encourage diet
        (7) Observe for change in color of stools or urine, mental confusion, coma
        (8) Destroy thermometer on recovery of patient
    i. Prevention—immune globulin for contacts, sanitation of food and water supply; avoid multiple-dose syringe; extensive use of blood and blood products complicates prevention of virus B hepatitis

3. Injuries of liver—rupture or stab wounds most common
    a. Characteristics
        (1) Shock
        (2) Hemorrhage
        (3) Pain
        (4) Possibly peritonitis, emboli, or liver abscess
    b. Treatment—surgical repair
4. Liver abscess—very hard to diagnose; patient extremely ill
    a. Symptoms
        (1) Severe pain

(2) Tenderness
(3) Chills and fever
b. Treatment and nursing care
(1) Drainage
(2) Antibiotics
(3) Meticulous nursing
5. Cancer of liver—usually secondary, following metastasis
a. Symptoms
(1) Weight loss
(2) Anemia
(3) Enlargement of liver
(4) Loss of strength
(5) Jaundice and ascites may or may not be present
b. Treatment—palliative only
6. Liver function tests
a. Icteric index—serum bilirubin concentration test
(1) Measures ability of liver to excrete bilirubin in bile
(2) Elevated concentration
(a) Either indicates mechanical obstruction to flow of bile to intestines
(b) Or indicates improper functioning of liver cells
(c) Eventually produces jaundice
b. Urobilinogen excretion
(1) Indicates amount of urobilinogen excreted in urine
(2) If no urobilinogen in urine, indicates no bile reaching intestinal tract
(3) High concentration urobilinogen in urine indicates liver cells damaged; not clearing blood of urobilinogen as it passes through liver
c. Bilirubin tolerance test
(1) Determines how rapidly liver clears bilirubin from bloodstream
(2) Serial determinations of serum bilirubin following injection done to determine rate of clearance
d. Plasma protein concentration—used to help determine liver insufficiency in chronic liver disease; in disease usually albumin decreased and globulin increased
e. Galactose tolerance test used to help determine liver's ability to utilize glycogen from simple sugars;

urine examined for galactose following test meal; increased amounts found with impaired liver function
C. Disease of gallbladder
1. Acute cholecystitis—acutely inflamed gallbladder almost always associated with calculi
a. Symptoms
(1) Begin with sudden, acute pain that radiates from right upper quadrant to tip of right scapula
(2) Nausea and vomiting
(3) Fever
(4) Jaundice may or may not be present
b. Treatment—surgery after acute symptoms subside
2. Chronic cholecystitis—characterized by attacks of acute symptoms with remissions and food intolerances; attacks milder than acute cholecystitis
3. Cholelithiasis—stones, multiple or single, blocking one of ducts
a. Symptoms
(1) Chronic indigestion
(2) Jaundice if stones in common bile duct
(3) Steady, constant pain if stones in cystic ducts
b. Treatment—surgical
4. Carcinoma of gallbladder—rare
a. Treatment—surgical or palliative
5. Cholecystogram—diagnostic test
a. Graham-Cole test—test in which radiopaque material given; 12 hours later x-ray films made of gallbladder
b. If no stones revealed, patient given fatty meal to determine ability of gallbladder to furnish bile for digestion
6. Conservative care of patients with gallbladder disease
a. Fat-free diet and avoidance of irritating foods
b. Bed rest during acute episodes
c. Sedatives (phenobarbital) after meals
d. Ice bag locally
e. Weight reduction of obese persons
f. Morphine and atropine for biliary colic
7. Nursing patients with biliary surgery
a. Preoperative care
(1) General surgical preoperative care

(2) Vitamin K

(3) Special skin care

(4) Fat-free, high-protein, and high-carbohydrate diet

(5) Sedatives as needed

b. Operations most frequently done

(1) Cholecystostomy for removal of stones or pus

(2) Cholecystectomy for removal of gallbladder

(3) Choledochotomy for removal of stones from common duct

(4) More radical procedure if carcinoma found

c. Postoperative care

(1) General care for major surgery

(2) Fat-free diet usually

(3) Intake and output record

(4) Stool noted for color daily

(5) If drainage tube, bile measured and charted

d. Principal complications — hemorrhage and pulmonary pathology

19. **Diseases of the pancreas—digestive disorders**

A. Acute pancreatitis—may be hemorrhagic or interstitial

1. Interstitial—edematous swelling of gland and escape of enzymes into surrounding tissues and peritoneal cavity

a. Symptoms

(1) Abdominal and back pain

(2) Nausea

(3) Vomiting

(4) Tenderness of upper abdomen

(5) Enzyme changes in blood, urine, peritoneal fluid

b. Treatment and nursing care—objective, decrease of enzyme production

(1) Parenteral fluids

(2) Anticholinergic and antispasmodic drugs

(3) Gastric suction

(4) Relief of pain

(5) Most attacks self-limiting

2. Hemorrhagic—may represent more advanced form of acute interstitial pancreatitis; high mortality rate

a. Symptoms—more severe, including also shock, elevated serum amylase and lipase

b. Treatment

(1) Same as for interstitial

(2) Shock—usual care for shock

c. Complications—severe may lead to abscess development

(1) Drainage required—may require close observation and constant nursing care for long time

B. Chronic pancreatitis—caused by repeated attacks of acute interstitial pancreatitis or prolonged use of alcohol in excessive amounts; occurs in adult; symptoms quite severe

1. Treatment and nursing care

a. Dependent on cause—surgery, if associated with gallbladder disease; nursing care same as for biliary tract surgery

b. Abstinence from use of alcohol

C. Tumors—may arise in any portion producing symptoms and signs that vary according to location of lesion and whether or not functioning, insulin-secreting pancreatic islet cells are involved

1. Treatment—usually limited to palliative measures

D. Cysts—most commonly are result of acute pancreatitis; produce symptoms through presence of secondary infection

1. Treatment and nursing care

a. Provide drainage

b. Protect skin

c. Make sure that drainage tube not dislodged

d. Give general postoperative care

NURSING PATIENTS WITH ENDOCRINE DISORDERS

1. **Basic principles of nursing**

A. Maintenance of professional, understanding attitude toward patient essential; often he is not responsible for his emotions or reactions

B. Emotional support necessary when undesirable changes develop in patient's appearance

C. Explanations and health education for patient and family basic so that patient encouraged to return to as normal life as possible

D. Careful observation extremely important, since patients may react to conditions or situations differently from other people

E. Remember that dysfunction of one endocrine gland affects, to some extent, functions of other endocrine glands

2. **Nursing care**

A. Accurate observation and recording, especially concerning results of medications

B. Awareness that much misinformation now present concerning endocrine dysfunction

C. Helping patient understand his illness
 1. Limitations
 2. Taking of prescribed medications regularly; may be either lifelong modification or temporary; patient should
   a. Keep 2-month supply on hand and use oldest first
   b. Know approximate length of time it will take for effects of hormone to become apparent
   c. Know signs of hypofunction and hyperfunction of the gland
 3. Carrying identification card with him at all times
 4. Avoiding stress
 5. Possible need for financial aid
 6. Encouragement to continue medical supervision

3. **Diagnostic tests and procedures commonly used**

A. Urine tests in diabetes reveal glucose (2% to 10%), increased specific gravity, increased ammonia, decreased urea, and albumin if acidosis present

B. Glucose tolerance test—used to determine body's ability to utilize carbohydrates
 1. In early A.M. patient voids and specimen saved; blood specimen taken for sugar determination
 2. 100 gm. glucose in 300 ml. lemon juice given by mouth, or 0.5 gm. glucose per kilogram body weight given intravenously
 3. Blood and urine specimens collected at stated intervals for 2 or 3 hours; specimens clearly labeled with patient's name and time collected
 4. Excessively high blood sugar level for prolonged period (over 2 hours) diagnostic for diabetes mellitus

C. Blood serum studies—amylase, calcium, glucose, insulin tolerance, lipase, phosphorus, potassium, Thorn, thyrotropin, protein-bound iodine (PBI)
 1. Protein-bound iodine
   a. Important that patient not receive any medications containing iodine during the week before the test
   b. Tests in which iodine preparations are used also interfere with accuracy of PBI results
    (1) X-ray series of gallbladder

   (2) Intravenous pyelogram
   c. Consent required

D. Tests on urine—amylase, calcium (Sulkowitch), 17-hydroxycorticosteroid, 17-ketosteroid excretion, and Thorn test

E. Basal metabolism test
 1. Important that patient be well-rested, calm, and physically relaxed
 2. N.P.O. after supper
 3. Sleeping medication withheld

F. Radioiodine uptake

G. Thyroid scan

H. Cortisone-glucose tolerance test—more sensitive than a glucose tolerance test
 1. Used when results of glucose tolerance test are inconclusive
 2. Frequently used to detect prediabetic states in pregnant women and relatives of persons with known diabetes

4. **Diseases of endocrine glands**

A. Effects of hormones so widespread that no organ or part of organ escapes influence; only more outstanding pathologic conditions mentioned here

B. Pathology of pituitary gland
 1. Hyperfunction of acidophilic cells of anterior lobe
   a. Giantism—symmetric overgrowth of body and early development; early adulthood usually brings mental and physical deterioration
   b. Acromegaly—occurs during adulthood, after puberty—excessive growth of short flat bones; progresses slowly and, unless self-limited, may result in visual disturbances, hypertrophy of heart, viscera, and in hyperthyroidism or diabetes
   c. Treatment not very satisfactory; radiation therapy of pituitary gland or surgery for relief of pressure on optic chiasm; mental distress very great
 2. Hypofunction of acidophilic cells of anterior lobe—dwarfism (i.e., pituitary dwarf as differentiated from Lorraine dwarf, just a small person); condition manifested by retardation of normal growth and development and premature aging
 3. Hyperfunction of basophilic cells of anterior lobe produces Cushing's syndrome—"buffalo-type" obesity; face and trunk become obese, extremities remain normal; hypertension, diabetes,

and/or osteoporosis may accompany condition
4. Hypofunction of basophilic cells of anterior lobe
  a. Fröhlich's syndrome—adipose genitalism or secondary hypogonadism
    (1) Symptoms
      (a) Obesity of torso
      (b) Hypogenitalism
      (c) Normal intelligence
      (d) Sensitivity to cold
      (e) Fine, scant hair
    (2) Treatment—replacement therapy
  b. Cryptorchism (undescended testicles)
    (1) Symptoms
      (a) Delay or failure of one or both testes to descend into scrotum—may be due to anatomic causes
    (2) Treatment
      (a) Gonadotropin early
      (b) Surgery before age 15
5. Hypofunction of both type cells of anterior pituitary gland
  a. Partial hypofunction
  b. Simmonds' disease—loss of function of all target glands
    (1) Characterized by profound, progressive emaciation
    (2) Replacement therapy continued indefinitely; small multiple feedings, and supportive care
6. Hypofunction of posterior lobe produces diabetes insipidus
  a. Characterized by excretion of enormous amounts of dilute urine
  b. Caused by failure of kidney tubules to reabsorb fluid
  c. Usual treatment—pituitary preparations (Pitressin tannate in oil) given as replacement therapy, fluids, and salt
C. Pathology of thyroid gland—may be toxic or nontoxic
1. Hypothyroidism
  a. Colloid goiter—large mass of colloid substance in thyroid due to iodine deficiency; treatment—administration of iodine
  b. Congenital myxedema or cretinism
    (1) Characteristics
      (a) Apathy
      (b) Subnormal temperature

      (c)
      (d) Dr
    (2) Treatment
  c. Myxedema (adul
    (1) Characteristics
      (a) Apathy
      (b) Change in perso
      (c) Puffiness of skin
      (d) Dullness
      (e) Constipation
    (2) Treatment—thyroid extract
2. Exophthalmic goiter (Graves' disease)—toxic hyperthyroid condition
  a. Symptoms
    (1) Exophthalmos
    (2) Increased activity of all organs of body
    (3) Increased appetite and weight loss
    (4) Irritability
    (5) Nervousness
    (6) Tachycardia
    (7) Enlarged, tender thyroid
    (8) Tremors
  b. Conservative treatment and nursing care
    (1) Rest
    (2) High-caloric, high-protein diet
    (3) Sedation
    (4) Calm environment
    (5) Iodine for some patients
    (6) Radioactive iodine used with limited success
  c. More usual treatment—subtotal thyroidectomy; usually reduces metabolism about 40%
    (1) Preoperative care
      (a) Administration of propylthiouracil to block formation of thyroxine
      (b) Iodine
      (c) Physical, mental, and emotional rest
      (d) Extra nourishment and diet
      (e) Extensive work-up
    (2) Postoperative care
      (a) Semisitting position; protect head from sudden movement
      (b) Tracheotomy set and calcium gluconate available
      (c) Oxygen tent
      (d) Observe patient for ability to speak, then discourage talking

edica-

Drooling
, wrinkled skin
—thyroid extract

nality

oms of

ge, or ex-

paralysis or
ue to section
ss of recurrent
nerve
eal obstruction due
esthesia, vocal cord
y, edema, or tracheitis
tany due to accidental
removal of parathyroids
 (e) Thyroid crisis—marked rise in temperature, nervousness, apprehension, and restlessness

3. Nodular or adenomatous goiter—may or may not produce excessive hormone; usually removed because may become malignant
4. Malignant tumors
 a. Metastasize to bones and lungs
 b. Removed if possible
 c. If inoperable, treated with radioactive iodine or radiation therapy
5. Thyroiditis—inflammatory condition of the thyroid gland
 a. Very rare and very serious
 b. Signs of inflammation and abscess formation
 c. If scarring and fibrosis result, iodine may be needed

D. Pathology of parathyroids (small glands situated on posterior capsule of thyroid)
1. Hypoparathyroidism—calcium and phosphorus not metabolized and stored in bones
 a. Symptoms
  (1) Decrease in blood calcium
  (2) Concentration of phosphorus in blood (Parathormone prevents reabsorption of phosphorus ion in kidney tubules)
  (3) Paresthesia of skin
  (4) Alkalosis
  (5) Hyperpnea
  (6) Tetany that may progress to carpopedal spasm, laryngospasm, and convulsions
 b. Treatment and nursing care
  (1) Intravenous administration of calcium gluconate

 (2) Calcium orally
 (3) Parathyroid hormone
 (4) Vitamin D
 (5) Dihydrotachysterol (AT-10)
2. Hyperparathyroidism—excessive excretion of phosphorus; increased blood calcium with resultant loss of bone calcium
 a. Symptoms
  (1) Anorexia
  (2) Weakness
  (3) Polydipsia
  (4) Pain in bones
  (5) Polyuria
  (6) In severe cases, renal stones and pathologic fractures
 b. Treatment and nursing care
  (1) Surgical removal of glands or tumor; subtotal may be done
  (2) Special care to avoid fractures
  (3) Large amounts of fluids
E. Pathology of adrenal gland
1. Hypofunction of adrenal cortex—Addison's disease
 a. Possible causes
  (1) Lack of stimulating adrenocorticotropic hormone from pituitary gland
  (2) Destruction of adrenal cortex
 b. Symptoms insidious and progressive
  (1) Weight loss
  (2) Muscular weakness
  (3) Anorexia
  (4) Gastrointestinal disturbances
  (5) Emaciation
  (6) Dark pigmentation of skin
  (7) Low blood pressure
  (8) Low blood sugar and blood sodium; high potassium
  (9) Low basal metabolic rate
 c. Treatment and nursing care
  (1) Adrenal steroid therapy
  (2) High-sodium, low-potassium diet
  (3) Prevention of infections
  (4) Adequate rest
  (5) Accurate recording of salt intake and urine output
  (6) Close observation; any symptoms such as nausea, vomiting, cyanosis, fall in blood pressure may be serious—addisonian crisis
2. Hypersecretion of cortical hormones (Cushing's syndrome)—usually due to tumors, sometimes hyperplasia

a. Symptoms—d e m o n s t r a t e some change in sexual characteristics, depending on age of person when pathology becomes manifest
   (1) Obesity
   (2) Hypertension
   (3) Weakness
   (4) Hirsutism
   (5) Amenorrhea
b. Treatment
   (1) Tumor removed if found
   (2) Low-sodium, high-potassium diet
   (3) Cortisone
   (4) Emotional support
   (5) Accurate records of fluid intake and output
   (6) Observation for complications
     (a) Renal insufficiency
     (b) Atelectasis
     (c) Hemorrhage
     (d) Anorexia
3. Hyperactivity of adrenal medulla
  a. Symptoms
   (1) Hypertension
   (2) Tachycardia
   (3) Excessive perspiration
   (4) Tremor
   (5) Nervousness
   (6) Hyperglycemia
   (7) High 17-ketosteroid excretion
  b. Treatment
   (1) Tumor (usually pheochromocytoma) removed if possible
   (2) Adrenergic blocking drugs such as phentolamine or benzodioxane sometimes used
4. Decreased medulla functions—Waterhouse-Friderichsen syndrome (rare, acute disease of children) or acute adrenal crisis
  a. Symptoms
   (1) Dehydration
   (2) Hypoglycemia
   (3) Low blood pressure
   (4) Low potassium and salt
   (5) Shock
   (6) Collapse
  b. Treatment and nursing care
   (1) Replacement therapy
   (2) Intravenous fluids
   (3) Sodium chloride
   (4) Glucose
   (5) Antibiotics
   (6) Rest
5. Replacement therapy

a. Includes administration of steroids
   (1) Cortisone—supplies most adrenal hormones; can be given intramuscularly, intravenously, or orally
   (2) DOCA—first synthetic drug produced; given deep intramuscularly or as pellets
   (3) Hydrocortisone—twice as potent as cortisone
   (4) ACTH (adrenocorticotropic hormone)—can be used when pathology not in adrenal gland
b. Principal action of replacement therapy
   (1) Suppresses inflammation
   (2) Impedes production of antibiotics and tissue repair
   (3) Suppresses ACTH formation
   (4) Retains sodium and water
   (5) Releases potassium
   (6) Increases blood sugar and use of nitrogen
c. Complications
   (1) Reactivation of tuberculosis, peptic ulcers, and other bacterial diseases
   (2) Slow healing of tissues
   (3) Heart damage through retention of sodium and water
   (4) Edema
   (5) Pigmented skin
   (6) Acne
   (7) "Moon facies"
   (8) Facial hair
   (9) Psychological disturbances
d. Nursing patients on replacement therapy
   (1) Daily record of weight
   (2) Examination for edema
   (3) 2 to 3 gm. potassium chloride daily
   (4) Restricted sodium intake usually necessary only in patients with diminished cardiac reserve
   (5) Observation for psychological aberrations
   (6) Reassurance
   (7) Weekly urinalysis
   (8) Daily blood pressure readings
F. Pathology of gonads*
  1. Premature sexual development in male

---

*This section will deal only with the endocrine secretions of the gonads.

—usually due to interstitial cell tumors of testes or tumors of adrenal cortex
2. Hypergonadism—increased production of testosterone; usually requires no treatment
3. Eunuchism—loss of testicular function due to castration, inflammation, or mechanical injury
   a. Symptoms
      (1) Depends on age when condition develops
      (2) Young person may grow tall with narrow chest and shoulders, be shy and high-strung, have infantile genitals, and be effeminate
      (3) Older person loses sexual desire but, usually, not sexual ability
   b. Treatment
      (1) Testosterone
      (2) Psychological help
4. Eunuchoidism—partial loss of testicular function
   a. Usually due to cryptorchism (undescended testes) and may produce almost any degree of dysfunction
   b. Treatment—replacement therapy
5. Complications of testosterone therapy
   a. Edema of ankles
   b. Acne
   c. Cardiac distress
6. Hypogonadism secondary to hypopituitarism (Fröhlich's syndrome)
   a. Characteristics
      (1) Obesity of thighs, lower abdomen, and breast
      (2) Low metabolism
      (3) Small genitals
   b. Treatment
      (1) Anterior pituitary gonadotropic factor
      (2) Testosterone preparations
7. Primary amenorrhea
   a. Cause—may be due to pituitary disease (dwarfism) or to ovarian deficiency
   b. Treatment — replacement therapy indicated
8. Secondary amenorrhea
   a. Possible causes
      (1) Menopause
      (2) Dietary insufficiency and psychic disturbances
      (3) Obesity

(4) Ovarian deficiency
   b. Treatment—ovarian deficiency treated with estrone or estradiol
9. Hypersecretion may cause precocious development in children or excessive menstrual flow in women
10. Excessive androgen secretion in female causes masculine characteristics (Cushing's syndrome)
G. Diseases of pancreas—beta cells of islands of Langerhans secrete insulin directly into bloodstream; insulin concerned with transporting glucose through cell membranes to be utilized or stored; production regulated by diabetogenic hormones of anterior pituitary gland
1. Hypersecretion of insulin—produces hypoglycemia; may be due to disease of pancreas (tumors, usually) or to hyposecretion of diabetogenic hormones
   a. Symptoms
      (1) Low blood sugar
      (2) Skin cool and moist
      (3) Weakness
      (4) Pallor
      (5) Hunger
      (6) Tremors
      (7) May progress to confusion, convulsions, and unconsciousness
   b. Treatment and nursing care
      (1) Removal of tumor or hypertrophic cells of pancreas
      (2) Sugar or glucose symptomatically
      (3) Epinephrine to raise blood sugar temporarily
      (4) Necessary physical care
2. Hyposecretion of insulin (diabetes mellitus)—causes increase in blood sugar, reduced liver glycogen, and negative nitrogen balance
   a. Symptoms in younger people
      (1) Rapid onset
      (2) Polyuria
      (3) Glycosuria
      (4) Loss of weight and strength
   b. Symptoms in older age group
      (1) Slow, insidious onset
      (2) Polyuria
      (3) Glycosuria (over 150 mg.%)
      (4) Polydipsia
      (5) Polyphagia
      (6) Itching, dry skin
      (7) Visual disturbances

c. Treatment and nursing care
  (1) Well-regulated diet
  (2) Education of patient
  (3) Avoidance of infections
  (4) If insulin required, instruction in use and administration of insulin
    (a) Short-acting insulins—regular and crystalline zinc
    (b) Slow-acting insulins—protamine zinc, globin, isophane (NPH), and lente
    (c) Complications—local allergic reactions, insulin lumps, lipodystrophy, transient presbyopia, insulin resistance, hypoglycemic reactions
    (d) Insulin required in children and in adults with excessive loss of weight, acute complications, or severe diabetes
  (5) Oral hypoglycemic agents— may act either to augment release of insulin from beta cells (e.g., sulfonylureas, chlorpropamide) or to aid peripheral tissues in burning carbohydrates (e.g., biguanides)

3. Complications of diabetes mellitus
  a. Susceptibility to infections: pyelonephritis, furuncles, carbuncles, tuberculosis
  b. Arteriosclerosis, gangrene, hemorrhage into retina, cataract of lens
  c. Polyneuritis due to thiamin deficiency
  d. Chronic acidosis: anorexia, headache, languor, fatigue
  e. Acute acidosis (diabetic coma)
    (1) Causes
      (a) Decreased glucose intake
      (b) Insufficient insulin
      (c) Infections of respiratory, genitourinary, or gastrointestinal tract; or pyogenic infections
      (d) Acute myocardial infarction
      (e) Gastrointestinal disturbances
    (2) Symptoms include
      (a) Anorexia, followed by nausea and vomiting
      (b) Weakness, malaise, and muscle aches

(c) Abdominal pain
(d) Kussmaul's respiration
(e) Fruity odor of breath
(f) Soft eyeballs
(g) Dry skin
(h) Slightly elevated temperature and leukocyte count
(i) Elevated NPN
(j) Tachycardia
(k) Slurred speech
(l) May lead to confusion, convulsions, and coma
  (3) Treatment and nursing care
    (a) Bed rest and warmth
    (b) Frequent blood and urine samples
    (c) Administration of short-acting insulin
    (d) Fluid and electrolyte therapy—glucose or fructose, isotonic saline, sodium lactate, sodium bicarbonate, potassium
    (e) Changing position frequently
    (f) Prevention of pressure
    (g) Gastric lavage if indicated
    (h) Treatment for circulatory collapse
    (i) Accurate intake and output records

4. Health teaching in diabetes
  a. Nature of disease
  b. Adequate medical supervision
  c. Factors that affect complications
    (1) Avoidance of exposure
    (2) Infections
    (3) Dietary indiscretions
    (4) Strenuous exercise
    (5) Emotional upsets
    (6) Eating so that same amount of carbohydrate is in stomach at all times
    (7) Care of skin and feet
    (8) Testing of urine
    (9) Use of insulin and other hypoglycemic agents
  d. Social agencies available and their functions

NURSING PATIENTS WITH ALLERGIC CONDITIONS

1. **Basic principles of nursing**
A. Observation for manifestation of allergic reaction to medication, emotions, or food

manifested by patient; first problem—to find allergen

B. Careful observation an essential part of nursing care of patients with allergies

C. All mental strain should be reduced and eliminated if possible

D. Patients with allergies usually apprehensive and need encouragement, understanding, and education regarding their allergic manifestations

E. When patients state that they are allergic to certain drugs, foods, or other things, they should be taken seriously

F. Prevention of recurrent attacks essential; important to know precipitating factors

2. **Nursing patients with allergies**

A. Terms commonly used in referring to allergies

1. Allergy—condition in which cells have at time of birth or develop property of reacting violently to certain stimuli that do not affect nonallergic cells

2. Allergen—substance that produces or generates allergy—usually protein, but not always

3. Antigen—any agent that, when introduced into body of susceptible person, produces antibodies

4. "Shock structures"—tissue groups in body, supplied with involuntary muscles; susceptible to allergic reactions

B. Tests used in allergic conditions

1. Skin tests to try to determine specific allergen

a. Patch test—suspected material applied to skin and reaction noted in from 2 to 7 days; results not conclusive

b. Scratch test—suspected material introduced into skin through scratch made in epidermis

c. Intracutaneous test—aqueous solution of suspected allergen introduced intradermally with 27-gauge needle, ¼ inch

2. Complement-fixation test—used to diagnose any disease, antigen of which is known or can be obtained

3. Precipitation test—used to determine identity of unknown protein

4. Agglutination test—used to determine presence and titer of specific or nonspecific agglutinins

C. Antihistaminic drugs—drugs that prevent release of histamine from stimulated allergic cells

1. Benadryl and pyribenzamine the basic antihistaminic drugs; many others

a. Help in many allergic conditions, but do not cure

b. Toxic effects

(1) Drowsiness

(2) Lassitude

(3) Less frequently, hyperactivity and insomnia

(4) Still less frequently, nausea, headaches, and diarrhea

2. Sedatives and hypnotics used with caution in patients receiving antihistaminic drugs

3. **Specific allergic diseases**

A. Spontaneous or familial allergies—allergies inherent in organism; have many inciting causes

1. Hay fever—many different clinical types

a. Local symptoms of mucous membranes of eye, nose, and pharynx

(1) Itching

(2) Edema

(3) Congestion

(4) Sneezing

(5) Discharge of thin mucus

(6) Increased eosinophils

2. Allergic asthma—characterized by "wheezy" type respiration due to obstruction of airflow

a. Symptoms

(1) Edema of bronchial mucosa

(2) Sticky mucus in bronchial lumen

(3) Spasm of bronchial muscles

(4) Disturbance in electrolytes

(5) Some degree of emphysema

b. Complications

(1) Emphysema

(2) Chronic and recurrent acute bronchitis

(3) Bronchiectasis

(4) Pulmonary hypertension

(5) Pulmonary heart disease

(6) Mental symptoms and personality changes

c. Treatment for acute attack

(1) Injection of epinephrine chloride

(2) Ephedrine

(3) Potassium iodide to dilute secretion

(4) Antihistaminics

(5) In severe cases, aminophylline I.V.

(6) Large amounts of fluids
d. Treatment for recurrent asthma
  (1) Prevention
    (a) Elimination of precipitating factor
    (b) Psychotherapy
3. Eczema, atopic—acute, subacute, or chronic polymorphous eruption in predisposed individual
  a. Characterized by patches of red, scaly, thickened skin covered with blood crusts or excoriations
  b. Most often found on face, neck, knees, or flexor surfaces of elbows
4. Contact dermatitis—acute or chronic epidermal condition characterized by vesicle formation
  a. Due to contact with allergen; blood vessels dilate and exude white blood cells and plasma
  b. Treatment consists in removing all allergen and treating itching and edema
5. Angioneurotic edema — characterized by transient, circumscribed, edematous swelling of skin or mucous membrane or, rarely, of viscera
  a. Symptoms seem to appear spontaneously
    (1) Swelling
    (2) Itching
    (3) Burning
    (4) May last for several days but usually subside in 2 or 3 days
  b. Treatment
    (1) Remove cause if it can be found
    (2) Tracheotomy for edema of glottis
    (3) Antihistaminics and sedatives
    (4) In some instances, epinephrine
6. Food and drug allergies may be manifested in many ways
  a. Those already mentioned
  b. Pruritus
  c. Migraine
  d. Nausea
  e. Ulcers
  f. Canker sores
B. Induced or acquired allergy—reaction due to union of foreign serum with precipitin produced during incubation period
1. Serum sickness—allergic reaction from parenteral administration of foreign serum

a. Characteristics
  (1) Incubation period from 6 to 12 days
  (2) Skin eruptions
  (3) Enlargement of lymph nodes
  (4) Fever
  (5) Edema
  (6) Polyarthritis
b. Symptoms—from few urticarial wheals to severe general involvement
c. Treatment and nursing care
  (1) Symptomatic
  (2) Lotions for pruritus
  (3) Epinephrine I.M. for transitory relief
  (4) Steroid therapy (hydrocortisone or dexamethasone)
2. Serum accident (anaphylactic shock)—immediate shocklike and sometimes fatal reaction to parenteral administration of foreign serum
  a. Symptoms
    (1) Very rapid onset
    (2) Local edema and itching
    (3) Apprehension
    (4) Edema of face, hands, and neck
    (5) Cyanosis
    (6) Choking
    (7) Violent asthma
    (8) Dilated pupils
    (9) Thready or imperceptible pulse
    (10) Convulsions may occur
    (11) If patient does not die, symptoms will become those of serum sickness
  b. Treatment
    (1) Prevention best—give a skin test
    (2) Sensitized person desensitized
    (3) Rapidity of treatment most important aspect
    (4) Specific for serum accident is epinephrine 0.3 to 0.8 ml. subcutaneously; larger dose if severe
    (5) For desensitization: 0.005 ml., double every half hour until 10 ml. given
3. Drug allergy—disorder, resulting from administration of chemical compound, that is in no way related to normal action of drug
  a. Drug reactions highly diversified
    (1) More usual reactions

(a) Fever
(b) Malaise
(c) Anorexia
(d) Muscle pain
(e) Nausea
(f) Abdominal pain
(g) Diarrhea
(2) Less frequent reactions
(a) Arthralgia
(b) Tender lymph nodes
(c) Rash
(d) Edema of face or generalized edema
b. Treatment—drug should be discontinued
c. Periarteritis nodosa—rare and serious form of drug allergy, manifested by multiple nodules along course of arteries
d. Agranulocytosis, thrombocytopenia, and aplastic anemia sometimes due to allergic reactions to chemicals

NURSING PATIENTS WITH DISEASES OF INTEGUMENTARY SYSTEM

1. **Basic principles of nursing**
A. Prevention
B. Institution of lifesaving measures in the severely burned person
C. Prevention of disability and disfigurement through early specialized, individualized treatment
D. Rehabilitation of the individual through reconstructive surgery and rehabilitative programs
E. Teach public dangers of home treatment or of treatment by anyone other than reputable physician
F. Never display attitude of horror, squeamishness, or repulsion toward patients with unattractive dermatologic manifestations
G. Treat all skin conditions as acute and contagious until diagnosed otherwise
H. Do not forget patient's general condition while caring for local manifestations
I. Never do anything that will further irritate already damaged skin; do not overtreat
J. Treat skin conditions early; much easier to manage during acute stage than chronic
K. Do not forget that internal disease may cause skin manifestations and severe skin diseases may affect general physiology
L. Help patient to participate actively in treatment

M. Psychological support of utmost importance
2. **Nursing patients with dermatologic conditions**
A. When bathing patients with skin conditions, use oil and soft cotton pledgets first, soap and water last
B. Be careful not to use ointments or lotions improperly made or too old
C. Moist dressings should be 2 or more layers thick and should be kept moist; dressings on open lesions should be sterile
   1. Bland oil or protective ointment should be used to protect skin around area
   2. Any number of solutions may be ordered
   3. Cold wet dressings ordinarily used on inflammations or serious lesions, warm dressings on suppurating lesions
D. Baths used extensively for dermatologic conditions
   1. Hospital patients should be seen by physician before being given bath
   2. Colloidal baths given for soothing purposes
   3. Medicated baths used as therapy; may be harmful if done improperly
E. Ointments and pastes should be fresh and smooth; they should smell pure and should be applied thickly; dressings with ointments should never be allowed to dry out
F. Corticosteroids are being widely used in the treatment of many dermatologic conditions
G. Dermatologic and plastic reconstructive surgery may be done for variety of reasons
   1. Disseminate information concerning availability of facilities for those in need of plastic or reconstructive surgery
   2. Help patient and family to know what to expect in terms of progress after surgery
3. **Symptoms**
A. Objective symptoms
   1. Primary lesions
      a. Macule—circumscribed skin discolorations, neither raised nor depressed
      b. Papule—small circumscribed solid skin elevations, from pinhead to pea in size
      c. Nodule—larger circumscribed solid

masses, even with or beneath surface of skin

d. Tumors—large, firm or soft, elevated or deeply seated masses, from walnut to egg size

e. Vesicles—small circumscribed elevations, containing free serous fluid

f. Bullae—larger epidermal elevations that contain serous or serosanguineous fluid

g. Pustules—small circumscribed elevations that contain free purulent fluid

h. Wheals—transitory, edematous, flat elevations—usually accompanied by itching; appear rapidly, disappear more slowly

2. Secondary lesions—modifications or alterations of primary lesions

a. Excoriation—discontinuity of skin, usually of epidermis only

b. Scales—dry or greasy laminated masses of epidermis; range from minute particles to dull sheets of horny material

c. Crusts (scabs)—masses of dried exudate, varying greatly in size, color, and shape

d. Fissures—linear breaks in continuity of skin caused by disease or injury; margins sharply defined with abrupt walls

e. Ulcers—excavations of integument, irregularly sized and shaped, due to loss of substance from necrosis

f. Scars—new formations of connective tissue that replace loss of substance in dermis and subcutaneous tissue

3. Residual lesions

a. Hyperpigmentation—excess coloration of skin due to deposition of pigment

b. Depigmentation—loss of color (pigment) from area of integument

B. Subjective symptoms

1. Pruritus (itching)—most common symptom of skin pathology; exact nature and intensity vary greatly

a. Symptoms

(1) Generally begins as localized condition

(2) May or may not become generalized

(3) If severe, secondary lesions

(a) Excoriations

(b) Fissures

(c) Pigmentation

(d) Lichenification

(e) Discomfort, ranging from mild to intolerable distress

b. Treatment

(1) Removal of cause

(2) Use of colloidal baths

(3) Antipruritic agents

(4) X-ray therapy

(5) Sometimes, nerve injections

c. Nursing care may be quite difficult

(1) Clothing and linen used should be soft and nonirritating

(2) Bathing should be limited to colloidal baths

(3) Antipruritics should be applied carefully, and patient noted for sensitivity reactions

(4) Scratching and rubbing must be prevented

(5) Warmth may increase discomfort

(6) Occupational or recreational therapy may lessen need for sedatives

2. Disorders of sensation

a. Soreness

b. Feeling of tenseness

c. Crawling or tingling sensation

d. Burning sensation

e. Hyperesthesia or anesthesia

f. Pain rare symptom

4. **Pathologic conditions of integument**

A. Metabolic manifestations

1. Comedo—mass of thickened secretions blocking excretory duct of sebaceous gland

a. Treatment—palliative

(1) Meticulous cleanliness

(2) Avoidance of trauma

(3) Healthful diet

(4) Warm packs

2. Acne vulgaris—chronic inflammatory disorder of sebaceous glands

a. Characteristics

(1) Development of papules

(2) Pustules

(3) Foreign body granuloma

b. Treatment—obstinate disease, to be treated only by physician to prevent permanent scarring

c. Nursing care

(1) Low-fat, low-carbohydrate diet

(2) Avoidance of trauma to skin

(3) Fresh air

(4) Sunshine
(5) Rest and sleep
(6) Sulfur preparations
(7) Success of nursing care dependent on psychological consideration of patient
3. Seborrhea—functional disorder of sebaceous glands, characterized by increase in amount of secretion and difference in consistency
a. Characteristics
  (1) On smooth skin
    (a) Oiliness
    (b) Large pores
    (c) Comedos
    (d) Dilatation of capillaries
    (e) Large sebaceous glands
  (2) On scalp, a severe dandruff
b. Treatment and nursing care
  (1) Selsun for dandruff
  (2) Low-fat diet
  (3) Vitamins
  (4) Sulfur ointments
  (5) Thorough cleansing with soap and water frequently
  (6) Attention to basic constitutional problem
4. Acne rosacea—disease of unknown etiology
a. Characteristics
  (1) Redness
  (2) Papules
  (3) Pustules
  (4) Permanent flushing of face
b. May produce fibrosis of nose known as rhinophyma
c. Treatment and nursing care
  (1) Same treatment as for acne
  (2) Large amounts vitamin B_{12}
  (3) Rest
  (4) Relaxation
  (5) Sometimes, cauterization
  (6) Treatment often unsatisfactory
B. Skin diseases due to metazoa
1. Scabies (7-year itch)—infestation due to itch mite—*Sarcoptes scabiei*
a. Symptoms
  (1) Intense itching, more severe at night
  (2) Tiny superficial whitish lines, anywhere on body
b. Treatment and nursing care
  (1) Isolation to prevent spread to others
  (2) Thorough cleansing bath
  (3) Application of scabicide

(4) Care of secondary infections
(5) Prevention of reinfection
2. Pediculosis—human infestation by lice
a. Principal varieties
  (1) Pediculosis capitis
  (2) Pediculosis corporis
  (3) Pediculosis pubis
b. Principal symptoms
  (1) Itching
  (2) Presence of louse and/or nits
c. Treatment and nursing care—chief factors
  (1) Public education regarding hygiene
  (2) Safeguarding others from being infested
  (3) Treatment with parasiticide
  (4) Antipruritic medications for comfort
C. Superficial fungous infections
Note: For further discussion see p. 434
1. Dermatophytids or "ids"—believed to be allergic manifestations to antigenic substance produced to combat specific fungus, dermatophytosis
a. Characteristics
  (1) Most common site, feet
  (2) Usually begins with very itchy clear vesicles
  (3) Later become scaly and eczematous or hyperkeratotic
b. Treatment
  (1) Fungicides never used on these lesions
  (2) Primary infection should be treated; ids will then heal
D. Viral infections of integument
1. Herpes simplex (fever blister)—group of vesicles on erythematous base
a. Characteristics
  (1) More often found on or near lips
  (2) May be found in many other locations
  (3) Usually will heal without scarring in 1 or 2 weeks
b. Treatment to alleviate
  (1) Aluminum acetate
  (2) Spirits of camphor
  (3) Ethyl chloride spray
  (4) Fractional x-ray used to alleviate severe conditions
2. Herpes zoster (shingles)—acute viral infection of nerve
a. Skin manifestations—vesicles or papulovesicles on elevated erythem-

atous base accompanied by considerable pain
  b. Lesions heal, leaving atrophic white scar
3. Verrucae (warts)—small circumscribed epidermal and papillary growths; several clinical types
  a. Warts benign, but may be disfiguring; plantar warts painful and incapacitating
  b. Most warts do not need to be removed; some will disappear spontaneously; may be removed by surgery, x-ray therapy, radium, freezing, or cauterization
E. Inflammations and bacterial skin manifestations
1. Erythema—due to venous stasis; characterized by erythematous lesions of various shapes
2. Erythema multiforme—acute inflammatory disease of unknown etiology
  a. Characteristics
    (1) Reddish macules
    (2) Papules
    (3) Vesicles symmetrically distributed
  b. Lesions bright or dark red; disappear on pressure; clear in center; no itching; heal with no scarring
  c. Treatment and nursing care
    (1) Fluids
    (2) Alkalies
    (3) Calamine lotion or aluminum acetate locally
    (4) Well-balanced diet
3. Erythema nodosum—dermatosis characterized by tender, nodular lesions of skin, accompanied by mild constitutional symptoms; lesions gradually disappear; rarely recur
4. Psoriasis—common, recurrent, inflammatory condition of skin characterized by rounded, dry, scaling patches
  a. Condition starts with erythematous papules covered with dry, silver scales that leave bleeding points if removed; seldom itches or burns, leaves no scars; exacerbations and remissions for years
  b. Treatment palliative, since neither cause nor cure known
    (1) Keratolytics containing sulfur
    (2) Salicylate acid and tars
    (3) Vitamin D
    (4) Low-fat diet

    (5) Sometimes, ultraviolet therapy
    (6) Alcohol, emotional disturbances, and extreme cold should be avoided
5. Pityriasis rosea—mild inflammatory disease of unknown origin, characterized by salmon-colored papules and macules
  a. Lesions usually oval, covered with dry crinkly epidermis; slightly itchy; arranged segmentally; begins with herald patch; disappears, leaving pigmented areas
  b. Treatment
    (1) Simple diet
    (2) Ultraviolet therapy
    (3) X-ray therapy
    (4) Sulfur ointment
6. Lichen planus—inflammatory condition of skin and mucous membrane; may be acute or chronic
  a. Characterized by small, shiny, intensely itchy papules with glistening scales
  b. Treatment symptomatic—x-ray therapy frequently helpful
F. Bacterial infections of integument
1. Cellulitis—infection of cells; may extend along lymphatics, veins, or by cells, fascial planes, or tendon sheaths directly; care should be taken not to injure cells at this stage
2. Felon (whitlow)—infection involving anterior, distal portion of finger
  a. Characterized by severe, throbbing pain in distal phalanx; edema; formation of pus
  b. Condition treated as local infection with elevation, rest, heat, and antibiotics; incision and drainage may be necessary
3. Paronychia (run-around) — infection around lateral border of nail bed
  a. Symptoms
    (1) Slight redness
    (2) Swelling
    (3) Tenderness
    (4) Pain
  b. Treatment and nursing care same as for felon
4. Ulcers of integument—many types
  a. Varicose ulcers—complication of varicose veins; ulcer may heal over scarred hard base and recur with slightest trauma

b. Trophic ulcers—due to interference of arterial blood supply

c. Diabetic ulcers—complication of diabetes

d. Neurogenic ulcers—secondary to diseases of nervous system

e. Decubitus ulcers—occur following pressure and reduced blood supply; infection usually present

5. Tenosynovitis—infection of flexor tendon sheath of finger; important condition because necrosis of tendon sheath leads to disability; early diagnosis and treatment vital

6. Gangrene—refers to death and degeneration of tissues in mass; directly due to loss of blood supply

a. Dry gangrene due to arterial obstruction without associated infection or venous obstruction, such as arteriosclerotic gangrene

b. Moist or wet gangrene due to venous obstruction or infection; characterized by edema

G. Conditions affecting appendages of skin

1. Hyperhidrosis—condition in which sweat glands markedly overactive; may be generalized or local condition

2. Bromidrosis — malodorous, excessive sweating; treatment unsatisfactory, but special attention to cleanliness may help temporarily

3. Hypertrichosis—excessive growth of hair in areas not usually hairy

4. Alopecia—loss of hair; may be diffuse or circumscribed and may be due to many factors

H. Benign and precancerous lesions of skin

1. Nevus (mole)—benign, congenital circumscribed tumor that may be present at birth or appear later; many types

a. Pigmented macules and patches—lentigines or congenital freckles that do not fade during cold weather; best left alone unless become coal-black

b. Soft, pigmented nevi—vary in size, color, and other factors; many potentially malignant, but may be eradicated safely

c. Hard, verrucose nevi—very rarely malignant

2. Hemangioma (vascular birthmark)—tumor of newly formed blood vessels; rarely malignant

a. Capillary hemangioma (port-wine mark)—flat, nonelevated, pink to purplish in color; treatment impracticable

b. Hemangioma simplex (strawberry mark)—flat papillary tumor that tends to grow slowly; treatment with sclerosing material, x-ray, or radium may leave scarring

c. Cavernous hemangioma—dark red elevated tumor of widely dilated vessels; superficial skin so very thin that serious hemorrhage may occur; radium or x-ray may give good results

d. Telangiectasis—spiderlike capillary mark; destruction of central point may eradicate entire mark

3. Clavus (corn)—tumor composed of cornified epithelium due to pressure

4. Seborrheic keratosis or warts—usually multiple, slightly raised, moist; may or may not itch; no treatment necessary unless disfiguring

5. Multiple benign cystic epithelioma—smooth, flesh-colored, shiny, firm or translucent nodules

6. Other benign tumors include lipomas (fat cell), neuromas (nerve tissue), myomas (muscle fibers), and fibromas (fibrous connective tissue)

7. Senile keratosis—precancerous tumor of skin, composed of atypical epithelial cells

a. Circumscribed flat dry harsh brownish slightly raised lesion, usually found on exposed skin of older people; should be removed as prophylactic measure

b. Simple removal adequate before changes occur; later must be removed with malignancy precautions

8. Cutaneous horn—elongated epidermal growth that frequently becomes malignant; care should be taken to excise completely to prevent recurrence

9. Keloid—dense fibrous scarlike tumor that usually develops on site of scar; may be painful and bleed easily; may recur following surgical removal

10. Steatoma (sebaceous cyst)—tumor arising from sebaceous gland; frequently becomes carcinomatous

a. Pea- to orange-sized, smooth, globular, multiple or single tumor

b. All should have complete surgical removal

11. Dermoid cyst of skin—congenital cyst containing squamous, stratified epithelium, sometimes hair, glands, or teeth; found in embryonic lines of closure; should be removed, as may become squamous cell carcinoma

I. Malignant lesions of skin—classified according to type of cells they resemble; differ in location, rapidity of growth, dissemination, and histology

1. Basal cell epithelioma (rodent ulcer)—slow-growing, nonmetastasizing tumor of epidermis, most commonly found on face, ear, and dorsum of hand

   a. Primary lesion consists of firm nodules that coalesce to form plaque with rolled, cordlike border; as lesion develops, center ulcerates and waxy border enlarges; eventually burrows deep into surrounding tissues, causing destruction and mutilation

   b. Early treatment most important; radiation therapy or excision gives good results and prognosis if tumor not too extensive

2. Squamous cell epithelioma (prickle cell carcinoma)—fairly rapidly progressing lesion that infiltrates, ulcerates, and metastasizes

   a. Usually begins as dry, wartlike growth with elevated, firm, red, indurated base that eventually becomes ulcer with elevated, rolled, hyperemic border; may begin under keratotic area or as benign lesion

   b. Treatment and nursing care
      (1) Deep, wide excision or radiation therapy
      (2) Psychological care
      (3) Application of principles of nursing care of patients with malignancies (p. 329)

3. Melanoma—one of embryonic tumors; arises from pigmented or nonpigmented mole, but usually from flat, hairless, coal-black, slightly elevated mole

   a. Characterized by extreme malignancy and resistance to irradiation, early metastasis by both blood and lymph, and smooth hard secondary lesions

   b. Prevention most important; black moles should be removed or closely watched for increase in size or in depth of color, formation of crust, bleeding, ulceration, peripheral nodules, and adenopathy of regional lymph glands; about 24% arise from improperly treated moles

   c. In early cases, deep, wide excision with removal of lymph vessels and glands may be effective, but they may recur many years later

4. Sarcoma—malignant connective tissue tumor infrequently found in skin

   a. Fibrosarcoma (spindle cell)—firm nodules that increase in size and number to form bluish, sclerotic plaques

   b. Neurogenic—nodules on nerve trunks or filaments that grow very bulky

5. Metastatic skin tumors—appear as multiple nodules or flat infiltrations; treatment of this stage supportive and palliative

J. Burns—cause approximately 8,000 deaths yearly in United States; over 75% could be prevented; causes—thermal, electrical, radioactive, or chemical agents

1. Classification of burns

   a. First-degree burns—characterized by redness, erythema, pain, and sometimes shock due to pain; no blisters and no scarring

   b. Second-degree burns—characterized by formation of blisters and blebs; separation of skin layers with loss of plasma, pain, shock, infection; toxemia may develop later; no scarring unless infection occurs

   c. Third-degree burns—characterized by complete destruction of skin, glands, and follicles; less pain, plasma loss, and later scarring

2. Paraphysiology of burns (stages of)
   a. Neurogenic shock
   b. Fluid-loss shock
   c. Burn slough and infection
   d. Stage of repair

3. Treatment and nursing care of patients with severe burns

   a. Treatment should be started immediately; greatest danger from shock
      (1) Plasma
      (2) Blood

      (3) Plasma expanders
      (4) Morphine to relieve pain
      (5) Sufficient fluids to maintain electrolyte balance
  b. Measures to prevent infection and toxemia begun at once
      (1) All objects coming in contact with patient sterile
      (2) Personnel masked
      (3) Antibiotics given
      (4) Tetanus antitoxin given
      (5) Fluids continued
  c. Method of treatment—physician's choice
      (1) Pressure dressing may be applied or an open method used
      (2) Stryker frames, Foster beds, or CircOlectric beds may be used in some cases
      (3) Treatment with 0.5% silver nitrate solution
      (4) Topical chemotherapy
      (5) Dressings and soaks
      (6) Skin grafts
  d. Kidney damage due to collection of hematin in tubules may lead to anuria or lower nephron nephrosis with uremia
      (1) NPN and urea nitrogen should be checked daily
      (2) Accurate intake and output record kept
      (3) Fluids given freely
      (4) Patient's cooperation obtained
  e. In addition to fluids, severely burned patient requires large amounts of protein (200 to 300 gm. daily) for tissue repair and to prevent anemia; anorexia or nausea may complicate problem; hematocrit should be watched closely
  f. Burned patient should be positioned to help prevent deformities; all parts of body moved and exercised as soon as pain permits; all third-degree burns leave scars and possible contractures
  g. Severe contractures need plastic or reconstructive surgery; procedures cannot be done successfully when infection present; postsurgically, area must be kept clean, blood supply to area unimpeded; trauma or movement of area prevented
4. Skin grafting
  a. Preoperative care

      (1) Area must be clean—no infection or granulating surface
      (2) Warm dressings, medicated dressings, and other measures may be used to prepare the area
      (3) Donor site must be thoroughly cleaned and shaved
  b. Types of grafts
      (1) Reverdin—pinch grafts, bits of skin
      (2) Thiersch—strips of superficial skin applied
      (3) Split-thickness—one-half skin thickness or dermatome grafts
      (4) Krause-Wolfe — full-thickness grafts
  c. Postoperative care
      (1) Wound must be kept clean
      (2) Oozing can be controlled temporarily by pressure; blood should not clot on area
      (3) Aseptic technique at all times
      (4) If flap becomes blue and congested, doctor may need to make small opening in it
      (5) Blood supply to area must not be impeded in any way
      (6) Various methods of treating area: adhesive, wet packs, open, dressing with paraffin or petrolatum gauze
      (7) High-protein diet
      (8) Cheerful, optimistic attitude helpful
K. Pathology of breast
  1. Mastitis—infection of one or more ducts with stagnation of milk in one or more lobes
    a. Characterized by dull pain and discharge of pus, serum, or blood
    b. Treatment and nursing care
      (1) Ice bags
      (2) Firm support
      (3) Rest
      (4) Antibiotics
  2. Mammary abscess—abscess of breast requires antibiotics, sedatives; when fluctuating, may require incision and drainage
  3. Chronic cystic mastitis
    a. Characterized by one or more small, hard, freely movable nodules in breast with uncomfortable feeling and/or shooting pains

b. Treatment often conservative, but simple mammectomy may be done
4. Tumors of breast
  a. Sarcoma grows very rapidly, may cause lump or retraction of skin, pain develops late; followed by edema and ulceration
  b. Acute inflammatory carcinoma resembles erysipelas, runs febrile course; usually causes death in 3 to 6 months
  c. Paget's disease of nipple (intraductal carcinoma) characterized by slow, progressive erosion of nipple and proliferation of epithelial cells into ducts
  d. Adenocarcinoma accounts for 95% of breast neoplasms; usually begins with microscopic lesion that becomes painless mass; early metastasis; connective tissue reaction that may change contour of breast, either increasing or decreasing its size; pain appears much later
5. Nursing patients with breast surgery
  a. Preoperative care
    (1) Psychological preparation, even in older patient
    (2) Cancer of breast will not affect menopause
    (3) Slightly higher incidence in women who have had no children
    (4) Can be diagnosed positively by biopsy
    (5) Many patients will not know until after surgery whether or not lesion malignant
    (6) Other preoperative care that is given for any major surgical procedure
  b. Radical mastectomy a major, lengthy operation—includes removal of
    (1) Breast
    (2) Skin over prominence
    (3) Pectoralis major and pectoralis minor muscles
    (4) Fat, fascia, lymphatic vessels, and glands of axilla all in one piece
  c. Postoperative care
    (1) Move patient gently (wound closed under tension)
    (2) Observe for
      (a) Shock
      (b) Hemorrhage
      (c) Edema
      (d) Respiratory difficulties
    (3) Diet as tolerated
    d. Movement and elevation of arm on affected side started on first postoperative day, continued until healing complete; patient reminded to hold shoulders evenly; prosthesis discussed
6. Inoperable carcinoma of breast treated with x-ray therapy, hormone therapy, or sterilization as palliative measure; palliative surgery also may be indicated; good nursing care vitally important

NURSING PATIENTS WITH PATHOLOGY OF EAR OR EYE

1. **Basic principles of nursing**
A. Nursing care emphasizes health teaching and prevention; often in area of public health nursing
B. Nursing care concerned with mental, social, and economic distress due to these diseases
C. Great emotional trauma; need for support and help
D. Early recognition and treatment of these conditions important factor; advocation of yearly medical examinations a nursing responsibility
E. Meticulous attention to details essential; nothing should be used as eye or ear medication unless ordered by competent physician
F. Instructions to patient and/or his family vital
G. Nursing care after acute stage includes helping handicapped person find help from social and rehabilitation agencies
H. Periodic examination should be emphasized
I. Rehabilitation of patients with problems involving eye or ear
2. **Special considerations**
A. Strength of any medication used in ears or eyes should be carefully noted
B. Diet often important in etiology or treatment of ear or eye diseases
C. Irrigations of ear or eye given with gentle, steady pressure not directed on eardrum or on cornea
D. When local anesthetic is used in eye, cornea should be protected against abrasions

E. Except in emergency, anything put into eye should be sterile
F. Hearing aid care
  1. Wash mold daily with soap and water with pipe cleaner
  2. Dry mold carefully
  3. Carry extra battery and cord at all times
G. Insufflation of eustachian tubes to test patency of tubes or to open them may be done in hospital or doctor's office; quite painful
H. Induced-fever therapy—used in severe infections of eye
  1. Usually bacterial antigen of typhoid bacilli used for inducing fever in adults; boiled milk often used for children
  2. After intramuscular injection, nursing care includes
    a. T.P.R. and B.P. every hour until temperature reaches 100° F., then every 15 minutes as long as elevation lasts
    b. Patient placed in bed after temperature reaches 99° F.; allowed up when temperature returns to normal
    c. Hot fluids encouraged; other food given if patient desires it
    d. Patient uncomfortable with chills and fever, but temperature of over 104° F. should be reported; after fever subsides, alcohol rub and dry linen given
I. Artificial eye care—eye should not be worn until irritation and fever gone
  1. To insert eye
    a. Lift upper lid; slide upper margin of eye under upper lid
    b. Hold in place
    c. Pull lower lid down; let lower margin of eye slide under
    d. Push lower lid up
  2. To remove eye
    a. Draw lower lid down with left hand
    b. Push up gently; slip eye out in front of lower lid
    c. Place thumb on upper lid; push down, forcing eye down and out
    d. Be careful not to drop eye; clean and place in normal saline solution or in clean dry place; do not scratch
J. Care of contact lenses

  1. Hand washing before and after removal
  2. Lens cleansed only with recommended sterile noncaustic solution
  3. Once removed, kept dry and stored
  4. Storage kit kept clean
  5. Worn no longer than prescribed time (maximal average 10 to 16 hours)
  6. Not worn when sleeping or eye infection is present
3. **Pathology of ear**
A. Diseases of external ear
  1. Acute or chronic eczema
  2. Perichondriosis
  3. Infection (external otitis)
  4. Cerumen
  5. Foreign bodies in canal
  6. Furuncles
B. Acute otitis media—acute inflammation of mucous lining of middle ear—caused by entrance of pathogenic bacteria
  1. Symptoms—vary with intensity of infection; may be mild and transient or very severe
    a. Feeling of fullness
    b. Drum red and may be retracted
    c. Cavity filled with fluid; may become purulent
    d. Pain
    e. Fever
    f. Deafness
    g. Ear noises
    h. Headache
    i. Anorexia, nausea, vomiting
    j. May become chronic
  2. Treatment
    a. Drum may be incised to release fluid, causing temporary loss of hearing
    b. Antibiotics and sedatives
    c. Prevention or avoiding recurrent attacks important
C. Mastoiditis—develops when above condition involves mastoid process
  1. Symptoms more severe; may include
    a. Vomiting
    b. Nystagmus
    c. Dizziness
    d. Chills
    e. Fever
  2. Treatment
    a. Mastoidectomy may be done
    b. Seldom necessary if adequate antibiotic therapy instituted
D. Perforations of eardrum—most frequent cause infections; trauma second

1. Treatment
   a. Medical—cauterization and use of prosthesis
   b. Surgical—tympanoplasty (several types)
E. Suppurative labyrinthitis—acute or chronic infection of inner ear or labyrinth
   1. Symptoms
      a. Loss of hearing
      b. Vertigo
      c. Nausea, vomiting
      d. Nystagmus
   2. Treatment
      a. Bed rest
      b. Antibiotics
      c. Adequate fluid intake
      d. Radical mastoidectomy if necessary
      e. Other care similar to that for Ménière's syndrome
F. Panotitis—suppurative involvement of both internal and middle ear
   1. Symptoms and complications
      a. Symptoms severe
      b. Deafness
      c. Meningitis
      d. Brain abscess
      e. Thrombosis of lateral sinus may develop
   2. Care and treatment—much the same as for acute purulent otitis media
G. Ménière's syndrome—dysfunction of vestibular branch of eighth nerve
   1. Characteristics
      a. Tinnitus
      b. Dizziness
      c. Nausea
      d. Staggering gait
      e. Deafness to external sound
   2. Treatment—brings no improvement in hearing
      a. Rest in bed
      b. Histamine I.V.
      c. Nicotinic acid I.M.
      d. Protection from falling
      e. Specific treatment of cause, if determined
      f. Surgery
         (1) Destruction of the membranous labyrinth
         (2) Ultrasonic surgery
         (3) Cryosurgery
H. Otosclerosis—conduction deafness due to interference of motion of stapes
   1. Starts in young adults with ringing in ears

2. Mobilization or fenestration operation often gives good results
3. Stapedectomy—operation of choice today
I. Hearing loss
   1. Possible causes
      a. Trauma or infection of ear
      b. Improper methods of cleansing
      c. Unskilled treatments
      d. Foreign bodies
   2. Loss of more than 30 decibels indicates need for hearing aid
   3. Hearing aid usually worn in good ear
   4. Classification
      a. Conductive—impairment of outer and/or middle ear
      b. Sensorineural—nerve pathways involved
      c. Combined—both conductive and sensorineural
      d. Psychogenic—nonorganic, functional
4. **Nursing patients with surgery of ear**
A. Nursing care of patient with mastoidectomy
   1. Preoperative care—patient prepared for major surgery
   2. Postoperative care
      a. Observation
         (1) For edema around dressing (bulky, tight dressing usual); may need to be adjusted
         (2) For indication of facial paralysis or cerebral irritation
      b. Fluids urged
      c. General postoperative care
B. Nursing care following labyrinth fenestration
   1. Position on back or on side having surgery
   2. Observation for and care of vertigo and nausea
   3. Activity encouraged as soon as nausea permits
   4. Later, patient instructed not to engage in activities that would get water in ear
   5. Restoration of hearing may cause nervousness at first
5. **The deaf person**
A. Deafness
   1. May be perceptive or conductive in origin
   2. Perceptive or nerve deafness seldom helped by surgery
B. Loss of 30 decibels or more, in range of

500 to 2,000 cycles per second, a handicapping deafness
C. For speaking to deaf person, normal tone of voice used, speaker directly facing listener
D. All deaf or partially deaf persons should learn to lip-read
E. Hearing aids cost from $150 to $500 and from $30 to $75 yearly to operate; wearer usually not completely satisfied; ability to hear not completely restored
F. Organizations concerned with welfare of deaf persons
   1. American Speech and Hearing Association
   2. American Hearing Society—publishes *Hearing News*

6. **Pathologic conditions of eye**
A. Abbreviations and terms commonly used in nursing patient with eye pathology

accommodation Involuntary process in which ciliary muscle affects zonule and lens to adjust eye to near or far distance
astigmatism Refractive error due to unequal curvature of one or more refractive surfaces of eye
cycloplegic Drug that paralyzes ciliary muscles and dilates pupil
D (diopter) Unit of measurement of strength or refractive power of lens
diplopia Double vision
E.O.M. Extraocular muscle
fusion Coordination, into single image, of separate images seen by 2 eyes
H (hyperopia) Farsightedness; focus of light behind retina
hemianopsia Blindness of ½ field of vision in one eye or in both
HT (hypertropia) Upward deviation of one eye
mydriatic Drug that dilates pupils
myopia Focus of light in front of retina—nearsightedness
O.D. (oculus dexter) or **R.E.** Right eye
O.S. (oculus sinister) or **L.E.** Left eye
O.U. (oculi unitas) or **O₂** Both eyes together
perimeter Instrument used to measure peripheral field of vision
photophobia Sensitivity to light
presbyopia Gradual loss of accommodation, "old sight"
refractive error Abnormal visual focusing
ST (estropia) Inward deviation of one eye
tonometer Instrument for measuring intraocular tension
+ Plus or convex
– Minus or concave

B. Infections of eye—may affect any part of eye and may be superficial or deep; some relatively mild; others may leave permanent damage
   1. Symptoms of eye infection
      a. Discomfort

      b. Lacrimation
      c. Burning
      d. Redness
      e. Interference with vision
      f. In some instances, purulent discharge
   2. Treatment and nursing care
      a. Depends on cause
      b. May include simple removal of cause
      c. Antibiotics locally
      d. Warm or cold packs
      e. Protection of uninfected eye
      f. Drastic treatment
         (1) Induced-fever therapy
         (2) Cortisone
   3. Conjunctivitis—inflammation or infection of conjunctiva—most common eye condition; may or may not be serious, depending on virulence of etiologic irritant
   4. Iritis—iris becomes swollen and dull in color; usually serious but may be mild
   5. Iridocyclitis—inflammation of ciliary body and iris; may resolve and leave no damage; often leaves adhesions between iris and lens; pupil small and irregular
   6. Retinitis—inflammation of retina; may be acute, mild, or peripheral; usually associated with other infections of eye; characterized by hemorrhage along retinal vein
   7. Choroiditis—inflammation of choroid; exudative type usually not too serious, but suppurative type, if not controlled, will cause blindness
   8. Keratitis—inflammation of cornea; usually leaves some permanent damage; characterized by vascularization and dullness of cornea
   9. Panophthalmitis—suppurative inflammation involving entire eye; severe eye symptoms and accompanying constitutional symptoms of infection usually present; condition usually leads to blindness of affected eye
   10. Uveitis—general term for inflammatory conditions of uveal tract (iris, ciliary body, choroid); may involve one or all parts; causative agents multiple
      a. Treatment essential to avoid serious complications and sequelae
C. Ulcers of cornea—may be due to infec-

tion, removal of foreign bodies, trauma, or inflammation; cause of 10% of all blindness

1. Symptoms begin with grayish infiltration, followed by usual symptoms of eye disease
   a. Severe pain
   b. Photophobia
   c. Lacrimation
   d. Blepharospasm
2. No scarring results if epithelium only is involved
3. Treatment
   a. Prevention
   b. Antibiotics and chemotherapeutic agents
   c. Mydriatics
   d. Relief of symptoms

D. Sympathetic ophthalmia—inflammation of uveal tract in one eye due to similar condition in other eye
1. Usually occurs after injury to ciliary body
2. Prompt treatment of injured eye helps in prevention
3. Corticosteroids administered locally and systemically; atropine locally
4. Enucleation of severely injured eye if warranted

E. Tumors of eye
1. Sarcoma—most usual tumor of choroid
   a. Displaces retina, resulting in detachment; disturbance of vision the first symptom
   b. Treatment—simple enucleation
2. Retinocytoma—glioma of retina
   a. Usually in children under 5 years of age
   b. Grows rapidly and extends along optic nerve to brain
   c. Unless enucleation done early, death ensues
3. Less usual tumors of eye
   a. Von Hippel's disease
   b. Malignancies of eyelids
   c. Malignancies of lacrimal glands

F. Muscular imbalance (strabismus)—inability of eyes to attain normal convergence required for fixation of near object, or deviation of one eye from parallelism with other
1. Unless condition rectified, child may lose ability to use one eye
2. Treatment—depends on severity of condition
   a. Corrective glasses
   b. Orthoptic training
   c. Surgical restoration of muscle balance

G. Cataract—condition characterized by opacity of crystalline lens
1. May be hard or soft; progressive or stationary
2. Often a disease of the elderly
3. Vision gradually fades
4. Lens may appear "smoky"
5. Surgery—only choice of treatment

H. Glaucoma—condition of increased intraocular tension, to point causing damage to visual apparatus; produces blindness if untreated
1. Acute (narrow-angle) glaucoma symptoms
   a. Very severe pain
   b. Malaise
   c. Vomiting
   d. Redness
   e. Swelling
   f. Dilated pupil
   g. "Steamy" cornea due to increased pressure
2. Chronic (wide-angle) glaucoma—symptoms slowly progressive; the most common form
   a. Headache
   b. Halo around lights
   c. Lessening periphery of vision
3. Treatment and nursing care
   a. Sedatives
   b. Miotics (pilocarpine, eserine or DFP)
   c. Carbonic anhydrase inhibitors (Diamox, Neptazane)
   d. Osmotic agents (urea, mannitol, glycerin)
   e. Surgery when indicated

I. Retinal detachment—separation of inner layers of retina from pigmental epithelium
1. Symptoms
   a. Sudden loss of vision in part of visual field
   b. Loss may come and go as though curtain flapping
2. Treatment
   a. Bed rest
   b. Sedative and tranquilizers
   c. Surgery as soon as possible usually indicated
   d. Mydriatic and steroid eyedrops continued from 4 to 6 weeks
   e. Psychological care and explanation

for posthospital care and follow-up visits of utmost importance

J. Traumatic conditions
1. Foreign bodies
2. Acid and alkali burns—emergency conditions; lids, conjunctiva, and cornea must be flushed copiously
3. Actinic—excessive sunlight or welder's arc light
4. Contusions and hematoma—frequent occurrence
5. Corneal abrasions—important to guard against development of corneal ulcer
6. Lacerations—not serious unless accompanied by injury to eyeball

K. Conditions of the eyelids
1. Blepharitis
2. Sty (external hordoleum)
3. Chalazion—cyst of meibomian glands
4. Trachoma—chronic, highly communicable disease; one of most common diseases in China, India, Japan and countries around Mediterranean; rare in the United States except among Indians and Mexicans
   a. Treatment—prevention best; antibiotic therapy

L. Eye manifestations of systemic diseases
1. Persistent systemic hypertension
2. Senile degeneration
3. Vascular accidents
4. Diabetes
5. Night blindness

M. Retrolental fibroplasia—rare since amount of oxygen administered to premature infants curtailed

7. **Nursing patients with surgery of eye**
A. Preoperative care
1. Complete explanation to patient of what to expect when returning from surgery
2. Have patient practice finding necessary articles and appliances if eyes are to be covered
3. Explain importance of being quiet after surgery, or of exercise
4. Nurse should wash hands carefully before doing any preoperative procedures
5. Often patient will have
   a. C.B.C.
   b. Urinalysis
   c. Eyelashes cut
   d. Tear sacs irrigated
6. Nurse may be instructed to cocainize eye
   a. 4% or 5% solution cocaine, and Adrenalin used
   b. Apply 3 drops cocaine and 2 drops of Adrenalin at 5-minute intervals for 6 applications
   c. Instruct patient to close eyes gently after each instillation and to keep them closed to prevent injury to cornea
   d. Be careful not to touch cornea when wiping away excess solution

B. Surgical procedures of eye frequently performed
1. Enucleation—removal of eye, either with or without its supporting structures
2. Iridectomy, iridencleisis, cyclodialysis and corneoscleral trephining—surgical procedures to create opening for aqueous fluid to drain from within eyeball and thus reduce intraocular tension
3. Cataract removal—lens removed from eye, either with or without its capsule
4. Surgery for reattachment of retina—various methods used, including electrocoagulation, electrodiathermy, cryosurgery, and scleral buckling

C. Postoperative care of patients with eye surgery
1. Postoperative orders should be checked very carefully, since great variation in postoperative care
2. Patient frequently returns from surgery with both eyes covered; allowed varying amounts of movement
3. Patient should not move suddenly, strain, or bend over
4. When dressing to be changed, nurse should arrange light so that no glare reaches patient
5. Any severe pain a danger signal

8. **The blind person**
A. Although the word "blind" means "without sight," various degrees of blindness
1. Vocational blindness
2. Legal blindness
3. Complete blindness

B. Legal blindness—central visual acuity of 20/200 or less in better eye with corrective glasses, or visual field of 20 degrees or less

C. Degree of rehabilitation of blind person depends on many factors
1. Age
2. Mental ability
3. Physical condition

4. Sex
5. Personality
6. Expertness and availability of rehabilitation experts and facilities

D. Beginning readjustment of newly blind starts in hospital
   1. Treat as normal person; explain strange places briefly, let patient hold your arm—do not push him
   2. Help him begin transition, both emotionally and physically, to role of blindness
   3. Let him be as independent as possible

E. Factors of total rehabilitation
   1. Vocational readjustment
   2. Recreational skills
   3. Living adjustment (mobility, protection, reading, writing)
   4. Physical reconditioning

F. Some helpful social agencies
   1. National Association for Prevention of Blindness, Inc.
   2. American Foundation for Blind
   3. Braille Evangel, Inc.
   4. Commissions or offices of social and rehabilitation service for blind in most states

G. Most states and communities have some type or types of financial aid for blind

H. Biggest problem enforced idleness and social isolation—learn not to associate blindness with shame

I. Talking books (records) can be obtained without charge from U. S. Library of Congress

NURSING PATIENTS WITH NEURAL SYSTEM PATHOLOGY

1. Basic principles of nursing

A. Psychological care and emotional support always vital, since loss of function traumatizing experience

B. Detailed observation necessary, since diagnosis and treatment necessarily determined by signs and symptoms displayed

C. Rehabilitation must be started immediately, since immobility leads to contractures and further disability; emotional and psychological rehabilitations often more difficult than physical rehabilitation

D. Prevention of decubitus ulcers if possible; enervation of muscles inevitably followed by atrophy and thin dry skin

E. All neurologic patients should be kept occupied physically and mentally as much as condition permits

F. Emotional stress should be avoided—neural disease symptoms greatly influenced by emotions

G. Therapeutic exercise and other physiotherapeutic devices for protection of joint function and neuromuscular rehabilitation should be used

H. Patient should be helped to overcome difficulty in communicating

I. Prevention of renal involvement if possible; immobility may result in formation of renal calculi and development of urinary tract infections

2. Special considerations

A. Diet high in protein

B. Daily massage and exercise—even 1 or 2 days of neglect may lose months of progress

C. For patients with various types of motor dysfunction
   1. Protect from decubiti
   2. Encourage patient to care for himself
   3. Guard against foot drop, wrist drop, and other types of deformity
   4. Guard against drafts, burns, and trauma
   5. Avoid bladder infection; tidal drainage may be indicated
   6. Give passive exercise if active exercise impossible
   7. Electrotherapy, physical therapy, massage, splints, and proper positioning also help prevent deformity

D. Degenerative conditions treated symptomatically
   1. Belladonna drugs (atropine, scopolamine, stramonium, etc.) may be used for spasticity
   2. Daily schedule of activities desirable
   3. Neatness and cleanliness very important
   4. Treat as human being
   5. Keep patient active as long as possible; ambulate if condition permits
   6. Keep extremities in most useful position
   7. Do not give sympathy but hope; mental hygiene most important aspect of nursing care

E. Patients with traumatic injuries should be observed closely and intelligently
   1. Should be kept quiet until extent of damage to central nervous system determined
   2. Observation for increased intracranial pressure vital

atropine
& scopolamine

3. Any motor, sensory, or mental changes should be noted
4. Oral foods should be given cautiously, if at all, until determined that vagus nerve not affected
5. Intake and output record should be kept and elimination maintained
6. Patient may vomit due to irritation of vomiting center in brain; good oral hygiene necessary to prevent aspiration
7. Asepsis very important—not only because central nervous system highly susceptible, but also because an infection often proves fatal
8. Patient must be protected from further injury from himself as well as from others
9. Headache often severe due to negative or positive pressure of dura
   a. Does not respond well to drugs
   b. Ice bags, slight elevation of head, and prevention of all strain may help
   c. Hypertonic glucose may be given I.V. to relieve edema
F. Patients with brain tumor paraplegia
   1. May be mentally unbalanced and require special care to maintain nutrition
   2. May be unable to care for self—family should be taught care of patient; family needs much emotional support
   3. Mental and physical pain alleviated as much as possible
G. Patients with cord paralysis particularly subject to bladder difficulties
   1. Types of bladder paralysis
      a. Spastic paralysis—some muscle tone under autonomic nerve control
      b. Flaccid paralysis—no muscle tone and complete incontinence
   2. Tidal drainage often used to maintain normal bladder tone and to encourage autonomic nerves to take over control of bladder function; bladder filled to predetermined degree of intervesicular pressure and empties automatically by combination of siphonage and gravity flow
   3. Patients should be ambulated if possible
   4. Massage and exercise should be done daily
   5. Deformities should be prevented if possible and extremities kept in most functional position

6. Hopeful, encouraging attitude most important
H. Hyperthermia or hyperpyrexia—markedly elevated temperature
   1. Due to irritation of temperature control center in brain
   2. Usually must be controlled by mechanical means
      a. Ice bags
      b. Cold sponges
      c. Hypothermia apparatus
   3. Care must be taken that temperature does not go too low
I. Some medications frequently used in neurologic conditions
   1. Anticonvulsants
      a. Dilantin sodium—for grand mal epilepsy
      b. Mesantoin—for grand mal epilepsy; quite toxic
      c. Tridione—for minor seizures
   2. Antispasmodics
      a. Belladonna group: stramonium, atropine, scopolamine — relaxes smooth muscles; toxic symptoms include dryness of mouth and skin and blurring of vision
      b. Curare—prevents transmission of nerve impulses; used to inhibit spasms of paraplegic patients; may cause respiratory embarrassment
   3. Vasoconstrictors
      a. Epinephrine (Adrenalin)—used in myasthenia gravis and allergic conditions and to elevate blood pressure
      b. Ergotamine tartrate (Gynergen)— used to relieve or prevent migraine; acts on smooth muscles

3. Neurologic signs and symptoms
A. Increased intracranial pressure—may be found in almost any neurologic condition including head injuries, cerebral vascular accidents (CVA), infectious diseases of structures within cranium, brain tumors, some developmental conditions such as hydrocephalus, and after central nervous system surgery
   1. Cardinal symptoms
      a. Increasing blood pressure (diastolic more sharply)
      b. Decreasing pulse rate
      c. Increasing headache
      d. Papilledema
      e. Decreasing mental alertness
   2. Other symptoms that may or may not develop

a. Tonic or clonic convulsions
b. Vomiting—may or may not be projectile
c. Enlarged pupil (side of pressure)
d. Incontinence
e. Paralysis of any part of body
f. Sensory disturbances of any part of body
3. Other localizing signs
  a. Frontal lobe
    (1) Aphasia
    (2) Changes in personality
    (3) Confusion
    (4) Jacksonian convulsions
  b. Parietal lobe
    (1) Convulsions
    (2) Sensory disturbances
    (3) Astereognosis
  c. Temporal lobe
    (1) Defects in visual field
    (2) Defects in taste or hearing
    (3) Smell of "burning rubber"
  d. Occipital lobe—visual disturbances
  e. Cerebellum
    (1) Ataxia
    (2) Tremors
    (3) Nystagmus
4. When there is evidence of increasing intracranial pressure, nurse should
  a. Watch blood pressure, pulse, temperature, and respiration carefully; report any major change
  b. Prevent straining of any kind—at stool, vomiting, emotional, at restraints or treatments
  c. Prevent aspiration by positioning or suctioning and good mouth care
  d. Avoid exciting patient in any manner

B. Common neurologic signs and symptoms
1. Astereognosis—inability to recognize familiar objects by manipulation
2. Aphonia—inability to speak due to dysfunction of larynx
3. Aphasia—inability to speak due to dysfunction of some part of central nervous system
4. Anesthesia—loss of sensation; hyperesthesia—exaggerated sensation; paresthesia—unusual or peculiar sensation
5. Nystagmus—"bouncing" eyeballs
6. Past-pointing—tendency to veer to one side of tip of nose when trying to touch it
7. Paresis—slight or incomplete paralysis
8. Hemianopsia—loss of one half the field of vision; homonymous hemianopsia—loss of one half the field of vision in both eyes
9. Anosmia—loss of sense of smell
10. Spastic paralysis—produced by injury or disease of upper motor neurons (in cerebral cortex or brainstem)
11. Flaccid paralysis—produced by disease in lower motor neurons (in ventral horns of commissure in spinal cord)

4. **Neurologic diagnostic procedures**
1. Lumbar puncture or spinal tap—subarachnoid space entered through lumbar interspaces with spinal needle
  a. Purposes
    (1) To secure fluid
    (2) To relieve pressure
    (3) To instill medications or dye
    (4) To determine pressure of spinal fluid
  b. Nursing care
    (1) Psychological care
    (2) Asepsis
    (3) Forcing fluids if not contraindicated
    (4) Usually keeping head low
2. Cisternal puncture—insertion of needle into cisterna magna just below foramen magnum
  a. Purposes
    (1) Same as for lumbar puncture
    (2) Often used for infants and when intracranial pressure very high
3. Queckenstedt test (spinal dynamics)—spinal tap done in conjunction with compression of jugular veins in neck to determine if any obstruction between site of entry and brain
  a. Nurse may be asked to compress jugular veins manually or with blood pressure cuff; aftercare same as for lumbar puncture
  b. If no obstruction, blood pressure will rise during jugular compression and return to normal 10 to 30 seconds after release of pressure
    (1) Slow rise and return indicate partial block
    (2) No rise indicates complete block
4. Pneumoencephalography — procedure in which air or gas is injected into cerebrospinal space, after fluid is re-

moved by means of spinal needle inserted in lumbar region, and then roentgenograms are made
  a. Procedure done to visualize cerebral ventricles for diagnostic and/or localization purposes
  b. Nursing care following procedure
    (1) Close observation
    (2) Noting vital signs often
    (3) Changing position frequently
    (4) Giving fluids freely
    (5) Administration of ice bags, aspirin, or codeine for headache
5. Myelography—procedure in which radiopaque dye introduced into subarachnoid space in spinal canal and roentgenograms made
  a. Purpose—to determine if any impingement on spinal cord
  b. If dye completely removed, patient treated as for lumbar puncture; if dye not completely removed, patient's head kept elevated because dye will cause meningeal irritation if it reaches meninges
6. Ventriculography—procedure in which air or gas injected directly into lateral ventricle with ventricular needle and then roentgenograms made
  a. Used as aid in diagnosis, especially in brain tumors; can be used when intracranial pressure very high
  b. Nursing care after procedure much same as for encephalogram; head will probably be elevated some, and sterile cannula should be available at bedside
7. Cerebral arteriography or angiography—radiopaque dye injected into internal carotid artery and cerebral arteries visualized by roentgenogram
  a. Used to discover abnormalities or aneurysms in cerebral arteries
  b. Nursing care after procedure includes observation for bleeding or respiratory distress; patient may have severe headache
8. Electroencephalography — procedure in which electrodes applied to scalp and graphic record made of electrical activity of brain
  a. Used to detect electrical abnormalities, especially in epilepsy, indicative of pathology or abnormal functioning
  b. No special nursing care except complete explanation and reassurances

9. Caloric test (vestibular, water)—injection of warm or cold water into external auditory canal to test vestibular (balance) function of eighth nerve
  a. Used to differentiate between lesions in brainstem and cerebellum
  b. Patient should be kept in bed for about 1 hour after procedure
10. Pitressin test—procedure in which Pitressin injected until patient convulses in order to observe pattern of seizure; used for localization of pathology
11. Paravertebral block — procedure in which sympathetic rami and ganglia anesthetized to alleviate pain in specific area or to determine value of contemplated sympathectomy
12. Sodium Amytal test—Sodium Amytal given; lowest blood pressure obtained indicates lowest blood pressure that can be expected from thoracolumbar sympathectomy
13. Radioisotope scanning—intravenous injection of certain radioactive compounds such as RISA or mercurial preparations and the application of a scintillation scanner
  a. Used to detect some intracranial lesions
    (1) Cerebral neoplasm
    (2) Hematoma
    (3) Abscess
    (4) Arteriovenous malformation
14. Echoencephalography — ultrasound echo used to measure midline structures in cranial vault
  a. Useful in detecting a shift in conditions precipitated by
    (1) Subdural hematoma
    (2) Intracerebral hemorrhage
    (3) Massive cerebral infarction
    (4) Cerebral neoplasms
  b. Not as accurate as carotid angiography or ventriculography
15. Discography—injection of a radiopaque substance directly into the intervertebral disc
  a. Useful in patients suspected of having herniated nucleus pulposus that is undiagnosed by myelography
5. **Diseases of neural system**
A. Developmental pathology of neural system (Chapter 11)
  1. Spina bifida—incomplete fusion of one or more vertebrae
  2. Meningocele—protrusion of meninges

through spina bifida; requires surgery soon after birth

3. Myelomeningocele—protrusion of spinal cord into meningocele; surgery not indicated

4. Rachischisis—incomplete closure of spinal vertebrae, meninges, and cord—all exposed to view; often associated with other anomalies

5. Hydrocephalus—excessive accumulation of cerebrospinal fluid in brain; followed by enlargement of head
   a. Internal hydrocephalus — obstruction of narrower pathways in cerebral ventricular system
   b. External hydrocephalus—probably due to faulty absorption of intracranial fluid by venous (arachnoid villa) system

6. Infantile cerebral palsy (congenital spastic diplegia)—congenital spastic paralysis of extremities, affecting lower extremities more severely; all degrees of severity; may or may not be impairment of mental faculties

B. Degenerative conditions of neural system
1. Disseminated (multiple) sclerosis—spotty degeneration of conducting pathways in brain and spinal cord
   a. Symptoms subject to remissions and exacerbations
      (1) Charcot's triad (ataxia, intention tremor, scanning speech)
      (2) Visual impairment
      (3) Emotional lability
      (4) Spasticity of extremities
   b. Treatment and nursing care symptomatic, but disease as whole progressive

2. Motor neuron disease—group of diseases characterized by muscle atrophy and spasticity; includes progressive muscular atrophy, bulbar palsy, amyotrophic lateral sclerosis

3. Syringomyelia — chronic progressive disease of spinal cord; may involve brainstem
   a. Characteristics
      (1) Loss of pain and temperature sensation in affected area

4. Subacute combined degeneration—progressive disease of peripheral nerves
   a. Characteristics
      (1) Paresthesia
      (2) Impaired muscular power
      (3) Spasticity
      (4) Frequently associated with pernicious anemia

5. Paralysis agitans (Parkinson's disease, shaking palsy)—loss of cells and fibers of corpus striatum and substantia nigra
   a. Characteristics
      (1) Progressive tremor
      (2) Stiffening of muscles
   b. Symptoms
      (1) Condition slowly progressive
      (2) Tremor (pin-rolling)
      (3) Rigidity
      (4) Masklike facial expression
      (5) Personality changes
      (6) Later, propulsion gait
   c. Present treatment
      (1) Symptomatic
      (2) Surgery of extrapyramidal tract being tried
      (3) Chemopallidectomy — destruction of globus pallidus with alcohol sometimes used
      (4) Electrocoagulation or chemothalamectomy—procedures for destruction of thalamus sometimes used
      (5) L-dopa offers some relief from symptoms

6. Huntington's chorea—familial, progressive disease of adults, characterized by violent choreiform movements and mental deterioration
   a. Treatment and nursing care protective and custodial at present

7. Athetosis—usually variant of infantile cerebral palsy
   a. Characteristics
      (1) Slow, writhing, purposeless movements of limbs
      (2) Bizarre posturing
      (3) Inability to perform coordinated movements

8. Myasthenia gravis—chronic but not degenerative disease due to deficiency of acetylcholine at myoneural junction, which causes muscle to receive weak or no motor impulses; muscle contracts poorly, if at all
   a. Characteristics
      (1) Extreme fatigability of muscles, so severe as to merge into paralysis
      (2) May have double vision, ptosis of eyelids, and difficulty in swallowing or breathing
   b. Treatment

(1) Neostigmine bromide (Prostigmin), pyridostigmine bromide (Mestinon)

(2) Excellent health care necessary adjunct

(3) During acute stages, tracheotomy may be necessary

C. Common infectious diseases of neural system

1. Sydenham's chorea (St. Vitus dance) —infectious disease of vascular and perivascular structures of brain manifested by involuntary, purposeless movements

    a. Symptoms

    (1) Involuntary movements that occur during sleep (symptom peculiar to this type of chorea only)

    (2) Fretfulness

    (3) Irritability

    (4) Emotional instability

    (5) Frequently, cardiac involvement

    b. Nursing care

    (1) Extremely important

    (2) Observations should be inclusive and exact; child should be kept quiet, given high-caloric, high-vitamin diet, large amounts of fluids, and be protected from any emotional and mental strain

    (3) Necessary for him to observe good health practices rest of life

2. Myelitis—acute inflammation of spinal cord substance

    a. Characteristics

    (1) Rapid onset of flaccid paralysis of extremities

    (2) Prognosis of life good, but may be residual effects such as paralysis

3. Poliomyelitis—infection and degeneration of anterior horn cells (Chapter 11)

4. Neuritis—infection of nerves and nerve roots (radiculitis); characterized by pain and weakness in individual muscles

    a. Infectious polyneuritis (Guillain-Barré syndrome)—fairly acute involvement of motor components of spinal and cranial nerve roots

    (1) Characteristics

    (a) Fever

    (b) Pain and weakness in muscle groups

    (c) No loss of sensation

    (d) Recovery with little or no residual damage

    (2) Treatment and nursing care

    (a) Palliative and symptomatic

    (b) Aim—to maintain comfort (heat and rest during acute stage) and prevent complications such as limited function

5. Herpes zoster (shingles)—(p. 392)

6. Neurosyphilis—complication of late syphilis; meningovascular, tabes dorsalis, general paresis

    a. Treatment and nursing care

    (1) Palliative and symptomatic

    (2) Procaine penicillin G biweekly for a total of 7 million units or 400,000 units of benzathine penicillin G weekly for 3 weeks

7. Encephalitis, endemic: 1,123 cases in 1972 in the United States

    a. Types most common in the United States

    (1) Eastern equine

    (2) Western equine

    (3) St. Louis

    (4) Japanese B

    b. Etiology—arbovirus; each type caused by its own specific virus; reservoir of infection: wild and domestic birds

    c. Transmission—bite of infected mosquito that has been infected by biting infected bird

    d. Incubation period—4 to 21 days, average 5 to 15 days

    e. Symptoms—similar for all types; onset abrupt, fever 104° to 105° F., pulse rapid, headache, nausea, vomiting, leukocytosis, neurologic signs, tremor of hand, tongue, lips, speech difficult, stiff neck, drowsiness, variation in level of consciousness, convulsions, death

    f. Diagnosis—serologic tests: complement-fixation test, hemagglutination-inhibition antibody test; isolation of virus on autopsy

    g. Complications—rare; sequelae: recurring convulsions, mental retardation, paralysis

h. Treatment—none; therapy similar to that for poliomyelitis

i. Nursing—no isolation; care as in febrile conditions, observing for convulsions

j. Prevention—elimination of breeding places of vector; no prophylaxis for humans; public education

D. Convulsive disorders

1. Causes
   a. Idiopathic
   b. Congenital defects in brain
   c. Brain injury
   d. Infectious diseases of central nervous system
   e. Brain diseases
   f. Uremia
   g. Fevers
   h. Asphyxia
   i. Drugs or poisons
   j. Electrical stimulation
   k. Hysteria

2. Jacksonian epilepsy
   a. Convulsions begin in one part of body and spread in orderly manner to all other parts of body
   b. Loss of consciousness rarely occurs
   c. Electroencephalogram characteristically shows very slow wave

3. Hysterical epilepsy
   a. Characteristics
      (1) No true loss of consciousness
      (2) No incontinence
      (3) No tongue biting
      (4) Bizarre thrashing about

4. Epileptic equivalent
   a. Characteristics
      (1) Amnesia
      (2) Bizarre behavior
      (3) Irresponsible actions
   b. Electrical discharge acts on mind instead of muscles
   c. Patients not responsible for actions at time

5. Petit mal epilepsy (little seizures, uncinate fit)
   a. Characteristics—may have one or several
      (1) Momentary lapses of consciousness
      (2) "Vacant look" for minute or two
      (3) Slight twitching for seconds
      (4) Automatic acts
      (5) Awareness of disagreeable taste or odor

      (6) Electroencephalogram showing fast, then slow waves
      (7) Medication with Tridione, Benzedrine, and others

6. Grand mal epilepsy (major seizures)
   a. Motor discharges from brain cells cause impairment of consciousness and paroxysms of convulsive movements
   b. Electroencephalogram shows fast type wave
   c. Symptoms
      (1) Aura in about 50% of cases
      (2) Tonic stage with extreme rigidity of muscles
      (3) Clonic stage which may include frothing at mouth or incontinence and stage of stupor
      (4) Patient awakens with no recollection of attack but may be exhausted, irritable, or confused
   d. Treatment
      (1) Removal of cause when possible
      (2) Psychotherapy
      (3) Good general health
      (4) No consumption of alcohol
      (5) Drug therapy—one or combination of drugs
         (a) Phenobarbital
         (b) Dilantin sodium
         (c) Mesantoin
         (d) Many others in use
   e. Nursing care
      (1) Accurate observation during attack
      (2) Protection of patient during attack; stay with patient, loosen tight clothing, screen, place pillow under head, prevent tongue biting
      (3) Helping patient adjust to disease; teach value of
         (a) Taking medications as ordered
         (b) Carrying card to make information available if seizure occurs
         (c) Avoiding alcohol and undue physical and emotional stress
         (d) Well-balanced diet

E. Tumors of central nervous system

1. Brain tumor—any expanding tumor within skull regarded as brain tumor;

all threaten life, encapsulated or not; location of tumor more important than type

a. Symptoms
(1) All show slowly developing intracranial pressure with
(a) Headache
(b) Dizziness
(c) Drowsiness
(d) Forgetfulness
(e) Progression to more definite symptoms, such as motor or sensory dysfunction

b. More common types
(1) Gliomas, arise from glia; very malignant
(2) Meningiomas, relatively benign
(3) Fibromas
(4) Pituitary adenomas
(5) Metastatic brain tumors

c. Nursing care
(1) Close observation
(2) Prevention of straining
(3) Keeping intake record (often cannot be trusted to eat enough)
(4) Keeping patient quiet (emotions often unstable)
(5) Keeping patient out of bed or head elevated
(6) Giving emotional support to patient and family

d. Treatment may be palliative or surgical

2. Spinal cord tumors—usually classified according to position: extradural, intradural, and intramedullary

a. Symptoms divided into 3 stages
(1) First stage
(a) Pain (intramedullary tumors relatively painless)
(b) Localized motor weakness and/or numbness or hyperesthesia
(2) Second stage comprises beginning of symptoms of cord compression below tumor
(3) Third stage—complete loss of motor and sensory function below compression

b. Types—meningiomas and gliomas most frequent types of cord tumors, meningiomas usually can be safely removed

c. Nursing care

(1) Comfort of patient
(2) Prevention of deformities
(3) Prevention of complications

F. Vascular pathology of neural system
1. Cerebral vascular accident (apoplexy, stroke) occurs more or less suddenly; pulse full and rapid; respirations labored; consciousness lost

a. Hemorrhage into the brain or meninges occurs instantaneously; unconsciousness develops rapidly; spinal fluid will contain blood

b. Cerebral thrombosis—narrowing of lumen of cerebral artery until occluded; symptoms
(1) Develop in matter of hours
(2) Convulsions frequent
(3) Patient may or may not lose consciousness

c. Cerebral embolism—clot lodged in cerebral artery; onset of symptoms rapid; coma develops

d. Treatment and nursing care
(1) Supportive and palliative
(2) At first, minimal handling important
(3) Aspiration, decubitus ulcers, and contractures must be prevented
(4) Later, ambulation and rehabilitation will be started
(5) Education for future health should be given

2. Cerebral aneurysm—dilatation of cerebral artery due to weakness in wall
a. If small, no symptoms unless rupture into subarachnoid space
b. If large, causes pressure on various structures; symptoms
(1) Intense headache
(2) Impaired vision
(3) Pain in face
(4) Symptoms of tumor
(5) Coma and death
c. Treatment—excision desirable if in favorable location

3. Cerebral arteriosclerosis
a. May or may not be part of general arteriosclerosis
b. May cause gradual deterioration of mental faculties
c. May be mistaken diagnosis for many other psychological conditions

4. Migraine—syndrome of paroxysmal, familial, recurring attacks of severe headache

a. Cranial arteries develop deep cranial pulsations, dilatation, and later thickening with edema
   (1) Chain of events starts in central nervous system
   (2) Pain increased by sustained muscle contraction of head and neck
b. Treatment and nursing care
   (1) Must be adjusted to individual
   (2) Helping patient relax and avoid distressing situations most important aspect of care
   (3) Ergotamine tartrate in some form specific for disease

5. Other vascular conditions
   a. Arteriovenous fistula
   b. Vascular spasm
   c. Ventricular hemorrhage
   d. Thrombosis of venous sinuses
   e. Ischemia or anemia of brain cells

G. Traumatic injuries of neural system
1. Traumatic injuries of head
   a. Fracture of skull—crack in skull with or without brain injury; seriousness depends entirely on amount of brain or cranial nerve damage
   b. Concussion—change in brain following blow or jar
      (1) Characteristics
         (a) Momentary or longer period of unconsciousness
         (b) May be followed by vertigo, nausea, headache, dizziness, or confusion
      (2) Must at first be regarded as serious
      (3) Patient must be observed for complications due to paralysis of vasomotor centers in medulla
   c. Extradural or epidural hemorrhage—bleeding beneath cranium and outside dura, frequently of middle meningeal artery
      (1) Symptoms of increasing intracranial pressure develop rapidly
      (2) Before surgery all movement or strain should be minimal
      (3) Early surgery mandatory to save patient's life
   d. Subarachnoid hemorrhage—bleeding between arachnoid and pia mater into cerebrospinal fluid
      (1) Typical symptoms of meningitis develop because blood irritating to meninges
      (2) Treatment protective and symptomatic
   e. Subdural hemorrhage or hematoma—hemorrhage between dura and arachnoid
      (1) Symptoms of increasing intracranial pressure develop slowly—hours to months later
      (2) Personality changes may be first noticeable sign
      (3) Treated conservatively or by aspiration or decompression

2. Traumatic injuries of spinal cord
   a. Lumbar cord injuries may affect any of motor or sensory functions below injury
      (1) Patient usually kept in hyperextended position to prevent further injury to cord
      (2) Bradford frame or Foster bed may be desirable
   b. Cervical cord injuries usually treated with Crutchfield tongs or other methods of traction to head
      (1) Patient may be turned carefully as long as traction on
      (2) Extremities should be put through range of motion exercises daily

3. Intervertebral pathology—may be evidenced in number of ways; intervertebral disc may be herniated, slipped, or bulging; may or may not be impinging on various spinal nerves
   a. Symptoms manifested in different ways
      (1) Pain in back or leg
      (2) Loss of reflexes
      (3) Disturbance of sensation in affected area
      (4) Excruciating pain on movement
      (5) Inability to bend back
   b. Treatment conservative or surgical
      (1) Conservative—orthopedic problem; traction, various types of back support usual
      (2) Surgical—laminectomy with removal of disc or spinal fusion
      (3) Nursing care depends largely on amount of damage to cord and of motor and sensory dysfunction

c. Complications of surgery rare, but quite serious
   (1) Sepsis
   (2) Phlebitis
   (3) Trophic ulcers
   (4) Toe drop
   (5) Paralysis of quadriceps
   (6) Headache
4. Peripheral nerve injury—must be immobilized for about 6 weeks after repair; peripheral nerves will regenerate to some degree under favorable circumstances

H. Cranial nerve pathology
1. Trigeminal neuralgia or tic douloureux —paroxysms of severe pain in one or more branches of fifth cranial nerve
  a. Pain appears periodically; lasts for a few weeks, increases in severity and duration until it becomes almost continuous; "trigger" point frequently on upper lip
  b. Treatment and nursing care
    (1) Injection or surgery of nerve (produces anesthesia of affected area)
    (2) Goggles over eyes immediately after surgery
    (3) Protection from hot foods and injury of affected area
    (4) Turning patient frequently and gently
2. Glossopharyngeal neuralgia—disturbance of ninth cranial nerve, affecting ability to swallow, talk, and breathe properly and to taste with posterior part of tongue
  a. Symptoms
    (1) Pain in posterior tongue and tonsil region
    (2) Mental depression
    (3) Respiratory failure
    (4) Regurgitation
    (5) Choking
3. Bell's palsy—loss of function of seventh cranial nerve that stimulates facial expression, maxillary and sublingual glands and is sensory for anterior tongue
  a. Symptoms indicating loss of function
    (1) Flaccid paralysis of one side of face
    (2) Inability to close one eye
    (3) Mouth drawn toward unaffected side

    (4) Drooling
    (5) Difficulty in swallowing and talking
  b. Treatment and nursing care
    (1) Treatment palliative and supportive: massage and electrotherapy
    (2) Nurse should help guard against
      (a) Emotional maladjustment
      (b) Stretching and loss of tone of weakened muscles
      (c) Trauma to eye or mucous membranes
      (d) Anorexia and weight loss
      (e) Facial contractures

6. **Nursing patients with surgery of the nervous system**
A. Preoperative care
1. Keep patient quiet physically and emotionally
2. Keep intake and output record; maintain nutrition
3. Atropine rather than morphine and derivatives usually given for central nervous system surgery
4. Cathartics contraindicated when increased intracranial pressure; small enemas may be given if indicated; in emergency brain surgery, usually nothing given
5. Excellent oral hygiene very important to help prevent aspiration later; bleeding ears or nostrils should not be cleaned inside
6. Routine bath given for scheduled surgery; in emergency central nervous system surgery, patient usually left quiet
7. Head shaved as much as necessary and hair saved
8. Patients with tumors and other conditions in which intracranial pressure is increased, except when hemorrhaging, should be kept out of bed or with head elevated
B. Some common operative procedures
1. Debridement—wound cleaned of all foreign material, including broken bones and tissues
2. Burr holes—small holes drilled through cranium and "hole" left in head; when trephine used, bone can be replaced; used for hematomas, hydromas, fifth nerve section, and many other procedures

3. Craniotomy—opening into cranium; bone may be replaced by "turning flap"; may be left open for decompression; or plate may be inserted
4. Decompression—removal or elevation of bone for relief of pressure
5. Ventricular drainage—drainage of ventricle by means of ventricular needle inserted into ventricle through burr hole
6. Frontal lobotomy or prefrontal leukotomy—surgical interruption of pathways between thalamus and frontal lobes to reduce emotional components of ideas; used in severe anxiety conditions and sometimes for intolerable pain; patient requires reeducation after surgery
7. Laminectomy—surgical procedure in which one or more laminae removed and spinal cord exposed; procedure done for many purposes—exploratory laminectomy, decompression laminectomy, etc.; dura may or may not be entered
8. Cordotomy—section of spinothalamic (anterolateral) tract of spinal cord for relief of intolerable pain; interrupts sensation of pain and temperature on opposite side below level of section
9. Tractotomy—section of nerve tract in brainstem
10. Neurectomy—injection or excision of peripheral or cranial nerve
11. Rhizotomy—excision of posterior roots of spinal nerve
12. Sympathectomy—section of spinal ganglion or preganglionic fibers; lumbar—for peripheral vascular disease; thoracolumbar—for malignant hypertension
13. Gastric vagotomy—section of gastric branches of vagus nerve
14. Cranial nerve surgery
    a. Section of fifth cranial nerve between ganglion and brain for relief of pain in trigeminal neuralgia
    b. Division of vestibular portion of eighth nerve for relief of Ménière's syndrome

C. Postoperative care of brain surgery or brain injury from any cause
1. Requires special techniques and special nursing care; diligence and most careful observation
    a. Side rails on bed and other protective devices as needed
    b. Move patient carefully—hold head; do not place on operative area; check orders to see if head to be elevated
    c. Turn frequently; guard against aspiration; use suction if cough reflex depressed
    d. Asepsis vital; central nervous system very susceptible to pathogenic organisms
    e. Patient usually fed intravenously or by gastric tube; check swallowing reflex before feeding orally; keep an intake and output record; may have retention or incontinence
    f. Fecal softener given instead of enema
    g. Observations
       (1) State of consciousness
       (2) Change in vital signs
       (3) Irregularity of pupils
       (4) Fresh bleeding
       (5) Convulsions or twitching
       (6) Clear fluid from ears, nostrils, or on dressing
       (7) Any marked change in mental state
       (8) Any disturbed motor or sensory functioning of any organ
2. Postoperative complications
    a. Emesis
    b. Internal hemorrhage
    c. Mental disturbances
    d. Hyperthermia
    e. Severe headache
    f. Shock
    g. Chest complications
    h. Periocular edema
    i. Convulsions
    j. Laryngeal spasm
    k. Sensory or motor dysfunction
3. Severe brain damage may leave residual damage; effects considered permanent between 3 and 4 months after injury
    a. Hemiplegia most common sequela
    b. Some loss of vision second most common
    c. Posttraumatic epilepsy, skull defects, scars, and brain abscesses may develop
4. Peripheral nerves will regenerate to some extent if neurilemma intact; such

injuries need physical therapy as soon as possible

5. In all cases, persistent aftercare mandatory; emotional and psychological rehabilitation may be more difficult than physical rehabilitation

6. After surgery on sensory nerve tracts, patient must be taught to protect himself; nurses must remember not to use hot-water bottles and must have patient change position frequently

NURSING PATIENTS WITH MUSCULOSKELETAL CONDITIONS

1. **Basic principles of nursing**
A to G. Similar to those for neural system pathology (p. 403)
H. Prevention best treatment
I. Helping patient with socioeconomic problems

2. **Orthopedic injury**
Includes injuries to bones and joints, fractures, dislocations, injuries to tendons and ligaments (soft tissue injuries), and others
A. Contusions, sprains, and dislocations
   1. Contusions—injury to soft tissues produced by blunt force, with hemorrhage (ecchymosis) resulting in discoloration; hematoma may develop
      a. Treatment and nursing care
         (1) Elevating affected part
         (2) Applying moist or dry cold for first 8 to 10 hours
         (3) Pressure bandage
         (4) Moist or dry heat and massage after hemorrhage stops
   2. Sprains—injury to ligamentous structures surrounding joint, caused by a wrench or twist
      a. Symptoms
         (1) Similar to contusions
         (2) Painful movement
         (3) Should have x-ray film to be certain no bone injury
      b. Treatment and nursing care
         (1) Cold compresses
         (2) Rest
         (3) Elevation
         (4) Support with temporary splint or elastic bandages
   3. Dislocations—articular surfaces of bones forming joint no longer in contact
      a. May be congenital, spontaneous or pathologic, or traumatic

   b. Symptoms
      (1) Change in contour of joint
      (2) Change in length of extremity
      (3) Loss of normal mobility
      (4) Change in axis of dislocated bones
      (5) May have associated fracture; x-ray examination required
   c. Treatment and nursing care
      (1) Immobilization best first-aid procedure
      (2) Reduction under general anesthesia
      (3) Nursing care after reduction essentially same as that after reduction of fractures
B. Fractures
   1. Classification
      a. Closed, simple—skin not broken
      b. Open, compound—skin broken
      c. Incomplete, greenstick—continuity of bone not entirely interrupted
      d. Complete—continuity of bone entirely interrupted
      e. Comminuted—fragments of bones broken into many small pieces
      f. Impacted—fragments are driven into the other so that break is stabilized
      g. Multiple—more than one separate fracture
      h. Articular—fracture of joint surface of a bone
      i. Pathologic—resulting from minor injury to a bone already weakened by disease
      j. Line of break—transverse, oblique, spiral
   2. Symptoms
      a. Pain
      b. Loss of function
      c. Deformity
      d. False motion
      e. Edema
      f. Spasm
   3. Treatment
      a. Principles of treatment
         (1) Obtain reduction of fracture
         (2) Maintain reduction in place until healing occurs (immobilization)
         (3) Regain normal function of affected part (rehabilitation)
      b. Methods used to obtain fracture reduction
         (1) Traction

(2) Closed reduction
(3) Open reduction
c. Methods used to maintain fracture reduction
(1) Plaster cast
(2) Splints
(3) Continuous traction
(4) Pin and plaster techniques
(5) Internal fixation devices
  (a) Nails
  (b) Plates
  (c) Screws
  (d) Wires
  (e) Rods
(6) Complications of fractures
  (a) Immediate—shock, fat embolism, pulmonary embolism
  (b) Delayed—delayed union, nonunion, avascular necrosis

C. Nursing the patient with a fracture
1. Prevention and emergency treatment
  a. Recognition and elimination of common home hazards that cause falls
  b. First aid
    (1) Treat every suspected fracture as fracture
    (2) Splint them where they lie, but not too vigorously if fracture compound
    (3) Transport in such a way as not to cause further injury—usually in position of full extension
2. Fracture of upper extremity
  a. When cast used
    (1) Check state of circulation for several days; report any signs of impairment without delay; do not cut windows in cast without instruction; do not cut cast back on foot or hand, since this will increase edema
    (2) Keep arm elevated; if sling worn, see that it supports wrist in extension and elbow at right angles; pin sling rather than tie it; if patient discharged wearing sling, instructions pertaining to shoulder exercise may be indicated
  b. If traction used
    (1) Observe for skin denudation pressure areas and circulatory disturbances
    (2) Make provision for counter-

traction by elevating side of bed of arm in traction
(3) Massage shoulders and cervical area frequently for relief of muscle strain
3. Fracture of femur
  a. Patient may be cared for in various types of apparatus
    (1) Hip spica cast
    (2) Well leg splint
    (3) Skin or skeletal traction with Thomas splint
    (4) Russell traction
    (5) Surgical procedure such as insertion of intramedullary nail; ambulation with crutches permitted when postoperative pain subsided and muscle strength sufficient; crutches used until bony union apparent on roentgenogram
  b. Expect considerable shock and disorientation during first 10 days after injury in elderly person
  c. Prevent chest congestion by frequent change of position, elevating head of bed, and deep breathing exercises
  d. Watch for signs of renal impairment; measure intake and output and report symptoms of suppression
  e. Nursing measures to prevent pressure areas must be started first day
  f. Provide overhead trapeze so patient may move himself; encourage bed activity—particularly of arms, shoulders, and uninvolved extremity
  g. Provide for good body alignment and functional positions
  h. Provide diversional therapy suitable to patient's interests
4. Nursing the patient with fracture of hip
  a. Major types of hip fracture
    (1) Those involving trochanteric region of femur—both fragments well supplied with blood; nearly always unite, if properly reduced and fixation adequate
    (2) Those involving intracapsular part of femoral neck—blood supply to proximal fragment may be disturbed resulting in avascular necrosis and degenerative process

b. Older age group—patients have other health problems such as cardiac, arteriosclerotic, arthritic, and hypertensive conditions

c. General nursing care
  (1) Older person often experiences severe pain in hip region with movement; involved limb externally rotated and slightly shorter than other extremity
  (2) Avoid unnecessary transfer of patient
  (3) Bed—provide firm support
  (4) Help patient adjust to hospital; explain routines
  (5) Use special skin care, foam rubber pads under sacrum and heels (distributing weight more evenly); maintain clean, dry, wrinkle-free bed; massage bony areas
  (6) Provide overhead trapeze; encourage change of position, active exercise of upper extremities and uninvolved lower extremity
  (7) Make meal time enjoyable, encourage self-feeding, fluids, and diet as tolerated and prescribed (adequate protein and vitamins); remember dentures (diet that patient can chew); record intake and output
  (8) Use nursing measures to prevent fecal impaction
  (9) Check for bladder distention (avoid use of catheter, if possible)
  (10) Give deep breathing exercise at scheduled intervals
  (11) Provide safety for confused patient (side rails, night-light, and adequate supervision)
  (12) Immobilization of limb
    (a) Traction—utilize appropriate nursing care
    (b) Sandbags—immobilize and maintain correct alignment or position preventing external rotation

d. Treatment—usually consists of closed reduction, with internal fixation as soon as patient's condition warrants surgical procedure

e. Postoperative nursing care
  (1) Amount of immobilization determined by surgeon
    (a) If hip unstable, traction may be applied and movement of patient restricted
    (b) If hip stable, encourage patient to change position
      (1) May roll on either side (more comfortable on unaffected side); place pillows between thighs and legs to prevent adduction of hip joint
      (2) Encourage active exercise and use of unaffected extremities
      (3) Active or passive exercise of involved extremity (as prescribed); dorsal and plantar flexion of ankle, flexion and extension of hip and knee
  (2) Maintain good body alignment and functional positions; prevent external rotation of involved limb, flexed knee, and drop foot deformity
  (3) Nursing care—pertaining to skin, diet, deep breathing, elimination, and maintenance of independence—same as given preoperatively
  (4) Up in chair (as ordered, first or second postoperative day); involved limb not weight bearing; have patient stand on good leg, pivot, and sit in chair; this encourages active exercise and helps patient's morale
  (5) Length of time patient is not to bear weight on involved extremity is determined by physician (may be up to 12 weeks); if patient's condition warrants, crutch walking taught —thus enabling limited ambulation; if crutch walking not feasible during nonweight-bearing period, an "active" bed-chair regimen should be provided
  (6) When partial weight bearing is permitted, patient taught to

ambulate with a walker or with crutches (three-point gait)

5. Hip prosthesis—may be used to replace head of femur when aseptic necrosis is a complication of hip fracture

   a. Postoperatively, patient placed in balanced-suspension traction or cast, or limb immobilized with sandbags for approximately 10 days

   b. Nursing care same as described for elderly patient with hip nailing; measures to prevent pressure sores, contractures, muscle atrophy, hypostatic pneumonia, and impactions; maintenance of good body alignment and functional positions; encouragement of active exercise of uninvolved extremities, self-help activities, and adequate diet

   c. Involved limb maintained in a neutral position, with slight abduction; functional position of foot maintained; active exercise of ankle and quadriceps-setting exercise encouraged

   d. After removal of traction or other supporting apparatus

     (1) Bed-chair activities

     (2) Ambulation with partial weight bearing (determined by doctor); walker or three-point crutch gait

6. Fracture of the spine

   a. Transportation of patient with back injury—avoid flexion, hyperextension, or rotation of the vertebrae

   b. Immediate care

     (1) Observe for

       (a) Respiratory difficulty (if injury in cervical area); maintain patent airway, keep equipment available for tracheotomy, suctioning, and administration of oxygen

       (b) Level of consciousness and signs of confusion—intracranial involvement

       (c) Hyperthemia, cause may be of central origin

       (d) Bladder distention—catheterize (if ordered); save specimen

     (2) I.M. drugs, parenteral fluids, and/or blood as ordered

     (3) Equipment for doing spinal puncture

   c. Type of bed (as prescribed)

     (1) Firm mattress

       (a) Sponge rubber

       (b) Alternating-pressure pad

       (c) CircOlectric bed—(facilitates turning of the paralyzed patient)

       (d) Stryker or Foster bed

     (2) Equipment for head traction

     (3) Protective bed covering to facilitate changes of linen

   d. Care of patient without cord damage under skeletal traction

     (1) Maintain cervical vertebrae in position of extension or hyperextension as prescribed

     (2) Diet—may have difficulty in swallowing; maintain high fluid and protein intake

     (3) Observe for loss of motion or muscle strength and change in skin sensation

     (4) Encourage deep breathing

     (5) Give special skin care for sacrum, heels, back of head, and elbows

     (6) Maintain good body alignment and functional positions

     (7) Provide change of position and passive or active exercises of extremities as prescribed

     (8) Observe for distention (paralytic ileus); relief provided with drugs or suctioning with stomach tube

     (9) Prevent fecal impaction

   e. Care of patient with neck brace

     (1) Roentgenograms satisfactory, patient fitted with neck brace

     (2) Brace worn continuously

     (3) Elevate head rest and utilize tilt table, to minimize orthostatic hypotension

     (4) Walking with assistance

   f. Fracture of the spine, with paraplegia or quadriplegia

     (1) Skin care and types of bed described previously

     (2) Prevention of deformity

       (a) Correct body alignment with frequent and regular change of position

       (b) Maintain functional positions

      (c) Maintain normal range of joint motion (actively or passively)

    (3) Mobilization should begin as soon as danger to life past

      (a) Encourage and teach self-help and self-care (activities of daily living, ADL)

      (b) Exercises to strengthen shoulder, arm, and back muscles—aid in performing ADL and in crutch walking

      (c) Tilt table

      (d) Bracing—to facilitate ambulation

      (e) Ambulation in parallel bars—progress to crutches

    (4) High-protein diet; high fluid intake

    (5) Elimination (bowel)

      (a) Prevent fecal impactions

      (b) Bowel training program

    (6) Bladder

      (a) Program for development of automatic bladder (if prescribed)

      (b) Catheter care, sterile technique, closed catheter drainage

      (c) Prevention of urinary tract infection and calculi

      (d) Use of antibiotics as ordered

    (7) Active life—wheelchair or crutches—goal for all patients

    (8) Teach patient and family all aspects of care

    (9) Help patient and family to accept situation and plan for realistic goals

    (10) Vocational planning and training

D. Nursing the patient in a cast

  1. Purposes of casts

    a. Correction and prevention of deformity

    b. Maintenance of position

    c. Immobilization (soft tissue or bone)

    d. Plaster models for braces

  2. General principles

    a. Bed to receive soft cast should have firm mattress and rubber or plastic-covered pillows

    b. Fingers and toes must be watched for circulatory or nerve impairment

      (1) Blueness

      (2) Swelling

      (3) Pallor

      (4) Coldness

      (5) Pain

      (6) Numbness or loss of motion

      (7) When pressure applied over great toe or thumbnail, blood should return to part immediately on release of pressure (blanching sign)

    c. Dry cast by exposing it to air; will set in few hours; not dry thoroughly for about 48 hours; heat-cradle or sunlight will hasten process

    d. Turn patient carefully on day cast applied and allow posterior surface to dry; use heat-cradle if necessary; turn patient toward unaffected side

    e. Trim cast as marked; after cast dry, pull stockinet lining out over edges and secure with adhesive or plaster splint; if not lined, seal edges with adhesive; if body cast or spica type, protect around groin and buttocks with waterproof material

    f. Casts made waterproof with shellac, lacquer, etc.; use only after cast dry; narrow strips of waterproof material secured about perineum; use adhesive and/or plaster splints to secure outer edges to cast; tuck inner edges under cast

    g. Patients in cast should be turned at least two times a day or oftener; see that toes of leg in cast do not dig into mattress as patient lies prone; encourage patient to lie on abdomen several hours daily

    h. Circle any bleeding area with pencil and check for spreading

    i. Inspect cast daily for musty odor—may indicate pressure area under cast; note every complaint about pressure or burning sensation, particularly over heel, ankle bones, dorsum of foot (instep), and iliac bones

    j. Inspect skin around cast edges frequently for signs of excoriation

    k. When cast removed, provide adequate support for all joints that have been in cast

    l. Guard against mishaps after removal, since bone very fragile from long immobilization

m. Protect other parts of body from deformity; encourage bed activity
n. All patients wearing casts should have definite directions given them about time to return to hospital
o. Broken casts or those worn threadbare or softened from secretions need attention at once
p. Parents must be instructed in care of cast and about danger of circulatory impairment and pressure sores; must be told to return at once if these occur even though time for return visit scheduled for later date

E. Nursing the patient in traction
1. Purposes of traction
   a. To promote or maintain alignment
   b. To reduce muscle spasm
   c. To reduce fractures or dislocations
   d. To correct deformities
   e. To immobilize
2. Types of traction
   a. Skin—Buck's extension or traction with suspension (Russell traction, Thomas, Hodgen or Keller-Blake splint; balanced traction with Balkan frame, Braun-Bohler inclined plane splint, etc.)
   b. Skeletal (with Kirschner wire or Steinmann pin, Crutchfield tongs, etc.)
   c. Manual
3. Nursing care of patient in traction: general principles
   a. Comfort measures—mental and physical
      (1) Patient should understand purpose of traction
      (2) Back care must often be given by lifting patient—provide overhead trapeze so patient may assist himself
      (3) Provide diversional activity also to exercise muscles of arms and shoulders
      (4) Narrow firm pad under lumbar area will often assist in eliminating backache
      (5) Provide adequate covers for warmth of patient; traction ropes often interfere with normal placement of bed linen
   b. Inspection of apparatus—frequent
      (1) Countertraction must be present
      (2) Weights must hang free; knots must be secure (square); pulleys in good working order; see that bedclothes do not impinge on traction
      (3) Eliminate friction (if hips, heels, or elbows dig into mattress, friction occurs)
      (4) Bandages may need reinforcing; if tape loose, traction may need to be reapplied
      (5) If hammocks used under limb, protect skin from pressure and grooving by use of felt pad
      (6) Weights should not be lifted at any time without specific instruction
      (7) Bradford frame and vest restraint may be necessary for child in traction to maintain alignment
   c. Prevention of pressure sores
      (1) Inspect body daily for signs of pressure
         (a) Base of spine
         (b) Skin over tendon of Achilles, dorsum of foot, ankle bones, and entire length of tibia
         (c) Back of head, chin, ears, and jaw in head traction
         (d) Iliac crests and sacrum in pelvic traction
         (e) Groin and ischial region when ring splint used with traction
      (2) Maintain clean, dry, wrinkle-free bed
      (3) Massage bony areas
      (4) Secure even distribution of body weight and/or change of pressure points by use of
         (a) Alternating-pressure mattress
         (b) Stryker, Foster, or CircOlectric bed (as prescribed by physician)
         (c) Foam rubber, polyurethane, or sheep's wool
         (d) Trapeze; patient can shift body weight within limits
   d. Prevention of joint contractures and muscle atrophy
      (1) Active exercise of uninvolved extremities
         (a) Overhead trapeze so patient may assist himself

(b) Encourage self-care (bathing, personal hygiene, feeding)
(2) Active muscle "settings"—for involved limb (quadriceps and gluteals) as prescribed
  (a) Active plantar flexion and dorsiflexion of foot
  (b) Passive hip flexion and extension (raising and lowering bed)
(3) Functional positions of involved extremity
  (a) Maintain foot at right angle to tibia
  (b) Prevent external rotation of limb
  (c) Keep knee in relaxed position, no pressure on popliteal space
  (d) Prevent flexion contracture at hip joint
e. Maintenance of adequate elimination
  (1) Prevent impactions—bulk-producing diet and/or medication, fecal softener, or mild laxative
  (2) Prevent urinary tract infection and calculi—adequate fluid intake
f. Prevention of hypostatic pneumonia
  (1) Change of position (within limit allowed by traction)
  (2) Deep breathing exercises
F. Nursing the patient on a frame
  1. Purpose of frames
    a. Hyperextension
    b. Immobilization
    c. Correction of deformities
    d. Facilitation of turning
    e. Relief of pressure
  2. Types of frames
    a. Bradford
    b. Whitman (curved Bradford)
    c. Balkan (overhead bars used with traction)
    d. Stryker or Foster (reversible paired Bradford frames with specially constructed turning device)—allows for horizontal turning of patient
    e. CircOlectric bed
      (1) Allows for vertical turning of patient
      (2) Patient may be placed in various positions—Trendelenburg, standing, supine, prone

(3) One nurse can turn patient
(4) Electric motor provides power
(5) Attachments permit application of traction
3. General principles
  a. Size—width should measure distance between tips of shoulders; length—length of patient's body plus 6 inches
  b. Frame cover of heavy canvas; tighten canvas daily
  c. Provide foot support; foot exercises beneficial for frame patients
  d. Side-lying and sitting on frame not permitted; for change of position, patient should lie prone; twin frames such as Stryker frame or Foster bed useful for this purpose; patient strapped sandwichlike between frames and turned
  e. Turning done all in one piece; patient rolled without twisting spine, in loglike fashion
  f. Patient should not reach out to side for tray while eating; provide table that can cross over bed, or feed patient
  g. Patient's clothes should open down back; avoid disturbing spinal rest by lifting patient to put garments over head or under buttocks; provide support to prevent foot drop and external rotation of the legs
G. Crutch walking
  1. Selection of crutches
    a. Proper length: with patient lying supine, measure from anterior fold of axilla to point 6 inches out from heel
    b. Rubber crutch tips—intact, of good quality
    c. Axillary bar not padded unless requested by physician
    d. Handbar should allow almost complete extension of arm when patient places weight on palms
  2. Preparation for using crutches
    a. Patient should have period of dangling before standing attempted; also push-up exercises, and other types of bed exercise to strengthen wrist extensors, elbow extensors, and shoulder depressors
    b. Shoes should be firm and well fitting; avoid bedroom slippers and mules

c. Guard patient so that he is not afraid; see that obstructions eliminated—throw rugs, light cords, etc.

d. Patient must learn to balance on crutches before attempting to walk; see that posture good—chest high, body in full extension—particularly hips and knees

e. Patient must learn to bear body weight largely on hands and should not lean on crutches with axillae—tendency causes crutch paralysis

3. Type of crutch walking will depend on disability

a. Four-point gait—right crutch, left foot, left crutch, right foot; for patients who can manipulate both extremities—as in poliomyelitis, arthritis

b. Two-point gait—more rapid version of above—right crutch and left foot advanced together

c. Three-point gait—when one leg unable to bear full weight of body (amputation, fractured hip, etc.); patient stands on good leg—places both crutches equal distance in advance; swings himself forward slightly ahead of crutches, places weight again on sound leg, regains balance before advancing crutches for another step

d. Swinging-to, or swinging-through gait—with crutches placed ahead, patient raises body off floor and up to or through crutches; for paraplegia, and other severe involvement of lower limbs

e. Tripod—for patients who cannot lift body off floor; tripod position assumed, patient drags body up to crutches

4. Common mistakes in crutch walking

a. Tendency to use body in poor mechanical fashion

b. Hiking of hip with abduction gait (common in amputee)

c. Trying to lift crutches while still bearing down on them

d. Tendency to bear body weight under arms

e. Hunching of shoulders (crutches usually too long) or stooping with shoulders (crutches usually too short)

f. Walking on ball of foot with foot turned outward, flexion at hip or knee level

H. Braces and splints

1. Purpose

a. Prevent and correct deformity

b. Support body weight, assist weak muscles, and provide joint stability

c. Relieve pain

d. Prevent further injury

e. Control involuntary movement

f. Provide immobilization and rest

g. Provide for improvement of function

2. General principles

a. Brace can be kept in good condition with saddle soap or naphtha; joints should be oiled each week; excess oil should be wiped off and lint eliminated; straps, laces, and elastic should be replaced when frayed or worn

b. Patient should be taught purpose and care of brace, and parent instructed as to when brace may be removed

c. Skin examined daily for abrasions, evidence of pressure; metal of brace should not rub the skin

d. Shoes kept in good repair

(1) Low-heeled, walking shoe desirable

(2) Shoe that opens over the toes, if spasticity present

(3) High-top shoe to hold heel down in shoe

e. Check alignment of brace—knee joint at level of the femoral condyles; hip joint opposite greater trochanter

f. Desirable to have an extra brace

g. Recognize signs that patient outgrowing brace

h. If there are loose pieces attached to brace, such as knee pads, secure when brace removed so that they do not become lost

i. Know purpose of each pad and apply correctly

j. Leg braces

(1) Attachment to shoe—caliper (prongs fit into shoe heel), stirrup (brace fastened to shoe), or foot plate (fits inside shoe)

(2) Ankle joint "stops" control ankle motion

(3) T straps at ankle control pronation and supination

(4) Knee lock allows for flexion of knee

(5) Leg cuffs and knee pads used to prevent "buckling of knee" (weak quadriceps), genu recurvatum (weak hamstrings), and genu varum or valgum

(6) Long leg brace with pelvic band designed to control hip joint movements

k. Back braces should grasp pelvis and trochanters firmly

(1) See that upright bars in center of back

(2) Begin lacing from below

(3) Do not save time by lacing in alternate holes, as this does not give proper support

(4) Allow patient to sit up in back brace before leaving him, to see that no metal pieces are pressing into groin or axilla

I. Orthotic appliances—provide for motion or change of position and improvement of function (help in performance of activities of daily living and in ambulation); these devices utilize an "outside force" to replace a weakened or paralyzed muscle; this force is of either active or passive nature and may be supplied by various means such as an electrical motor, cylinder of carbon dioxide under pressure, or spring and cables that are attached to the appliance and body in a specific manner

3. Other considerations

A. Nursing the patient with arthritis—types of arthritis (arthritis means inflammation of the joint)

1. Osteoarthritis (degenerative, nonankylosing)

a. Symptoms

(1) Associated with aging process and the "wearing out" of articular cartilage; more common in middle age or old age

(2) Roughened cartilage causes trauma to synovium and joint capsule

(3) Muscle spasm and inflammation result in swelling and pain

(4) Weight-bearing joints more frequently involved

(5) Obesity increases joint stress

b. Treatment

(1) Relief of pain

(a) Drugs—salicylates usually adequate

(b) Rest of joint

(2) Physical therapy

(a) Maintain muscle strength (prevent contractures and maintain range of motion)

(b) Correct poor body mechanics (faulty weight bearing)

(c) Encourage activity (alternate with short rest periods)

(3) Use of cane or crutches—can relieve pain by decreasing amount of weight borne by joint

(4) Diet—limit in calories if patient overweight

(5) Maintain shoe corrections

(6) Provide reassurance; eliminate worry and other emotional disturbances

(7) Surgical procedures (usually arthroplasty) may be necessary when severe joint destruction, pain, or limitation of motion is present

2. Arthritis, rheumatoid (Still's disease, infectional form, polyarthritis, ankylosing, Marie-Strümpell)—involvement of back, sacroiliac joints, and shoulders

a. Cause unknown

(1) Theories of causes include emotional stress, hereditary tendency, virus, development of antibodies that attack body tissues

(2) Occurs in all age groups (most frequent in fourth decade)

(3) More frequent in women

b. Symptoms

(1) Inflammatory process of joint tissue

(2) Early morning stiffness

(3) General weakness, fatigue, loss of appetite and weight

(4) Deformity and loss of joint motion caused by the inflammatory process, synovial membrane changes, pain and muscle spasm

(5) Usually more than one joint involved

(6) May show inflammation of the eyes, nodules under the skin, and anemia

c. Diagnostic procedures (not specific for arthritis)
  (1) Latex agglutination
  (2) Erythrocyte sedimentation rate
  (3) X-ray films

d. Treatment—based on recognition that arthritis is a systemic disease
  (1) Adequate diet; avoid overweight condition
  (2) Improvement in posture and prevention of deformity; muscle spasm holds joint in position of greatest comfort (flexion and adduction); joints may ankylose in these positions if provision for relieving muscle spasm is not made; provide for functional positions, maintaining good body alignment with regular change of position
  (3) Heat—used to relax muscles, relieve pain and stiffness; given by means of electric pad, baths, hot packs, paraffin wax
  (4) Exercise—may include active, passive, resistance
    (a) Build and maintain muscle strength and range of joint motion (should be carefully prescribed)
    (b) Avoid fatigue and pain
  (5) Drug therapy
    (a) Salicylates (aspirin most commonly used)—relieve pain, tend to lessen joint inflammation
    (b) Phenylbutazone—relieves pain, stiffness; may have undesirable side effects
    (c) Indomethacin—anti-inflammatory drug
    (d) Hydroxychloroquine—antimalarial drug; periodic eye examinations necessary
    (e) Corticosteroids—decrease inflammation, pain, stiffness; patient may experience recurrence of pain as drug decreased or discontinued; toxic reactions may be severe
    (f) Hydrocortisone—injected directly into joint; used with varying degrees of success in controlling pain in specific joint, thus enabling patient to continue joint motion and prevent ankylosis
    (g) Gold salts—be familiar with toxic symptoms
  (6) Help patient understand condition, lessen worry and anxiety; prevent self-pity and apathy
  (7) Use of braces and splints
    (a) Give support, protect joint, and increase activity
    (b) Prevent contractures
  (8) Use of cane or crutches—protect weight-bearing joints
  (9) Properly fitted shoes essential
  (10) Encourage therapeutic and diversional crafts, particularly those that promote functional use of hands, arms, and legs
  (11) Surgical procedures (not necessary to wait till disease "burned out")
    (a) Prophylactic surgery—to prevent destruction of joint
    (b) Reconstructive surgery—to restore joint motion and correct deformities
    (c) Surgical procedures include synovectomy, arthroplasty, osteotomy, arthrodesis, and soft tissue procedures
  (12) Rehabilitation plans need to be encouraged and developed

3. Gouty arthritis
  a. Cause—disturbance in purine metabolism
  b. Occurs more frequently in men than in women
  c. Metatarsophalangeal joint of great toe usually affected first
  d. Urates deposited in periarticular structures
  e. Treatment
    (1) Drugs to increase output of urates (p. 246)
    (2) Diet low in purines
    (3) Increased fluid intake

B. Nursing the patient with scoliosis (lateral curvature of spine)
1. Types

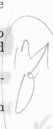

a. Functional or postural (usually left total curve) most frequently result of temporary postural influences; with treatment can be completely cured

b. Structural or rigid (S curve) caused by poliomyelitis, rickets, empyema, congenital defects; large group called idiopathic—cause unknown

2. Prophylactic treatment—earlier treatment is begun, greater is chance of complete recovery

3. Early symptoms
   a. Uneven height of shoulders
   b. Prominent hip
   c. Tendency to habitual poor posture
   d. Projecting shoulder blade
   e. Constant fatigue

4. Functional scoliosis
   a. Corrective exercises to strengthen muscles to maintain corrected position
   b. Good general hygiene .
      (1) Well-balanced diet (high in animal protein)
      (2) Rest
      (3) Fresh air
   c. Elimination of causes of faulty posture
      (1) Clothing that pulls unevenly on shoulders
      (2) Improper school furniture
      (3) Bad habits of carrying books
      (4) Long periods of reading in poor positions
      (5) Poor vision
      (6) Defective hearing
   d. Temporary supports such as corset *or* light body brace for more severe cases

5. Structural scoliosis
   a. Corrective plaster jackets or braces (Risser cast, Milwaukee brace) may be used to correct curvatures
   b. Spinal fusion, muscle transplants, or back brace may be used to maintain correction
   c. Continual medical supervision through entire period of growth to prevent further curvature

C. Nursing the patient with joint tuberculosis
   1. Prevention
      a. Pasteurization of milk
      b. Protection of children from contact with infected adults
      c. Early diagnosis, segregation, and treatment of known cases
      d. Improvement in housing conditions, nutrition, and general hygiene of low-income groups
   2. Treatment as systemic disease
      a. Building up resistive powers of patient
         (1) Rest—local and general
         (2) Adequate diet
         (3) Freedom from infection
      b. Local treatment to hasten recovery
         (1) Immobilization of affected joint (cast, frame, traction, or brace)
         (2) Surgical fusion of joint
      c. Observation for complications
         (1) Abscess formation
         (2) Cord compression
         (3) Tuberculous meningitis
         (4) Secondary focus of infection
         (5) Pulmonary involvement
         (6) Renal complications
      d. Drugs for bone and joint tuberculosis include streptomycin, isoniazid, and para-aminosalicylic acid
         (1) Most effective when given early in course of disease
         (2) Help to shorten convalescent period
         (3) Prevent secondary complications such as
            (a) Kidney involvement
            (b) Joint deformity
      e. Most common sites of skeletal tuberculosis—spine and hip (p. 342)

D. Nursing the patient with osteomyelitis
   1. Nonsurgical treatment
      a. Osteomyelitis may result from compound fractures or from bloodstream infection
      b. Immobilization of affected area—usually joint above and joint below site of infection
      c. Hot fomentations may be ordered; *Staphylococcus* organism most frequent cause of osteomyelitis; *Streptococcus* next most common
      d. Antibiotics will be ordered
      e. Intravenous therapy and blood transfusions
   2. Surgical treatment
      a. Incision and drainage followed by instillation of antibiotic and administration of antibiotics by oral, intramuscular, or intravenous route
      b. Handle joint with utmost gentle-

ness; support adjacent joints when moving extremity

  c. Prevent deformity of injured extremity; common sequelae of osteomyelitis
    (1) Drop foot
    (2) Flexion of hip and knee
  d. Provide diet high in protein and vitamins for tissue repair

E. Nursing the patient with poliomyelitis
1. Symptoms similar to those of acute infection, gastrointestinal disturbance, or respiratory infection (Chapter 11)
2. Cause—filtrable virus that attacks anterior horn cells of spinal cord (three strains)
3. Transmission; diagnosis; prevention (Chapter 11)
4. Nursing care in early stages of disease
  a. Isolation
  b. Careful observation for signs of respiratory difficulty or inability to swallow
  c. Hot packs to relieve spasm and tenderness
  d. Keeping body in good alignment as soon as muscle spasm relieved
  e. Range of motion exercises to prevent joint contractures
5. Convalescent care
  a. Continue with good body alignment, packs, functional positions, and range of motion
  b. Stretching exercises started early (within limits of pain)
  c. Tightness of muscles and tenderness should be overcome before ambulation is permitted
  d. Bracing may be necessary to prevent deformity, provide for greater activity, and prevent stretching of involved muscles
  e. Crutches are used when patient permitted up (lower limb involvement)
  f. Education as well as a continued intensive program of social, vocational, and physical rehabilitation should be carried on for involved patients to prevent lifelong dependency on others
6. Chronic stage (after 18 months)
  a. Reconstructive surgery to eliminate use of apparatus, prevent deformity, increase patient's activity
  b. Surgical procedures consist of tendon and muscle transplants, arthrodesis, osteotomy, epiphyseal arrest, tenotomy

F. Nursing the patient with an amputation
1. Orthopedic considerations
  a. Prevention of flexion contracture of hip and of knee
    (1) See that bed does not sag under hips
    (2) Eliminate pillow under stump as soon as danger of hemorrhage passed
    (3) Encourage patient to lie prone and to extend hip several times during day
    (4) When patient begins to walk, note particularly that he does not keep the hip in slight flexion; teach him to avoid hiking of shoulder and abduction of artificial leg
  b. Provide support and exercise for remaining leg—to maintain muscle strength
  c. Teach patient to avoid too constant dependence on crutches
  d. Beware of psychological factors; promote healthy attitude toward disability
  e. Assume responsibility as member of health team working toward rehabilitation of amputee
  f. Teach care of stump
    (1) Compression bandage may be used to prepare the stump for prosthesis
    (2) For thigh amputation, several cotton elastic bandages will be necessary; 2 sets needed so can be washed between applications
    (3) Apply bandages snugly, compressing the end of the stump into smooth, rather conical shape
    (4) For thigh amputation use spica type bandage
    (5) When patient begins to wear prosthesis, will need several all-wool stump socks
      (a) Must be kept in good condition by frequent washing
        (1) Warm soft water
        (2) Mild soap
        (3) Thorough rinsing

(b) Patient should be discouraged from wearing several stump socks at one time to make prosthesis fit better

(c) Limbmaker (orthotist) should be consulted for adjustment of apparatus

(6) Toughening of stump and preparation for wearing prosthesis should be taught by physical therapist if at all possible

(7) Instruct patient to report to physician any skin irritation or other abnormality that occurs in stump

G. Nursing the patient with tumor of the bone

1. Benign tumor
   a. Osteocartilaginous exostosis, enchondroma, chondroblastoma, osteoid osteoma, giant cell tumor
   b. Usually grow slowly, do not destroy surrounding tissue, and do not spread to other parts of body
   c. Diagnosis made by roentgenogram and surgical biopsy
   d. Treatment usually consists of surgical removal
   e. Nursing care consists of routine postoperative care of patient with soft dressing or plaster cast
   f. Prognosis good

2. Malignant tumor
   a. Osteosarcoma, fibrosarcoma, chondrosarcoma, Ewing's sarcoma, multiple myeloma
   b. Usually rapid in growth, spread to other parts of body through bloodstream
   c. Diagnosis made from history, roentgenograms, and surgical biopsy (laboratory findings helpful in some types)
   d. Patient usually complains of intermittent pain, worse at night, limp, tiredness, and swelling
   e. Treatment
      (1) Surgical removal—wide local resection or amputation
      (2) X-ray or radioactive cobalt irradiation
      (3) Chemotherapy
   f. Nursing care includes
      (1) Care of patient with amputation or other surgical procedure

(2) Care of patient receiving radiation therapy (p. 331)
   (a) Help patient understand treatment and what to expect
   (b) Importance of not missing treatment (outpatient)
   (c) Care of involved skin area
   (d) Medication to relieve nausea helpful
   (e) Routine and frequent blood counts

(3) Care of patient receiving chemotherapy
   (a) Knowledge of drugs, method of administration, and the equipment used
   (b) Observations—toxic reactions or other side effects

(4) Provision for diet high in calories, protein, and vitamins

(5) Protection of patient from respiratory tract infections

(6) Awareness of possibility of metastasis to lungs—chest pain, coughing, expectoration of blood

(7) Promoting optimistic and hopeful attitude toward condition and providing comfort measures and support for the patient and family

3. Metastatic lesions from other tissues or organs
   a. Metastasize most commonly from breast, prostate, lung, kidney, thyroid, cervix
   b. Bone marrow has rich blood supply, and cancer cells spread easily through bloodstream
   c. Sites commonly involved—pelvis, vertebrae, femur, skull, ribs, and humerus
   d. Treatment usually consists of surgical biopsy and irradiation

NURSING PATIENTS WITH COMMUNICABLE DISEASES

1. Definitions

carrier A person who harbors within his body the organisms of a specific disease and, although asymptomatic, transmits the disease to other persons

communicable disease A disease caused by an infectious agent that can be transmitted from one person to another through either direct or indirect contact

contact A person who has been in close proximity to a person with a communicable disease

droplet nuclei Minute, dried droplets that remain suspended in the air

endemic Disease is continuously present in a community, but in a small number of cases

epidemic Disease is present, with a large number of cases in the community at the same time and with a tendency to spread rapidly

immunity Ability of the host, the body, to resist the infectious agent

pandemic Disease is widespread throughout the world

nosocomial Disease occurring within a hospital

surveillance Keeping under continuous observation

vector Animal or insect that carries a disease from person to person

virulence Ability of infectious agent to overcome defenses of the body

zoonosis Disease of animals that may be transmitted to humans

2. Principles of communicable disease control

A. What the nurse should know
   1. Nature of the organism and its capacity for survival within and outside of the body
   2. Most effective methods for its destruction
   3. Route of invasion and escape from the body
   4. Incubation period, prodromata, period of communicability
   5. Current methods of prophylaxis and duration of their effectiveness
   6. Fundamental basis for control measures
   7. How to protect herself and others
   8. Clean versus contaminated areas

B. Abilities needed include competence to
   1. Establish effective isolation
   2. Be alert to conditions contributory to nosocomial infection
   3. Provide skilled physical, psychological, and rehabilitative nursing care

C. Isolation—separation from others for period of infectiousness
   1. Order for, duration, and termination of the responsibility of physician
      a. Varies with specific disease—strict or modified
      b. May be affected by chemotherapeutic therapy
      c. Bacteriologic release required in some diseases
   2. Patient and family must understand need for isolation
   3. May be private room, ward, cubicle, intensive care unit
      a. Special hospitals being discontinued

   4. Reverse isolation—keeping all environmental pathogenic organisms from patient

D. Medical asepsis
   1. Gown—purpose to protect uniform
      a. Completely cover uniform and lap 12 inches in back
      b. To be worn by all who enter unit
      c. Clean gown for each contact with patient
      d. Overalls, hooded mask, goggles, gloves in pneumonic plague
   2. Mask—according to hospital policies
      a. Change every hour
      b. Discard same as gown
   3. Handwashing—to prevent transfer of organisms
      a. After each contact with patient or contaminated article
      b. Use warm water, liquid soap, bar soap in drainable dish
      c. Thorough drying with paper towels or warm air blower
   4. Concurrent disinfection—the immediate destruction of infectious organisms after escape from body (p. 304)
   5. Terminal disinfection—depends on adequacy of concurrent disinfection, specific disease, and hospital policy; routine cleaning usually all that is necessary

E. Common diseases controlled by immunization
   1. Bacterial diseases
      a. Diphtheria
      b. Pertussis
      c. Tetanus
      d. Typhoid fever
   2. Viral diseases
      a. Measles
      b. Mumps
      c. Poliomyelitis
      d. Smallpox

F. Diseases for which immunization is available
   1. Limited to high-risk groups
      a. Anthrax
      b. Cholera
      c. Rabies (Chapter 11)
      d. Rocky Mountain spotted fever
      e. Tuberculosis (p. 341)
      f. Typhus fever, louse-borne
      g. Yellow fever

G. Disease partially controlled by immunization
   1. Influenza—advised for high-risk groups

H. Diseases for which there is no immunization
   1. Control of socioeconomic factors important
      a. Deep mycoses
      b. Encephalitis
      c. Hepatitis
      d. Parasitic infections
      e. Pneumonia
      f. Venereal diseases
I. Immunization for foreign travel
   1. May vary with prevalence of disease in each country
   2. May affect travel into or out of country
   3. Specific immunizations
      a. Smallpox required by most countries, but not everywhere in United States
   4. Requirements may include
      a. Cholera
      b. Typhus
      c. Yellow fever
      d. Immune serum globulin for hepatitis
      e. Duck embryo vaccine for preexposure immunization to rabies
   5. Other immunizations that may be advised by U. S. Public Health Service
      a. Diphtheria
      b. Influenza
      c. Plague
      d. Measles
      e. Malaria-suppressive medications
3. **Communicable diseases caused by bacteria**
A. Anthrax—primarily a disease of animals transmitted to humans; an occupational disease; in 1972, 2 cases in the United States
   1. Etiology—*Bacillus anthracis*
   2. Forms of disease
      a. Cutaneous
      b. Inhalation type, rare
      c. Gastrointestinal type, rare
   3. Transmission—handling contaminated animal hair, hides, wool, and animal tissue; inhalation of spores; ingestion of meat contaminated by organism
   4. Incubation period—2 to 7 days
   5. Symptoms
      a. Cutaneous form—macule and vesiculation; vesicle ruptures leaving necrotic lesion, healing by granulation; lymph node tenderness, fever, leukocytosis

      b. Pulmonary form—pulmonary edema, hemorrhage, pneumonia, death
      c. Intestinal form—lesions in ileum and cecum, hemorrhage
   6. Diagnosis—stained smears of material from beneath unopened vesicle
   7. Treatment—procaine penicillin G 300,000 units
   8. Nursing measures—isolation, strict medical asepsis, bacteriologic release; because of spores, autoclaving of nondisposable equipment and linens
   9. Prevention—anthrax vaccine for high-risk persons; prevention of disease in animals, epidemiologic investigation of cases, international control of some animal products
B. Cholera (Asiatic)—rare in the United States, endemic in many countries, incidence increasing
   1. Etiology—*Vibrio cholerae (Vibrio comma)*; El Tor strain causes paracholera
   2. Transmission—anal-oral route; vehicles for transmission: contaminated water, milk, fruit, vegetables; convalescent carriers and asymptomatic persons
   3. Incubation period—24 hours to 5 days
   4. Symptoms—abrupt onset, profuse vomiting and diarrhea, dehydration, cramping of extremities, hypotension, subnormal temperature, cold clammy skin, oliguria, collapse
   5. Diagnosis—bacteriologic examination of stools
   6. Treatment—no specific therapy; intravenous isotonic saline solution, chemotherapeutic drugs
   7. Nursing—isolation, strict medical asepsis, gown and gloves, only the essential nursing procedures
   8. Prevention—WHO requires reporting, examination and immunization of contacts, quarantine of contacts for 5 days, clothing of patient autoclaved or disinfected
C. Leprosy (Hansen's disease)—rare in the United States; 122 cases in 1972
   1. Etiology—*Mycobacterium leprae* (Hansen's bacillus)
   2. Forms of disease
      a. Lepromatous—most infectious
      b. Tuberculoid
   3. Transmission—method unknown, believed to be direct or indirect contact

with lesions; socioeconomic factors and social customs believed important

4. Incubation period—variable, 5½ months to 8 years
5. Symptoms—early symptoms unrecognized
   a. Lepromatous type—thickening of skin with granulomatous condition, anesthesia and gradual destruction of peripheral nerves, atrophy of skin and muscles, absorption of small bones, ulceration of mucous membranes, negative lepromin skin test
   b. Tuberculoid form—skin test positive, elevated macules, anesthesia of skin, peripheral nerve involvement more rapid
6. Diagnosis—difficult; serologic test, biopsy of lesions, smears from lesions
7. Treatment—sulfone therapy that must be continued for life; physical therapy, occupational therapy, rehabilitation
8. Nursing—isolation in general hospital; no danger to nurse
9. Prevention—no specific measures

D. Meningitis (meningococcic)—about 1,329 cases (including influenzal and pneumococcal types) in the United States in 1972
1. Etiology—*Neisseria meningitidis* (meningococcus)
   a. Serologic groups
      (1) Group A causes most epidemics
      (2) Groups B and C cause sporadic cases
      (3) Group D rare in the United States
2. Transmission—respiratory tract, by direct and indirect contact with droplet infection or droplet nuclei; person-to-person contact usually necessary; carriers unconfirmed
3. Incubation period—estimated 2 to 10 days
4. Symptoms—onset variable; headache, nausea, vomiting, resistance in posterior neck, opisthotonos, spasms may occur, reflexes exaggerated, fever 100° to 103° F., pulse rapid, respiration irregular, positive Kernig and Brudzinski signs, petechiae, convulsions in infants
5. Complications—acute bacteremia, meningococcemia (Waterhouse-Friderichsen syndrome), congestive heart failure, pneumonia

6. Diagnosis—laboratory examination of blood, spinal fluid, nasopharyngeal material
7. Treatment—chemotherapy: tetracyclines, penicillin, sulfisoxazole, sulfadiazine, sulfadimetine, antipyretics, parenteral fluids
8. Nursing—isolation and medical asepsis; isolation may be terminated after 24 hours of chemotherapy; take temperature, pulse, respiration every 2 hours during acute period, administer parenteral fluids carefully, keep intake-output records, observe for intracranial pressure, urinary retention or incontinence
9. Prevention—no immunization, chemoprophylaxis during epidemics and in institutions

E. Shigellosis (bacillary dysentery)—incidence increasing
1. Etiology—*Shigella dysenteriae, Shigella flexneri, Shigella boydii, Shigella sonnei*
2. Transmission—anal-oral route, contaminated food and water, improper disposal of excreta, unhygienic habits, food handling by infected persons, carriers possible
3. Incubation period—variable, 1 to 7 days
4. Symptoms—acute onset: abdominal pain, diarrhea, griping, mucus and blood in stools, tenesmus, fever 100° to 103° F., leukocytosis, vomiting, headache, prostration
5. Diagnosis—clinical signs, bacteriologic examination of stools; serologic tests of doubtful value
6. Treatment—disease self-limiting; sulfonamides, antibiotics, camphorated tincture of opium, electrolyte replacement, low-residue diet, no milk and cream
7. Nursing—isolation, medical asepsis, care for as in typhoid fever; bacteriologic release from isolation, 2 negative stool cultures
8. Prevention—pasteurization of milk, safe water, screening homes, washing fruits and vegetables, personal hygiene, proper disposal of excreta

F. Tetanus—about 118 cases in 1972 in the United States; endemic worldwide
1. Etiology—*Clostridium tetani* (tetanus bacillus) organism produces lethal toxin, causing toxemia

2. Transmission—spore-forming organism widely distributed in soil; enters tissue through wound; in tetanus neonatorum, organism enters through unhealed umbilicus; other pathways—contaminated syringes and needles used by drug addicts, burns, and criminal abortions

3. Incubation period—variable, from few days to several weeks

4. Symptoms—restlessness, irritability, stiffness of jaw, neck, and extremities, pain and tingling at site of wound, opisthotonos, fever 101° to 104° F., diaphoresis, risus sardonicus due to spasm of facial muscles; severe muscle spasms precipitated by
   a. Exteroceptive stimuli—noise, bright lights
   b. Proprioceptive stimuli—moving or turning patient
   c. Interoceptive stimuli—flatus, bladder distention

5. Diagnosis—clinical signs and history of injury

6. Treatment—not uniform, based on
   a. Neutralization of toxin in circulation; tetanus antitoxin or homologous (human) serum antitoxin; sensitivity tests prior to giving horse serum
   b. Destruction of *Clostridium tetani* spores; long-acting penicillin or tetracycline
   c. Supportive therapy, sedation with thiopental sodium, tribromoethanol by rectum, methocarbamol, chlorpromazine, and others; attention to fluid and electrolyte balance, nutritional needs

7. Nursing—care of tracheotomy, retention catheter in urinary bladder, automatic cycling respirator, nasogastric feedings; close monitoring of vital signs; observation for rise in temperature, cyanosis, convulsions, twitching of muscles

8. Prevention—immunization with tetanus toxoid (DPT) for infants beginning at second month of age, 3 injections at 4- to 6-week intervals with booster doses; for adults, 2 injections of tetanus toxoid, with reinforcing dose in case of injury if more than 1 year since series; for adults with no prior immunization, human tetanus immune globulin or homologous human serum antitoxin

G. Tularemia—about 142 cases in the United States in 1972; sporadic cases in many countries; primary source is rabbit
   1. Etiology—*Pasteurella tularensis*
   2. Forms of infection
      a. Cutaneous ulceroglandular form
      b. Septicemic form
      c. Typhoidal—from ingestion of infected rabbit meat
      d. Pneumonic form—secondary to disease, or by inhalation of the organism
   3. Transmission—mechanical inoculation through skin by bite of infected vector, handling infected animal, eating infected rabbit meat, drinking contaminated water; laboratory workers at risk
   4. Incubation period—1 to 10 days
   5. Symptoms—headache, fever 102° to 104° F., vomiting, aching, diaphoresis, chills, prostration, regional lymph nodes tender with bubo formation, papular lesion at site of inoculation, which breaks down with ulceration and necrosis
      a. Typhoidal form—necrotic ulcers in gastrointestinal tract, hemorrhage, abscesses in mouth and pharynx, toxemia; disease serious
      b. Pneumonic form may resemble tuberculosis
   6. Diagnosis—history, clinical signs, serologic tests; fluorescent antibody technique used to identify organism; sputum examination and gastric washings
      a. Tests that aid in diagnosis
         (1) Polysaccharide antigen test
         (2) *Pasteurella tularensis* antibody test
         (3) Protein antigen test
   7. Treatment—streptomycin, chloramphenicol, tetracycline
   8. Nursing—concurrent disinfection if suppurating lesions; other care as for febrile patient
   9. Prevention—use of rubber gloves when handling wild rabbits, avoiding bites from vectors, thorough cooking of rabbit meat, interstate control of rabbits for food, no drinking from streams in infected areas; antitularemia vaccine with live strains of organism available; aerogenic tularemia

vaccine to be used by inhalation recently developed

H. Typhoid fever—about 377 cases in the United States in 1972; worldwide distribution

1. Etiology—*Salmonella typhi*
2. Transmission—anal-oral route, ingestion of contaminated water, milk, food products; most cases result from carriers
3. Incubation period—10 to 14 days
4. Symptoms—headache, anorexia, malaise, joint pains, abdominal discomfort, vomiting, cough with bronchitis, gradual rise in temperature to 104° F., pulse rate slow, splenomegaly, leukopenia, rash (rose spots) on abdomen and chest, lymphoid follicles (Peyer's patches) in lower ileum; hemorrhage or perforation of intestine possible; mental confusion and delirium may occur
5. Diagnosis—stool and urine cultures, blood cultures positive first week, agglutination tests; accurate diagnosis depends upon isolation of *Salmonella typhi*
6. Treatment—chloramphenicol, mild sedation, fluid and electrolytes
7. Nursing—isolate, with release based on bacteriologic examination of stools; strict medical asepsis, skin care important, tepid or alcohol sponges, no antipyretic drugs; use care in administering parenteral solutions, feed patient, do not allow to sit up; guard against abdominal distention, observe stools for blood, observe for retention of urine; report immediately chills, increase in pulse rate, abdominal pain, or chest pain
8. Prevention—epidemiologic investigation of all cases; control of water supply, excreta disposal, pasteurization of milk; control of typhoid carriers; immunization of contacts and persons traveling abroad; typhoid vaccine weekly for 3 weeks, 1 ml. injected; reinforcing dose at 1- to 2-year intervals if traveling abroad

4. **Diseases caused by viruses**

A. Infectious mononucleosis (glandular fever)

1. Etiology—unknown; believed to be of viral origin
2. Transmission—unknown; believed to be direct contact with salivary secretions
3. Incubation period—present evidence indicates 33 to 49 days for adults, less than 14 days for children
4. Symptoms
   a. Fever 100° to 102° F.
   b. Sore throat
   c. Enlarged cervical, inguinal, and axillary lymph nodes
   d. Splenomegaly
   e. Jaundice in about 10% of cases
5. Diagnosis—no specific tests; leukocyte count, heterophil agglutination antibody test, liver function, and SGOT tests
6. Treatment—no specific therapy; treatment symptomatic and supportive
7. Complications—rare
8. Nursing—no special care; care as in febrile illness
9. Prevention—none; isolation unnecessary

B. Influenza—occurs in sporadic cases, epidemics, and pandemics; worldwide distribution

1. Etiology—viruses A, A prime, A-2, C, A2/Hong Kong/68, A/England/42/72; most prevalent virus throughout the world in 1972
   a. Widespread epidemics by all except C
2. Transmission—respiratory route; evidence suggests direct contact; spreads rapidly in crowds
3. Incubation period—24 to 48 hours
4. Symptoms—onset sudden
   a. Headache
   b. Malaise
   c. Aching
   d. Chilliness or chills
   e. Fever 101° to 104° F.
   f. Cough and laryngitis
5. Complications—primarily among high-risk groups: infants, elderly persons with chronic disease, and pregnant women
   a. Staphylococcal or pneumococcal pneumonia
   b. Bronchitis
6. Diagnosis—clinical signs or on isolation of the virus by laboratory techniques
7. Treatment—no specific therapy; bed rest, hydration, sedative cough mixture, analgesics

8. Nursing—same as in febrile illness; protect from bacterial infection, observe for increase in pulse and respiration rates, cyanosis, character of sputum; good nursing may prevent complications

9. Prevention—immunization with 1 ml. of chicken cell agglutination vaccine I.M. for high-risk groups and hospital personnel; immunize early in fall before influenza season

C. Psittacosis (ornithosis)—worldwide, as sporadic cases; 35 cases were reported in 1972 in the United States

1. Etiology—a viral disease of birds transmitted to humans; virus may be atypical

2. Transmission—inhalation of virus; handling or bites of infected birds; man-to-man transfer possible

3. Incubation period—5 to 28 days; usually 10 days

4. Symptoms—sudden onset
   a. Headache, malaise, aching back, anorexia, sore throat, chills, fever 100° to 105° F., cough that may be productive, slow pulse rate; may be nausea and vomiting, epistaxis, abdominal distention, skin rash; symptoms vary
   b. If fatal, cyanosis, hypotension, and circulatory collapse occur

5. Diagnosis—clinical signs, history of contact with birds; chest x-ray film, isolation of virus, complement-fixation tests; inoculation of mice with specimens of blood, sputum, vomitus, or throat washings

6. Treatment—tetracycline, Achromycin or Declomycin; oxygen in cyanosis, vasopressor drugs for hypotension; steroids have been used

7. Nursing—isolation with medical asepsis; wear well-fitting mask; give care as in febrile illness; recovery slow, extreme fatigue

8. Prevention—control of disease in birds; international regulations for importing birds, quarantine of pet shops when disease occurs; no immunizing agent available

D. Rocky Mountain spotted fever (tick fever—52.2 cases in the United States in 1972

1. Etiology—*Rickettsia rickettsii*

2. Transmission—the bite of any of several species of ticks that may be infected

3. Incubation period—3 to 10 days

4. Symptoms
   a. Mild or severe: malaise, headache, anorexia, fever 103° to 104° F., chills, aching, joint and muscle pain, nausea, vomiting, maculopapular skin rash
   b. If severe, weak rapid pulse rate, hypotension, increased respiration, photophobia, oliguria, azotemia, nonproductive cough, neurologic symptoms with delirium, convulsions, coma

5. Diagnosis—history of tick bite, complement-fixation test, positive Weil-Felix reaction

6. Treatment—antibiotic therapy: chloramphenicol, chlortetracycline, oxytetracycline; parenteral fluids

7. Nursing—no isolation; inspection of body for ticks; patient very sick and to have care as for febrile illness; parenteral fluids must drip very slowly; high-protein diet; observation for anuria, convulsion; continuous care necessary

8. Prevention—avoid tick-infested areas, use protective clothing, persons at risk may be immunized with *Rickettsia rickettsii* vaccine, 3 injections of 1 ml. at 7- to 10-day intervals

E. Typhus fever—endemic in many parts of world, sporadic cases in the United States

1. Etiology—caused by a *Rickettsia*
   a. Epidemic typhus—*Rickettsia prowazeki*
   b. Brill-Zinsser disease—*Rickettsia prowazeki*
   c. Murine typhus—*Rickettsia mooseri*

2. Transmission
   a. Epidemic typhus transmitted by vector *Pediculus humanus corporis* (human body louse)
   b. Brill-Zinsser disease—history of prior epidemic typhus; louse infestation absent
   c. Murine typhus—transmitted by vector *Xenopsylla cheopis* (rat flea)

3. Incubation period—10 to 14 days

4. Symptoms—abrupt onset; malaise, headache, chills, aching, fever 104° to 106° F., pulse and respiration rapid, hypotension, nonproductive cough, maculopapular skin rash turning from pink to reddish purple; neurologic

symptoms—stupor, delirium, coma; symptoms same for all forms

5. Diagnosis—clinical diagnosis difficult; laboratory serologic tests, blood cultures, and Weil-Felix reaction; new bedside test with results in few minutes

6. Treatment—antibiotic therapy: chlortetracycline, chloramphenicol, oxytetracycline; paraldehyde and chloral hydrate for sedation, analgesics; oxygen for cyanosis; electrolyte balance to be maintained

7. Complications — bronchopneumonia, otitis media, furunculosis, necrotic skin lesions with gangrene of toes, fingers, earlobes, nose; cardiovascular and renal complications

8. Nursing—wear surgical gown and gloves while delousing patient, bathe patient with 1% Lysol solution, dust with 10% DDT; dust bed every week while patient hospitalized; no isolation after delousing; other care as in Rocky Mountain spotted fever

9. Prevention—immunization of contacts with Cox-type vaccine; 2 injections of 1 ml. at 10- to 14-day intervals; booster may be required; quarantine contacts 15 days, delouse, and dust garments with DDT; not required in murine typhus; control of fleas difficult; rodent eradication best

F. Yellow fever—endemic in some countries; southeastern United States a receptive area
1. Etiology—filtrable virus of arbovirus group
2. Forms
   a. Classic yellow fever
   b. Sylvatic (jungle) yellow fever
3. Transmission
   a. Classic yellow fever—bite of infected vector Aedes aegypti, semidomestic mosquito
   b. Sylvatic form, bite of infected mosquito, any of several genera
   c. Inhalation of aerosols containing virus in laboratory
   d. Aedes aegypti widely distributed in parts of southeastern United States
4. Incubation period—3 to 6 days
5. Symptoms—abrupt onset; fever 104° F., pulse slow, headache, aching, nausea, vomiting, dizziness, prostration, jaundice with hemorrhage, urine scan-

ty, hypotension, weak pulse, collapse, neurologic delirium, restlessness, death

6. Diagnosis—laboratory isolation of virus from blood early in disease, serologic tests for antibody, examination of liver tissue on necropsy

7. Treatment—none; therapy symptomatic; analgesics, blood transfusion, fluid and electrolytes

8. Nursing—no isolation or medical asepsis; continuous care same as other febrile illness; careful determination of blood loss

9. Prevention—destruction of breeding places and vector; immunization with 1 injection of 0.5 ml. of 17D yellow fever virus vaccine; the United States requires immunization of international travelers whose destination is yellow fever–receptive areas of the United States, if they come from areas where endemic yellow fever exists

5. Infections caused by helminths
A serious problem in many parts of world
A. Partial classification
   1. Flatworms
      a. Flukes
      b. Tapeworms
   2. Roundworms
      a. Ascaris
      b. Hookworm
      c. Pinworm
      d. Trichinella
B. Etiology—metazoa of the animal kingdom
C. Transmission—varies with specific parasite
   1. Ingestion of infected uncooked plants or inadequately cooked or raw beef, pork, and fish
   2. Inoculation through skin by wading in contaminated water or contact with contaminated soil
   3. Anal-oral transmission of eggs
   4. Possible inhalation of eggs of pinworm
D. Incubation period—depends on maturation of adult worm in body; may be several months
E. Symptoms variable—depend on specific parasite; may include diarrhea, dysentery, nausea, vomiting, pulmonary lesions, cough, hemoptysis, abdominal discomfort, ascites, anorexia, splenomegaly, fever, headache, anemia, urinary tract

disease, allergic manifestations, increased eosinophils
F. Diagnosis—microscopic examination of feces and sputum; observation of worms in stools; precipitin tests, complement-fixation test, recently fluorescent antibody test for trichinosis
G. Treatment—varies with specific parasite; many drugs in current use (Chapter 7)
H. Prevention
   1. Public education
   2. Improved sanitary disposal of excreta
   3. Control of pollution of streams and lakes
   4. Thorough cooking of beef, pork, and fish
   5. Interstate control of infected animals
   6. Teaching principles of personal hygiene
6. **Infections caused by fungi**
   More than 50 species may cause disease in man
A. Systemic mycoses
   1. Etiology—saprophytes or parasites found in decaying organic matter, especially in soil and dust enriched by animal and bird fecal matter
   2. Most common forms
      a. Blastomycosis
      b. Candidiasis—also superficial infections
      c. Coccidioidomycosis (valley fever)
      d. Cryptococcosis
      e. Histoplasmosis
   3. Transmission—inhalation of spores from saprophytes growing in soil; transmission from person to person not confirmed
B. Superficial mycoses
   1. Etiology—specific species of dermatophytes
   2. Common forms
      a. Dermatophytosis (athlete's foot)
      b. Tinea (ringworm) of skin, beard, scalp
   3. Candidiasis
      a. Cutaneous
      b. Vulvovaginal
      c. Oral, thrush
   4. Transmission—direct and indirect contact; long-continued therapy with broad-spectrum antibiotics
   5. Diagnosis—direct microscopic examination of infected skin and culture of offending organism
   6. Treatment

   a. Systemic mycoses—amphotericin B (Fungizone), sulfonamides, 2-hydroxystilbamidine, X5079C
   b. Superficial mycoses—griseofulvin; benzoic and salicylic acid ointment (Whitfield's ointment)
   7. Nursing in systemic mycoses
      a. Understanding of both disease and patient
      b. Knowledge of the drug therapy, its toxicity
      c. Some patients isolated
      d. Emotional support of patient very important
      e. Not believed transferred from person to person
   8. Nursing in superficial mycoses
      a. Ringworm of scalp causes exclusion from school
      b. Good foot care should be taught
      c. Clothing and bedding should be boiled
      d. Disinfection of shoes, showers, tubs, etc.
      e. Toxic manifestations from drogs to be observed
7. **Agencies contributing to communicable disease control**
A. International
   1. World Health Organization
      a. Expert Committees
   2. United Nations International Children's Emergency Fund
   3. Pan-American Sanitary Bureau
   4. National Malaria Eradication Service
   5. Pan-American Health Organization
   6. South Pacific Commission
   7. Agency for International Development
B. United States—governmental
   1. Department of Health, Education and Welfare
      a. Bureau of States Services
      b. National Institutes of Health
      c. Center for Disease Control
      d. Bureau of Medical Services
      e. International Research Act of 1960
      f. National Library of Medicine
   2. Department of Agriculture
C. State—official
   1. State Department of Public Health
      a. May be divided into specific areas—tuberculosis, venereal disease, etc.
      b. Environmental sanitation
      c. Food sanitation
      d. Public health education
      e. Laboratory services

f. Vital and health statistics
2. State Department of Agriculture
   a. Control of animal diseases
   b. Some aspects of food inspection
   c. Public education
D. Local—official
   1. City Public Health Department
   2. City-County Health Department
      a. Activities coincide with those of State Department of Public Health
E. Agencies—voluntary
   1. American Red Cross
   2. National Foundation–March of Dimes
   3. National Tuberculosis Association
   4. American Social Health Association
F. Private foundations
   1. W. K. Kellogg Foundation
   2. Rockefeller Foundation
G. Many other local, state, and national agencies and foundations

EMERGENCY NURSING

1. Basic principles of nursing
A. Prevention best; teaching public accident prevention essential responsibility of professional nurse
B. Awareness of own psychological defenses in order to cope with and to control own anxieties in an emergency situation
C. Prevention of further injury by improper first aid care important aspect of emergency nursing
D. Medical aid should be obtained as soon as possible
E. Professional people should be prepared for intelligent action in emergency situations
2. Nursing patient in emergencies
A. Maintain respiration
B. Control bleeding
C. Prevent and treat shock
D. Protect wound with sterile dressing or as clean a dressing as possible
E. Keep injured person lying down and covered
F. Allay anxiety, and keep patient as comfortable as possible
G. Effort should be made to determine extent of injury or cause of emergency condition
H. Observe and reevaluate the patient at frequent intervals
I. With motor vehicle accident victims, always remember possibility of a "whiplash" injury to spinal cord
3. Specific emergency conditions

A. Accident patient—accidents first cause of death for young people from 1 to 24 years of age, second cause for those 25 to 44 years of age
B. Food poisoning
   1. Acute gastroenteritis due to food infected with certain bacteria or *Staphylococcus* toxin
      a. Symptoms
         (1) Short incubation period
         (2) Headache
         (3) Nausea
         (4) Vomiting
         (5) Abdominal cramps
         (6) Diarrhea
         (7) Occasionally muscle aches
         (8) Fever
         (9) Prostration
      b. Treatment and nursing care
         (1) Rest in bed
         (2) Nothing by mouth while nauseated
         (3) Intravenous fluids to prevent dehydration
         (4) Later, warm bland fluids and foods may be given
      c. Condition may be prevented by sanitary habits and taking proper care of foods in warm weather; canned meat, salads, and pastries common agents for these bacteria
   2. Botulism—acute intoxication manifested by neuromuscular disturbances, after ingestion of food containing toxin elaborated by *Clostridium botulinum*
      a. Symptoms
         (1) Incubation period of 1 to 3 days
         (2) Lassitude
         (3) Fatigue
         (4) Visual disturbances
         (5) In severe cases, difficulty in swallowing, difficulty in talking, and muscle incoordination
         (6) About 65% of cases fatal
      b. Treatment and nursing care
         (1) Keeping patient quiet in darkened room
         (2) Prevention of aspiration and choking
         (3) Administration of polyvalent antiserum
         (4) Maintenance of nutrition and electrolyte balance
      c. Prevention

(1) Use of pressure-cooking method of home canning
(2) Cooking food for 10 to 15 minutes makes it safe for consumption
3. Mushrooms—poisonous type most common cause of death from poisoning by food
  a. Symptoms
    (1) Severe abdominal pain
    (2) Nausea
    (3) Vomiting
    (4) Diarrhea
    (5) Prostration
  b. Treatment
    (1) Prevention—eat only those grown under cultivation
    (2) Give fluids
    (3) Induce vomiting
    (4) Keep patient warm
    (5) Notify doctor
    (6) One ounce of magnesium sulfate, orally
    (7) Enemas
C. Electric shock—injury produced by passage of electricity through body
  1. In addition to burns, electricity through human body produces respiratory arrest or cardiac fibrillation; other manifestations, tremors or vomiting
  2. Current should be broken by shutting off power or removing contact, using long dry stick; next step to give artificial respiration; rescue (mouth-to-mouth) breathing currently considered to be most efficacious
D. Drowning—respiratory obstruction due to laryngeal spasm resulting from effort to breathe under water; victim should be placed in prone position and rescue breathing given; victim should be kept warm and given oxygen when available
E. Acute poisoning
  1. Poisoning from inhalation and ingestion of toxic materials, both accidental and intentional, a major health hazard
  2. One half of all poisonings involve drugs; other products commonly implicated include household preparations, pesticides, and petroleum distillates
  3. Prevention best; see p. 438
  4. Barbiturates—one of most common of drug poisons
    a. Symptoms
      (1) Sleep
      (2) Slow respirations
      (3) Cyanosis
      (4) Moderately dilated pupils
      (5) Low blood pressure
      (6) May include fever
      (7) Anuria
      (8) Circulatory collapse
    b. Treatment and nursing care
      (1) Lavage if discovered in time
      (2) Rescue breathing if indicated
      (3) Oxygen
      (4) Suctioning
      (5) Respiratory stimulants
      (6) Efforts to prevent pulmonary edema and/or pneumonia (positioning, suctioning, penicillin)
  5. Carbon monoxide gas
    a. Symptoms
      (1) Elevated blood pressure
      (2) Dilated pupils
      (3) Dusky red skin
      (4) Muscular rigidity
      (5) Bounding pulse
    b. Treatment and nursing care
      (1) Fresh air
      (2) Rescue breathing
      (3) Warmth
      (4) Rest
      (5) Oxygen
      (6) Stimulants if indicated
  6. Corrosive poisons (acids or alkalies)
    a. Symptoms
      (1) Corrosion of mucous membranes
      (2) Dysphagia
      (3) Nausea and vomiting
      (4) Pain in gastrointestinal tract
      (5) Shock
      (6) Difficult respiration
      (7) Later, inflammations and ulcerations
    b. Treatment—demulcents should be given
      (1) Oil
      (2) Milk
      (3) Starch water
      (4) Flour water
      (5) Avoid chalk and alkaline carbonates
  7. Aspirin and other salicylates
    a. Symptoms
      (1) Vomiting
      (2) Epigastric pain
      (3) Perspiration
      (4) Headache
      (5) Dizziness

(6) Visual disturbances
(7) Rapid pulse
(8) Low blood pressure
(9) Dyspnea
(10) Restlessness
b. Treatment
(1) First step to remove drug from stomach
(2) Then give sodium bicarbonate
(3) Give stimulants
8. Skin contamination
a. Important to drench and cleanse skin with water thoroughly and rapidly to reduce extent of injury
9. Eye contamination
a. Hold eyes open, wash eyes with gentle stream of running water immediately
b. Wash until physician arrives
c. Do not use chemicals
10. Injected poisons (scorpion and snake bites)
a. Make patient lie down as soon as possible
b. Apply tourniquet above injection site; tourniquet should be loosened for 1 minute every 15 minutes
c. Apply ice pack to site of bite
d. Take patient to physician or hospital
11. Chemical burns
a. Wash with large quantities of H_2O (except those caused by phosphorus)
b. Cover immediately with loosely applied clean cloth
c. Avoid use of ointment, grease, powder, or other drugs in first aid treatment of burns
d. Treat shock
F. Heat disorders
1. Heat exhaustion or prostration—syndrome resulting from exposure to excessive heat
a. Symptoms
(1) Varying degrees of circulatory collapse
(2) Listlessness
(3) Apprehension
(4) Perspiration
(5) Low blood pressure
(6) Dizziness
(7) Headache
(8) Mild muscular cramps
(9) In severe cases, unconsciousness

b. Treatment and nursing care
(1) Place patient in cool environment
(2) Provide rest
(3) Give fluids with sodium chloride
(4) Patient may be prone to heat exhaustion during rest of life
2. Heat stroke—severe disturbance of heat-regulating mechanism
a. Symptoms
(1) Sudden onset
(2) Hot dry skin
(3) Headache
(4) Vertigo
(5) Nausea
(6) Precordial distress
(7) Very rapid pulse
(8) Markedly elevated temperature
(a) Temperature of over 106° F. by rectum—grave prognostic sign
(b) Temperature of over 108° F.—indicates irreversible brain damage
b. Treatment should be immediate and vigorous
(1) Mechanical methods of lowering temperature (ice baths, ice packs, etc.) used at once
(2) Precautions must be taken that sudden drop in temperature does not occur and produce collapse
(3) Patient will need close observation and symptomatic care for some time
(4) Should be warned to avoid excessive heat, fatigue, and alcohol in the future
3. Heat cramps—sudden muscle pains caused by excessive loss of sodium chloride in perspiration during strenuous exercise in hot weather
a. Prevention best—taking extra salt when severe exertion is anticipated
b. Immediate treatment
(1) Salty fluids and foods
(2) Extra water
(3) Rest
4. Sunburn
a. Prevention best
(1) Careful, gradual exposures to sun's rays, avoiding the midday hours when the rays are hottest

(2) Use of trade preparations, or olive oil, cocoa butter, creams, ointments, etc., helpful

b. Treatment

(1) Compresses of magnesium sulfate or sodium bicarbonate

(2) Advise to see physician if chills, fever, edema, or blistering occurs

G. Cold injury

1. Hypothermia—extreme depression of metabolic processes, resulting from exposure to excessive cold

a. Symptoms

(1) Progressive deterioration with ataxia, dysarthria, drowsiness, and eventually coma

(2) Cardiac irregularities if body heat below 30° C.

b. Treatment and nursing care

(1) Check pupillary light reflex and tendon reflexes

(2) Rewarm slowly to raise temperature to 30° to 32° C.

(3) Observation for 20 to 30 days may be necessary because of considerable instability in thermoregulation and vasomotor control

2. Local cold injury—of two types: nonfreezing cold injury (immersion foot or trench foot) and frostbite

a. Symptoms—dependent on exposure; may vary from mild to severe (i.e., from hyperemia, swelling, redness, and mild cyanosis to destruction of entire area involved and gangrene)

b. Treatment and nursing care

(1) Do not allow walking if lower extremities are involved

(2) Remove constrictive clothing

(3) Rewarm affected part by immersion in comfortably warm water for 10 minutes

(4) Blot skin dry and apply sterile, dry, loose dressings

(5) Follow with active physical therapy

(6) Keep body warm and encourage sleep and rest

H. Foreign bodies in the ear

1. Identify object—use flashlight if necessary

2. Remove if object readily seen or has free ends

3. Irrigation not advised

4. Drop a little oil or a strong alcohol into ear canal in case of insects

I. Foreign bodies in the eye

1. Eye should not be rubbed

2. Hands should be thoroughly washed

3. Examine to locate

4. Remove with small applicator

5. If unable to remove or if object present in eye for long period of time, send patient to doctor

J. Radiation exposure—not immediately recognizable

1. Exposed persons should be decontaminated and given bed rest and fluids

2. Later, nausea, vomiting, and malaise may appear

3. Radiation sickness occurs several hours or days after exposure

K. Environmental poisons—detergents, pesticides, radioactive substances, injurious drugs ingested by animals

1. Treatment—education, legislation, etc.

L. Fractures—see nursing the patient with a fracture

4. **Measures to prevent poisoning accidents**

A. Keep drugs, poisonous substances, and household substances out of reach of children

B. Do not store nonedible products on shelves used for storing food

C. Keep all poisonous substances in original containers

D. Destroy discarded medications

E. When giving flavored and/or brightly colored medicine to children, always refer to it as medicine—never candy

F. Have sufficient light when giving or taking medications

G. READ LABELS before using chemical products

5. **Nursing in major disasters**

Unlike usual nursing because nurse must take more responsibility and assume degree of authority when physician not available; number of adjustments to be made

A. Victims with chance of survival but needing immediate emergency treatment cared for first

1. Priorities of treatment

a. First priority—immediate attention

(1) Any wound interfering with patent airway

(2) Any wound requiring immediate pressure

(3) Shock due to major hemorrhage
b. Second priority—early surgery
(1) Visceral injuries, wounds of genitourinary tract, thoracic wounds without asphyxia
(2) Vascular injuries requiring repair—includes all injuries in which tourniquet is necessary
(3) Closed head injuries with increasing loss of consciousness
c. Third priority—surgery required but can be delayed
(1) Spinal injuries in which decompression required
(2) Soft tissue wounds in which debridement necessary but not involving major muscle damage
(3) Lesser fractures and dislocations
(4) Injuries of the eyes
(5) Maxillofacial injuries without asphyxia
B. Food and water supplies may be contaminated; should be used with caution; in natural disasters, epidemics must be prevented; in bombing, water and food may contain radiation dust
C. Patients manifesting shock and/or hemorrhage should be given first aid care; when tourniquet applied, patient's forehead should be marked with large "T"
D. Open chest wounds should be closed or "plugged" with cleanest material available
E. Severe emotional reaction major problem; ranges from acute panic to paralysis of part of body; since all reactions due to fear, only friendly understanding will help; if at all possible, give emotionally disturbed person definite task
F. Burns—classified into three groups: hopelessly burned, severely burned, and moderately burned; prevention of infection by giving antibiotics; alleviation of pain; severely burned victims should be covered with clean, dry cloth if available; tight clothing loosened; treatment given for shock, including warm fluids if possible
G. Obstetric emergencies—many women may abort and many may deliver babies prematurely; improvisation and resourcefulness needed; identification of mother and baby and time of birth important;

help baby with mother if possible; antibiotic if necessary
H. Nerve gas damage—atropine sulfate should be given in large doses; clothing should be removed and skin washed with water or sodium bicarbonate in water; since clothing highly contaminated, care to avoid contamination of others with such clothing
I. Necessity to keep in mind that person may be suffering from effects of many stressors, which complicates treatment
J. Further information can be obtained from local Civil Defense organization

REVIEW QUESTIONS FOR MEDICAL-SURGICAL NURSING
Multiple choice

Read each question carefully and consider all possible answers. When you have decided which answer is best, blacken in the corresponding space on the answer sheet. There is only one best answer for each question or implied question.

Situation: Mrs. Grey is a 45-year-old woman who has been admitted to the hospital with a diagnosis of open-angle chronic glaucoma. (See questions 1 to 10.)

1. Which of the following symptoms is Mrs. Grey most likely to exhibit first?
   1. A sudden, complete loss of vision
   2. Impairment of peripheral vision
   3. Sudden attacks of acute pain
   4. Constant blurred vision
2. The chief aim of medical treatment in chronic glaucoma is
   1. Controlling intraocular pressure
   2. Dilating the pupil to allow for an increase in the visual field
   3. Allowing for healing process by resting the eye
   4. Preventing secondary infections that may add to the visual problem
3. Mrs. Grey should be instructed to
   1. Use mydriatrics regularly
   2. Restrict fluid intake
   3. Avoid bright lights or darkness
   4. Exercise in moderation
4. The patient with glaucoma needs assistance in learning to accept his disease because
   1. There is usually restriction to the use of the eyes
   2. Vision lost cannot be restored
   3. Total blindness is inevitable, even with treatment
   4. Surgery will preclude the need for any further care
5. Which of the following would not prove dangerous for Mrs. Grey?
   1. Use of sedatives
   2. Release of emotions by crying

3. Use of atropine in any form
4. Severe bouts of constipation
6. Mrs. Grey should be advised to
   1. Use eyewashes
   2. Use laxatives
   3. Keep an extra supply of eye medication on hand
   4. Have prescriptions filled when necessary
7. When the nurse is asked to instill 1 drop of 2% homatropine hydrobromide o.d. in preparation for refraction, the most appropriate action for the nurse would be to
   1. Instill the drug in the right eye
   2. Recall that hospital policy necessitates a written order
   3. State that the patient's age contraindicates use of this drug
   4. Remind the physician that her condition may contraindicate use of this drug
8. A systemic drug that may be prescribed to produce diuresis and inhibit formation of aqueous humor is
   1. Acetazolamide (Diamox)
   2. Bendroflumethiazide (Naturetin)
   3. Chlorothiazide (Diuril)
   4. Demecarium bromide (Humorsol)
9. Drugs instilled in the eye are said to be administered by which of the following methods?
   1. Topical   3. Injection
   2. Intraocular   4. Insufflation
10. Which one of the following drugs is likely to be prescribed to relieve symptoms if Mrs. Grey develops an inflammatory reaction in the eye?
    1. Nitrofurazone (Furacin)
    2. Sulfisoxazole (Gantrisin)
    3. Neomycin
    4. Cortisone

Situation: Mrs. Smith, a 45-year-old, rather obese mother of 5 children, is admitted to the emergency room of M. B. Hospital, complaining of nausea, belching, gas, and right upper quadrant pain that was not relieved by Alka Seltzer. She states that she has had these attacks for the past several years, especially after eating fatty or fried foods. The attacks have also been more frequent since the birth of her youngest child, age 2. On the basis of findings from a physical examination and some laboratory work, the doctor had advised immediate hospitalization. After a series of diagnostic tests, the patient was prepared for surgery. A cholecystectomy and choledochotomy were performed. Mrs. Smith was reluctant to cough or move. A wound dehiscence necessitated further surgery. Mrs. Smith was discharged 2 weeks later with printed instructions for her care at home and a clinic appointment to return 6 weeks later for a checkup. (See questions 11 to 23.)

11. Mrs. Smith experienced discomfort after ingesting fatty foods because
    1. The liver was manufacturing inadequate bile
    2. Fatty foods are hard to digest
    3. Obstruction of the common bile duct prevented emptying of the bile into the intestine

4. She did not eliminate fatty foods from her diet
12. For the Graham-Cole test that was performed, an important nursing action was
    1. Providing emotional support
    2. Noting whether all the fat-free supper was eaten
    3. Ascertaining if the patient had taken and retained the tablets
    4. Providing a fatty meal for supper
13. Cholecystography was performed to
    1. Detect obstruction at the ampulla of Vater
    2. Observe patency of the common bile duct
    3. Determine the concentration ability of the gallbladder
    4. Distinguish stone formation from other types of obstruction
14. Symptoms of surgical jaundice include
    1. Dark-colored urine, clay-colored stools, itchy skin
    2. Straw-colored urine, putty-colored stools, yellow sclera
    3. Inadequate absorption of fat-soluble vitamin K
    4. Light amber urine, dark brown stools, yellow skin
15. Severe postoperative hemorrhage may occur in any jaundiced patients because of
    1. Deficient formation of prothrombin
    2. Decreased synthesis of vitamin K
    3. Inadequate absorption of fat-soluble vitamin K
    4. Increase in serum bilirubin
16. Mrs. Smith had a prolonged bleeding and clotting time because of
    1. Absence of bile salts in the intestine
    2. Accumulation of bile in the blood
    3. Inadequate intake of menadione
    4. Decreased synthesis of vitamin K by intestinal bacteria
17. Patients with biliary tract surgery are prone to upper respiratory tract complications because of
    1. Lowering of resistance due to bile in the blood
    2. Invasion of the bloodstream by infection from the biliary tract
    3. Proximity of the incision to the diaphragm
    4. Length of time required for the surgery
18. A T tube was inserted into the common duct in order to
    1. Divert the flow of bile to outside
    2. Drain the gallbladder bed
    3. Prevent peritonitis
    4. Prevent production of cholecystokinin
19. When rupture of a wound occurs, the nurse should first
    1. Place patient in low Fowler's position
    2. Apply a firm Scultetus binder
    3. Cover the viscera with sterile gauze moistened in saline
    4. Provide emotional support to allay the patient's fears
20. To promote healing of the large incision, the physician may ask that Mrs. Smith receive daily doses of which of these vitamins?
    1. Ascorbic acid
    2. Mephyton

3. Vitamin B$_{12}$ complex
4. Vitamin A

21. After Mrs. Smith returned to the surgery ward from the recovery room following her surgery, the nurse made frequent checks of the wound area to note any tendencies toward excess bleeding or hemorrhage. She made these observations because
    1. Mrs. Smith was exceedingly anxious about her incision
    2. Her temperature was slightly elevated
    3. Blood clotting may be hindered by lack of vitamin K absorption due to interference with normal bile flow
    4. Mrs. Smith was complaining of much pain

22. When Mrs. Smith was able to eat solid food, which of the following special diets was ordered?
    1. High in protein and calories to help her regain her strength
    2. Low in fat to avoid painful contractions in the wound area
    3. Low in protein and carbohydrate to avoid excess calories and help her lose weight
    4. High in fat and carbohydrate to meet energy demands

23. When Mrs. Smith was ready to be discharged, the dietitian instructed her to remain on her prescribed diet for several more weeks. Afterward Mrs. Smith asked her nurse, "Will I have to stay away from fat for the rest of my life?" Which of the following responses would be most appropriate?
    1. "You'll have to remain on a fat-free diet from now on, to avoid a return of your previous symptoms."
    2. "It's too early to say. Later, when we see whether your operation is successful, we'll know the answer."
    3. "Only your doctor can answer that. Why don't you ask him about it before you are discharged from the hospital?"
    4. "After you have fully recovered from surgery, you'll probably be able to eat a normal diet, avoiding excessive fat."

Situation: A small urban community in the western area of the country is flattened by a severe, widespread tornado. (See questions 24 to 33.)

24. Immediately after the storm has passed the rescue team with which you are working is searching for injured people. You split up to search, and you find a man lying next to a broken natural gas main. He is not breathing and is bleeding heavily from a wound on the foot. Your first step would be to
    1. Remove him from the immediate vicinity
    2. Apply surface pressure to the foot wound
    3. Start rescue breathing immediately
    4. Treat him for shock

25. In the event a decision is made to apply a tourniquet to control the bleeding from the wound on the foot, you should
    1. Be sure someone will be available to loosen it at 15-minute intervals
    2. Assume that eventually an amputation will be necessary
    3. Apply the tourniquet tightly to the wound

4. Keep the patient informed of your actions

26. You find a young boy under the wreckage of a frame house. He is conscious, breathing satisfactorily, and lying on his back. He complains of pain in his back and is unable to move his legs. First you would
    1. Gently raise him to a sitting position to see if the pain either diminishes or increases in intensity
    2. Leave him lying on his back, giving him instructions not to move, and seek additional help
    3. Roll him on his abdomen, place a pad under his head, and cover him
    4. Gently lift him onto a flat piece of lumber and, using any available transportation, rush him to medical help

27. You find another injured person, obviously in shock. You would keep him lying on his back and
    1. Elevate the head higher than the rest of the body; give stimulants in small sips
    2. Surround the body with hot-water bottles or chemical heating pads if available
    3. After evaluation, allow the patient to walk around if injuries permit
    4. Place the head lower than the rest of the body, prevent chilling, and give fluids if possible

28. All the following problems will be important. Which will be of primary urgency within the first 2 hours after the storm?
    1. Food supply
    2. Flies and pest control
    3. Water supply
    4. Identification of the dead

29. When a disaster occurs, you may have to treat the mass hysteria first. The person or persons to be cared for immediately would be those in
    1. Depression   3. Panic
    2. Euphoria   4. Comatose state

30. In any disaster concerning a number of people, the function that contributes most to saving of lives is sorting, or triage. This requires clinical judgment based on "greatest good for the greatest number." Assume that you are the nurse who has to determine this priority of needs. The patients who need immediate care are those with
    1. Second-degree burns of 10% of the body
    2. Severe lacerations involving open fractures of major bones
    3. Closed fractures of major bones
    4. Significant penetrating or perforating abdominal wounds

31. The patients who need minimal care are those with
    1. Second-degree burns of 10% of the body
    2. Hemorrhage from an easily accessible site
    3. Noncritical central nervous system injuries
    4. Closed fractures of major bones

32. A crushing injury to the chest may cause "sucking wounds." After you have closely bandaged the wound, to prevent further air from entering the lung you would place the patient in which of the following positions?
    1. Trendelenburg   3. Sims'
    2. High Fowler's   4. Slight Fowler's

triage - sorting of people

33. Local health officials concerned with food damage and contamination after the tornado would contact which of the following agencies for help in food inspection and removal of contaminated items?
    1. National Red Cross
    2. National Research Council
    3. Food and Drug Administration
    4. Federal Trade Commission

Situation: Mr. Smith is a 60-year-old man who is admitted to the hospital with a diagnosis of idiopathic trigeminal neuralgia. He is complaining of severe pain in the right side of the face. (See questions 34 to 42.)

34. In planning the nursing care for Mr. Smith, the nurse would
    1. Emphasize the importance of mouth care
    2. Be alert to prevent dehydration or starvation
    3. Initiate exercises of the jaw and facial muscles
    4. Apply iced compresses to the affected area
35. Which of the following symptoms would Mr. Smith be likely to demonstrate?
    1. Exhaustion and fatigue due to extreme pain
    2. Excessive talkativeness due to apprehension
    3. Hyperactivity due to medications received
    4. Prolonged periods of a sleep broken only by external stimuli
36. Surgery, with cutting of the nerve, is performed. Which of the following would be an unusual occurrence after surgery?
    1. Development of a painless rash in the area
    2. Recurrence of the pain, which will gradually decrease
    3. Development of a crawling or tingling sensation in the area
    4. Loss of muscle power in the area
37. Postoperatively, which of the following precautions should be taught to Mr. Smith?
    1. Exercise extreme care when eating
    2. Carefully avoid any stimulation of the area
    3. Drink only very hot fluids
    4. Avoid mouth care for at least a week
38. Which of the following symptoms would be a particular danger signal for Mr. Smith?
    1. Pain due to a cavity in a tooth
    2. Slight drooping of the mouth
    3. Inability to blink
    4. Redness of the eye
39. To avoid the above complication, Mr. Smith should be advised not to
    1. Touch or rub his eye
    2. See his dentist regularly
    3. Eat hot or cold foods
    4. Blink at frequent intervals
40. The cause of idiopathic trigeminal neuralgia is
    1. Genetic
    2. Autoimmune reaction
    3. Unknown
    4. Infections
41. The most serious complication of resection of this nerve is caused by resection of which branch?
    1. Mandibular   3. Ophthalmic
    2. Maxillary   4. Facial

42. The physician prescribes amyl nitrite inhalations. The presumed action of this drug in the relief of pain due to trigeminal neuralgia is
    1. Primarily psychological
    2. To lower the blood pressure and relax the bronchi
    3. Dilate small blood vessels in the affected region
    4. Exert an antagonistic action on acetylcholine

Situation: Mrs. J A is a 59-year-old patient who for the past few days has been experiencing colicky pain, referred down the thigh and to the genitalia, frequency, and oliguria. Since home treatment was ineffective, she is now hospitalized with a diagnosis of recurrent ureteral colic. (See questions 43 to 52.)

43. The physician performs several renal function tests. All the following might be expected except:
    1. Retrograde pyelography
    2. Phenolsulfonphthalein test
    3. Intravenous urogram
    4. Bromsulphalein test
44. Active treatment must immediately be instituted for Mrs. A's ureteral colic. Assuming the doctor's orders have been written, the nurse would first administer
    1. The prescribed pain medication
    2. Large amounts of fluid per os
    3. A hot bath
    4. Infusion of 5% dextrose and water with 20 mEq. KCl
45. Atropine (0.4 mg. I.M.) and morphine (10 mg. I.M.) are ordered stat. The major effect of atropine is to
    1. Relax smooth muscle
    2. Reduce frequency of bladder contractions
    3. Potentiate parasympathetic control of the bladder
    4. Dilate ureters
46. The expected effect of the morphine is
    1. Respiratory depression
    2. Sedation and sleep
    3. Pain reduction
    4. Control of cough
47. The diagnosis was confirmed and Mrs. A was taken to the operating room for a ureterolithotomy. A frequently encountered complication after this operation is
    1. Urine draining from wound
    2. Hemorrhage
    3. Paralytic ileus
    4. Hydronephrosis
48. Mrs. A has an indwelling catheter attached to straight drainage. To keep a secondary bladder infection from developing, the nurse should
    1. Keep the drainage bottle emptied
    2. Have the area around the meatus and the catheter cleansed frequently
    3. Use measures to acidify the urine
    4. Irrigate the catheter b.i.d.
49. Inasmuch as urinary calculi may recur, it is necessary for the nurse to teach Mrs. A that she may eat liberal amounts of
    1. Sardines   3. Apples
    2. Cheese   4. Nuts

50. Since Mrs. J A's urine had an alkaline reaction, the following acidifying agent might be used:
1. Mandelamine
2. Ammonium chloride
3. Sodium bicarbonate
4. Sodium acid phosphate

51. The ureteral stones were most likely composed of which of the following substances?
1. Uric acid
2. Calcium
3. Cystine
4. Phosphate

52. Special nursing measures may be needed past a ureterolithotomy to
1. Care for the draining urinary fistula
2. Maintain fluid and electrolyte balance
3. Lavage the bladder
4. Prevent hemorrhage

Situation: Mrs. Giles has been admitted to the hospital after having a seizure. She is a 33-year-old housewife and mother of 3 children. (See questions 53 to 61.)

53. Mrs. Giles was interviewed and examined by the doctor on call. Which of the following statements in regard to the etiology of epilepsy is not correct?
1. Epilepsy has been proved to be an inherited disease
2. Epilepsy may be manifested after head trauma
3. The epileptic may have a history of petit mal seizures in childhood
4. There is no known cause for certain forms of epilepsy

54. The term epilepsy signifies
1. A specific disease entity
2. Loss of consciousness and involuntary movements
3. Occurrence of irregular brain waves
4. Emotional instability accompanied by seizures

55. Mrs. Giles questions the nurse regarding the scheduling of her medication. The nurse informs her that the medications
1. Can usually be stopped after one year's absence of seizures
2. Need to be taken only in periods of emotional stress
3. Will probably have to be continued for life
4. Will prevent the occurrence of seizures

56. Mrs. Giles expresses concern about her ability to do her housework and care for her children. The nurse bases her reply on which of the following factors?
1. Limiting the activity level of the brain will limit seizures
2. Physical and mental productivity will help to limit seizures
3. Physical activity must be limited if seizures are to be controlled
4. A strict adherence to a regimen of physical exertion is necessary to prevent seizures

57. In observing Mrs. Giles for seizures, the nurse should be aware that
1. Accurate reporting of a jacksonian seizure will aid in localizing the affected area of the brain

2. Petit mal seizures are generally preceded by a loud vocal aura
3. Psychomotor seizures last for a rather prolonged period
4. A period of confusion after a grand mal seizure is indicative of permanent brain damage

58. A ketogenic diet most likely will not be prescribed because
1. The low carbohydrate tends to produce acidosis
2. The high fat causes ketosis
3. It is unpalatable and lacks bulk
4. Of the age factor in this instance

59. Symptoms Mrs. Giles may exhibit after an electroencephalogram are
1. Temporary memory loss, nausea, and vomiting
2. Fall in blood pressure, dysphagia
3. Rise in temperature and blood pressure
4. None of these

60. The physician prescribes diphenylhydantoin (Dilantin) to control the seizures. The expected effect of this drug is to
1. Alter the permeability of the cell membrane to potassium
2. Control nerve impulses to the skeletal muscles
3. Prevent depression of the central nervous system
4. Produce an antispasmodic action on the muscles

61. Mrs. Giles also has petit mal epilepsy. The drug that is likely to be used to control this condition is which of the following?
1. Diphenylhydantoin (Dilantin)
2. Mephenytoin (Mesantoin)
3. Phenobarbital (Luminal)
4. Trimethadione (Tridione)

Situation: Mrs. Black was in a serious auto accident. She suffered internal injuries and deep lacerations with hemorrhage. When she was admitted via ambulance to the hospital, she was in severe shock and was rushed to the operating room. She was given a blood transfusion that proved to be incompatible with her blood type. (See questions 62 to 69.)

62. Initial sign of such transfusion reaction would be
1. Dyspnea
2. Backache
3. Cyanosis
4. Shock

63. As a result of this transfusion reaction she suffered kidney damage. The most significant clinical response for determining kidney damage is
1. Acute pain over kidney area
2. Decreased urinary output
3. Hematuria
4. Polyuria

64. Laboratory tests revealed
1. Elevated BUN, NPN, and K levels
2. Albuminuria, high specific gravity
3. Elevated BUN; lowered NPN and K levels
4. Albuminuria, low specific gravity

65. Hemodialysis was ordered immediately for Mrs. Black. This therapy was instituted to
1. Permit use of extracorporeal radiation

2. Provide an emergency substitute for the action of normal renal tissue
3. Provide oxygenation of body tissue
4. Permanently take over kidney function

66. Chemical assay of electrolyte balance is important during dialysis to determine patient status. Nurses' observations can be just as vital. The most important sign to be observed in a patient with uremia is
   1. Condition of skin   3. Mental status
   2. Fluid intake   4. Respiratory rate
67. Dialysis was repeated every 2 weeks for Mrs. Black. During this time it would be important to watch for
   1. Pressure sores
   2. Uremic frost
   3. Hemorrhage at cut-down sites
   4. Increased anxiety
68. Mrs. Black's urinary function returned to normal with this care. She was happy that she would soon be discharged. She should understand prior to discharge that
   1. She will need dialysis periodically for the rest of her life
   2. Medical supervision and avoidance of infection are important
   3. Measuring of intake and output is important
   4. She will never need dialysis again
69. One of the first indications that Mrs. Black was approaching a uremic stage would be
   1. Shaking chills
   2. Temperature of 103° F.
   3. Headache
   4. Severe pain

Situation: Mr. X, 39, is seen in his doctor's office for treatment of angina pectoris. He hopes that his condition is not serious, since his business needs him right now. He has nitroglycerin tablets that he takes when he feels pain, and he knows not to overexercise. (See questions 70 to 79.)

70. Angina pectoris is
   1. A serious cardiac disorder of unknown etiology
   2. A coronary artery disease
   3. Atherosclerosis of the heart vessels
   4. Pain caused by lack of oxygen to the myocardium
71. On experiencing pain, Mr. X should
   1. Phone his doctor for help
   2. Cease effort immediately
   3. Not worry about his condition, since he probably is not having a heart attack
   4. Make preparations to go into the hospital
72. For some patients with angina, nitroglycerin tablets are most helpful for their
   1. Placebo effect
   2. Action on the myocardium
   3. Effect on respiration
   4. Moderate to fast action in the system
73. The nurse in counseling Mr. X might be wise to help him see the importance of
   1. Finding work involving less emotional strain
   2. Having regular checkups
   3. Finding a job involving more experience
   4. Staying with the job he has, since it does not involve physical exertion

74. The doctor says Mr. X may drink an ounce of whiskey several times during the day. This is probably to
   1. Allay apprehension
   2. Dilate blood vessels
   3. Avoid Mr. X's having to change his social habits
   4. Increase his appetite
75. As in the case of Mr. X, one might expect that the
   1. Variations of the location and severity of pain occur infrequently
   2. Same pattern of pain occurs repeatedly in a given individual
   3. Frequency and severity of the attacks remain the same over a period of years
   4. Increasing exertion over a period of years may cause an attack
76. In accordance with the physician's orders, a supply of nitroglycerin tablets is obtained and they are kept at Mr. X's bedside. During morning care Mr. X points to the bottle of nitroglycerin tablets that has been placed on his bedside table and asks, "What is in that bottle?" Which of the following might the nurse best reply?
   1. "Did the doctor not tell you?"
   2. "Tell me if you take a nitroglycerin tablet."
   3. "Don't you remember what those tablets are for?"
   4. "The doctor wants you to take one of these tablets if you feel pain in your chest."
77. After a few days the nurse learns that Mr. X is taking a tablet of nitroglycerin every 20 minutes. Mr. X tells the nurse that they relieve the discomfort in his epigastric region. The nurse's action will be guided by knowledge of which of the following?
   1. Cardiac pain never begins in the epigastrium
   2. Tolerance to nitroglycerin is readily acquired
   3. Few drugs should ever be given at intervals of 20 minutes
   4. Habituation to this drug is apparent
78. For which of the following purposes was nitroglycerin ordered?
   1. To reduce the frequency of attacks of angina pectoris
   2. To control acute attacks of angina pectoris
   3. To produce vasoconstriction
   4. To relieve smooth muscle spasm of the gastrointestinal tract
79. A daily dose of pentaerythritol tetranitrate (Peritrate) is prescribed. It is expected to produce which of the following effects?
   1. Sedation
   2. Dilatation of the coronary arteries
   3. Potentiation of the effects of digitoxin
   4. Relief of anxiety and apprehension

Situation: Mary Jane Lee, age 33, was admitted from the emergency room of General Hospital to the neurological service with a diagnosis of myasthenia gravis. (See questions 80 to 91.)

80. Because of the involvement of the ocular muscles a common early symptom is
    1. Nystagmus   3. Blurring
    2. Diplopia   4. Tearing
81. The person with myasthenia gravis may be compared to the person with hypoglycemic diabetes in that both will have the following modification to make in life patterns:
    1. Medication   3. Rest
    2. Diet   4. Sleep
82. Mary Jane Lee will be advised to avoid fatigue because the one great symptom of this disease is
    1. Progressive weakness and muscle atrophy
    2. Muscular fatigue
    3. Muscle atrophy
    4. Muscular twitching
83. During the acute stage of this disease it is advisable for the nurse to
    1. Have a tracheotomy set at the bedside
    2. Administer narcotics as ordered
    3. Keep padded side rails in place
    4. Permit bathroom privileges only
84. The prognosis of this disease is most likely to be
    1. Poor, with termination in a few months
    2. Chronic, with exacerbations and remissions
    3. Slowly progressive, without remissions
    4. Excellent, with proper treatment
85. The sex and age most frequently affected are
    1. Males, age 15-35
    2. Females, age 10-30
    3. Both sexes, ages 20-40
    4. Children, age 5-15
86. The physician orders ambenonium (Mytelase) and pyridostigmine bromide (Mestinon). These drugs are expected to relieve the symptoms of myasthenia gravis by producing which of the following actions?
    1. Blocking neural transmission at the axon terminals
    2. Preventing acetylcholine from concentrating at the myoneural junction
    3. Inhibiting cholinesterase and stimulating skeletal muscle
    4. Decreasing muscle contractions and promoting enzyme activity
87. When she goes home, Mary Jane is to take a timed-release form of pyridostigmine bromide (Mestinon) at bedtime. Which of the following ought to be taught to at least one member of her family?
    1. Administration or injection of drugs that act against myasthenia gravis
    2. Intubation and its use in giving oral medication if dysphagia occurs
    3. Establishment of a method for reminding Mary Jane to take her medicine
    4. Awaken Mary Jane every 4 hours to take her medicine
88. In the event that Mary Jane develops symptoms of myasthenic crisis or cholinergic crisis, the nurse can anticipate that the physician will probably administer edrophonium (Tensilon) intravenously to establish definitive diagnosis. The reason that edrophonium is more useful for this purpose than any other drugs is that it
    1. Produces a pronounced, long-lasting effect
    2. Causes minimal but visible effects on muscle strength
    3. Causes no known toxic effects
    4. Has a rapid onset and a short duration of action
89. If the physician prescribes atropine, its purpose will be to control which of these groups of symptoms?
    1. Sweating, bradycardia, excessive salivation
    2. Constipation, urinary retention, nausea
    3. Aching, fatigue, lassitude
    4. Respiratory tract secretions, tingling, nervousness
90. Mary Jane states that the doctor injected medicine into her vein to make the diagnosis of myasthenia gravis and that she was immediately able to raise her eyelids and focus her eyes. The nurse knows that the drug she described was probably
    1. Neostigmine (Prostigmin)
    2. Pyridostigmine bromide (Mestinon)
    3. Ambenonium (Mytelase)
    4. Edrophonium (Tensilon)
91. During the development of a therapeutic regimen, it is important that the nurses teach Mary Jane to do which of the following?
    1. Take the exact dose prescribed precisely ½ hour before meals
    2. Take the drugs regularly, adjusting the dose according to her needs
    3. Ask a relative or friend to remind her to take her medicine on schedule
    4. Use a check-list and alarm clock to maintain a correct dosage schedule

Situation: Mr. L, age 55, a highly reputable criminal lawyer, states he has had increasing chest discomfort for the past 2 weeks but did not mention this to anyone because of the magnitude of work and severe mental strain involved in preparing the defense for a client. He now enters the hospital with a diagnosis of acute coronary occlusion. Admission orders include complete bed rest, coronary precautions, 1,500-calorie bland diet as tolerated, morphine sulfate gr. ¼ q. 4 h.p.r.n., nasal oxygen 6 L./min. p.r.n., ECG, urinalysis, ESR, CBC stat., LDH, SGOT × 3, daily prothrombin time monitoring, Lee-White clotting time q. 4 hr. until discontinued, VS q. 30 min., I.V. 1,000 ml. 5% G/DW to keep vein open, if BP drops below 90 systolic, start 500 ml. 5% G/DW with 2 ampules of Levophed, heparin 5,000 units I.V. stat., further doses to be ordered by attending physician only, no visitors except wife, special nurses round the clock. (See questions 92 to 118.)

92. The pain in coronary occlusion is due primarily to
    1. Arterial spasm
    2. Irritation of nerve endings in cardiac plexus
    3. Ischemia of the heart muscle
    4. Blocking of the coronary veins
93. Caution should be exercised in administering large doses of morphine because the
    1. Problem of addiction developing is great
    2. Pain of the acute infarct is very difficult to relieve

3. Problem of development of intolerance is likely
4. Pain is antagonistic to morphine

94. In the event of a fall in BP, Levophed will be used primarily for its
    1. Action on the heart
    2. Peripheral effects on blood vessels
    3. Ability to increase cardiac output
    4. Depression of the vasomotor center in the medulla

95. A temperature of 102° F. on the second day indicates that
    1. Mr. L is developing an upper respiratory tract infection
    2. Necrotic changes are occurring in the myocardium
    3. The body is responding to the necrotic process in the myocardium
    4. Phlebitis may be occurring as a complication of the strict bed rest

96. Anticoagulant therapy was used in order to
    1. Improve coronary circulation
    2. Hasten the clotting time of blood
    3. Delay the clotting time of blood
    4. Retard coronary circulation

97. The results of the ECG indicated a posterior wall infarct; one of the physiologic adaptations made by the body after coronary occlusion is
    1. The autonomic conservation of oxygen
    2. The development of collateral circulation
    3. A decrease in the metabolic rate
    4. A decrease in the carbon dioxide level of the blood

98. Mr. L was ordered to stop smoking by his physician. The primary reason for his action is that nicotine causes
    1. Dilatation of the peripheral vessels removing blood from the heart
    2. Cancer of the lung
    3. Constriction of the blood vessels
    4. Alteration of the clotting time

99. Mr. L received oxygen, primarily to
    1. Relieve his dyspnea
    2. Relieve the cyanosis
    3. Increase oxygen concentration in myocardium
    4. Supersaturate the red blood cells

100. Subsequent heart attacks, with scarring, dilatation, and hypertrophy could cause Mr. L to progress to cardiac decompensation; this would result in
    1. Decreased cardiac output
    2. Rapid emptying of left ventricle
    3. Rapid emptying of right auricle
    4. Increased cardiac output

101. Mr. L voices concern about returning to his job as criminal lawyer. The nurse's answer should be made with the understanding that
    1. A person who has had a coronary should have a sedentary job
    2. The functional capacity of the patient does not always determine the amount of physical activity permitted
    3. Most patients with cardiac disorders are reduced to permanent inactivity
    4. Employers can make modifications in jobs for the cardiac patient

102. The primary rationale for Mr. L's initial special diet—1,500 calorie, bland—is
    (a) To reduce the metabolic work load associated with digestion, absorption, and utilization of food and consequent cardiac output demand
    (b) To reduce his weight and make him more comfortable
    (c) To avoid effort in eating and pressure from a volume of food at meals
    (d) To avoid gastric irritants and control acidity
       1. a and d   3. b and d
       2. a and c   4. b and c

103. A substance that may be kept at hand for use as an antidote for Coumadin because of its effective coagulant action as an antimetabolite to the drug is
    1. Phytonadione (vitamin K_1)
    2. Calcium lactate
    3. Ascorbic acid
    4. Ferrous sulfate

104. The effects of bishydroxycoumarin Warfarin sodium (Coumadin) can be expected to be
    1. Rapid and persistent for several days
    2. Delayed and persistent for several days
    3. Delayed and effective for a few hours
    4. Rapid and effective for several hours

105. During the time Coumadin is administered to Mr. L, provision will probably be made for which of the following daily determinations?
    1. Blood sedimentation rate
    2. Intake and output
    3. Prothrombin time
    4. Electrocardiographic readings

106. Which of the following groups of symptoms would indicate untoward action of Coumadin?
    1. Bleeding from the mouth, ears, rectum, and bladder
    2. Increased salivation, hyperhydrosis, restlessness
    3. Decreased alimentation, hot, dry skin, stupor
    4. Dyspnea, precordial pain, slow, weak pulse

107. Which of the following drugs would you expect the physician to order if symptoms of overdosage from Coumadin are observed?
    1. Dicumarol
    2. Iron-dextran complex (Imferon)
    3. Heparin
    4. Vitamin K

108. During the early hospitalization period, the physician is likely to want Mr. L to be given morphine
    1. More frequently to promote rest and comfort
    2. Sparingly to prevent addiction
    3. When an impending attack is apparent
    4. Every 4 hours without fail

109. The multiple-dose vial is labeled to indicate that 1 ml. of solution contains 15 mg. of morphine. To give a dose of gr. ¼, the nurse would prepare how much solution?
    1. 1 ml.   3. 1½ ml.
    2. ⅔ ml.   4. ½ ml.

110. Morphine is classified as belonging in which of the following groups of substances?
    1. Glycosides   3. Tannins
    2. Alkaloids   4. Resins

111. Because Mr. L receives morphine often, the nurse will need to be alert to the symptoms of early morphine poisoning, which include the following:
   1. Profuse sweating, pinpoint pupils, deep sleep
   2. Slow pulse, pinpoint pupils, stupor
   3. Slow pulse, slow respirations, stupor
   4. Slow respirations, constricted pupils, deep sleep

112. Two hours after receiving pain medication, Mr. L develops excruciating chest pain that is unrelieved by currently ordered medications. The physician, after examining Mr. L, writes this order: morphine sulfate gr. ¾ stat. Which of the following describes the best action for the nurse to follow?
   1. Give the drug as prescribed
   2. Adjust the dose to gr. ¼
   3. Request clarification of the order
   4. Refuse to give this dose

113. When the physician does not indicate the route of administration by which he wishes the morphine given, which of the following actions is preferred?
   1. Give the drug orally because this is the least expensive and the most comfortable route of administration
   2. Give the drug intramuscularly to promote its rapid absorption
   3. Administer the drug subcutaneously because this is the method most frequently ordered
   4. Request clarification of the order for legal reasons

114. Which of the following actions of heparin is crucial to Mr. L's health status?
   1. Its role in immunologic reactions
   2. Its ability to reduce coagulation of blood
   3. Its cumulative effect that is predictable
   4. Its inability to cause adverse effects

115. If Mr. L develops signs of hemorrhage that may indicate heparin overdosage, the nurse can anticipate that the physician may order which of the following therapeutic agents to neutralize the action of heparin?
   1. Phytonadione (vitamin K₁)
   2. Protamine sulfate
   3. Whole human blood
   4. Fresh blood plasma

116. The purpose of Levophed is to help in the treatment of
   1. Pain and discomfort
   2. Loss of body fluid
   3. Cardiogenic shock
   4. Kidney dysfunction

117. When Levophed is being administered by intravenous infusion, the primary nursing action is to
   1. Observe the patient for a diastolic blood pressure below 50 or above 90
   2. Regulate the rate of flow to maintain the blood pressure at the desired level
   3. Observe the patient for flushing, sweating, tremor, and nausea
   4. Regulate the flow of the solution so that blood volume is restored

118. If Levophed extravasates into the tissues, the nurse should recognize this promptly and immediately
   1. Interrupt the flow of the solution and notify the physician
   2. Reduce the rate of flow and apply warm, moist packs
   3. Inject phentolamine and heparin into the affected tissues
   4. Elevate the involved extremity and call the supervisor

Situation: Mr. S, a 55-year-old, tall, thin, unemployed Negro house painter, was transferred from the County Sanatorium to the General Hospital for workup and surgery. Admitting diagnoses were (a) pulmonary tuberculosis, (b) bronchogenic carcinoma. Admission orders included room isolation, isoniazid 100 mg. t.i.d., pyridoxine 25 mg. O D, PAS 3 Gm. t.i.d., Crysticillin 600,000 units q. 6 h. I.M., streptomycin 0.5 Gm. I.M. t.i.d., regular diet, extensive diagnostic studies. Sputum examinations were negative for *Mycobacterium tuberculosis* and malignant cells. Mr. S had few visitors prior to surgery, since his wife worked and other relatives lived out of the state. He seemed depressed and lonely and could not understand why he had to be confined to a room alone, since he had been able to move about freely at the sanatorium. He was also tired of waiting for the surgery, which could not be performed until sufficient blood was available. Finally, after a waiting period of 3 weeks, a right upper lobectomy was performed for atelectasis. Postoperatively, he did well except for urinary problems developing after the temporary use of an indwelling Foley catheter. Prior to surgery he denied any problems with urination, and the physical examination was not remarkable. After an extensive GU workup a transurethral prostatectomy (TUR) for benign prostatic hypertrophy was performed. (See questions 119 to 137.)

119. A negative sputum examination for *Mycobacterium tuberculosis* most likely indicated that
   1. Mr. S had not been instructed properly in the collection of the specimen
   2. Mr. S no longer has active tuberculosis
   3. Repeated examinations are necessary for conclusive evidence
   4. This test should be used in conjunction with other tests

120. In helping Mr. S understand why room isolation is necessary, the nurse should
   1. Explain the mode of transmission of tubercle bacilli
   2. Inform him that isolation will be discontinued, since he no longer has active tuberculosis
   3. Recognize that Mr. S may not be verbalizing his major problems
   4. Explain that it is necessary because he is now in a general hospital

121. Nursing implications for patients on isoniazid include observation for symptoms of
   1. Numbness, tingling, weakness
   2. Dyspepsia, diarrhea, fever
   3. Tinnitus, deafness, unsteady gait
   4. Urticaria, fever, polyarthritis

122. After surgery Mr. S had a closed (underwater) drainage for a few days to provide drainage and to

1. Maintain aseptic condition in the cavity
2. Maintain a negative pressure in the cavity
3. Provide gentle suction
4. Equalize internal and external pressures

123. Exercise was started early to prevent loss of function in shoulder and arm on the affected side. This was accomplished best by having Mr. S in a
    1. Prone position
    2. Supine position
    3. Fowler's position
    4. Orthopneic position

124. Mr. S experienced difficulty in voiding after the catheter was removed, because of
    1. Interruption in normal voiding habits
    2. Nervous tension
    3. Remaining effects of anesthetics
    4. Toxic symptoms from antituberculosis chemotherapy

125. The definitive diagnosis of benign prostatic hypertrophy was arrived at by
    1. Serum phosphatase studies
    2. Rectal examination
    3. Papanicolaou smear of prostatic fluid
    4. Biopsy of prostatic tissue

126. If Mr. S had complained of persistent discomfort in the bladder and urethra, the nurse most likely did which of the following first?
    1. Checked the patency of the catheter
    2. Notified the doctor at once
    3. Milked the tubing gently
    4. Irrigated the catheter with prescribed solutions

127. After the removal of the catheter Mr. S should have been instructed to
    1. Measure and record the time and amount of each voiding
    2. Attempt to void every hour for the next 24 hours
    3. Force fluids equal to the amount of output
    4. Expect difficulty in voiding

128. From her basic observations and background knowledge, which of the following facts are important to the nurse's understanding of Mr. S's postoperative nutritional needs?
    (a) Optimum protein and vitamin C are necessary to support wound healing and combat negative nitrogen balance
    (b) Sufficient calories are needed to spare protein for tissue synthesis
    (c) A rapid return to oral feedings is unnecessary because I.V. therapy with 5% dextrose solution will meet his energy needs
    (d) Mr. S's general nutritional status appears good, so he should have sufficient reserves to meet the stress of surgery
    1. a and b   3. b and c
    2. c and d   4. a and d

129. The label on the para-aminosalicylic acid indicates that each capsule contains 500 mg. of drug. To prepare each daily dose ordered, the nurse would use
    1. 3 capsules   3. 15 capsules
    2. 6 capsules   4. 18 capsules

130. The nurse takes the prepared dose of para-aminosalicylic acid to Mr. S who states, "I had more capsules than this yesterday." Which of the following replies would be most appropriate?

1. "I am certain this dose is the amount the doctor feels will be most beneficial to you."
2. "This is the number of capsules the doctor ordered for you."
3. "Permit me to recheck the order."
4. "This must be a new order."

131. Which of the following actions would be most appropriate if the nurse feels reasonably certain a medication error has occurred?
    1. Tell Mr. S he may have thought he received a different number of capsules but the chart proves otherwise
    2. Check the chart and relate the facts to the nurse in charge, who may investigate this situation
    3. Contact the other nurse involved so she can take the necessary steps to protect herself
    4. Recognize that no error is ever truly rectified, a principle that will guide her in discussing this situation

132. During the period of prescribed drug therapy, the nurse should be alert to which of these symptoms that may occur with para-aminosalicylic acid and streptomycin and produce permanent disability?
    1. Gastrointestinal upset
    2. Dermatitis
    3. Hearing loss
    4. Painful joint motion

133. The preferred site for injection of Crysticillin, a penicillin preparation, is the
    1. Anterior thigh
    2. Gluteal region
    3. Inner aspect of the gluteus maximus
    4. Triceps or deltoid muscle

134. Which of the following conditions must be considered first in determining the effectiveness of penicillin?
    1. Adequate concentration of the drug is maintained in the bloodstream
    2. Intramuscular method of administration is employed
    3. Infective organism is sensitive to the drug
    4. Treatment is continued a few days after the patient's temperature returns to normal

135. The chief disadvantage that may be encountered with the use of penicillin is that
    1. Bone marrow may become depressed
    2. Patient may be desensitized
    3. Organism may develop resistance
    4. Rate of absorption may vary

136. Side effects appearing after the injection of penicillin that may warrant emergency treatment include which of the following symptoms?
    1. Dyspnea   3. Palpitation
    2. Abdominal pain   4. Aphasia

137. The expected effect of pyridoxine hydrochloride is to
    1. Stimulate appetite and decrease nausea and vomiting
    2. Increase protein anabolism and amino acid catabolism
    3. Reverse peripheral neuritis if it occurs with isoniazid therapy
    4. Provide replacement therapy of an essential dietary nutrient

Situation: Mr. S J, age 45, who has smoked 3 to 4

packs of cigarettes per day for the last 25 years, was treated with irradiation of his larynx 3 months ago for squamous cell carcinoma of the larynx. For the past 2 weeks he has noted recurrent hoarseness that has progressively worsened. He now enters the hospital for evaluation and further therapy. He plays the harmonica professionally. Except for findings of hoarseness and a small mass in the left vocal cord, the remainder of his physical examination was unremarkable. Total laryngectomy with block dissection of the cervical lymph nodes was performed after appropriate diagnostic studies and preparation for surgery had been carried out. Mr. S J was discharged 14 days after surgery. (See questions 138 to 149.)

138. An important aspect of preoperative nursing care includes
1. Adequate explanation of the nature of surgery to be performed
2. Instruction in breathing exercises and/or equipment used postoperatively to prevent complications
3. Basing instruction on the needs of the patient
4. Having the speech therapist visit Mr. S J

139. Mr. S J is unable to sleep prior to surgery despite sedation and spends most of the time smoking and pacing his room. Nursing intervention should be aimed at
1. Providing further explanations to him
2. Informing his physician that the sedative is not effective
3. Having a laryngectomized patient visit him
4. Finding out what is bothering him

140. Nasogastric feedings will be required
1. For the rest of Mr. S J's life
2. Until healing has occurred
3. Until Mr. S J develops the ability to belch
4. Until Mr. S J can tolerate oral feedings

141. On the day Mr. S J was being discharged, he exhibited concern about the possibility of his laryngectomy tube becoming dislodged. The nurse should
1. Notify the doctor at once
2. Recognize that there is no immediate emergency
3. Recognize that prompt closure of the tracheal opening may occur
4. Reinsert another tube immediately

142. Immediate postoperative management would not include
1. Placing the patient in a high semi-Fowler position
2. Removing the outer tube p.r.n.
3. Application of suction to the tube at least every 10 to 15 minutes
4. Instructing the patient not to talk

143. Preoperatively, Mr. S J expresses concern about being able to return to his job. The nurse could best help Mr. S J by replying:
1. "Don't worry, esophageal speech is quite like regular speech."
2. "I can understand your concern. What has the doctor told you about esophageal speech?"
3. "Now is not the time to worry about returning to work. Let's take one thing at a time."

4. "Don't worry, the Musician's Society takes care of their members. They'll have a job for you."

144. Since Mr. S J's tracheostomy will be permanent, which of the following factors should be included in the teaching plans?
1. The sterile technique necessary for care of his tracheostomy tube
2. The establishment of a regular pattern for suctioning the tube
3. The importance of cleanliness around the site
4. The importance of covering the tube opening while bathing and swimming

145. The nurse can best help the patient communicate after surgery by
1. Teaching the patient to cover the tube while speaking
2. Teaching the patient preoperatively some simple signals to be used to express his needs postoperatively
3. Attempting to meet the patient's needs without his expressing them
4. Providing the patient with a slate board and chalk

146. On the second postoperative day the physician orders prochlorperazine (Compazine), 10 mg., to produce which of the following effects?
1. Increased rate of healing
2. Relief of pain
3. Relief of vomiting
4. Prevention of infection

147. Mr. S J's initial feedings were by nasogastric tube. Soon afterward he began to develop diarrhea. A possible solution to this problem would be to
1. Increase the carbohydrate content of the formula to give it more energy value
2. Decrease the protein content to make it easier to digest
3. Dilute the formula with water to give it more volume
4. Decrease the carbohydrate content of the formula and give it more slowly

148. Prior to dismissal from the hospital, Mr. S J asks the nurse to recommend a good laxative. She would most appropriately recommend which of the following?
1. Castor oil because it is considered "foolproof"
2. Glycerin suppositories, which act only on the rectal mucosa
3. The laxative that he has found works best for him
4. Consulting his physician so that he may evaluate Mr. S J's needs

149. If the physician wishes to prescribe bulk-forming laxatives for Mr. S J, which of the following agents is he likely to choose?
(a) Bran
(b) Magnesium sulfate
(c) Psyllium hydrophilic muciloid (Metamucil)
(d) Methylcellulose (Cellothyl)

1. c only
2. a and b
3. c and d
4. a, c, and d

Situation: Mrs. Jones, a 35-year-old mother of 4

...been diagnosed as having Cushing's... (See questions 150 to 158.)

...n planning her care, the nurse would take into consideration the fact that Mrs. Jones would
1. Be bothered by frequent urination
2. Probably be hypotensive
3. Have muscle weakness due to protein depletion
4. Probably have a high potassium blood level

151. Mrs. Jones would probably demonstrate which of the following symptoms?
1. Lability of mood
2. Decrease in the growth of hair
3. Thin body build with a hollowness of the face
4. Increased resistance to bruising

152. An adrenalectomy is performed. Postoperatively, until she is regulated on steroid therapy, Mrs. Jones may show symptoms of
1. Hyperglycemia
2. Sodium retention
3. Potassium excretion
4. Hypotension

153. In teaching Mrs. Jones about her medications, the nurse would stress the fact that
1. Once she is regulated, her dosage will remain the same for life
2. Taking her medications late in the evening may cause sleeplessness
3. While she is taking medications, her salt intake may be restricted
4. Steroid therapy should be given only in conjunction with insulin

154. After discharge from the hospital, Mrs. Jones returns home. If her children become ill with one of the communicable diseases, she should visit her doctor because
1. She will have lost all of her acquired immunities
2. The dosage of her medication should be decreased
3. Her ability to handle stress is decreased despite steroid therapy
4. Stress will cause feelings of exhaustion and lethargy

155. The most common cause of Cushing's syndrome is
1. Deprivation of cortical hormones
2. Excess of cortical hormones
3. Hyperplasia of adrenal cortex
4. Neoplasm of the pituitary gland

156. Intake and output measurements and recordings are important after surgery in this instance because
1. Hypofunction of the posterior pituitary gland may occur
2. Hyperfunction of the isles of Langerhans may occur
3. Neurogenic bladder may develop
4. Of the proximity of the incision to the bladder

157. Mrs. Jones' therapy included a low-sodium, high-potassium diet because
1. She began gaining too much weight
2. Excessive secretions of aldosterone and cortisone caused renal retention of sodium and loss of potassium

3. Her excessive habit of salt use had contributed to her disease
4. She was losing excess salt in her urine and required less renal stimulation

158. Mrs. Jones began to develop signs of diabetes mellitus, and her diet was further modified to provide adequate protein and control carbohydrate. The diabetes developed because
1. She had begun to eat excessive sweets because of her depression
2. The excessive glucocorticoids secreted by the adrenal gland caused excess tissue catabolism and consequent gluconeogenesis
3. A negative nitrogen balance resulted from the tissue catabolism
4. She had recently been losing weight rapidly

Situation: Mrs. B J Thompson, age 39, was admitted to the hospital with a diagnosis of Addison's disease. She exhibited the following signs and symptoms: muscular weakness, anorexia, emaciation, gastrointestinal symptoms, generalized dark pigmentation, hypotension, hypoglycemia, low sodium and high potassium, as well as a loss of libido. (See questions 159 to 169.)

159. The hypotension can be explained by the fact that Addison's disease involves a disturbance in the production of
1. Glucocorticoids
2. Androgens
3. Mineralocorticoids
4. Estrogens

160. The nurse should observe this patient closely for signs of infectious complication because there is a disturbance of function in
1. Proinflammatory effect
2. Anti-inflammatory effect
3. Metabolic effect
4. Electrolytic effect

161. The emaciation, muscular weakness, and fatigue are due to disturbance of function in
1. Protein anabolic effect
2. Electrolytic effect
3. Metabolic effect
4. Masculinizing effect

162. Where the patient shows concern about the fact that she is developing signs of masculinity, the nurse will most probably
1. Explain that it is a further sign of the illness she has
2. Explain that this is due to the therapy
3. Tell her not to worry, since it will disappear with therapy
4. Tell her that this is not important so long as she gets better

163. An important aspect of nursing care for Mrs. Thompson is
1. Encouraging exercise
2. Providing a variety of diversional activities
3. Permitting as much activity as the patient desires
4. Protecting from exertion

164. Therapy in Addison's disease is aimed chiefly at
1. Restoring electrolyte balance
2. Improving carbohydrate metabolism
3. Increasing lymphoid tissue
4. Increasing eosinophils

165. Mrs. Thompson's husband was quite disturbed when she developed a psychiatric disturbance following the steroid therapy. To alleviate his anxiety, the nurse will most probably tell him
1. The time for patients to respond to this therapy varies
2. Psychiatric complications of steroid, unlike its other complications, are irreversible
3. The prognosis for Mrs. Thompson's psychological integrity is related to her premorbid status
4. Mrs. Thompson may require surgery if the present therapy does not alleviate these symptoms

166. Mrs. Thompson's treatment included a high-protein, high-calorie diet with extra salt. As a means of encouraging her patient to eat, the nurse explained the reasons for this diet therapy as follows:
(a) Extra salt is needed to replace the amount being lost due to lack of sufficient aldosterone to conserve sodium
(b) Increased calories are needed to supply energy to help her regain lost weight
(c) Increased protein is needed to heal the adrenal tissue and hence cure the disease
(d) Increased amounts of potassium are needed to replace renal losses
1. a and b   3. c and d
2. a and d   4. b and c

167. Prior to dismissal, the physician prescribes hydrocortisone, 10 mg. t.i.d., and fludrocortisone, 0.1 mg. q.d. The purpose of hydrocortisone is to
1. Prevent hypoglycemia and permit Mrs. Thompson to respond to stress
2. Increase amounts of angiotensin II to raise Mrs. Thompson's blood pressure
3. Control excessive loss of potassium salts
4. Decrease cardiac arrhythmias and dyspnea

168. In order to help Mrs. Thompson remember to take her medicine as prescribed, which of the following suggestions is preferable?
1. Place each day's medicine in a dish on the kitchen table
2. Post a dosage schedule daily and cross through each dose after taking it
3. Keep the medicines on the dresser in her bedroom so she will take a dose when she awakens
4. Keep the medicine on the windowsill above the kitchen sink

169. Mrs. Thompson should be instructed to consult her physician immediately if she experiences which of these symptoms related to fludrocortisone?
1. Fatigue, particularly in the afternoon
2. Increased frequency of urination
3. Rapid weight gain and dependent edema
4. Unpredictable changes in mood

Situation: Mr. Greene, a 56-year-old married construction worker, has been in the hospital for 2 weeks with a diagnosis of cerebral thrombosis. His symptoms include aphasia, right-sided paresis, and loss of the gag reflex. (See questions 170 to 178.)

170. Due to the location of the lesion, Mr. Greene has effective aphasia. As part of the long-range planning, the nurse would

1. Help the family to accept the fact that Mr. Greene cannot be verbally communicated with
2. Wait for Mr. Greene to verbalize his needs regardless of how long it may take
3. Begin associating words to their physical objects
4. Help Mr. Greene accept this disability as permanent

171. Mr. Greene is still on bed rest and, even though his doctor has not ordered physical therapy for him, the nurse may institute
1. Active exercises of all extremities
2. Passive range of motion exercises
3. Light weight-lifting exercises of the right side
4. Exercises that would actively capitalize on returning muscle function

172. Mr. Greene's emotional responses to his illness would probably be determined by
1. His premorbid personality
2. The location of his lesion
3. The care he is receiving
4. His ability to understand his illness

173. Mr. Greene's wife insists on doing everything for him when she visits. After she leaves, Mr. Greene seems to be quite depressed. The nurse could assume
1. That Mr. Greene feels guilty about being a burden to his wife
2. This depression is a natural outcome of his illness
3. Mr. Greene feels the loss of his independence
4. Mr. Greene is losing faith in the future

174. Mrs. Greene seems unable to accept the idea that her husband must be encouraged to do things for himself. The nurse may be able to work around these feelings by
1. Telling Mrs. Greene to let her husband do things for himself
2. Letting Mrs. Greene know that the nursing staff has full responsibility for the patient's activities
3. Letting Mrs. Greene assume the responsibility as she sees fit
4. Asking Mrs. Greene for her assistance in planning the activities most helpful to the patient

175. Mr. Greene's position should be changed
1. Every hour   3. Every 4 hours
2. Every 2 hours   4. Every 6 hours

176. Since one of the primary nursing objectives is the maintenance of the airway, the nurse should place Mr. Greene in which of the following positions?
1. Sims' or semiprone
2. Prone
3. Semi-Fowler's
4. Orthopneic, or Fowler's

177. Since Mr. Greene was comatose on admission, the nurse would expect him to
1. Not be able to react to painful stimuli
2. Be incontinent
3. Be capable of spontaneous motion
4. Have twitching or picking motions

178. To support Mr. Greene's optimum nutrition, the nurse may find that he needs assistance with his eating. To accomplish this goal, the nurse may

(a) Explore with Mr. Greene and his family his food preferences and attempt to have them served for him

(b) Encourage him to participate in the feeding process to the extent of his capacity

(c) Do all the feeding for him so Mr. Greene can rest

(d) Feed him rapidly to get in as much as possible before he tires

(e) Leave the feeding entirely to a nursing aide

1. a and b   3. a and d
2. c and d   4. c and e

Situation: Mr. Ray is admitted to surgical unit with a diagnosis of cancer of the colon. His doctor plans to do a colon resection with a permanent colostomy. During the 3 days prior to surgery, Mr. Ray is very cooperative in all preoperative procedures, responds pleasantly when approached by the nurses, and does not question them about what is being done to him. (See questions 179 to 190.)

179. From his behavior the nurse recognizes that Mr. Ray most likely
1. Is totally denying his illness
2. Has been fully informed by his doctor on what to expect
3. Is not verbalizing his feelings about what will happen to him
4. Feels reassured by his frequent contacts with the nurses

180. The night before Mr. Ray's surgery the nurse notices that each time she makes rounds he is awake despite adequate sedation. He has no requests but invites her to have a cigarette with him. The nurse realizes that most likely Mr. Ray
1. Is responding to her friendly interest in him
2. Knows that he can't smoke at night without supervision
3. Is aware that the nurse might like to rest a moment
4. Is offering a cigarette as an attention-seeking device

181. Based on her understanding of Mr. Ray's behavior, the nurse's response would be to
1. Send in a nurse's aide to keep him company while he smokes
2. Point out to him that nurses cannot smoke in patients' rooms
3. Light his cigarette and tell him to call her again if he still can't sleep
4. Light his cigarette and indicate she has noticed his inability to sleep

182. During the rehabilitation period, when the nurse is discussing with Mr. Ray the regaining of some measure of bowel control, she would emphasize
1. Having a set time each day for his colostomy irrigation
2. The importance of a soft low-residue diet
3. The importance of limiting his fluid intake
4. The necessity for a high-protein diet

183. The most effective way of helping Mr. Ray to accept his colostomy would be to
1. Give him literature containing factual data about colostomies

2. Point out to him the number of important people who have had colostomies
3. Teach him self-care of his colostomy
4. Contact a member of Colostomies, Inc., to speak with him

184. During a colostomy irrigation, if Mr. Ray complains of abdominal cramps, the nurse should
1. Raise the irrigating can, so that the irrigation can be completed quickly
2. Reassure Mr. Ray and continue the irrigation
3. Pinch the tubing so that less fluid enters the colon
4. Clamp the tubing and allow Mr. Ray to rest

185. As a result of several catheterizations, Mr. Ray developed a mild cystitis. Which of the following is not a symptom of cystitis?
1. Pain in the region of the bladder
2. Inability to begin micturition
3. Pus and blood in the urine
4. Frequency in urination

Situation: To prepare Mr. Ray for colon surgery, the physician writes these drug orders: Terramycin 250 mg. four times daily; neomycin 0.5 Gm. four times daily; phospho-soda drams ii at 7 P.M. (See questions 186 to 190.)

186. The generic name for Terramycin is
1. Achromycin   3. Oxytetracycline
2. Chlortetracycline   4. Tetracycline

187. Which of the following groups of symptoms is indicative of side effects to Terramycin therapy?
1. Nausea, vomiting, loose stools
2. Dizziness, lack of coordination, deafness
3. Urticaria, dermatitis, pruritus
4. Leukopenia, anemia, ecchymoses

188. For which of the following reasons is neomycin especially useful prior to colon surgery?
1. It is effective against many organisms
2. It acts systemically without delay
3. It will not affect the kidneys
4. It is poorly absorbed from the gastrointestinal tract

189. Phospho-soda is classified as which of the following types of cathartics?
1. Drastic purgative
2. Saline cathartic
3. Emollient cathartic
4. Surface tension–lowering agent

190. Mr. Ray's postoperative diet order reads "diet as tolerated." Principles that should guide food choices include
(a) A low-residue diet should be followed indefinitely to avoid overstimulating the intestine
(b) A return to a regular diet as soon as possible gives psychological support and more rapid physical rehabilitation
(c) Those few foods that caused individual discomfort before the colostomy will likely continue to do so and can be avoided
(d) More rigid dietary rules limiting food choices are needed to provide security

1. a and d   3. a and c
2. b and c   4. b and d

Situation: Mrs. Smith is admitted to the hospital with an acute attack of ulcerative colitis. She has been very worried about her 2 small children and calls her mother frequently for help. She recently pleaded with her mother to come and live with them. Mr. Smith objects to this, goes out alone quite often, and does not seem to take an interest in the children. (See questions 191 to 199.)

191. The nurse will understand the organic aspects of psychosomatic disease more readily if she recognizes the "stress" functions of the
  1. Cerebral cortex and thyroid gland
  2. Sympathetic nervous system and the pancreas
  3. Autonomic nervous system and the adrenal glands
  4. Parasympathetic nervous system and the hypothalamus

192. The nurse observes that Mrs. Smith has many requests and rings often for the bedpan, cold drinking water, etc. When the nurse answers her call for the fifth time, Mrs. Smith states, "I'm an awful pest aren't I? You don't like taking care of me." The nurse replies:
  1. "No, you're not a pest. I know you're sick and not your usual self."
  2. "I want to take care of you, that's why I'm here."
  3. "Why do you say that? You know we understand how you feel."
  4. "You do seem to have a lot of requests. You must not be feeling well."

193. In order to give complete nursing care to Mrs. Smith, it would be most important for the nurse to
  1. Understand the patient's emotional conflict
  2. Recognize her own feelings toward this patient
  3. Talk with the patient's husband and mother
  4. Develop rapport with the patient's doctor

194. The prognosis for Mrs. Smith will remain guarded until
  1. A surgical procedure is performed to remove the somatic factor
  2. Her husband accepts her desire to have her mother move in with them
  3. Her emotional conflicts are resolved
  4. She reaches her 40's and endocrine activity is decreased

195. Which of the following symptoms most accurately describe this condition?
  1. Diarrhea, anorexia, weight loss, abdominal cramps, anemia
  2. Anemia, nausea and vomiting, weight loss, abdominal cramps
  3. Fever, anemia, nausea and vomiting, leukoptosis, diarrhea
  4. Leukocytosis, anorexia, weight loss

196. A serious complication of this disease is
  1. Hemorrhage   3. Obstruction
  2. Perforation   4. Ileus

197. Mrs. Smith's initial hospital diet is residue-free during the acute stage. Which of these food combinations would be the best choice for her?
  1. Lean roast beef, buttered white rice with egg slices, white bread with butter and jelly, tea with sugar
  2. Cream soup and crackers, omelet, mashed potatoes, roll, orange juice, coffee
  3. Stewed chicken, baked potato with butter, strained peas, white bread, plain cake, milk
  4. Baked fish, macaroni with cheese, strained carrots, fruit jello, milk

198. After she begins to improve, Mrs. Smith's diet is increased to supply her need for
  (a) High calories (3,000 calories) with ample fat to supply energy
  (b) Frequent feedings of milk and cream to soothe the gastrointestinal lining
  (c) High protein (150 gm.) to replace loss from intestinal lesions and poor absorption and to support healing
  (d) High calories, mostly of easily digested and absorbed carbohydrate, to restore nutritional deficits and spare protein for tissue synthesis
  (e) Low-residue foods to avoid irritation to the colon
    1. a, b, and e   3. c, d, and e
    2. a, b, and c   4. b, c, and d

199. Potassium chloride, 40 mEq., is to be added to each liter of intravenous solution. Parenteral preparations of potassium are administered slowly and cautiously to prevent which of the following conditions?
  1. Acidosis
  2. Cardiac arrest
  3. Edema of the extremities
  4. Psychotic-like reactions

Situation: Mr. Brown is a 68-year-old retired widower who lives alone. He has a 10-year history of arthritis and has just been admitted to the hospital in an acute episode. (See questions 200 to 209.)

200. In planning the nursing care for Mr. Brown, the nurse would take into consideration the fact that
  1. If redness and swelling of a joint occurs, it signifies irreversible damage
  2. Bony ankylosis of the joint is irreversible and causes immobility
  3. Inflammation of the synovial membrane will rarely occur
  4. Complete immobility is desired during the acute phase of inflammation

201. Range of motion exercises are ordered for Mr. Brown. In planning his nursing care, you would take into consideration the fact that
  1. The exercises would be discontinued if they caused even slight pain
  2. Passive exercises should be done to all his joints
  3. Exercises are done only to the joints that are actually inflamed
  4. The joints need protection against overuse, wobbling, and partial dislocations

202. A regimen of rest, exercise, and physical therapy will
  1. Help prevent the crippling effects of the disease

2. Prevent arthritic pain
3. Provide for the regaining of joint motion that has been lost for a prolonged period
4. Halt the inflammatory process

203. The most important factor to be considered in the motivation of a patient is his
1. Age and occupation
2. Role in the family and society
3. Lifetime values and attitudes
4. Physical capacity and ability

204. The occurrence of a chronic illness that limits major activity is
1. Present to the same degree in every group
2. Greatest in children because of the prevalence of congenital defects
3. Greatest in the older age group
4. Greatest in the middle years of life

205. Mr. Brown reports that over the years the following diet suggestions have been given him for his arthritis. Which of these recommendations for his daily diet intake is valid?
1. Yogurt and blackstrap molasses
2. Wheat germ and yeast
3. A variety of meats, fruits, vegetables, milk, cereal grains
4. Multiple vitamin supplements in large doses

206. Drug therapy includes large doses of acetylsalicylic acid and sodium bicarbonate. Acetylsalicylic acid is prescribed and expected to produce which of the following systemic effects when gout is present?
(a) Analgesic
(b) Antipyretic
(c) Decreased renal threshold of uric acid
(d) Increased excretion of uric acid
1. a and c   3. a, c, and d
2. b and d   4. All the above

207. Which of the following dosage forms of acetylsalicylic acid is preferable for Mr. Brown, who has a past history of gastric ulcers?
1. Dulcets
2. Gelatin capsules containing powdered aspirin
3. Enteric-coated tablets
4. Rectal suppositories

208. For which of the following purposes might sodium bicarbonate be prescribed concomitant with large doses of acetylsalicylic acid?
1. To help prevent gastrointestinal irritation
2. To change the pH of urine
3. To increase the secretion of uric acid
4. To lower the serum level of acetylsalicylic acid

209. One of the drugs that may be prescribed and that has long been known to be of value in the prevention and treatment of acute attacks of gout is
1. Hydrocortisone
2. Colchicine
3. Phenylbutazone (Butazolidin)
4. Probenecid (Benemid)

Situation: Mrs. Rifkin is a 33-year-old housewife who is admitted to the hospital with an acute episode of bronchial asthma. She has a long history of asthma dating back to her childhood. (See questions 210 to 218.)

210. Mrs. Rifkin is experiencing difficulty in breathing due to
1. Spasms of the bronchi, which trap the air
2. A too rapid expulsion of air
3. An increase in the vital capacity of the lungs
4. Hyperventilation due to an anxiety reaction

211. Treatment in asthma is aimed at
1. Raising mucus secretions from the chest
2. Limiting pulmonary secretions by decreasing fluid intake
3. Curing the condition permanently
4. Convincing the patient that her condition is emotionally caused

212. It will be important for Mrs. Rifkin to understand that
1. She can control and limit her asthmatic attacks if she wants to
2. She should try to limit coughing, since this causes distention of the chest
3. By controlling her anxiety she will decrease the severity of future attacks
4. She will be quite prone to other respiratory tract infections

213. Mrs. Rifkin is found to be allergic to dust. The teaching plan for her should include the fact that
1. She will probably be unable to do her own housework in the future
2. It is imperative that her entire house be redecorated, since she must live in a dust-free environment
3. Damp-dusting her house will help limit dust particles in the air
4. She may as well accept her condition, since dust cannot be avoided

214. One of the most common complications of chronic asthma is
1. Atelectasis
2. Emphysema
3. Pneumothorax
4. Pulmonary fibrosis

215. The physician ordered aminophylline to be given in the form of a suppository at the hour of sleep. The most desirable effect of this therapy is
1. Rest and relaxation
2. Evacuation of lower bowel
3. Relaxation of bronchial muscles
4. Mild diuresis

216. Inhalation of isoproterenol (Isuprel), 1:200 p.r.n., is prescribed. For which of the following reasons was isoproterenol prescribed?
1. To increase bronchial secretions
2. To decrease blood pressure
3. To produce sedation
4. To relax bronchial spasm

217. Mrs. Rifkin should be instructed to
1. Inhale the vapors until all the drug has been nebulized
2. Stop inhaling the vapors as soon as she obtains relief
3. Never to inhale more than 0.3 ml. during any 20-minute period
4. Not to repeat the dose more frequently than every 4 hours

218. During therapy with isoproterenol, Mrs. Rifkin complains of palpitation, chest pain, and

a throbbing headache. In view of these symptoms, which of the following statements represents the most appropriate nursing action?

1. Reassure Mrs. Rifkin that these effects are temporary and will subside as she becomes used to the drug
2. Withhold the drug until additional orders are obtained from the physician
3. Tell her not to worry; she is experiencing expected side effects from the medicine
4. Ask her to relax; then instruct her to breathe slowly and deeply for several minutes

Situation: Mr. O is 68 years old. He is recovering from a herniorrhaphy. He also has chronic pulmonary emphysema. He tells the nurse it will soon rain. (See questions 219 to 225.)

219. The nurse
1. Determines his orientation to reality
2. Checks his chart to see if he has arthritis
3. Notes the quality of his respirations
4. Begins to question his ability to expectorate
220. This is because
1. Humidity affects the viscosity of secretions
2. Many patients with pulmonary emphysema are senile
3. Arthritis may often accompany emphysema
4. Anxiety can cause physiologic changes in respiration
221. Emphysema causes a failure in oxygen supply because of
1. Infectious obstructions
2. Respiratory muscle paralysis
3. Pleural effusion
4. Loss of aerating surface
222. The nurse should be aware of complications involving
1. Kidney function
2. Peripheral edema
3. Cardiac function
4. Joint inflammation
223. Respiratory acidosis may occur as a result of a long-term problem in oxygen maintenance when
1. The carbon dioxide is not excreted
2. Any localized tissue necrosis occurs as a result of poor oxygen supply to the area
3. Hyperventilation occurs, even if the cause is not physiologic
4. There is a loss of carbon dioxide from the body's buffer pool
224. When she is caring for a patient who has a problem with hyperventilation, the most significant factor the nurse should consider is that
1. Respiratory alkalosis may occur because of a fall in the carbon dioxide content of the blood
2. The patient may very well be approaching congestive heart failure
3. The patient is probably experiencing a great deal of anxiety
4. The patient will experience giddiness and euphoria
225. When the alveoli lose their normal elasticity, exercises that lead to effective use of the diaphragm should be initiated because

1. The patient has an increase in the vital capacity of his lungs
2. The residual capacity of the lungs has been increased
3. Inspiration has been markedly prolonged and difficult
4. Abdominal breathing is an effective compensatory mechanism that is spontaneously initiated

Situation: Jane Bond, a 15-year-old young lady, is brought into the emergency room after being found unconscious in the locker room at school. There is a strong odor of acetone to her breath and her face is flushed. (See questions 226 to 243.)

226. When Jane regains consciousness, she refuses to talk to the staff about her condition. Her mother states she has been a known diabetic for 3 years. The nurse without further information could assume that Jane may
1. Be rejecting her illness
2. Be feeling guilty about taking an overdose of insulin
3. Be mentally retarded due to diabetic anoxia
4. Be uncooperative and resistive with authority figures
227. After developing a relationship with the nurse, Jane tells her that she has not been adhering to her diabetic regimen. As a first step in attempting to help Jane develop some understanding of the importance of a diabetic regimen, the nurse would
1. Give her printed material about diabetes in teen-agers
2. Impress the mother with duty of helping and understanding Jane
3. Allow Jane to express her feelings about diabetes
4. Assume that Jane has not been properly taught previously
228. In talking with the nurse, Jane states she will never marry because of her diabetes. Which of the following responses by the nurse would be most helpful?
1. "You may feel that way now but when Mr. Right comes along you'll feel different."
2. "You seem to be quite concerned about the future."
3. "Aren't you a bit young to be thinking such serious thoughts?"
4. "Why? Are you afraid diabetes is hereditary?"
229. The cause of Jane's symptoms is a
1. Sudden increase in the concentration of cholesterol in the extracellular compartment
2. Physiologic phenomenon following the ingestion of too much highly acidic food
3. Rise in the pH of the blood to a point above 7.5
4. Decrease in the pH of the blood to a point below 7.3
230. Several laboratory tests were done. Jane's symptoms would cause one to expect the blood test to reveal
1. Low sugar, decreased acidity, low CO_2 combining power

2. Elevated sugar, normal acidity, high CO_2 combining power
3. Low sugar, increased acidity, high CO_2 combining power
4. Elevated sugar, increased acidity, low CO_2 combining power

231. In the exchange system of dietary management, which of the following is not equivalent?
1. 1 scoop ice milk = 1 slice bread
2. 1 oz. cheese = 1 cup milk
3. 1 egg = 1 oz. meat
4. 1 slice bacon = 2 tbsp. cream

232. Jane and her mother should be instructed about
1. Weighing all her food on a gram scale
2. Eating all her meals at home
3. Preparing her food separately from the rest of the family
4. Always carrying some form of sugar with her

233. After initial treatment to correct the acidosis, Jane is moved to the medical ward. She is average height and weight (5′ 3″, 114 lb.), and the diet ordered for her is 2,200 calories, 75 gm. protein, 250 gm. carbohydrate, and 100 gm. fat. She is receiving NPH insulin mixed with regular insulin, according to need. In planning a menu pattern for a juvenile diabetic such as Jane, principles to consider include
1. Limit calories to encourage weight loss
2. Allow for normal growth and development needs
3. Avoid using potatoes, bread, and cereal
4. Discourage substitutions on the menu pattern

234. The diet for a juvenile diabetic should be
1. Restricted only in carbohydrate
2. A detailed pattern of special foods
3. A list of specific foods to be eaten regularly
4. A basic menu pattern that can be varied by substituting different foods of equal nutrient content

235. A night feeding planned for Jane included milk, crackers, cheese. This will provide
1. High carbohydrate nourishment for immediate utilization
2. Nourishment with latent effect to counteract late insulin activity
3. Encouragement for her to stay on her diet
4. Added calories to help her gain weight

236. The type of insulin that will be used during the emergency treatment of the acidosis and until Jane is eating regularly is
1. Isophane insulin suspension (NPH insulin)
2. Protamine zinc insulin suspension
3. Insulin zinc suspension (lente insulin)
4. Insulin injection (regular insulin)

237. Jane's hypotensive state helps the nurse to anticipate early institution of intravenous fluid therapy. Which of the following solutions would be most appropriate?
1. 5% dextrose in water
2. Hyperalimentation solution
3. 0.9% sodium chloride
4. Dextran

238. A diagnosis of diabetic ketoacidosis is established, and 50 units of insulin is given intravenously. The physician also orders 50 units of insulin to be given subcutaneously immediately. The label on the insulin bottle reads 40 u = 1 ml. The amount of solution needed to give the dose subcutaneously will be
1. 1.25 ml.   3. 2.5 ml.
2. 0.8 ml.   4. 4.0 ml.

239. In order to rehydrate Jane, it is desirable to increase the rate of flow of the intravenous solution as increases occur in
1. Central venous pressure
2. Blood hematocrit readings
3. Glycosuria
4. Urinary volume

240. After blood studies and observation of urinary volume, the physician orders KCl, 20 mEq., to be added to the intravenous solution. The primary purpose for administering this drug to Jane is
1. Replacement of potassium deficit
2. Treatment of hyperpnea
3. Prevention of flaccid paralysis
4. Treatment of cardiac arrhythmias

241. Jane and her family members should be taught the use of glucagon. The primary use of glucagon is to treat
1. Diabetic acidosis
2. Insulin-induced hypoglycemia
3. Idiosyncratic reactions to insulin
4. Hyperinsulin secretion related to neoplasm

242. The usual amount of glucagon that is administered is
1. 1 mg.   3. 0.4 mg.
2. 2.5 mg.   4. 1.2 mg.

243. The methods that may be used to administer glucagon are
1. Inhalation, sublingual, injection
2. Intramuscular, intravenous, subcutaneous
3. Orally, rectally, injection
4. Intramuscular, subcutaneous, intradermal

Situation: Mr. S Z, age 35, is an architectural engineer, married and the father of 5 children. His wife states that she has noted several outstanding changes in her husband's behavior during the past few months. He no longer shows any interest in his family or home, he uses obscene language, and he is extremely untidy and careless in his appearance. Since brain tumor was suspected, Mr. Z was immediately hospitalized. (See questions 244 to 250.)

244. The symptoms exhibited by Mr. Z indicate that there is probably involvement of the
1. Motor cortex   3. Frontal lobe
2. Occipital lobe   4. Cerebellum

245. Mr. Z is given a complete neurologic workup. On the basis of this it was decided that surgery should be performed immediately. The test that most likely would just precede the surgery, if it is to be done, would be
1. Electroencephalogram
2. Ventriculogram
3. Cerebral angiogram
4. Pneumoencephalogram

246. Postoperatively the earliest complication the nurse should watch for is

1. Shock   3. Aphasia
2. Respiratory failure   4. Paralysis
247. In the rehabilitation of Mr. Z, nursing care would include
1. Helping the patient to recover
2. Making the patient comfortable and as happy as possible
3. Keeping Mrs. Z informed of the progress of her husband
4. Helping Mrs. Z accept her responsibility in the care of her husband
248. The question of whether or not a patient is told that he has cancer is dependent on the
1. Feelings of the physician
2. Distress of the patient
3. Cooperation of the patient
4. Needs of the patient
249. Orders included "observation of vital signs for increased intracranial pressure." Which of the following would the nurse consider significant?
1. Increase in BP, increase in P, decrease in R
2. Falling BP, increase in P and R
3. Decrease in BP, increase in P and R
4. Rise in BP, decrease in P and R
250. When she is observing for an increase in intracranial pressure, the aspect of pulse pressure that the nurse should note is the
1. Difference between the normal pulse rate of the patient and his present pulse rate
2. Diastolic reading as recorded by the sphygmomanometer
3. Perceptible intensity of pressure felt when counting the radial pulse
4. Difference between systolic and diastolic pressures

Situation: Miss R, 32 years old, is admitted to the emergency room with second-degree burns over 40% of her body and face, which she received when her nightgown caught fire. (See questions 251 to 268.)

251. Her condition would be considered
1. Good   3. Poor
2. Fair   4. Critical
252. Which of the following would not be a problem during the first few hours after the incident?
1. Edema of the larynx and trachea
2. Maintenance of blood volume
3. Rapid decrease in leukocyte count
4. Pain
253. Which of the following behaviors displayed by Miss R during her convalescent period would most concern the nurse?
1. Removal of the mirror from the room
2. Requesting each of her visitors to bring her facial makeup
3. Crying and saying "Why did this happen to me?"
4. Refusing to see visitors
254. Intravenous fluid replacement therapy is important to the patient with burns. Which of the following would be expected in the first 24 hours?
1. Intake 8,000 ml.   output   480 ml.
2. Intake 12,000 ml.   output 4,500 ml.

3. Intake 3,000 ml.   output 2,400 ml.
4. Intake 6,000 ml.   output 1,200 ml.
255. Fluid shifts are a great danger to the patient with burns. Which of the following would be expected to occur?
1. Increased fluid shifts after 2 hours, which result in irreversible shock
2. Loss of sodium and increase in blood potassium
3. Decreased capillary permeability
4. Rise in blood volume
256. After the "turning point," when Miss R begins to recover, the nurse should
1. Help her maintain complete immobility
2. Prevent her from picking or scratching newly formed scales
3. Help her overcome the emotional trauma by forcing her to talk about the incident
4. Make her take fluids by mouth even if nausea is present
257. To maintain Miss R's nutrition during convalescence, which of the following measures would be most important?
1. Reduce protein intake so as not to overtax the kidneys
2. Limit caloric intake so as to decrease the work of the body
3. Encourage the intake of orange juice or other fluids containing vitamin C
4. Encourage excessive intake of sodium
258. Which of the following statements is true of the recovery and convalescent period for the patient with extensive burns?
1. Death may still occur from septicemia
2. The danger of physical complications is past
3. Diversional therapy cannot be initiated as yet, due to the need for rest
4. All mirrors should be removed from the room to decrease the patient's anxiety about her appearance
259. In the immediate shock period after Miss R's injury, nutritional care centered on replacement therapy by I.V. fluids. These initial fluid replacements included
(a) Colloid (protein) through blood or plasma transfusions or by use of plasma expanders such as dextran
(b) Electrolytes sodium and chloride by use of a saline solution such as lactated Ringer's solution
(c) Potassium added to replace losses
(d) Water (dextrose solution) to cover additional insensible losses
1. a, b, and d   3. b, c, and d
2. All of these   4. a, b, and c
260. In the secondary feeding period after recovery from the shock and balance of circulating fluids and electrolytes, vigorous nutritional therapy is mandatory because
(a) Tissue destruction by the burn has caused large losses of protein and electrolytes
(b) Tissue catabolism follows, with continuing nitrogen losses
(c) Energy needs require extra protein and vitamin D
(d) Infection and fever may require reduction in calories

(e) Tissue regeneration in the healing process requires extra protein and vitamin C
1. a, b, and e
2. a, b, and c
3. c, d, and e
4. b, c, and d

261. Miss R's diet program should be planned to include
(a) High-protein, low-calorie feedings
(b) A high-protein, high-calorie, high-vitamin intake
(c) Concentrated oral liquids using protein hydrolysates to ensure adequate intake
(d) A careful record of protein and calorie value in the amount of food consumed
1. a and c
2. b and d
3. b, c, and d
4. a and d

262. It can be anticipated that the physician will wish to prevent tetanus from developing. If it is impossible to determine whether Miss R has been immunized against tetanus, which of the following preparations would produce passive immunization for several weeks with minimal danger of allergic reactions?
1. Tetanus antitoxin
2. Tetanus toxoid
3. Tetanus immune globulin
4. DPT vaccine

263. An antacid is prescribed to prevent this condition which tends to occur 2 weeks after the burn
1. Curling's ulcer
2. Gastric ulcer
3. Colitis
4. Gastritis

264. An indwelling catheter is inserted and Gantanol, 0.5 Gm., is to be administered 2 times daily. The nurse who finds only Gantrisin in Miss R's individual supply of medications would most appropriately
1. Call the pharmacist's attention to his error in filling the prescription
2. Ask the physician to correct the written order
3. Request the head nurse to correct the medication card
4. Inquire if a preparation called Gantanol exists

265. Sulfisoxazole (Gantrisin), which is often used to combat urinary infections, belongs to which of the following groups of drugs?
1. Antibiotics
2. Analgesics
3. Sulfones
4. Sulfonamides

266. Sometimes Azogantrisin rather than Gantrisin is prescribed. Azogantrisin contains phenazopyridine (Pyridium). The latter agent will act to produce which of the following effects?
1. Enhance the activity of Gantrisin
2. Sterilize the urine
3. Anesthetize the bladder
4. Relieve symptoms of frequency and burning

267. Which of the following systemic drugs is most likely to be ordered to treat urinary infection due to strains of Escherichia coli that are insensitive to the action of Gantrisin?
1. Nitrofurantoin (Furadantin)
2. Protargol (strong silver protein)
3. Penicillinamine
4. Chloramphenicol (Chloromycetin)

268. When the catheter is removed, Miss R continues to be unable to empty her bladder.

Drugs used to relieve urinary retention include which of the following?
(a) Bethanechol (Urecholine)
(b) Pilocarpine hydrochloride
(c) Carbachol injection
(d) Neostigmine (Prostigmin)
1. a and c
2. b and d
3. a and d
4. c and d

Situation: Mr. A M, age 84, was admitted to the hospital with the following signs and symptoms: severe dyspnea, marked generalized edema of lower extremities, penis, scrotum, back and abdomen, confusion, irritability, and frequent complaint of low back pain. Three months earlier he had been hospitalized for acute urinary retention, at which time a transurethral prostatectomy (TUR) was done, followed by bilateral orchidectomy and hormonal therapy when the pathology report revealed carcinoma of the prostate. Laboratory findings indicate markedly elevated chemistries. Corticosteroids are presently being administered. (See questions 269 to 274.)

269. In cancer of the prostate it is possible to follow the course of the disease through the study of
1. Serum acid phosphatase
2. Creatinine
3. Blood urea nitrogen
4. Nonprotein nitrogen

270. The confusion and irritability are probably due to
1. Brain metastasis
2. Uremia
3. Drug therapy
4. Senility

271. Mr. A M requests the urinal at frequent intervals but either does not void or voids in very small amounts. This is most likely due to
1. Renal failure
2. Edema
3. Retention
4. Suppression

272. Nursing care is primarily
1. Palliative
2. Preventive
3. Therapeutic
4. Rehabilitative

273. An important aspect of nursing care for this patient would be
1. Keeping the patient in Fowler's position
2. Avoiding pressure areas
3. Avoiding injection of medications into edematous tissue
4. Taking and recording a daily weight

274. The low back pain is due to cancerous tissue causing
1. Displacement of vital organs
2. Ulceration and infection
3. Compression of vital tissues or organs
4. Replacement of healthy tissue

Situation: Mrs. J H, age 30, a chemist, is the mother of 2 young children. For the past few months she has noticed that she tires easily, has painless swelling of the lymph nodes, and has been running a low-grade fever with excessive diaphoresis at night. She also has anorexia with loss of weight. She does not recall having any serious illness except that once during the winter she experienced what she believed was a virus infection. On her admission to the hospital the doctor ordered a complete medical examination for Mrs. J H. On the basis of diagnostic tests, Mrs. J H is said to have Hodgkin's disease. (See questions 275 to 280.)

275. The lymph nodes usually affected first are the
1. Inguinal   3. Cervical
2. Axillary   4. Mediastinal

276. The nature of the above symptoms would seem to indicate that Mrs. J H has systemic involvement; therefore the choice of treatment will probably be
1. External irradiation therapy
2. Internal irradiation therapy
3. Surgery
4. Chemotherapy

277. The highest incidence of Hodgkin's disease is in
1. Children
2. Young adults
3. Middle-aged persons
4. Elderly persons

278. In etiology, this disease is believed due to
1. Genetic causes
2. Infectious process
3. Precancerous conditions
4. Chronic irritation

279. An important supportive and protective measure for Mrs. J H is
1. Correction of anemia
2. Relief of pain
3. Hydration and nutrition
4. Control of infection

280. Common symptoms that might be expected after therapy for Mrs. J H are
1. Chills and fever
2. Nausea and vomiting
3. Pruritus and sensitive skin
4. Fatigue and weakness

Situation: Mr. Clark has had a history of Buerger's disease for 2 years. He now enters the hospital for further evaluation and treatment. (See questions 281 to 285.)

281. Common symptoms of this disease are
(a) Burning pain precipitated by exposure to cold
(b) Intermittent claudication
(c) Easy fatigue of the part
(d) Blanching of the skin of a lower extremity
1. a, b, and c   3. c, d, and a
2. b, d, and a   4. d, c, and b

282. Although Mr. Clark has been told to discontinue smoking, he persists in his habit. The most effective nursing intervention would be
1. Controlling his purchasing of cigarettes
2. Having other patients who are in various stages of this disease visit him
3. Satisfying his oral needs in another manner
4. Providing him with filter tip cigarettes

283. In an effort to help increase collateral circulation, Mr. Clark will be instructed to
1. Engage in passive and active exercises as indicated
2. Use only warm clothing to keep his feet warm
3. Abstain completely from tobacco
4. Prevent injury and infection

284. When teaching Buerger-Allen exercises to this patient it is most important that the nurse include in her instructions

1. The effects and symptoms of tissue anoxia
2. That the exercises should not exceed a period of 15 minutes
3. The fact that the exercises should be repeated 5 times, at least 3 times a day
4. That fatigue and pain are important symptoms to be aware of

285. Postoperatively, Mr. Clark's most important intake needs include all of the following except:
1. High-protein diet
2. Increased potassium
3. Supplemental vitamin B_{12}
4. Carbohydrate

286. In a disaster situation a victim having the following symptoms would receive priority in care:
1. Cold, clammy skin
2. Bleeding from femoral artery
3. Expectoration of pinkish sputum
4. Decerebrate rigidity

287. Treatment could not be delayed for a patient with
1. Head injury
2. Ventricular fibrillation
3. Penetrating abdominal wound
4. Fractured femur

Situation: While returning from his job as department manager for an NYC store, Mr. Smith was conscious he again had a headache. By the time he reached home he felt slightly dizzy and had a sudden severe episode of epistaxis. On his last annual physical examination, it was noted that Mr. Smith was 57 years old, weighed 195 pounds, was 5 feet 9 inches tall, smoked 1 pack of cigarettes per day, and had a BP of 168/96. A slight enlargement of the heart was noted on x-ray film, and his ECG was normal. The doctor at that time told him he had hypertension and should "take it easy." (See questions 288 to 297.)

288. At the time of Mr. Smith's episode of epistaxis, headache, and dizziness, one knowing he had cardiac enlargement with hypertension might consider that he is on which adaptive level?
1. Maintenance of homeostasis without undue effort
2. Maintenance of homeostasis under stress, with effort required
3. Damage or loss at any level of organization, which requires development of compensatory adaptive mechanisms
4. Compensatory adaptive mechanisms as a problem

289. To help Mr. Smith follow his doctor's direction to "take it easy," the nurse would need to know
(a) The nature of his job
(b) Mr. Smith's attitude concerning expectations of himself
(c) How much sleep he gets
(d) The relationship of stress and his condition
1. b, c, and d   3. a, c, and b
2. a, b, and d   4. c, d, and a

290. In talking with the nurse he voiced concern that he may have a stroke "since his father had died of a stroke and he had high blood

pressure, too." The nurse's response could be based on her knowledge that
1. Heredity plays a large part in incidence of hypertension and stroke
2. The overweight male who smokes is prone to stroke
3. Therapy is directed toward assisting the patient's adaptive capacity
4. Stroke is inevitable; therefore, she should give emotional support

291. To anticipate any further complications of Mr. Smith's condition on future visits to the health department, the nurse should be aware that hypertension may cause
(a) Changes in patient's vision
(b) Congestive heart failure
(c) Coronary artery disease
(d) Renal changes
   1. a, b, and c   3. c, d, and a
   2. b, c, and d   4. All of these

292. The physiology of arterial hypertension involves
1. Increased cardiac output
2. Increased peripheral resistance
3. Thickening of walls of arterioles
4. Hypertrophy of muscle of left ventricle

293. A wise weight reduction diet for Mr. Smith would be based on the following principles:
(a) Sufficient calorie reduction in relation to energy expenditure to effect a gradual weight loss
(b) Nutritional adequacy ensured by large amounts of extra vitamins
(c) A balanced ratio of protein, carbohydrate, and fat, supplied by a variety of foods
(d) A food plan suited to Mr. Smith's living situation and personal desires, one that can form the basis for permanent reduction of his eating habits
   1. a, c, and d   3. a, b, and c
   2. b, c, and d   4. a, b, and d

294. A realistic goal for Mr. Smith in terms of overall weight loss and rate of loss would be
1. A 60 lb. loss in the next 2 months
2. A loss of about 35 lb. at the rate of 1 or 2 lb. a week
3. About a 10 lb. loss during the next year
4. Maintaining present weight and avoiding any further gain

295. Mr. Smith is advised to build an exercise component into his weight reduction program. The best way he could accomplish this goal is by
(a) Taking a rapid walk each day during his lunch hour
(b) Doing 50 push-ups before breakfast every morning
(c) Playing two rounds of golf every Saturday
(d) Riding a bicycle or swimming daily
(e) Actively working out in a nearby gym several times a month
   1. a and d   3. a and b
   2. b and c   4. c and d

296. Mr. Smith is also advised by his physician to restrict the amount of sodium in his diet to 1 gm. daily. To accomplish this, he will need to make all the following modifications except one. Which is it?
1. Eliminate all salt in cooking or seasoning

2. Eliminate foods processed with salt
3. Use less milk and meat daily
4. Avoid fruits and fruit juices
5. Omit canned vegetables and certain fresh ones such as leafy greens, carrots, beets, celery

297. To impove the flavor of his food, Mr. Smith may season it with all of these except
1. Lemon juice or vinegar
2. Celery, onion, or garlic salt
3. Salt substitute
4. Herbs and spices
5. Onion and garlic

Situation: Plans are being made for survival in the event of thermonuclear warfare. (See questions 298 to 303.)

298. Realize that radiation can best be detected by
1. Observing a dust cloud in the air
2. Special measuring instruments
3. A pricking sensation on the skin
4. Observing that people around you suddenly become ill

299. Since a supply of water or other liquids safe for drinking is a basic requirement for survival, what is the approximate daily amount to be provided, per adult?
1. 1 to 2 pints   3. 6 to 8 quarts
2. 1 to 2 quarts   4. 1 gallon

300. If you were planning treatment of persons with possible radiation exposure and one developed nausea, you would
1. Give him a remedy to settle his stomach
2. Undress and bathe him and keep him in bed
3. Listen for emergency instructions on the radio
4. Remove him from the presence of other people

301. In planning for shelter living, with limited water supply, the most important use of water is for drinking. Second in importance of the uses of water is
1. Flushing toilets   3. Washing hands
2. Washing clothes   4. Washing dishes

302. In nursing patients with radiation sickness, the nurse recognizes that
1. Radiation sickness is contagious
2. Food and water exposed to fallout radiation are contaminated
3. People who have fallout particles on their clothing probably would not carry enough to endanger other people
4. Fallout radiation can make everything radioactive

303. Which of the following is most vital for life?
1. Water   3. Air
2. Food   4. Shelter

Situation: Mr. H V, age 39, was admitted to the hospital with the following diagnosis: rheumatic heart disease, inactive, with enlarged heart, mitral stenosis and aortic insufficiency, atrial fibrillation, congestive heart failure, Class III D. Therapy instituted included that specific for patients in heart failure. (See questions 304 to 318.)

304. The symptom(s) that this patient most likely presented on admission is (are)

1. Dyspnea, edema, and fatigue
2. Weakness, palpitations, and nausea
3. Fatigue, vertigo, and headache
4. A feeling of distress when breathing

305. According to the therapeutic classification, this patient will most probably be
   1. Placed on complete bed rest
   2. Given bathroom privileges only
   3. Out of bed ad lib.
   4. Out of bed in chair b.i.d.

306. The nurse's most important responsibility in relation to the digitalized patient is
   1. Administration of the drug at the time and in quantities prescribed by the physician
   2. Observation of effects on the patient
   3. Stopping the drug if the patient's pulse is 60 or less
   4. Correlation of the fluid intake with the output

307. The marked salt retention that occurs will most probably be treated by
   1. Administration of salt-free diet and fluids ad lib.
   2. Restriction of salt intake and fluids
   3. Administration of salt intake and fluids as desired
   4. Restriction of salt intake and fluids ad lib.

308. Mr. H V's bed position should be
   1. Flat, to decrease edema formation in the extremities
   2. Semi-Fowler, to ease the dyspnea
   3. Upright, to decrease pulmonary edema
   4. Position of comfort, to relax the patient

309. Careful hygiene for Mr. H V is
   1. Contraindicated because of need for rest
   2. Of great importance, since edematous tissue is not as well nourished as healthy tissue
   3. Of little importance, since edematous tissue serves as a padding for bony areas
   4. Aimed at utilizing the deeper veins for venous return

310. Mr. H V's increasing cardiac edema is caused by
   (a) An imbalance in the capillary fluid shift mechanism due to rising venous pressure, causing fluid that normally would flow between interstitial spaces and blood vessels to be held in tissue spaces
   (b) Increased aldosterone secretion in response to decreased renal circulation and resulting renin-angiotensin cycle, causing increased sodium retention and potassium loss
   (c) Increased ADH secretion in response to cardiac stress and reduced renal flow, causing increased water reabsorption
   (d) Increased cellular free potassium due to depressed cell metabolism and release of protein-bound potassium, causing increase in sodium ions in surrounding extracellular fluid to maintain osmotic balance, hence more water retention
   1. a and b only   3. c and d only
   2. b and c only   4. All of these

311. The most effective diet therapy for congestive heart failure and subsequent cardiac edema is
   1. Low saturated fat   3. Bland
   2. Low sodium   4. Low cholesterol

312. To help counteract potassium loss from Mr. H V's diuretic therapy, extra food sources of potassium are recommended. These include
   1. Orange juice, bananas, dried fruit
   2. Refined cereals and breads
   3. Corn oil and special margarine
   4. Cheese and eggs

313. Soon after Mr. H V's admission, the physician orders digitoxin to be given stat. and daily thereafter. The most important precaution for the nurse to observe prior to administering the daily dose of digitoxin is which of the following?
   1. Establish the apical pulse rate and the rate of respirations
   2. Make certain that Mr. H V has eaten food before the drug is given to him
   3. Withhold this medication if Mr. H V has fewer than 14 respirations per minute
   4. Withhold the drug if the pulse rate has slowed a substantial amount in the last 24 hours

314. Mr. H V asks who discovered this drug (digitoxin) that makes him feel so much better. The nurse can truthfully reply
   1. Alexander Fleming
   2. William Morton
   3. Philip Hench
   4. William Withering

315. Mr. H V receives digitoxin, 1.2 mg. daily, on each of the first days of his hospitalization. These early and large doses will be referred to appropriately as which of the following kinds of dose?
   1. Initial   3. Maintenance
   2. Digitalizing   4. Therapeutic

316. Prior to the administration of each dose of digitoxin, the nurse should determine if which of the following significant groups of toxic symptoms are apparent?
   (a) Anorexia, nausea, vomiting
   (b) Diarrhea, abdominal pain, slow pulse
   (c) Irregularity in rate and rhythm of pulse
   (d) Headache, malaise, visual disturbances
   1. a and b   3. a, b, and c
   2. c and d   4. All of the above

317. Digitoxin, like other preparations of digitalis, will produce which of the following effects?
   (a) Accumulation   1. a and c
   (b) Slower heartbeat   2. a and b
   (c) More forceful   3. b, c, and d
       contraction of   4. All of the above
       the heart
   (d) Diuresis

318. On the third day the physician reduces the daily dose of digitoxin to 0.1 mg. and states that Mr. H V is digitalized. Which of the following statements best describes the meaning of digitalization?
   1. Mr. H V has developed symptoms of overdosage and continues to exhibit them to some extent
   2. Mr. H V's condition is now characterized by the absence of cardiac symptoms
   3. Maximum therapeutic effects have been achieved, and a smaller dose of digitoxin will maintain this therapeutic state
   4. Maximum dosage of digitoxin is no longer warranted

mild toxicity has occurred

Situation: Mr. B L, age 45, has been aware of a mass in his right cheek and upper neck for several years. Although the mass had become increasingly noticeable, he did not seek medical attention. As a result of an extensive campaign in his community, he made an appointment at a local hospital for a cancer detection examination. Mr. B L was informed by the doctor that he should be hospitalized for surgery immediately for a tumor involving the parotid gland. (See questions 319 to 324.)

319. Although the doctor had explained the possible extent of surgery, the patient was still quite anxious. Nursing intervention should be aimed at
    1. Attempting to discover what is bothering the patient
    2. Elaborating on what the doctor has already told the patient
    3. Planning for postoperative communication, since a tracheotomy is likely to be performed
    4. Teaching the patient to use the suction equipment preoperatively

320. On surgical intervention, the tumor proved to be malignant, and right total parotidectomy was performed. The most distressing complication from the patient's point of view is
    1. Tracheostomy
    2. Facial nerve dysfunction
    3. Frey syndrome
    4. Salivation

321. Postoperatively, Mr. B L was kept in a high semi-Fowler's position to
    1. Promote drainage of the wound
    2. Avoid venous oozing from the incision
    3. Avoid strain on the incision
    4. Provide comfort for the patient

322. When Mr. B L complained of his dressings being too tight, the best nursing intervention involved
    1. Checking the dressings for signs of bleeding
    2. Checking the dressings for signs of constriction
    3. Informing the patient that the tight dressings serve a purpose
    4. Altering the dressings to relieve this sensation

323. When Mr. B L is able to tolerate liquids orally, the physician orders Darvon, 65 mg. q. 3-4 h. p.r.n., for pain. Propoxyphene (Darvon) is considered to be equivalent in analgesic potency to which of the following narcotics?
    1. Codeine   3. Methadone
    2. Morphine   4. Meperidine

324. If the nurse finds the supply of Darvon Compound-65 is depleted, but Mr. B L needs this medication urgently, she would most appropriately
    1. Give two capsules of Darvon Compound
    2. Borrow a capsule of Darvon Compound-65 from the supply belonging to another patient
    3. Ask the pharmacist to refill the prescription immediately
    4. Ask Mr. B L if he can wait another hour when the next delivery from the pharmacy is scheduled

Situation: Miss Doe, a senior student nurse, is on duty in the emergency room on an extremely hot summer day. Two unconscious male patients were admitted during her tour. Mr. S, age 64, was brought to the hospital from a nearby iron foundry. His skin was hot and dry and he had a rectal temperature of 105° F. Mr. M, age 40, was doing road construction work when he collapsed. His skin was pale and moist, and his temperature normal. (See questions 325 to 327.)

325. Treatment for Mr. M would include
    1. Reduction of shock
    2. Reduction of body temperature
    3. Replacement of body fluids
    4. Stimulation of central nervous system

326. Treatment for Mr. S is aimed at
    1. Reduction of body temperature
    2. Reduction of shock
    3. Replacement of body fluids
    4. Stimulation of the central nervous system

327. Mr. S will most likely be
    1. Admitted to the hospital
    2. Advised to plan his living so that repeated long exposures to heat are avoided
    3. Have his temperature checked at frequent intervals until it has been lowered to 102° F.
    4. Advised to avoid strenuous exertion in the future

Situation: Mrs. T McC, a 93-year-old widow, has been admitted to M. S. Hospital from a nursing home, complaining of severe lower abdominal pain, anorexia, nausea, and vomiting for the past 24 hours. History and physical examination revealed a thin, elderly white woman in remarkably good physical and mental condition except for the present complaints. The most likely cause of Mrs. T McC's illness was thought to be sigmoid diverticulitis. After the appropriate diagnostic work-up and preparation for surgery, an exploratory laparotomy and subtotal gastrectomy (Billroth I) were performed. Surgery confirmed the admitting diagnosis but also revealed a large silent giant ulcer in the stomach. Mrs. T McC did well past surgery but on the fifth postoperative day developed severe abdominal pain with distended abdomen, a markedly elevated w.b.c., and temperature of 103° F. rectally. She was taken to O.R. once again where plication for a leak in the duodenostomy was performed. (See questions 328 to 335.)

328. Diagnostic procedures commonly used in patients with problems of this type include
    1. Radiography   3. Blood counts
    2. Sigmoidoscopy   4. All of these

329. The primary reason for surgery being performed in the first instance was most likely because
    1. Diverticulitis in some instances is difficult to differentiate from carcinoma except at surgery
    2. Of the symptoms presented by the patient on admission
    3. The complication, perforation, had occurred with resultant abscess formation or generalized peritonitis
    4. Surgery is usually indicated in patients with this diagnosis

330. One of the major problems after this type of surgery is the prevention of pulmonary complications. The nurse can best achieve this by
   1. Encouraging deep breathing and coughing to counteract voluntary diaphragm splinting
   2. Promoting frequent turning and moving to mobilize bronchial secretions
   3. Ambulating to increase respiratory exchange
   4. Administering I.P.P.B. q. 4 h.

331. Because Mrs. McC's skin is extremely dry, flaky, wrinkled, sagging, and sallow, an important nursing measure is to
   1. Avoid daily bathing but use emollients
   2. Bathe her once or twice a week and use emollients
   3. Bathe when necessary and use emollients
   4. Use emollients for skin care

332. In caring for a patient with a nasogastric tube attached to the suction, the nurse should
   1. Irrigate the tube frequently with physiologic saline or Ringer's solution
   2. Allow the patient to have small chips of ice or sips of water unless nauseated
   3. Use clean technique in irrigating the tube
   4. Withdraw the tube quickly when decompression is terminated

333. The wisest guideline for Mrs. T McC's diet would be
   1. No oral feedings for a prolonged period
   2. Very gradual resumption of small, easily digested feedings, according to her tolerances
   3. At her age allow her anything she wants at any time
   4. Give nothing by mouth and depend on I.V. indefinitely

334. After several days of inactivity, Mrs. T McC has developed a decubitus ulcer. Which of the following drugs is likely to be used to treat this lesion?
   1. Chymotrypsin
   2. Hyaluronidase
   3. Penicillinase
   4. Streptokinase-streptodornase (Varidase)

335. When she returns from surgery, Mrs. T McC has a nasogastric tube that is connected to intermittent suction. During this period of decompression, therapy fluid and electrolyte therapy will be maintained by the intravenous administration of solutions of
   1. Sodium bicarbonate
   2. Dilute hydrochloric acid
   3. Normal saline
   4. Distilled water and glucose

Situation: Mr. S K, age 59, a construction supervisor presently stationed at Kennedy Airport, was admitted to the I.C.U. with severe chest pain that occurred on the job. Mr. S K's work has caused him to travel extensively. His most recent assignment was in Viet Nam. His home is in Philadelphia, but at present he and his wife are living in a motel near the airport. Mrs. S K, a thin, nervous appearing woman, states she is in good health except for a nervous stomach and insomnia. She states she always travels with Mr. S K on his assignments. They have one son age 25, who is scheduled to leave for an assignment with the Merchant Marine in 2 days. An ECG revealed that Mr. S K has had an acute myocardial infarction, anterior wall. 1,000 ml. of 5% D/DW was started I.V. to keep the vein open, with 500 ml. of 5% G/DW with Lidocaine to be kept on hand. Mr. S K states that nothing is wrong with his heart and that he isn't going to be treated by any young interns. He has pulled out all I.V. attachments, removed leads from the monitor, and refuses all tests, medicines, and treatments. He states he will go to seek medical help in Philadelphia and has signed himself out against the advice of physicians. (See questions 336 to 340.)

336. In caring for Mr. S K you should try to
   1. Help him understand why it is unwise to sign himself out of the hospital at this time
   2. Explain that the hospital will not be responsible if his condition worsens
   3. Allow the patient to ventilate his feelings and give whatever care he is willing to accept
   4. Ask to be assigned to another patient, since you are unable to help Mr. S K

337. A serious arrhythmia that can develop in acute myocardial infarction is
   1. Atrial flutter
   2. Ventricular tachycardia
   3. Atrioventricular block
   4. Atrial fibrillation

338. Mrs. S K is likely to develop serious illness unless she
   1. Is hospitalized immediately for diagnostic services and/or treatment
   2. Stops traveling with her husband on his assignments and stays home
   3. Recognizes that her problems may be related to her manner of handling unpleasant situations
   4. Is able to convince Mr. S K to retire

339. The most likely reason behind Mr. S K's behavior is that
   1. Inadequate explanations have been given to help him understand his illness
   2. No one has taken time to explain the role of the various doctors assigned to the I.C.U. unit
   3. He would rather be hospitalized in his hometown
   4. He is denying that he is sick and is not accepting his illness

340. After the chief-of-staff had convinced Mr. S K of the seriousness of his condition and persuaded him to remain in the hospital, continuing diagnostic studies revealed an underlying lipid disorder, type IV hyperlipoproteinemia, with elevated pre-beta lipoproteins, triglycerides, and blood glucose. He is moderately overweight. Thus, his diet therapy includes:
   (a) 135 gm. of carbohydrate, 1,500 calories
   (b) 300 mg. of cholesterol, low saturated fat
   (c) Low protein and salt
   (d) Alcohol as desired
   1. a and b   3. b and c
   2. a and c   4. b and d

Situation: Mrs. A B, a 35-year-old housewife and

the mother of 5 young children, ages 6 months to 15 years, was involved in a serious auto accident on the highway when her car skidded on the wet pavement, striking the concrete partition. She was taken to M. B. Hospital where it was determined that she had multiple trauma: possible fractured skull, fractures of the fifth and sixth cervical and the tenth, eleventh, and twelfth vertebrae as well as ruptured spleen and hematuria. Mrs. A B's husband, a mechanical engineer, recently lost his job. (See questions 341 to 347.)

341. A splenectomy was necessary because
   1. The spleen is a highly vascular organ
   2. Rupture of the spleen is frequently associated with diseases of the liver and blood
   3. The spleen is the largest lymphoid organ in the body
   4. Enlarged spleen causes such discomfort or disability as to justify its removal

342. The most frequent complications after splenectomy are
   1. Hemorrhage, abdominal distention
   2. Peritonitis, pulmonary complications
   3. Shock, infection
   4. Intestinal obstruction, bleeding

343. The patient who has a possible fractured skull is
   1. Observed for signs of brain injury
   2. Placed in Trendelenburg position if in shock
   3. Hemorrhaging from oral cavity
   4. Observed for decreased intracranial pressure and temperature

344. The most frequent complaint of a patient with fractures of the ribs is
   1. Pain on expiration
   2. Pain on inspiration
   3. Difficulty in breathing
   4. Breathing rapidly and ineffectively

345. Mrs. A B should be observed for shock primarily because of
   1. The possibility of brain injury
   2. Associated injuries
   3. Frequency of occurrence after surgery
   4. Possible impairment of her level of consciousness

346. Hematuria in this instance probably means that there has been injury to the
   1. Kidneys   3. Bladder
   2. Ureters   4. Urethra

347. Since Mrs. A B has hematuria, the nurse should observe for
   1. Anuria
   2. Symptoms of peritonitis
   3. Gross or increasing hematuria in each urine specimen
   4. All of these

Situation: Mr. J D, age 39, single and an executive producer with one of the major television networks, enters the hospital for peritoneal dialysis. He tells the nurse that he has only 10% function of his kidneys and that he expects to go to Boston soon to have a renal transplant. His twin brother Bill is in good health and is going to donate one of his kidneys. (See questions 348 to 353.)

348. Peritoneal dialysis once instituted
   1. Is largely a nursing responsibility
   2. May be maintained from 12 to 48 hours
   3. Requires checking of vital signs every 15 minutes
   4. Should be discontinued if patient complains of severe abdominal pain

349. If Mr. J D is observed to have severe respiratory difficulty, the most immediate nursing action would be to
   1. Change the patient's position
   2. Drain fluid from the peritoneal cavity
   3. Notify the doctor
   4. Discontinue the treatment

350. The purpose of peritoneal dialysis is to
   1. Aid in removal of toxic substances and metabolic wastes
   2. Remove excessive body fluid
   3. Assist in regulating the fluid balance of the body
   4. All of these

351. In caring for Mr. J D, the nurse should
   1. Determine if he is aware of the advantages of hemodialysis
   2. Discuss the problems involved in renal transplant
   3. Begin preoperative preparation
   4. Implement nursing actions based only on evaluation of patient's present nursing needs

352. A patient who is going to have a renal transplant should know that
   1. He will require immunosuppressive drugs daily for the rest of his life
   2. He will be unable to follow a full program of work and recreation, including sports
   3. Symptoms of rejection include fever, proteinuria, hypotension, and edema
   4. All of these

353. Between dialysis treatments, Mr. J D is maintained on a modified Giodorano-Giovanetti diet. Which of the following statements is *not* true of this dietary regimen?
   1. Protein is low (15 gm.) and composed only of essential amino acids, causing the body to use its excess urea nitrogen to synthesize the other "nonessential" amino acids needed for tissue protein synthesis
   2. Potassium is high to replace losses
   3. Sodium is allowed according to need
   4. Calories are allowed as needed within designated food lists

Situation: Mr. and Mrs. B L, a retired Jewish couple who spent the winter in Florida, flew back to New York to see their newest grandson. On returning to their apartment after a family dinner, Mrs. B L, age 72, tripped over a rug in the foyer. X-ray films at the hospital reveal a fracture of the acetabulum of the femur. Mrs. B L's general state of health appears good except for the necessity to take enemas periodically. (See questions 354 to 358.)

354. A fracture of the acetabulum of the femur most likely involves the following part:
   1. Head
   2. Shaft
   3. Neck
   4. Trochanteric region

355. The treatment of choice in this instance will probably be
    1. Insertion of hip prosthesis with traction
    2. Hip pinning or nailing
    3. Application of spica cast
    4. Skeletal traction
356. To prevent pulmonary and circulatory complications, Mrs. B L should be
    1. Turned from side to side every 5 hours
    2. Ambulated as soon as the effects of anesthesia are gone
    3. Turned on the unaffected side every 2 hours
    4. Permitted to be up in a chair as soon as the effects of anesthesia are gone
357. Since Mrs. B L is accustomed to taking enemas periodically to avoid constipation, the nurse should
    1. Arrange to have enemas ordered
    2. Realize that enemas will be necessary because the normal conditioned reflex has been lost
    3. Offer Mrs. B L a large glass of prune juice in warm water each morning
    4. Arrange to have laxatives ordered
358. Elderly patients have a high incidence of hip fractures because of
    1. Carelessness
    2. Fragility of bone
    3. Associated medical diseases
    4. Sedentary existence and disease

Situation: Dr. L K was found in a coma in his room at the large hospital where he had begun his residency. There was a strong odor of acetone on his breath. He is married and 28 years of age. His wife, Jane, states he is a diabetic and recently switched to Orinase on his own instead of taking insulin as prescribed. Health records submitted did not reveal that Dr. L K had diabetes mellitus. Emergency measures were instituted immediately. (See questions 359 to 368.)

359. Oral hypoglycemic agents may be used for diabetic patients with
    1. Ketosis or impending coma
    2. Mature onset
    3. Juvenile onset
    4. Obesity
360. Dr. L K has omitted pertinent information from his health record because
    1. M.D.'s with diabetes are not accepted for residency in many hospitals
    2. He is unable to handle the psychological stress related to alteration in body functioning
    3. He needs assistance in developing a more favorable adaptation to this stress
    4. All of these
361. The most common cause of diabetic ketoacidosis is
    1. Infection
    2. Failure to take prescribed insulin
    3. Inadequate food and fluid intake
    4. Additional stress
362. Early treatment of Dr. L K's condition will include administration of
    1. Potassium
    2. Intravenous fluids
    3. Regular insulin
    4. All of these

363. An independent nursing action in the care of this patient is
    1. Regulating insulin dosage according to the amount of ketones found in the urine
    2. Withholding glucose in any form until the ketoacidosis is corrected
    3. Observing for signs of hypoglycemia
    4. Giving fruit juices, broth, and milk as soon as the patient is able to take fluids orally
364. As the patient recovers
    1. The precipitating cause of the coma must be investigated to prevent a recurrence
    2. The cause of his condition should be reviewed with him so that he understands how to avoid such a recurrence
    3. Teaching will be necessary in order to help him accept his disease
    4. He will need assistance in obtaining a clear conception of the general character of diabetes
365. Diabetic coma results from an excess accumulation in the blood of
    1. Nitrogen from protein catabolism, causing ammonia intoxication
    2. Ketones from rapid fat breakdown, causing acidosis
    3. Glucose from rapid carbohydrate metabolism, causing drowsiness
    4. Sodium bicarbonate, causing alkalosis
366. Emergency treatment for diabetic acidosis includes administration of
    (a) Insulin to regulate metabolism of the glucose
    (b) Glucose to supply energy and restore glycogen reserves
    (c) Fluids and electrolytes to counteract dehydration and restore acid-base balance
    (d) Potassium replacement to facilitate entry of glucose into cell and its storage as glycogen in liver and muscle
    1. a and b
    2. b and c
    3. a and c
    4. All of these
367. Important to both Dr. L K and his wife Jane is an understanding that his diet for management of his diabetes
    (a) Is based on his own individual nutritional requirements
    (b) Can be planned around a wide variety of commonly used foods
    (c) Should be rigidly controlled to avoid similar emergencies
    (d) Must avoid combination dishes and processed foods, since they have too many variable seasonings
    1. a and b
    2. c and d
    3. a and c
    4. b and d
368. Dr. L K needs to understand and accept the fact that Orinase, like other oral hypoglycemic agents, is useful only if the diabetic person
    1. Has an unstable blood glucose level
    2. Is experiencing a fever or surgical trauma
    3. Tends to develop ketoacidosis
    4. Has a stable, mild form of diabetes

Situation: Dr. B E, a single 25-year-old professor of mathematics at a major university, is hospitalized for bleeding gastric ulcers. A conservative regimen is being followed at present. Dr. B E is one of two children of Mrs. E who was widowed 3 years after the birth of her second son, T E. At an early age it became apparent that B E was a genius. His capabilities were encouraged to develop to their fullest potential by his mother. He graduated from high school at the age of 13 *summa cum laude* and at the age of 19 had received a Ph.D. in mathematics. His brother is now married and has a 20-month-old son. Dr. B E lives at home with his aging mother. (See questions 369 to 379.)

369. Peptic ulcer disease is a psychosomatic disorder in which it is believed that
    1. Structural changes have occurred as a result of psychological conflicts
    2. Illness is a defense against psychological conflicts
    3. Structural changes have occurred as a result of physiologic changes caused by psychological conflict
    4. All of these

370. Analysis of factors resulting in psychological conflict for Dr. B E reveal
    1. Unconscious concern with independence, success, and activity
    2. The drive to excel in whatever he does
    3. Conversion of emotional tension due to chronic repressed hostility
    4. Many feelings that are unconscious but near the surface

371. Characteristic physiologic changes in peptic ulcer include
    (a) Hypermotility
    (b) Ulceration of the gastric mucosa
    (c) Excessive production of secretions
    (d) Hypotonicity
        1. a, b, and c   3. b, c, and d
        2. a, c, and d   4. All of these

372. To differentiate between a gastric ulcer and gastric carcinoma, which one of the following diagnostic tests may be performed?
    1. Gastric analysis
    2. Gastrointestinal series
    3. Gastroscopy
    4. Stool examination

373. Dr. B E is vomiting thick coffee-ground material in small amounts and appears very restless and apprehensive. Therapy that will most likely be instituted immediately includes
    (a) Administration of fluids and/or transfusions
    (b) Small frequent feedings of milk and cream
    (c) Complete rest
    (d) Opiates or sedatives q. 4 h. p.r.n.
        1. a, b, and c   3. a and d
        2. a, c, and d   4. b and c

374. Despite initiation of therapy, Dr. B E continues to be apprehensive and restless. Nursing action will include
    1. Assuring him that every effort is being made to control the bleeding and replace the lost blood
    2. Explaining the importance of resting quietly in bed
    3. Administering sedatives as ordered by the doctor
    4. All of these

375. Dr. B E's conservative dietary regimen has which basic goals?

    (a) To neutralize gastric acidity
    (b) To eliminate chemical, mechanical, and thermal irritation
    (c) To provide optimum amounts of all nutrients
    (d) To provide psychological support by offering a wide variety of foods
        1. a and d   3. a and b
        2. b and c   4. c and d

376. After the acute stage subsided, a more liberal, individual approach to diet therapy was ordered. Dr. B E responded well to the following plan of nutritional care:
    (a) A careful history of food attitudes, reactions, and tolerances
    (b) Feedings liberalized according to his individual tolerances
    (c) A variety of food offered to support nutritional needs for healing and emotional outlook
    (d) A pattern of frequent, small, unhurried meals
        1. b and c   3. c and d
        2. a and b   4. All of these

377. When cardiovascular disease is a concern, reduction of the saturated fat in an ulcer diet may be desired, and substitutes made of polyunsaturated fat. In such a case, which of the following foods would *not* be allowed?
    1. Whole milk
    2. Special soft margarine
    3. Corn oil
    4. Fish

378. If Dr. B E has lost enough blood to develop a mild anemia, which of the following drugs may be used in treatment of this condition?
    1. Dextran
    2. Carbacrylamine resins (Carbo-Resin)
    3. Salts of iron
    4. Vitamin B$_{12}$

379. Aluminum hydroxide gel (Amphojel) is prescribed for Dr. B E. For which of the following purposes was this medication prescribed?
    (a) To systemically neutralize gastric acidity
    (b) To chemically neutralize hydrochloric acid of the stomach
    (c) To inhibit the secretion of hydrochloric acid
    (d) To exert a rapid, prolonged antacid effect
        1. b only   3. b and d
        2. a and c   4. All of the above

Situation: Mr. E, 50 years old, recently came from Italy with his wife to visit with American relatives. While here, he was admitted to the hospital complaining of anorexia, loss of weight, abdominal distention, and passage of abnormal stools. The most likely diagnosis on the basis of history and physical examination was cancer of the esophagus or malabsorption syndrome. Neither Mr. E nor his wife speaks any English. Their trip to America was sponsored by relatives. (See questions 380 to 387.)

380. To determine the corrected diagnosis, extensive diagnostic studies were performed. Tests in connection with cancer of esophagus included
    (a) X-ray examination
    (b) Biopsy

(c) Esophagoscopy
(d) Bronchoscopy
   1. a and b   3. a, b, and c
   2. a and c   4. All of these

381. Since Mr. E's nutritional status is poor, the nurse should
(a) Maintain I.V. therapy as ordered
(b) Encourage the patient to take whatever food and/or fluids he will take
(c) Keep an accurate record of intake and output
(d) Keep the patient n.p.o., since he has diarrhea
   1. a and b   3. a, b, and c
   2. a and c   4. a, c, and d

382. A 72-hour collection of stool for fat has been ordered. To assist in this examination, the nurse should
1. Realize that the patient must ingest 90 to 100 gm. of fat per day during its collection
2. Discontinue the stool collection if the patient has difficulty in tolerating the diet
3. Know that no special requirements are indicated for this collection
4. Discontinue the stool collection if any specimens are lost

383. It is essential that you develop some form of communication with the patient and his wife in order to
1. Help them to participate actively in his care as much as is feasible
2. Eliminate psychological stress
3. Explain any problems he may have in relation to his illness
4. Ensure accuracy in diagnostic studies being done

384. Differential diagnosis established that Mr. E has nontropical sprue. Striking clinical improvement was noted in condition after administration of
1. A gluten-free diet   3. Corticotropin
2. Folic acid   4. Vitamin B_{12}

385. Because malabsorption syndrome seemed to be present, a trial period on a gluten-free diet was ordered for Mr. E. He was not allowed to have
1. Wheat, rye, or oats
2. Rice or corn
3. Milk or cheese
4. Fruit or fruit juices

386. A typical food combination served to Mr. E on his gluten-free diet was
1. Creamed turkey on toast, rice, green peas, milk
2. Roast beef, baked potato, carrots, tea
3. Cheese omelet, noodles, green beans, coffee
4. Baked chicken, mashed potatoes with gravy, zucchini, Postum

387. Since fat absorption was a problem, a special form of fat was used because it could be absorbed directly into the portal blood instead of the lacteals. This fat substance was
1. Lecithin
2. MCT (medium chain triglycerides)
3. Linoleic acid
4. Lipoprotein
5. Glycerol

Situation: Mrs. E W, a 40-year-old housewife, is admitted to the hospital with a history of vomiting, tarry stools, ascites, and long-standing poor nutrition due to excessive alcoholic intake. Her admitting diagnosis is bleeding esophageal varices. After emergency treatment the plan of therapy involves preparing Mrs. E W for a portal caval anastomosis. (See questions 388 to 398.)

388. The pathophysiologic problem in cirrhosis of the liver causing esophageal varices is
1. Dilated veins and varicosities
2. Portal hypertension
3. Ascites and edema
4. Loss of regeneration

389. Medical management that may be used to control the hemorrhage includes
(a) Pituitrin S
(b) Balloon tamponade
(c) Gastric suctioning
(d) Application of cold
   1. a and b   3. a, b, and c
   2. b and c   4. All of these

390. Neomycin may be administered to prevent
1. Absorption of urea
2. Absorption of ammonia
3. Formation of urea
4. Formation of ammonia

391. If intubation is used, the type of tube most likely to be used is
1. Sengstaken-Blakemore
2. Devine
3. Andersen
4. Levin

392. Dangers that may result as a use of this tube are
(a) Asphyxiation
(b) Ulcers in stomach
(c) Erosion
(d) Necrosis
   1. a, b, and c   3. a, b, and c
   2. a, b, and d   4. b, c, and d

393. Characteristic signs that are a direct result of liver insufficiency may include
(a) Neurological disturbances
(b) Ascites
(c) Edema
(d) Fetor hepaticus
   1. a and b   3. a, b, and c
   2. a and d   4. b, c, and d

394. In an effort to prevent hepatic coma, it may become necessary to
(a) Eliminate protein from diet
(b) Eliminate carbohydrate from the diet
(c) Give colonic washouts
(d) Prepare for emergency surgery
   1. a and c   3. b and c
   2. a and d   4. All of these

395. Assuming that Mrs. E W eventually does have a portal caval anastomosis performed, she should know that
1. The surgery will alleviate the cirrhosis
2. Strict adherence to the medical regimen prescribed will still be necessary
3. The ascites will be cured
4. All of these

396. Mrs. E W's long-standing poor nutrition, especially her deficiency of protein, has led to
(a) Ascites due to low plasma protein levels

(b) Fat accumulation in the liver tissue, since lipoproteins are not formed
(c) Impaired blood clotting due to inadequate production of prothrombin and fibrinogen
(d) Tissue catabolism and negative nitrogen balance
   1. a, b, and c   3. b, c, and d
   2. a, c, and d   4. All of these

397. When Mrs. E W was able to eat, the diet ordered for her was
   1. High-protein, low-carbohydrate, low-fat
   2. Low-sodium, protein to tolerance, moderate-fat, high-calorie, high-vitamin, soft
   3. High-carbohydrate, low-saturated fat, 1,200 calories
   4. Low-protein, low-carbohydrate, high-fat, soft

398. Mrs. E W began to develop slurred speech, confusion, drowsiness, and a flapping tremor. With these evidences of impending hepatic coma, her diet was changed to
   1. 20 gm. protein, 2,000 calories
   2. 80 gm. protein, 1,000 calories
   3. 100 gm. protein, 2,500 calories
   4. 150 gm. protein, 1,200 calories

Situation: Mr. A P, a 56-year-old mechanical engineer, was discharged from the hospital 3 weeks ago after a mitral valve replacement. He lives with his wife, Ann, who has been under psychiatric treatment for a nervous disorder. He experienced no difficulty at home since discharge and has seen his doctor as specified. Yesterday he went to the pharmacist to refill his prescription for Coumadin. The pharmacist remarked that Mr. A P should see his doctor immediately because his skin and sclerae appeared to have a yellow color. His doctor advised hospitalization immediately. (See questions 399 to 403.)

399. It was suspected that Mr. A P most likely had serum hepatitis, which was probably caused by his receiving infected blood or blood derivatives during his hospitalization for mitral valve replacement. In helping Mr. A P understand how this may occur, you tell him that
   1. Persons known to have had serum or infectious hepatitis are asked not to donate blood to the Red Cross or other blood programs
   2. Infective blood cannot be always identified with certainty
   3. Supplies of gamma globulin are not sufficient to permit its routine use in conjunction with every transfusion
   4. All of these

400. Prophylaxis includes
   1. Enteric precautions applied to infected cases
   2. Screening of blood donors
   3. Case finding and treatment of infection
   4. Patient isolation

401. The earliest indication of parenchymal damage to the liver usually is
   1. Elevation in transaminase
   2. Rise in bilirubin
   3. Alteration in proteins
   4. Rise in alkaline phosphatase

402. Treatment in serum hepatitis
   1. Utilizes chemotherapeutic agents
   2. Is symptomatic in nature
   3. Requires isolation of the patient for 7 days
   4. Requires active immunization

403. Nursing action for meeting the emotional needs of Mr. A P will include
   (a) Utilization of knowledge of patient from all relevant sources
   (b) Observing the patient and interpreting the meaning of his feelings and thought
   (c) Recognizing that Mr. A P, on the basis of his adaptation to surgery, will not need assistance
   (d) Providing for periods for the patient to express his feelings and thoughts
      1. a and b   3. a and d
      2. a and c   4. All of these

Situation: Mr. M L, a 26-year-old lawyer, is admitted from the emergency unit with the following symptoms: headache, anorexia, malaise, fever, and swelling of the parotid gland. He recalls visiting his married sister and her family within the past two weeks but states that at this time her 2 children, Debbie and John, were recuperating from one of their frequent (at least he thought) acute respiratory tract infections. (See questions 404 to 409.)

404. Uncertainty exists as to whether Mr. M L had mumps as a child or whether he has been exposed to it recently. Which of these diagnostic studies may be performed?
   (a) Specific serologic tests
   (b) Skin test
   (c) Tissue culture
   (d) Blood culture
      1. a, b, and c   3. a and c
      2. a and b   4. All of these

405. Commonly occurring complication(s) of mumps in the adult male include
   1. Orchitis   3. Impotence
   2. Sterility   4. All of these

406. Mumps vaccine should be used as prophylaxis in
   1. Military forces
   2. Pregnant women
   3. Anyone who has not had the disease
   4. All of these

407. In planning appropriate nursing intervention for Mr. M L, the nurse should know that
   (a) Bed rest will help to prevent complications
   (b) It may be necessary to restrict the diet
   (c) Isolation will be necessary
   (d) Astute nursing care will prevent complications
      1. a and b   3. b and c
      2. a and c   4. All of these

408. If Mr. M L develops orchitis, treatment will include
   (a) Antibiotics
   (b) Application of cold
   (c) Cortisone
   (d) Scrotal support
      1. a, c, and d   3. b, c, and d
      2. a, b, and c   4. All of these

409. The physician prescribes mumps immune globulin. This drug is expected to do which of the following for Mr. M L?

1. Prevent mumps
2. Reduce severity of mumps and prevent orchitis
3. Treat the complication, meningoencephalitis
4. Confer lifetime immunity

Situation: C A, a 31-year-old private in the Marines, recently returned from South Viet Nam after a 13-month tour of active duty. On the basis of the history and physical examination, the doctor believes the most likely diagnosis is malaria. (See questions 410 to 420.)

410. The most important diagnostic test in malaria is
1. Smear of peripheral blood
2. Blood leukocyte count
3. Erythrocyte sedimentation rate
4. Splenic puncture

411. An important finding in malaria is
1. Splenomegaly
2. Leukocytosis
3. Elevated sedimentation rate
4. Erythrocytosis

412. Prophylaxis for the control of malaria include
1. Vaccination
2. Patient isolation
3. Prompt detection and effective treatment of case
4. All of these

413. Complications of malaria of any type include
1. Relapses
2. Black-water fever
3. Splenomegaly and hepatomegaly
4. Anemia and cachexia

414. Complications of acute malaria are
(a) Anemia and cachexia
(b) Congested and enlarged spleen
(c) Changes in viscosity and water and electrolyte regulation
(d) Gastrointestinal disturbances
   1. a and b   3. a, b, and c
   2. c and d   4. All of these

415. In caring for C A, the nurse should know that
(a) Care during a paroxysm is similar to the care of any patient exhibiting these symptoms
(b) Patient should be awakened only for nourishment after a paroxysm
(c) Attention should be focused on rest and nourishing food between paroxysms
(d) Isolation is necessary
   1. a and b   3. a, b, and c
   2. a and c   4. All of these

416. Whenever quinine is used, the nurse should be alert to symptoms of *severe* cinchonism, which are
1. Tinnitus, decreased auditory acuity, nausea
2. Deafness, vertigo, severe visual, gastrointestinal, and central nervous system disturbances
3. Pruritus, urticaria, and difficulty in breathing
4. Leg cramps, fever, swollen and painful joints

417. Because C A is experiencing an acute attack of malaria, the physician orders 650 mg. of quinine dihydrochloride to be given over an 8-hour period of time by I.V. drip in 1,000 ml. of normal saline. He further specifies that the drug must not be injected more rapidly than 50 mg. per minute. The intravenous equipment is calibrated at 20 drops per milliliter. To avoid exceeding a dosage of 50 mg. per minute, the solution must never flow at the rate of
1. 12 ml. per minute
2. 80 ml. per minute
3. 10 ml. per minute
4. 5 ml. per minute

418. To regulate the rate of flow so that the solution would be infused over an 8-hour period, the nurse would select which of these rates of flow?
1. 160 gtt. per minute
2. 60 gtt. per minute
3. 20 gtt. per minute
4. 40 gtt. per minute

419. When the danger of the acute attack has passed, the physician replaces the intravenous injection with quinine sulfate, 2 Gm. per day in divided doses. The nurse should administer this medication after meals in order to
1. Delay its absorption
2. Minimize gastric irritation
3. Decrease stimulation of appetite
4. Decrease its antiarrhythmic action

420. Which of the following statements is true concerning successful drug therapy against *P. falciparum* infections?
1. The infections can be completely eliminated
2. Transmission by the *Anopheles* mosquito can occur
3. The infections are controlled
4. Immunity will prevent reinfection

Situation: Mr. D J, an 87-year-old salesman, is admitted to the I.C.U. with a pulse rate of 40. Temporary cardiac pacing was subsequently begun by inserting a cardiac electrode into Mr. D J's right ventricle through the jugular vein and attached to an external battery. Mr. D J, although appearing chronically ill, still worked part-time and lived alone in a hotel. He stated he was all alone, since his wife had been dead for 5 years and his family physician for 2 years. Mr. D J denies having any adverse symptoms except for fainting spells, although on admission, it was revealed that he had a greatly enlarged prostate and signs of long-standing renal failure. The regimen planned for Mr. D J is to implant a permanent pacemaker, assuming his medical problems can be corrected; otherwise, Mr. D J must be sent to a nursing home. (See questions 421 to 429.)

421. Mr. D J is a poor risk for surgery primarily because of
1. The existence of several chronic diseases that may have developed gradually
2. Normal physiologic changes that occur with aging processes
3. Greater susceptibility to infection
4. His age

422. The decision as to operability should be based on assessment of the patient's
(a) Cardiovascular and urinary reserves

(b) Nutritional status
(c) Age and apparent infirmities
(d) Physiologic status
   1. a and b   3. a, b, and c
   2. a and d   4. All of these

423. On giving Mr. D J back care, you observe that his bed is wet. Although he requests the urinal frequently and voids in small amounts, you should
   1. Have the patient keep the urinal in place to avoid accidents
   2. Realize that the patient is not emptying his bladder
   3. Inform the doctor so that an indwelling catheter may be inserted
   4. All of these

424. Long-term pacing with a transvenous catheter electrode and an external battery pacemaker generally has been abandoned because of
   (a) Limitations on patient's movements
   (b) Bathing difficulties
   (c) Skin infection
   (d) Bacteremias
     1. a and b   3. a and d
     2. a, b, and c   4. All of these

425. The nurse may best assist in the decision on operability by
   1. Observation of the patient and reporting his responses
   2. Using preventive nursing measures to prevent systemic infection
   3. Preventing anxiety of the patient by providing constant reassurance
   4. Forcing fluids to prevent dehydration

426. Mr. D J does not understand why the doctors seem concerned about his voiding pattern. He states, "It is no different that it has been for the past few years. When my regular doctor was alive, I saw him once a month for a check-up. My work did not interfere with my being able to go to the men's room." To help Mr. D J understand the situation, you should
   (a) Explain that all patients with an enlarged prostate have increased frequency of voiding in small amounts
   (b) Explain that since he is voiding in small amounts, he may not be emptying his bladder
   (c) Explain that backup of urine in the bladder over a prolonged period of time can result in inflammation of the bladder and damage to the kidney
   (d) Inform the doctor of your plans prior to talking with the patient
     1. a   3. a, b, and c
     2. b and c   4. All of these

427. Diagnostic studies in relation to Mr. D J's urinary problems will include
   1. NPN, hemoglobin   3. Blood grouping
   2. BUN, hemoglobin   4. Cystography

428. Prostatectomy will be performed only if
   (a) The patient requires a prostatectomy
   (b) There is no infection in the urinary tract
   (c) Diagnostic blood studies are normal
   (d) Diagnosis has been confirmed
     1. a and c   3. a, b, and c
     2. a and b   4. All of these

429. If prostatectomy is contraindicated, Mr. D J will require

(a) A prolonged period of rest
(b) Bladder drainage
(c) Limited salt intake
(d) Increased fluid intake
   1. b and c   3. a, b, and c
   2. a and b   4. All of these

Situation: Mrs. A W, age 49, was recently admitted to a large city hospital with cyanosis, anasarca, pain in the right upper chest, and shortness of breath. There was also a weight loss from 140 to 100 pounds in the course of a year. Extensive diagnostic studies revealed that there was a mass in each breast, a mass in the mediastinum and finally extensive inoperable cancer of the chest. Mrs. A W had lived until recently with her widowed, 83-year-old invalid mother and 18-year-old daughter. Her mother died a few months ago. Mrs. A W's husband lives in Washington, D. C., where he is employed as a truck driver for a major soda firm. He sends $40 weekly to his wife. The other source of income has now been cut off since the death of her mother. The chosen course of therapy for Mrs. A W was that she would receive 30 treatments in radiation therapy on an outpatient basis. Taxicab fare would average $10 round trip. Mrs. A W was advised to see the hospital social worker. Although the resident states Mrs. A W is aware of her diagnosis, she has never once admitted this. (See questions 430 to 434.)

430. After an interview with the patient, the social worker
   (a) Informed the doctor that the patient should remain in the hospital because of insurmountable family problems at this time
   (b) Arranged for a volunteer taxi service to pick up Mrs. A W at her home at designated times on the days of treatment
   (c) Stated that she would assist the 18-year-old daughter find some type of work immediately
   (d) Referred the patient to welfare for financial assistance
     1. a, b, and c   3. b and c
     2. b, c, and d   4. a and d

431. Mrs. A W should remain in the hospital
   (a) Because of the extent of her disease
   (b) Since radiation will have a marked systemic effect upon the patient
   (c) Since her 18-year-old daughter cannot assume responsibility for her care
   (d) If there is a bed available
     1. a and b   3. None of these
     2. a, b, and c   4. All of these

432. Since the patient undergoing radiation therapy may have some form of skin reaction, Mrs. A W should be
   1. Instructed in the care to be given to the area being radiated
   2. Informed of the possible side reactions that may occur
   3. Given information only if she requests it
   4. Advised to discuss the problem with the radiologist

433. In an effort to determine why Mrs. A W has never admitted that she has cancer, the nurse should

1. Realize that Mrs. A W is handling this problem according to her customary lifestyle
2. Realize that the patient must have assistance in adapting to the psychological stresses imposed on her by this diagnosis
3. Observe and interpret the meaning of the patient's feelings and behavior for appropriate nursing action
4. Seek validation from the patient prior to nursing action

434. Radiotherapy has been prescribed for Mrs. A W in hope that it may accomplish
    1. Cure   3. Resolution
    2. Palliation   4. All of these

Situation: The topic of discussion for the high school assembly meeting at which you are scheduled to appear is "Dependence on, and Abuse of, Tobacco, Alcohol, and Drugs." (See questions 435 to 444.)

435. Characteristics of drug habituation include
    1. A compulsion to continue the drug for the sense of improved well-being that it engenders
    2. A tendency to increase the dose
    3. Detrimental effect on the individual and on society
    4. Some degree of psychic dependence on the effect of the drug

436. Dependence on drugs, alcohol, and tobacco have the following characteristics in common:
    (a) They are examples of dependence on harmful substances
    (b) Discontinuing the use of these substances is difficult
    (c) They may lead to a variety of personal and social problems
    (d) They impair one's judgment
    1. a and b   3. a, b, and c
    2. a and c   4. All of these

437. In helping people to succeed who wish to stop smoking, the nurse should
    (a) Stress the dangers of disease in relation to smoking
    (b) Recognize that smoking is a complicated pattern of behavior
    (c) Recognize that her attitude in relation to the person who is attempting to become an ex-smoker is of prime importance
    (d) Support the person in his resolve to stop smoking
    1. a and b   3. a, b, and c
    2. b, c, and d   4. All of these

438. Lou Ann states she has tried to give up smoking by chewing gum and eating candy but finds she is gaining weight. She should be advised to
    1. Try to stop using candy and chewing gum, since she is aware of the consequences

2. Eat candy or chew gum that are artificially sweetened even though she may not like the taste
3. Lose the weight she gains after the need for cigarettes has lessened
4. Find another substitute to aid her in losing weight now

439. The dangerous time for taking the wheel of a car for anyone has already arrived when the following effects of alcohol ingestion are present:
    1. Euphoria and confidence
    2. Loss of digital dexterity and muscular coordination
    3. Speed of motor response decreased
    4. All of these

440. Which of the following statements are true?
    (a) Drug abuse is primarily a problem of persons who are economically, socially, and educationally disadvantaged
    (b) Low self-esteem is a significant characteristic of persons who misuse and become dependent on drugs
    (c) Drug use is of particular significance among young people of high school and college age
    (d) LSD, which alters a person's perception, is reputed to assist him to achieve insight that may help him experience life more fully
    1. a, b, and c   3. a, c, and d
    2. b, c, and d   4. All of these

441. The use of marijuana
    1. May produce lasting physical or mental damage
    2. Does not lead to physical dependence and tolerance
    3. May incite its users to criminal behavior, violence, etc.
    4. All of these

442. Particularly dangerous is the use of alcohol in combination with
    (a) Amphetamines
    (b) Barbiturates
    (c) Tranquilizers
    (d) Hypnotics
    1. a, b, and c   3. a, c, and d
    2. b, c, and d   4. All of these

443. Harmful effects from the use of tobacco occur as the result of
    1. Smoking   3. Using snuff
    2. Chewing tobacco   4. All of these

444. Heroin may be tried for various reasons
    1. In a conscious or unconscious effort to hurt oneself or another
    2. As a method of producing unnatural wakefulness and alertness
    3. As a method of controlling nervousness
    4. For its "consciousness-expanding" properties

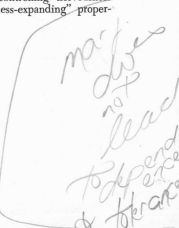

SCORES

1	5
2	6
3	7
4	8

NAME _____ LAST _____ FIRST _____ MIDDLE _____ DATE _____

SCHOOL _____ CITY _____

DATE OF BIRTH _____ AGE _____ SEX M OR F

GRADE OR CLASS _____ INSTRUCTOR _____

NAME OF TEST _____ PART _____

DIRECTIONS: Read each question and its numbered answers. When you have decided which answer is correct, blacken the corresponding space on this sheet with the special pencil. Make your mark as long as the pair of lines, and move the pencil point up and down firmly to make a heavy black line. If you change your mind, erase your first mark completely. Make no stray marks; they may count against you.

SAMPLE:
1. Chicago is
1—1 a country
1—2 a mountain
1—3 an island
1—4 a city
1—5 a state

BE SURE YOUR MARKS ARE HEAVY AND BLACK.
ERASE COMPLETELY ANY ANSWER YOU WISH TO CHANGE.

Printed by the International Business Machines Corporation, Endicott, N. Y., U. S. A.   IBM FORM I.T.S. 1000 B 108

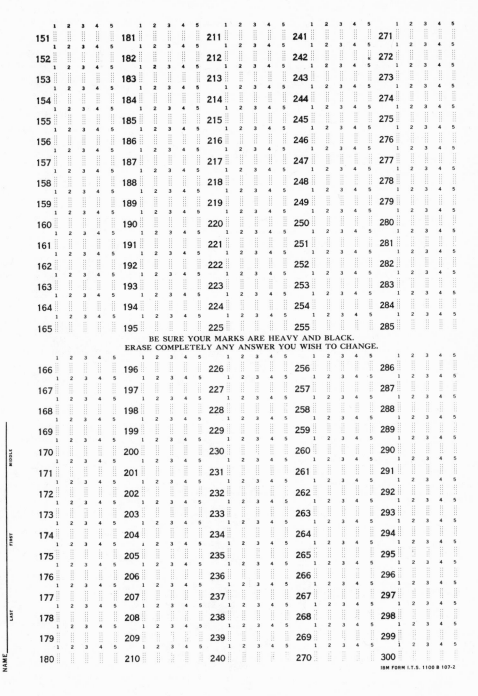

BE SURE YOUR MARKS ARE HEAVY AND BLACK.
ERASE COMPLETELY ANY ANSWER YOU WISH TO CHANGE.

SCORES

1
2
3
4
5
6
7
8

NAME

LAST

FIRST

MIDDLE

IBM FORM I.T.S. 1100 B 107-2

	1	2	3	4	5		1	2	3	4	5		1	2	3	4	5		1	2	3	4	5		1	2	3	4	5
301						331						361						391						421					
302						332						362						392						422					
303						333						363						393						423					
304						334						364						394						424					
305						335						365						395						425					
306						336						366						396						426					
307						337						367						397						427					
308						338						368						398						428					
309						339						369						399						429					
310						340						370						400						430					
311						341						371						401						431					
312						342						372						402						432					
313						343						373						403						433					
314						344						374						404						434					
315						345						375						405						435					

BE SURE YOUR MARKS ARE HEAVY AND BLACK.
ERASE COMPLETELY ANY ANSWER YOU WISH TO CHANGE.

	1	2	3	4	5		1	2	3	4	5		1	2	3	4	5		1	2	3	4	5		1	2	3	4	5
316						346						376						406						436					
317						347						377						407						437					
318						348						378						408						438					
319						349						379						409						439					
320						350						380						410						440					
321						351						381						411						441					
322						352						382						412						442					
323						353						383						413						443					
324						354						384						414						444					
325						355						385						415						445					
326						356						386						416						446					
327						357						387						417						447					
328						358						388						418						448					
329						359						389						419						449					
330						360						390						420						450					

OBSTETRIC AND GYNECOLOGIC NURSING

Abramson, H.: Resuscitation of the newborn infant and related emergency procedures: principles and practice, ed. 3, St. Louis, 1973, The C. V. Mosby Co.

Aldrich, A. C.: Babies are human beings, ed. 2, New York, 1955, The Macmillan Co.

August, R. V.: Hypnosis in obstetrics, New York, 1961, McGraw-Hill Book Co., Inc.

Babson, S. G., and Benson, R. C.: Management of high-risk pregnancy and intensive care of the neonate, ed. 2, St. Louis, 1971, The C. V. Mosby Co.

Ball, T. L.: Gynecologic surgery and urology, ed. 2, St. Louis, 1963, The C. V. Mosby Co.

Bell, N. W., and Vogel, E. F., editors: Modern introduction to the family, New York, 1960, The Free Press of Glencoe.

Benedek, T.: Psychosexual function in women, New York, 1952, The Ronald Press Co.

Bing, E.: Six practical lessons for an easier childbirth, New York, 1963, Bantam Books, Inc.

Bonner, D. M.: Heredity, Englewood Cliffs, N. J., 1961, Prentice-Hall, Inc.

Bookmiller, M. M., and Bowen, G. L.: Textbook of obstetrics and obstetric nursing, ed. 5, Philadelphia, 1967, W. B. Saunders Co.

Bradley, R. A.: Husband-coached childbirth, New York, 1965, Harper & Row, Publishers.

Buxton, C. L.: A study of psychophysical methods for relief of childbirth pain, Philadelphia, 1962, W. B. Saunders Co.

Caplan, G.: Concepts of mental health and consultation, U. S. Department of Health, Education, and Welfare, Children's Bureau Pub. no. 373, U. S. Government Printing Office, 1959.

Chabon, I.: Awake and aware: participating in childbirth through psychoprophylaxis, New York, 1966, Dell Publishing Co.

Clyne, G. W.: A textbook of gynecology and obstetrics, Boston, 1963, Little, Brown & Co.

Davis, E. M., and Rubin, R.: De Lee's obstetrics for nurses, ed. 18, Philadelphia, 1966, W. B. Saunders Co.

Eastman, N. J., and Hellman, L. M., editors: Williams' obstetrics, ed. 13, New York, 1966, Appleton-Century-Crofts.

Ewy, D., and Ewy, R.: Preparation for childbirth—a Lamaze guide, Boulder, Colo., 1970, Pruett Publishing Co.

Fitzpatrick, E., Reeder, S., and Mastroianni, L.: Maternity nursing, ed. 12, Philadelphia, 1970, J. B. Lippincott Co.

Flanagan, G. L.: First nine months of life, New York, 1962, Simon & Schuster, Inc.

Gibert, H.: Love in marriage, New York, 1964, Hawthorne Books, Inc.

Greenhill, J. B.: Clinical obstetrics and gynecology, New York, 1963, Harper & Row, Publishers.

Gruenberg, S. M.: The wonderful story on how you were born, Garden City, N. Y., 1952, Hanover House.

Guttmacher, A., and others: Planning your family, New York, 1963, The Macmillan Co.

Hamilton, J. A.: Postpartum psychiatric problems, St. Louis, 1962, The C. V. Mosby Co.

Hutton, I. G.: The sex technique in marriage, New York, 1961, Emerson Books, Inc.

Iorio, J.: Principles of obstetrics and gynecology for nurses, ed. 2, St. Louis, 1971, The C. V. Mosby Co.

Kroger, W.: Psychosomatic obstetrics, gynecology, and endocrinology, Springfield, Ill., 1963, Charles C Thomas, Publisher.

Mead, M.: Family, New York, 1965, The Macmillan Co.

Meeting the childbearing needs of families in a changing world, New York, 1962, Maternity Center Association.

Mendelson, C. L.: Cardiac disease in pregnancy, Philadelphia, 1960, F. A. Davis Co.

Montagu, M. F. A.: Human heredity, ed. 2, Cleveland, 1964, The World Publishing Co.

Newton, N.: Maternal emotions, New York, 1955, Harper & Brothers.

Parker, E.: The seven ages of woman, Baltimore, 1960, The Johns Hopkins Press.

Pryor, K.: Nursing your baby, New York, 1963, Harper & Row, Publishers.

Psychological preparation for childbirth: guidelines for teaching, ed. 2, New York, 1969, Maternity Center Association.

Read, G. D.: Childbirth without fear, ed. 2, New York, 1953, Harper & Brothers.

Ribble, M.: The rights of infants, ed. 2, New York, 1965, Columbia University Press.

Silverman, W.: Premature infants, New York, 1961, Harper & Row, Publishers.

Te Linde, R. W.: Operative gynecology, ed. 3, Philadelphia, 1962, J. B. Lippincott Co.

The womanly art of breast-feeding, Franklin Park, Ill., 1961, La Lèche League Internationale.

Trends and techniques in parent education, New York, 1964, Child Study Association.

Vincent, C.: Unmarried mothers, New York, 1961, The Free Press of Glencoe.

Wallace, Helen M.: Health services for mothers and children, Philadelphia, 1964, W. B. Saunders Co.

Willson, J. R., Beecham, C. T., and Carrington, E. R.: Obstetrics and gynecology, ed. 4, St. Louis, 1971, The C. V. Mosby Co.

Periodical journals related to maternal child health

American Journal of Nursing, New York, American Nurses' Association.

American Journal of Obstetrics and Gynecology, St. Louis, The C. V. Mosby Co.

American Journal of Public Health, Albany, N. Y., American Public Health Association.

Briefs, New York, Maternity Center Association.

Child and Family, St. Meinrad, Ind., Abbey Press.

Children, Department of Health, Education, and Welfare, Children's Bureau, U. S. Government Printing Office.

Journal of Marriage and the Family, Chicago, Rand McNally & Co.

Nursing Forum, Hillsdale, N. J., Nursing Publications, Inc.

Nursing Outlook, New York, National League for Nursing.

Nursing Science, Philadelphia, F. A. Davis Co.

Obstetrics and Gynecology, New York, Harper & Row, Publishers.

R. N. Magazine, Oradell, N. J., Medical Economics, Inc.

The cumulative index to nursing literature, published by the Glendale Sanitarium and Hospital, P. O. Box 871, Glendale, Calif., lists many more nursing and medical journals for research study.

THE NURSE AND THE FAMILY

1. Role of the nurse

A. Member of the health team
  1. Collaborates with physicians, nutritionists, social workers, and others in the care of patients and families during childbearing and child-rearing cycles

  2. Cares for women during the maternity cycle and for newborns and families
    a. Gives direct nursing care
    b. Relieves or reduces physiologic and psychological stresses
    c. Counsels and instructs prospective parents and families
    d. Acts as "advocate" for parents and families

B. Member of the community
  1. Participates in community planning for maternal and child health
  2. Utilizes available community resources to best advantage
  3. Assists prospective parents and families in finding and utilizing necessary community resources

2. Goals and objectives of maternity care

A. Promotion of optimum health and well-being of women during the maternity cycle, and of the newborns and the total families
  1. Preparation of young people for marriage and parenthood
    a. Premarital health examinations
    b. Early medical supervision during pregnancy
    c. Health supervision and health teaching throughout the maternity cycle
    d. Nutrition education for women, during and prior to maternity cycle, and for families
    e. Childbirth education for couples
  2. Continued family health supervision
    a. Family planning as integral part of maternity care
    b. Health supervision through infancy and childhood

3. Trends in family development

A. Early-age marriages
B. Jobs held by both husband and wife
C. Change in attitude toward marriage and family
D. Three-generation families living together very rare
E. Marriages occurring more and more frequently between people of differing cultural, social, and socioeconomic backgrounds

4. Problems to be considered

A. Prematurity—low birth weight
B. Congenital anomalies
C. Birth injuries
D. Complications of the maternity cycle
E. "High-risk" pregnancies

F. Abortions

G. Maternal morbidity and mortality

H. Perinatal mortality

ANATOMY AND PHYSIOLOGY OF REPRODUCTIVE ORGANS

Reproductive organs well developed at birth

1. **Male reproductive system**

A. External genitalia

1. Penis, male organ of copulation, transports sperm and urine
2. Scrotum—contains testes, which produce sperm; the testes are 2 ovoid bodies composed of seminiferous tubules suspended by a spermatic cord

B. Internal structures

1. Spermatic cord, seminal vesicles, ejaculatory duct
2. Base of prostate gland just below the bladder and spermatic cord; surrounds urethra; spermatogenesis occurs in male from puberty into old age

2. **Female reproductive system**

A. External genitalia

1. Mons veneris, fat pad over symphysis, is covered with hair
2. Labia majora, large outer tissue flaps extending downward parallel to the side of both thighs
3. Labia minora, smaller inner tissue flaps, contain sebaceous glands, protect delicate structures, rich in nerve and blood supply, sensitive
4. Clitoris, at junction of extreme upper end of labia, sensitive erectile tissue
5. Urinary meatus, opening directly below clitoris
6. Skene's glands, one on each side of urinary meatus
7. Vagina, directly below urinary meatus, opening into internal reproductive system
8. Hymen, membranous tissue partially covering vaginal opening
9. Bartholin's glands, lateral distal vaginal wall; secrete lubricating substance
10. Perineum, muscles and fascia (includes levator ani); supports pelvic structures; extends from ischial and pubic bones down and back to sacrum and coccyx

B. Internal reproductive organs

1. Vagina, musculomembranous canal extending into uterus; rugated, having great power of stretching and dilating; bladder lies anterior and rectum posterior; function: path for release of menstrual flow, organ of copulation, birth canal at time of delivery

2. Uterus, hollow muscular organ (entirely nonstriated), suspended by ligaments between bladder and rectum in pelvic cavity

a. Covered with peritoneum; layers: perimetrium, outer layer; myometrium, middle layer; endometrium, inner layer
b. Divisions: fundus, upper rounded portion above insertion of tubes, contractile muscle power; body, from tube insertion to cervix; cervix, lower portion, great power of effacement and dilatation (internal os leads into uterus, external os leads into vagina)
c. Fornices, blind vaults where cervix extends downward into vaginal canal; deeper in posterior portion
d. Blood supply directly from uterine and ovarian arteries, ultimately from hypogastrics and aorta
e. Nerve supply principally from sympathetic and also from parasympathetic and cerebrospinal nervous systems
f. Ligaments suspend uterus in pelvic cavity: broad—lateral walls of uterus; round—either side of uterus; insert beneath tubes and terminate in labia majora
g. Function of uterus: receives and houses fertilized ovum, nourishes baby, contracts, and propels baby through birth canal at term

3. Fallopian tubes, convoluted muscular canals, insertion at upper cornua of uterus, below fundus; narrow at insertion, wider at distal fimbriated end

4. Ovaries, small almond-shaped organs on either side of uterus, attached to posterior wall of broad ligament; function: produce and develop ova, and produce hormones during pregnancy

5. Mammary glands, in anterior chest wall that extends from second to seventh rib

a. External structures: nipple ducts, nipple, and milk secretions; areola with tubercles of Montgomery secretes sebaceous substance; protects and lubricates nipple

b. Inner structures: tissue—glandular, adipose, and connective; divided into lobes, terminates into milk ducts in nipple
c. Breasts develop during puberty
d. Function: nourish infant following birth

C. Pelvis
1. Two-storied bony structure, basinlike, made up of 4 united bones: 2 innominate bones laterally and in front and the sacrum and coccyx in back; innominate bones divided into three parts—ilium, ischium, and pubic bone—and joined in front by the symphysis pubis; upper flaring part, false pelvis; lower part, true pelvis—the birth canal through which the baby must pass during labor and delivery
2. True pelvis divided into three parts
   a. Inlet or brim, bounded by upper border of the symphysis in front, ridge of the 2 iliac bones on the sides, and promontory of the sacrum in back; the inlet is slightly heartshaped, widest from side to side, narrowest front to back
   b. Midpelvis or pelvic cavity, bounded by inlet above, walls of the pelvis laterally, and outlet below; the midpelvis is cylindric in shape
   c. Outlet, bounded by lower border of symphysis pubis arch in front, ischial tuberosities laterally, and coccyx and greater sacrosciatic ligaments in back; the outlet is roughly triangular in shape; angle of the pubic arch is important in determining ease of delivery—the wider the angle, the larger the outlet, the easier the delivery

Puberty

1. **Physical and physiologic changes**
A. Male, 14 to 20 years of age—deepening of voice, growth of body hair over face, axillae, and genitalia; spermatogenesis with periodic erection and emission of mature sperm
B. Female, 11 to 18 years of age—pelvis widens, mammary glands develop, pubic and axillary hair growth and the production of ova herald menarche with beginning of menstruation
2. **Psychological changes**
Heterosexual interest, with girls matur-

ing earlier than boys; detachment from parental influence; development of identity

3. **Menstrual cycle**
A. Hormones produced by anterior pituitary (gonadotropins) interact with ovarian hormones (estrogen and progesterone), resulting in menstruation
B. Follicle-stimulating hormone (FSH) from anterior pituitary produces changes in graafian follicle, ovum matures; follicular phase, proliferation of cells in endometrium; ovulation occurs with formation of corpus luteum in cavity of ruptured follicle
C. Luteinizing hormone (LH) from the anterior pituitary causes graafian follicle to secrete estrogen and progesterone to prepare uterine lining for implantation should fertilization occur; absence of sperm and fertilization heralds menstruation with rhythmic cycle every 26 to 35 days until menopause

MATERNITY CYCLE
Antepartal period

1. **Maturation, fertilization, and implantation**
A. Maturation of ovum and spermatozoon by mitosis and meiosis; reduction in chromosomes from 46 to 23
B. Sexual union—uniting of ovum and sperm in distal portion of fallopian tube
C. Rapid division by cleavage without increase in size of cell cluster in 6 days (morula stage)
D. Implantation by 6 to 9 days in upper fundal portion of uterus
E. Blastocytic stage—rearrangement of cells into three layers: ectoderm, mesoderm, entoderm
F. Trophoblastic stage—projection of villi into maternal tissue later to become placenta, vehicle for exchange of nutriments and wastes
2. **Growth and development of baby (cephalocaudal)**
A. 14 days—heart begins to beat, brain, early spinal cord, muscle segments
B. 26 days—tiny buds for arms
C. 28 days—tiny buds for legs
D. 30 days—¼ to ½ inch in length, embryo has definite form, beginning of umbilical cord
E. 31 days—arm buds divide into hand, arm, and shoulder

F. 33 days—finger outlines

G. 46 to 48 days—first bone cells replace cartilage, upper arms

H. 5 to 7 weeks—amniotic fluid surrounds baby, discernible face

I. 12 weeks—weighs 1 ounce, moves parts of body, swallows, practices exhaling and inhaling

J. 16 to 20 weeks—weight increases six times (6 ounces), 8 to 10 inches in length, movements felt by mother

K. 20 to 24 weeks—weight 1 pound, 12 inches in length, hair growth on head, eyelashes, and brow, eyelids closed, skeletal frame hardens, fetal heart sounds heard with fetoscope

L. 24 to 28 weeks—eyelids open, weighs 1¼ pounds, amniotic fluid increases to 1 quart daily, exchange 6 gallons, cannot survive more than 24 hours outside uterus

M. 28 to 34 weeks—fat deposits, weighs 1 to 1½ pounds

N. 34 to 40 weeks—weight gain of 4 pounds, stores protein for extrauterine life

3. **Fetal circulation**

A. Structures
1. Placenta and cord (1 vein, 2 arteries)
2. Foramen ovale, opening between auricles
3. Ductus arteriosus—connects aorta and pulmonary arteries
4. Ductus venosus—between umbilical vein and ascending vena cava

4. **Physical and physiologic changes during pregnancy**
All body systems affected

A. Endocrine and reproductive systems
1. Fatigue—increased hormonal levels
2. Amenorrhea—corpus luteum persists, ovulation inhibited
3. Breast changes—tingling, fullness, soreness, later darkening of areola and nipple due to increase in hormonal levels
4. Leukorrhea—activation of glandular tissue in lower uterine segment, increased acidity a protection from bacterial invasion
5. Changes in uterus—hormonal and circulatory
   a. Goodell's sign, softening of cervix
   b. Hegar's sign, softening of lower uterine segment
   c. Chadwick's sign, purplish hue to vaginal mucosa
   d. Position of uterus—first trimester,

pelvic cavity; second and third trimesters, abdominal cavity before lightening occurs

B. Digestive system
1. Nausea and vomiting—reduction in hydrochloric acid, interferes with gastric motility
2. Constipation—pressure of baby in uterus against rectum, common early and late pregnancy

C. Excretory system
1. Frequency—early and late pregnancy, proximity of uterus and bladder
2. Lower specific gravity—increase in urinary output, excretion of wastes
3. Lower renal threshold—common in last trimester, sugar in urine (diabetes always ruled out)
4. Gonadotropins in urine—significant for diagnosis of pregnancy

D. Circulatory system
1. Blood volume—increase due to excretion of baby's wastes, resulting in lowered hemoglobin, physiologic anemia
2. Cardiac output—highest level at 24 to 32 weeks, declines to 40 weeks
3. Edema of extremities—stasis of blood, pressure on peripheral vascular system in last trimester
4. Leg cramps—calcium depletion by fetus, or increased phosphorus intake in mother's diet

E. Respiratory system
1. Dyspnea—at 36 to 38 weeks, pressure of growing fetus on diaphragm and lungs
2. Vital capacity increased, lung width increased, more air inspired

F. Integumentary system
1. Diaphoresis—excretion of wastes through skin
2. Skin changes—darkening of areolae, face (chloasma), striae due to skin stretching

G. Skeletal system—softening of all ligaments and joints; due to increased hormonal action

H. Nervous system—no changes unless related to prepregnant state

I. Metabolic—total weight gain—20 to 24 pounds; first trimester—2 pounds, second trimester—6 pounds, third trimester—12 pounds

5. **Duration and positive signs of pregnancy**

A. Estimated date of delivery—Nägele's

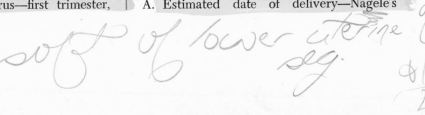

rule, count back 3 months and add 7 days from first day of last normal menstrual period; from 270 days (9 calendar months) to 290 days (10 lunar months)

B. Positive signs of pregnancy—hearing fetal heart sounds, palpating fetal parts, x-ray visualization of fetal skeleton

C. Pregnancy tests—Aschheim-Zondek, Friedman, induced progesterone, ortho test (chemical)

Prenatal care

1. Objectives

A. Early prenatal care to ensure optimum health of mother and baby

B. Medical supervision includes physical and psychological needs of family

C. Education for parents in preparation for childbearing

D. Continued health supervision of family

2. Components of adequate prenatal care

A. Complete examination by doctor—history, including medical, surgical, gynecologic, and obstetric data; family history of hereditary and transmittable diseases such as diabetes or heart disease

B. Physical examination—temperature, blood pressure, weight, examination of skin, thyroid, teeth, lungs, heart, breasts, abdominal palpation, auscultation, height of fundus, and vaginal examination (prior to last 4 weeks of pregnancy; smears taken for monilial and trichomonal infections, Papanicolaou test for cancer; size and position of uterus, palpation of adnexa

C. Pelvic estimation
1. Diagonal conjugate—diameter from symphysis pubis to promontory of sacrum
2. Transverse diameter of outlet
3. Pelvic contour—promontory of sacrum, coccyx, ischial spines, pubic arch, tuberosities

D. Blood work—standard test for syphilis (STS), Rh factor, blood typing and crossmatching, complete blood count

E. Urinalysis—routine and microscopic

3. Hygiene during prenatal period

A. Digestion—nutritional status
1. Importance of nutritionally well-balanced diet to ensure mother and baby's health
2. Start with what mother is eating daily, considering cultural and economic factors

3. Discuss basic 4 food groups; stress importance of added protein, iron, and vitamins during last trimester
4. Weight gain during various trimesters; discuss diet accordingly

B. Circulation
1. Adequate exercise without resultant fatigue
2. Importance of rest during day preventing stasis in extremities (especially last trimester)
3. Loose clothing to prevent constriction around waist and legs

C. Integumentary system
1. Cleanliness for comfort and proper elimination of wastes

D. Excretory system
1. Bowels—adequate fluid and fruit for roughage intake
2. Urine—increase in urinary output, elimination of wastes

E. Respiratory system
1. Fresh air essential to keep lungs aerated for sufficient oxygen consumption

F. Nervous system
1. Adequate rest and social activities for relaxation of mind and body

G. Reproductive system
1. Proper care and support of breasts in preparation for lactation
2. Skin care includes daily washing, using soap sparingly on nipple to prevent excessive drying
3. Supportive brassiere to facilitate adequate blood supply to breast
4. Well-fitted abdominal support if needed

4. Preparation for childbirth

A. Objectives of teaching program for parents
1. To increase understanding of anatomy and physiology of pregnancy and labor
2. To discuss emotional changes occurring during pregnancy (emphasis on normal)
3. To prepare mother for physical work during labor by improving muscle tone of abdominal and perineal muscles
4. To encourage exercises that aid in relaxation such as positioning, breathing, and body mechanics
5. To alleviate fears associated with childbearing, through individual and group discussion

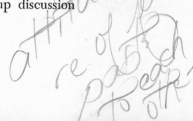

6. To acquaint parents with facilities available to them in hospital and community for continued optimum health care and for supervision of new family

Intrapartal period

1. **Labor**

Physiologic and mechanical process in which the baby, placenta, and membranes are expelled through the pelvis and birth canal

2. **Bony pelvis**

A. Composition—ischium, ilium, sacrum, and coccyx

B. Bones joined by fibrous cartilaginous tissue, which becomes elastic and softened during pregnancy

C. Cavity protects reproductive organs

D. Entrance into true pelvis downward and curved backward as in letter J

E. Transverse diameter greatest at inlet

F. Anteroposterior diameter greatest at outlet

G. Normal pelvis—curved sacrum, movable coccyx, blunt ischial spines, curved side walls, ample pubic arch

H. Conjugate diagonal diameter—most important diameter, from promontory of sacrum posteriorly to symphysis pubis anteriorly

I. Classification of pelves—gynecoid, android, anthropoid, platypelloid

3. **Attitude, presentation, position of baby**

A. Attitude—relationship of fetal parts to each other

B. Presentation—position baby engages into true pelvis

   1. Cephalic—vertex, brow, or face

   2. Breech—frank, complete, single or double footling

C. Position—relationship of presenting part to four quadrants

   1. Vertex—occiput, LOA, LOP, ROA, ROP

   2. Face—chin (mentum) LMA, LMP, RMA, RMP

   3. Breech—sacrum, LSA, LSP, RSA, RSP

D. Station—relationship of presenting part to false and to true pelvis

   1. Floating—presenting part movable above the pelvic inlet

   2. Engaged—suboccipitobregmatic diameter through pelvic inlet

   3. True pelvis—presenting part at ischial spines, station 0

   4. Levels below ischial spines, +1, +2, +3

   5. Levels above ischial spines, -1, -2, -3

4. **Labor process**

A. Prior to true labor—lightening, settling of baby into true pelvis; Braxton Hicks' contractions, in preparation for true labor; increased vaginal secretions; softening of cervix

B. Muscular uterine contractions increase in frequency, strength, and intensity, with resistance of cervix and perineal floor muscles

C. Pressure on cervix causes effacement and dilatation, and expulsion of baby through birth canal

5. **Mechanisms and rotation of baby with vertex presentation through pelvis**

A. At onset of labor, baby's head descends, chin flexes on chest as engagement occurs in true pelvis

B. Uterine contractions move baby downward, internal rotation occurs as baby's head passes ischial spines

C. Occiput impinges under symphysis as baby's head is borne by extension

D. Shoulders meet resistance of symphysis and smallest diameter presents itself through birth canal; one shoulder delivered at a time

E. Baby's body delivered by lateral flexion due to pelvic contour

6. **Evaluating labor status on admission**

A. Parity

B. Time contractions began, frequency, duration, and strength

C. Occurrence of membrane rupture, bloody show

D. Temperature, pulse, respiration, blood pressure, fetal heart sounds

E. Perineal shave and cleansing (optional; in many labor and delivery units not done)

F. Previous obstetric, gynecologic, and medical-surgical history

G. Evaluation by physician

7. **Stages of labor**

A. First stage—onset of true labor to complete effacement and dilatation

B. Second stage—complete effacement and dilatation until birth of baby

C. Third stage—birth of baby until expulsion of placenta

D. Fourth stage—first hour after delivery; astute observation of fundus, lochia, blood pressure, and pulse for signs of bleeding

8. **Behavior during labor**

A. Phases of first stage
   1. Entertainment—irregular contractions, cervix dilated 0 to 2 cm.; mother excited and happy labor has started, yet apprehensive
   2. Relaxation—moderate to strong regular contractions 5 to 8 minutes or 3 to 5 minutes, cervix dilated 2 to 6 cm., bloody show, membranes may rupture; abdominal breathing lifts abdominal wall away from contracting uterus, medication to elevate pain threshold and aid in relaxation, supportive measures by nurse such as encouragement, praise, reassurance, "thereness"; informing patient of progress, restlessness during contractions but rest in between
   3. Transition—strong contractions 1 to 2 minutes apart, bloody show, mother irritable, restless, highly emotional, cannot follow instructions, face flushed and perspiring, belching, tremors of legs, pale white ring around mouth, sudden nausea and vomiting
B. Beginning second stage—full dilatation, perineum bulges, desire to push with each contraction, grunting sounds
9. Nursing care during labor and birth of the baby
A. Strict asepsis
B. Timing of frequency, duration, strength of contractions
C. Checking of fetal heart sounds—rate, regularity, and tone
D. Frequent observation of perineum for show, rupture of membranes, presenting part
E. Frequent checking of blood pressure and pulse
F. Emergency equipment such as oxygen, blood, oxytocic, stimulant drug available on labor unit
G. Preparation and checking of sedation before administration, for safe care of mother and baby
H. Recognition of mother's basic needs in relation to body fluids, excretion, etc.
I. Support by nurse or husband
10. Danger symptoms during labor
A. Tonic contractions, strong, continuous, sudden sharp pain with boardlike abdomen
B. Variation in rate, regularity, and tone of fetal heart sounds
C. Excessive amniotic fluid, meconium-stained amniotic fluid
D. Increase or decrease in blood pressure
E. Increase in pulse and temperature
F. Sudden excessive fetal movements
G. Bleeding, expulsion of umbilical cord or placental fragments
11. Immediate care of mother and baby following delivery
A. Mother
   1. Check fundus as to firmness and height
   2. Check for open airway if anesthesia has been administered
   3. Check blood pressure and pulse, report fluctuations
   4. Check perineum for bleeding; check suture line of episiotomy or laceration
B. Baby
   1. Ensure patent airway, free of mucus; frequent observation of respiratory effort (Apgar scoring method)
   2. Quick appraisal for anomalies (keep warm)
   3. Eye care to prevent ophthalmia neonatorum
   4. Check identification band with that of mother before leaving delivery room

Postpartal period

1. Puerperium and family planning
   Period following delivery, during which the organs of reproduction undergo physical and physiologic changes; process called involution, usually takes 6 weeks
2. Systemic changes during puerperium
A. Digestive system
   1. Organs of digestion return to normal state
   2. Nutrients essential in preparation for lactation
   3. Fluid intake and roughage relieve constipation
B. Circulatory system
   1. Blood volume and plasma unstable, slight rise
   2. Increase in blood fibrinogen first week
   3. Leukocytes may increase to 15,000 or higher if labor long
   4. Hemoglobin and red blood cell count low on fourth postpartal day
C. Excretory system
   1. Increase in urinary output second to fifth postpartal day; 3,000 ml. excreted daily

2. Retention with overflow may occur; bladder capacity increased during pregnancy
3. Lactose in urine not uncommon—activation of lactogenic hormone
4. Nitrogen excreted—replenish with high-protein diet to rebuild body tissue

D. Integumentary system
1. Profuse diaphoresis; replace fluid intake

E. Reproductive system
1. Uterus—contractions bring about involution, may also cause afterpains; analgesics helpful
2. Vaginal flow—regeneration of uterine lining with new epithelium 2 or 3 days after delivery; entire endometrium and ovulatory cycle restored by end of third postpartal week; vaginal discharge, lochia, changes from rubra to serosa in 1 week, then becomes alba by 12 days
3. Vagina—returns to near-nonpregnant state; cicatrization, healing of soft tissues
4. Abdominal wall—soft and flabby but regains tone
5. Breasts
   a. Delivery of placenta activates luteinizing hormone in the anterior pituitary
   b. Posterior pituitary secretes oxytocin; "let-down reflex" occurs with ejection of milk as baby suckles
   c. Colostrum, forerunner of milk
   d. Engorgement of breast on second or third day due to increase in blood supply prior to lactation

3. **Nursing care during puerperium**
A. Aseptic technique used in giving care to genital area
B. Breast—daily washing (use soap sparingly to prevent nipple breakdown) and support with well-fitted brassiere; frequent changes prevent bacterial growth due to milk leakage
C. Importance of hand washing in caring for self and baby
D. Emphasis on hand washing by personnel to avoid cross-contamination
E. Daily observations of vital signs; temperature of 100.4° F. for any 2 consecutive days (excluding first 24 hours) considered sign of beginning puerperal infection; pulse lower following delivery

F. Checking fundus for firmness—process of involution
G. Meeting mother's needs enables mother to meet the infant's needs
H. Adequate nutritious diet to restore body with proteins, added nutrition for lactation
I. Careful attention to bladder and bowel function
J. Early ambulation, when condition permits prevents blood stasis
K. Postpartal blues not uncommon on fourth or fifth day, due to drop in hormonal level
L. Teaching of mother as need arises in relation to self-care and care of baby
M. Group discussions prove favorable on breast feeding, infant care, etc.

4. **Principles in teaching and learning**
A. Learner must be ready and willing to learn
B. Begin with what learner already knows (this strengthens teaching relationship)
C. Wait for opportune time to teach (e.g., when baby is with mother)
D. The more senses used in process of learning, the quicker learning occurs (demonstrating baby bath, instead of just discussing, and then allowing mother to practice soon afterward is ideal)
E. Behavior changes when learning occurs (apprehensive mother becomes calmer, feels more secure in her role)

5. **Family planning**
A. Objectives
1. Combined effort on part of both parents
2. Health of mother enhances the care of family
3. Nurse's role—knowledge of methods, referral of parents, with due respect to religious beliefs
B. Methods of contraception
1. Rhythm method, only method sanctioned by Roman Catholic Church, abstinence from coitus during fertile period
2. Coitus interruptus—withdrawal of the penis during coitus, prior to ejaculation
3. Vaginal douches—follow sexual contact
4. Jellies, creams, suppositories—spermicidal effect prevents conception
5. Condom—rubber sheath that covers penis

6. Diaphragm—mechanical device that covers cervix
7. Intrauterine contraceptive devices (IUCD)—mechanical devices inserted into uterus; cause excessive tubal motility, prevent conception
8. Oral progestins—hormones taken orally, suppressing ovulation
9. Intramuscular progestins—3-month, 6-month doses

THE NEWBORN

1. Needs of newborn
A. Open airway, clear of mucus, observation
B. Warmth and comfort
C. Nutrition
D. Love and security (for establishing sense of trust)

2. Systems in newborn
A. Circulatory
  1. Own circulation after cord tied and cut
  2. Liver immature, with hyperbilirubinemia—may cause jaundice on third day due to red cell destruction
  3. Clotting mechanism poor; vitamin K essential, given intramuscularly
  4. Hemoglobin—14 to 20 grams per 100 ml. (grams) of blood
  5. Red blood cell count—4.5 to 5.5 million per 100 cu. mm. of blood
  6. White blood cell count—6,000 to 22,000 per cu. mm. of blood
B. Respiratory—irregular abdominal respirations, 30 to 40 per minute
C. Renal
  1. Kidneys immature, excrete urine first 24 hours
  2. Bladder empties 20 times daily by 2 weeks
  3. Urates—brick red stain on diaper; increase in fluid intake
D. Digestive
  1. Digests simple carbohydrates, fats, and proteins
  2. Needs very little in first few days, since he has stores from intrauterine life
  3. Sucking and rooting reflex present
E. Metabolic—10% of birth weight lost
F. Integumentary
  1. Lanugo—fine downy hair, first month of life
  2. Milia—small sebaceous cysts over nose
  3. Mongolian spots—bluish black discoloration on buttocks, back, and sacral region
G. Hormonal reactions

1. From transmission to fetus in utero; normal, rapidly disappear
2. Breast changes—enlargement, "witch's milk"
3. Bloody mucoid vaginal discharge

3. Infant feeding
A. Objectives
  1. To supply adequate nourishment for growth and development toward maintenance of optimum health
  2. To satisfy the infant's sucking reflex, oral phase, development of sense of trust and security
B. Breast-feeding
  1. Care of breasts during prenatal period, cleanliness and support
  2. Desire to breast-feed
  3. Mother's comfort prior to feeding is essential
  4. Stimulating both breasts establishes an increased milk supply
  5. Encourage feeding infant on demand
C. Advantages of breast-feeding
  1. Psychological value, closeness of mother and baby is a satisfying and rewarding experience in beginning mother-infant relationship
  2. Easily accessible, clean, optimum nutritional value, digested well by baby
  3. Stimulates uterine contractions, hastens involution in mother
  4. Economical
  5. Develops jaws and nasal passages
  6. Protects infant from development of allergies
D. Artificial feeding
  1. Terminal-heat method or aseptic method, lowers bacterial count
  2. Composition of formula: protein and fat diluted with water and added carbohydrate
  3. 45 to 50 calories per pound adequate for newborn
  4. 2 to 3 ounces of fluid per pound of body weight
  5. One-fifth of total daily caloric intake carbohydrate
  6. Formula feedings take longer to digest, infant takes fewer feedings than by breast
  7. Adjust nipple holes to satisfy baby's sucking needs (20 minutes' sucking time per feeding)

4. Reflexes present at birth
A. Rooting and sucking
B. Tonic neck

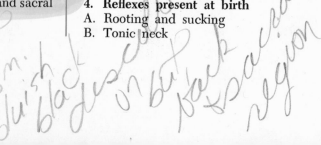

C. Grasp
D. Moro
E. Dance

5. Appraisal of newborn
A. Open airway; breathing—abdominal, shallow, irregular
B. Good muscle tone
C. Skin color
D. Frontal and occipital fontanels
E. Symmetry of face
F. Equal distance from ear to shoulder, left and right
G. Unrestricted movements of arms and legs
H. Abduction of legs; rule out dislocation
I. Check feet to rule out clubbing
J. Check genitalia for normalcy, patency of rectum
K. Check spine for abnormal openings
L. Check fingers and toes for webbing
M. Check reflexes listed above
N. Listen to character of cry
O. Measure circumference of head and of chest and measure crown to rump; all practically equal at birth in full-size infants

6. Mother-infant relationship
A. Contact with one person (mother or mother substitute)
B. Inborn impulse of mothering in women
C. Biologic changes enhance and develop motherliness
D. Biologic separation of mother and infant at birth
E. Gratification a two-way process between mother and infant
F. Nurse's role in support of mother and infant in beginning relationships
G. Husband's role in mother-infant interaction

DEVIATIONS FROM THE NORMAL MATERNITY CYCLE

1. Toxemias of pregnancy—peculiar to third trimester
A. Triad of symptoms
   1. Edema
   2. Elevation in blood pressure
   3. Proteinuria
B. Classification (American Committee of Maternal Welfare)
   1. Acute toxemia of pregnancy
      a. Preeclampsia—mild and severe
      b. Eclampsia—convulsions associated with above triad of symptoms
   2. Chronic hypertensive disease with pregnancy

a. Without superimposed acute toxemia
   (1) Hypertension known to have antedated pregnancy
   (2) Hypertension discovered during pregnancy, before twenty-fourth week, and continuing after delivery
b. With superimposed acute toxemia
   3. Unclassified toxemia
C. Prevention
   1. Adequate nutrition
   2. Early and adequate prenatal care
   3. Education during prenatal period
D. Treatment and nursing care of preeclampsia
   1. Hospitalization and treatment determined by degree of symptoms
   2. Bed rest with sedatives
   3. Diet—high-protein, low-salt
   4. Frequent revisits to physician or visits to clinic
   5. Diuretics to relieve edema
   6. Blood chemistry (danger signs—rise in blood serum proteins, increase in cell volume and hemoglobin, rise in uric acid concentration)
   7. Qualitative urinalysis
E. Treatment and nursing care of eclampsia
   1. Strict bed rest
   2. Observations for irritability, restlessness, signs of labor, epigastric pain
   3. Emergency equipment available—tongue blade, oxygen, sedatives, hypertensives, glucose solution, central nervous system depressants such as magnesium sulfate and morphine sulfate (calcium gluconate and Lorfan available for latter two drugs, respectively, as antidotes)
   4. Equipment in readiness for induction of labor or emergency cesarean section
   5. Careful check of vital signs and fetal heart tones

2. Bleeding during maternity cycle (and associated complications)
A. Classification
   1. First-trimester bleeding during pregnancy
      a. Abortions—(complete or incomplete); spontaneous (habitual or missed); induced (therapeutic or elective)
      b. Ectopic pregnancy
      c. Hydatidiform mole

2. Third-trimester bleeding during pregnancy
   a. Placenta praevia—marginal, partial, complete
   b. Abruptio placentae—afibrinogenemia
3. Postpartal hemorrhage
   a. Atony of uterus
   b. Tears and lacerations
   c. Retained placental fragments
4. Outside uterus
   a. Cervix
   b. Lacerations
   c. Erosions
   d. Polyps
   e. Carcinoma in situ
5. Inside uterus
   a. Placental site
   b. Defective germ plasm
   c. Improper implantation site
   d. Detachment of placenta
B. Bleeding during first trimester of pregnancy
   1. Abortion—interruption of pregnancy before 28 weeks (7 months)
      a. Classification
         (1) Threatened—spotting; bed rest and observation for 24 hours
         (2) Inevitable—continued bleeding after 24 hours
            (a) Complete — contractions, expulsion of entire products of conception
            (b) Incomplete—contractions, expulsion of fragments of products of conception; hospitalization, dilatation and curettage done
         (3) Missed—spotting each month, death of fetus in uterus, eventual complete or incomplete expulsion of fetus
         (4) Habitual—repeated abortion, following three pregnancies
         (5) Therapeutic—interruption of pregnancy for safety of mother's health
         (6) Criminal—obsolete term, better stated as extrahospital or extraclinic: termination of pregnancy outside of medical facilities, frequently by nonphysician abortionists, regardless of the validity of indication
      b. Causes
         (1) Defective germ plasm (ovum or sperm)

(2) Poor nutritional status of mother
(3) Physiologic maternal causes
   (a) Infection
   (b) Endocrine disturbances
   (c) Anomalies of reproductive organs
(4) External causes
   (a) Radiation
   (b) Trauma
2. Ectopic pregnancy—implantation outside uterus
   a. Causes—obstruction in fallopian tube, cicatrization in tube from infections, growths obstructing fallopian tube, abnormal growth of fertilized ovum in tube, causing immobilization, previous plastic surgery of tube
   b. Danger signals—pain radiating to shoulder after activity; pain during cervical manipulation on pelvic examination; as pregnancy advances, death of fetus and rupture of tube occur
3. Hydatidiform mole—abnormal pregnancy—benign growth of chorion
   a. Clinical course
      (1) Continuous or intermittent brownish-colored bleeding commencing at 12 weeks' gestation
      (2) Excessive uterine enlargement, inconsistent with gestational weeks
      (3) Toxemia symptoms prior to third trimester
      (4) Fetal parts difficult to palpate
      (5) High chorionic gonadotropin level at 12 weeks (ruling out true pregnancy)
   b. Dangers
      (1) Hemorrhage
      (2) Infection
      (3) Uterine perforation
      (4) Susceptibility to choriocarcinoma
   c. Treatment
      (1) With severe bleeding, evacuation with ovum forceps or hysterectomy
      (2) Blood replacement
      (3) Antibiotics
      (4) Avoid early subsequent pregnancy
      (5) Follow-up care: weekly chori-

onic gonadotropin levels for
2 months
  (6) Continued rise in blood serum
levels warrant hysterectomy
  (7) Follow-up care: blood serum
levels indicated for a year to
rule out chorionic carcinoma
C. Bleeding during latter part of pregnancy
  1. Placenta praevia—low implantation of
placenta
    a. Variations
      (1) Marginal—along lower uterine
segment
      (2) Partial—partially covers inter-
nal os
      (3) Complete—completely covers
internal os
    b. Causes—unknown
    c. Predisposing factors
      (1) Multiparity
      (2) Endometritis
    d. Symptoms
      (1) Painless bleeding during last
trimester
      (2) Recurrent hemorrhage
    e. Treatment
      (1) Hospitalization
      (2) Strict bed rest
      (3) Blood typing, crossmatching,
blood available
      (4) No rectals or enemas
      (5) Strict asepsis
      (6) Management of delivery either
vaginal or by cesarean section;
depends on amount of bleeding, condition of baby and
mother, and condition of cervix
and labor process
  2. Abruptio placentae—premature separation of normally implanted placenta,
occurring in last trimester or during
labor; may be partial or complete
    a. Cause—unknown
    b. Predisposing factors
      (1) Short cord
      (2) Multiparity
      (3) Toxemia
    c. Symptoms
      (1) Sudden severe sharp pain over
fundus
      (2) Uterus boardlike and rigid
      (3) Hemorrhage, mostly concealed
      (4) Fetal distress
      (5) Sudden symptoms of shock
    d. Treatment
      (1) Immediate treatment for shock

      (2) Emergency cesarean section
  3. Incompetent cervix
    a. Course—early rupture of mem-
branes and abortion in middle of
second or beginning of third trimester
    b. Causes—congenital, acquired (re-
sult of birth injury to birth canal,
especially cervix, trauma during
cervical dilatation)
    c. Treatment—Shirodkar: purse-string
closure of cervix; removal of purse-
string prior to onset of labor is followed by vaginal delivery or cesarean section when indicated
D. Bleeding during delivery and immediate
postpartal period
  1. Causes
    a. Tear or laceration of cervix
    b. Atony of uterus
  2. Predisposing factors
    a. Difficult delivery
    b. Long labor
    c. Polyhydramnios—overdistention of
uterus
    d. Faulty uterine musculature
    e. Grandmultiparity
  3. Treatment
    a. Tear or laceration—immediate su-
turing to prevent hemorrhage
    b. Atony of uterus—holding fundus
firmly above symphysis and administration of oxytocics intravenously and replacement of fluids
with plasma expander or whole
blood
    c. Retention of placental fragments—
removal manually and administration of oxytocic
E. Nursing care for excessive bleeding
  1. Apprehension, anxiety, and fear result in physiologic increase in epinephrine with resulting constriction of
vessels; when replacement therapy is
life-sustaining, reassurance keeps
mother calm
  2. Blood work-up: typing and crossmatching, Rh factor, with availability
of whole blood
  3. Frequent checking of vital signs and
fetal heart tones
  4. Availability of oxygen for mother,
should fetal distress occur
  5. Treatment for shock: Trendelenburg
position, blood replacement, etc.
F. Dangers associated with bleeding

1. Hemorrhage
2. Infection
3. Rupture of uterus
4. Sterility
5. Debilitation of optimum health

G. Spiritual care of mother and infant
1. Spiritual attendance prior to surgery
2. Baptism of infant—Roman Catholics and Protestants (exclusion of Baptists and Disciples of Christ)
3. Emergency delivery—reassure mother; support perineum with clean hand or towel; instruct mother to pant, prevent rapid delivery; provide airway for infant, milk trachea; check fundus; after delivery of placenta put baby to breast—stimulates uterine contractions

3. **Pathology of labor**
A. Dystocia—long, difficult labor
1. Mechanical—contracted pelvis; obstructive fibromyoma; abnormal size, malformation, or malpresentation of baby
2. Functional—patterns of uterine contractions deviating from the normal, either hypertonic or hypotonic
a. Causes: anomalies of uterus, overdistention of uterus (multiple pregnancy or polyhydramnios), postmaturity, fibromyomas, scar tissue of cervix from delivery or gynecologic surgery, maternal debilitating disease
3. Management of mechanical and functional dystocia
a. Trial labor—specified number of labor hours allotted
b. Roentgen-ray examination—cephalopelvic disproportion warrants surgical intervention

B. Precipitate labor—a labor of 2 hours or less
1. More frequent in multigravidas with history of rapid labor and delivery
2. Dangers
a. Mother—lacerations of cervix and external genitalia and postpartal hemorrhage
b. Infant—anoxia and asphyxia, possible intracranial damage

C. Desultory and prolonged labor—labor extending beyond 18 to 24 hours
1. Causes
a. Distention and distortion of myometrium

b. Polyhydramnios
c. Fibromyomas
d. Multiple pregnancies
e. Malpresentations and malpositions of baby
f. Higher incidence in elderly primigravidas and grandmultigravidas

2. Treatment
a. Course of treatment considers mother and infant
b. Prophylactic antibiotics to prevent infection
c. Uterine stimulants (oxytocics given)
d. Replacement of body fluids parenterally
e. Forceps delivery with full effacement, dilatation
f. Surgical intervention with cephalopelvic disproportion

3. Nursing care with prolonged labor
a. Observe for signs of maternal exhaustion and elevation in body temperature, fruity odor to breath, diminished urinary output, positive acetone reaction
b. Observe for signs of fetal distress, changes in rate, regularity, and strength of fetal heart tones, excessive movements, and meconium staining of amniotic fluid
c. Oxygen availability
d. Equipment for aspiration and resuscitation
e. Parenteral fluids and availability of blood

D. Induction of labor
1. Indications for induction
a. Medical—diabetes, pyelonephritis
b. Obstetric—toxemia, sensitization to Rh factor and blood incompatibility, polyhydramnios, premature rupture of membranes at term without contractions, abruptio placentae

2. Contraindications for induction
a. Cephalopelvic disproportion
b. Malpresentation
c. Grandmultigravida
d. Previous cesarean section
e. History of uterine surgery in which danger of rupture of uterus exists
f. Reconstructive surgery of cervix or uterus

3. Obstetric criteria for safe induction
a. No evidence of cephalopelvic disproportion

b. Cervix must be "ripe" (partially effaced) and 1.5 to 2 cm. dilated
c. Vertex presentation with engagement
d. No abnormal distention of uterus
4. Medical methods for induction—posterior pituitary extracts such as oxytocin, sparteine sulfate administered by buccal, intramuscular, or intravenous route
5. Mechanical methods of induction—artificial rupture of membranes done with vertex well engaged in true pelvis and some effacement and dilatation of cervix
6. Nursing care during induction
   a. Preparation of mother; explaining treatment
   b. Constant timing of contractions
   c. Vital signs and fetal heart tones
   d. *Constant attendance* during induction
   e. With drip induction, astuteness as to rate of flow
   f. Blood typing and crossmatching, Rh factor, and blood availability prior to induction
   g. Preparation of mother for emergency cesarean section when warranted
   h. Availability of oxygen for mother and for aspiration and resuscitation of infant
E. Abdominal delivery by cesarean section
   1. Indications—cephalopelvic disproportion; placenta praevia, abruptio placentae, uterine inertia; toxemia; fetal distress; malpresentation; Rh isoimmunization; diabetes; postmaturity; uterine growths that block birth canal; maternal risks—cranial aneurysms and brain tumors
   2. Contraindications—fetal death (no other complication); major fetal anomaly, eclampsia, infection of peritoneal cavity
   3. Types of cesarean section
      a. Low-segment—midline incision below umbilicus to symphysis on skin transverse incision into lower uterine segment
      b. Classic—same as above on skin, longitudinal into uterus up to peritoneal flap
      c. Extraperitoneal—dissecting bladder downward, exposure and incision into uterus without entering peritoneal cavity
   4. Nursing care
      a. Psychological preparation
      b. Physiologic preparation—abdominal, perineal, rectal shave, blood typing and crossmatching, Rh factor, catheterization, vital signs
      c. Spiritual
      d. Postoperative care—vital signs, incisional drainage, abdominal distention, early ambulation, deep breathing, and leg motion, intake and output records
F. Vacuum extractor
   1. Suction device used on baby's head to facilitate delivery
   2. Maternal risks—cervical lacerations, increased incidence of retained placenta, postpartal hemorrhage
   3. Infant risks—intracranial hemorrhage, brain damage

4. **Medical-surgical diseases in pregnancy**
A. Prevention
   1. Premarital physical examination—family history
   2. Genetic counseling
B. Heart disease
   1. 1% of pregnant women have organic heart disease
   2. 90% of these are of rheumatic origin
   3. 10%, congenital lesions and syphilis
   4. Hemodynamics during maternity cycle
      a. Increased oxygen needs for growing fetus
      b. Accelerated heart rate, 14,000 extra beats in 24 hours (latter half of pregnancy)
      c. Blood volume and cardiac output greatest at 24 to 32 weeks
      d. Fall in cardiac output, after twenty-seventh week, to term
      e. Blood volume reaches peak at thirty-sixth week; declines to term
      f. Oxygen consumption rises with contractions of labor
      g. Heart rate accelerated at beginning of contraction, slower at height of contraction
      h. Tachycardia during delivery
      i. Bradycardia following delivery
   5. Review functional and therapeutic classification
   6. Management and treatment
      a. Extra bed rest

b. Weekly prenatal visits by cardiologist
c. Hospitalization for patient with class III or IV disease until after delivery
d. Hospitalization with history of cardiac failure
e. Low-sodium diet
f. Report immediately fatigue, dyspnea, hemoptysis, edema
g. Minimal analgesia and anesthesia with decreased cardiac reserve; forceps used to shorten second stage
h. Inhalation anesthesia contraindicated
i. Scopolamine contraindicated
j. Oxytocins contraindicated; if necessary, given in intravenous solution, slowly
k. Observation of vital signs following delivery imperative
l. Antibiotics given to prevent infection
m. Digitalis and diuretics to strengthen heart muscle and increase circulation time—prevent heart failure and pulmonary edema
n. Continued medical supervision following discharge
7. Nursing care
a. Prenatal period—health teaching, rest and diet, referral to community agencies such as homemaker service, avoidance of emotional stress, physiologic and psychological preparation for labor and delivery, prevention of infection
b. Intrapartal period—early admission for rest prior to labor, vital signs, signs of heart failure and pulmonary edema, Fowler's position, oxygen equipment available, added support and observation, delivery in bed under aseptic technique if necessary
c. Postpartal period—30% increase in cardiac output, decrease on fifth day; vital signs, watch for tachycardia and respiratory distress; sedation and rest, referral to public health, homemaker and social agencies for continuity in care
C. Diabetes mellitus
1. Incidence—0.25% to 1%, of all pregnancies; history of repeated stillbirths, fetal deaths, excessively large infants (over 4000 grams); neonatal deaths due to hypoxia and hypoglycemia, congenital anomalies, premature labor, stillbirth, toxemia, and hydramnios greater
2. Physiology of pregnancy related to diabetes mellitus
a. Pregnancy—vomiting decreases carbohydrate intake; danger of acidosis; increased activity of anterior pituitary decreases tolerance for sugar; therefore larger quantities of insulin required; elevated BMR and decrease in CO_2 combining power increase tendency toward acidosis; sugar in urine in early pregnancy due to lowered renal threshold
b. Labor—muscular activity during labor depletes glycogen; therefore carbohydrate with insulin coverage needed
c. Puerperium—hypoglycemia as involution and lactation occur
3. Nursing care
a. Prevention of acidosis and toxemia, prenatal period
b. Weekly prenatal supervision visits to internist and obstetrician
c. Dietary regimen
d. Teaching and guidance in relation to signs of hypoglycemia and acidosis, diet, exercise, urinalysis, personal hygiene, avoidance of emotional stress
e. Identification card on person
f. Referral to public health nursing service for continuity in care
D. Acute and chronic pyelonephritis
1. Acute pyelonephritis—diffuse inflammatory process of interstitial connective tissue of kidney (nephron involved when infection is extensive)
2. Organism most common—Escherichia coli; occasionally Staphylococcus and Streptococcus
3. Signs and symptoms—chills, fever, severe backache, tenderness over kidney region, rise in nonprotein nitrogen, decrease in phenolsulfonphthalein excretion and dye excretion on pyelography
4. Nursing care
a. Adequate diet and rest
b. Chemotherapy; force fluids and record intake and output

c. Sims' position—relieve pressure on ureters

d. Teaching importance of health supervision

e. Medical follow-up after delivery

f. Family planning to avoid risk of early reoccurrence of pregnancy

5. **Complications of the newborn**

A. Causes

1. Placenta praevia or abruptio placentae
2. Umbilical cord malformation, knotting
3. Infectious agents, viruses
4. Abnormal presentations
5. Prolonged rupture of membranes
6. Precipitate or instrument delivery
7. Prolonged labor with oversedation
8. Maternal disease

B. Neonatal respiratory distress

1. Asphyxia neonatorum—respirations not well established 60 seconds after birth
   a. Asphyxia livida—cyanosis, muscle tone good
   b. Asphyxia pallida—marked pallor, loss of muscle tone
   c. Causes—anoxia, cerebral damage, narcosis
   d. Prevention—early prenatal care, early management of deviations from normal, prenatal education, good medical management during labor and delivery
   e. Treatment—observation first 24 hours of every newborn by qualified personnel, intubation equipment, respiratory stimulants

2. Atelectasis—incomplete expansion of lung or portion of lung
   a. Causes—prematurity, oversedation, damage to respiratory center, inhalation of mucus or amniotic fluid
   b. Symptoms—cyanosis, rapid irregular respirations, flaring nostrils, intercostal or suprasternal retraction, audible expiratory grunt
   c. Treatment—patent airway, oxygen administered with high humidity, stimulation of respirations, frequent change of position, carbon dioxide under pressure, antibiotics to prevent infection

3. Hyaline membrane disease—protein material in alveoli, preventing lung aeration
   a. Causes—prematurity, cesarean section
   b. Symptoms—cyanosis, dyspnea, ster-

nal retraction; symptoms occur few hours following birth

c. Treatment—patent airway, Isolette with humidity and oxygen, antibiotics

C. Birth injuries

1. Caput succedaneum—edema with extravasation of serum into scalp tissues due to molding during birth process; no treatment, subsides in few days

2. Cephalohematoma—edema of scalp with effusion of blood between bone and periosteum, reabsorption occurs in a few days

3. Intracranial hemorrhage—tearing of tentorium cerebelli with bleeding into cerebellum, pons, and medulla oblongata; occurs following prolonged labor, difficult forceps delivery, precipitate delivery, version, breech extraction
   a. Symptoms—abnormal respirations, cyanosis, sharp shrill or weak cry, flaccidity, spasticity, restlessness, wakefulness, convulsions, poor sucking reflex
   b. Prevention—medical supervision during labor and delivery
   c. Treatment—Isolette with oxygen and humidity, elevation of infant's head, vitamins C and K to control and prevent further hemorrhage, gavage if sucking reflex is impaired, support of parents

4. Facial paralysis—asymmetry of face due to damage of facial nerves, difficult forceps delivery; temporary, disappears in a few days

5. Erb-Duchenne paralysis (arm paralysis)—result of difficult forceps delivery or breech extraction; treatment depends upon severity; massage and exercise prevent contractures, splinting and casting done when severe

6. Dislocations and fractures—crepitation, immobility, and variations in range of motion on appraisal of newborn; treatment depends upon site of fracture; swaddling, positioning, splints, slings, and casts; referral to public health agency for continuity in care and support of parents; report to Crippled Children's Commission for rehabilitation

7. Infections—prevention by medical

asepsis in care of newborn and isolation of all suspects in nurseries

  a. Thrush—mouth infection caused by *Candida albicans;* transmitted through organisms in vaginal canal of mother, trauma to mouth tissues, unclean feeding utensils, improper hand-washing techniques

    (1) Symptoms—white patches on tongue, palate, inner cheek surfaces, which bleed on examination; poor sucking reflex

    (2) Treatment—application of 1% gentian violet, oral Mycostatin, care of equipment by boiling; prevent transmission

  b. Impetigo—infectious skin eruptions, characterized by vesicles or pustules caused by *Staphylococcus* or *Streptococcus*

    (1) Prevention—adequate hand washing and medical asepsis in nurseries

    (2) Treatment—isolation, pHisoHex baths daily, alcohol, gentian violet, bacitracin, neomycin, local application, antibiotics

D. Ophthalmia neonatorum—eye infection caused by *Neisseria gonorrhoeae*

  1. Source—genital tract during delivery, infected hands of personnel

  2. Prevention—prophylactic treatment of eyes at birth of all newborns

  3. Treatment—antibiotic therapy; strict hand-washing technique and boiling of all equipment; prevent transmission

E. *Staphylococcus* infections

  1. Prevention—reduce number of personnel in nurseries, allow adequate crib spacing, eliminate carriers of organisms from nurseries, use medical asepsis

F. Epidemic diarrhea—organism in stool (*Escherichia coli*)

  1. Prevention—(as above)

  2. Symptoms—frequent forceful watery yellow-green stool; dry skin, rapid drastic weight loss; acidosis

  3. Treatment—oral neomycin, Coly-Mycin, penicillin, or streptomycin to prevent other infections; replacement fluids parenterally, electrolytes; isolation, boiling all equipment, care of linens

G. Syphilis—spirochetal infection

  1. Prevention—STS during early and late pregnancy, immediate treatment of mother if reactive

  2. Symptoms—maculopapular lesions of palms of hands and soles of feet, restlessness, rhinitis, hoarse cry, enlargement of spleen and palpable lymph nodes, ends of long bones enlarged on x-ray examination

  3. Treatment—penicillin 1 to 2 years; follow-up

6. **Congenital malformations**

A. Birth defects—structural or metabolic disorders present at birth, genetically determined or a result of environmental interference during intrauterine life (birth injuries not included)

B. Incidence—1 infant in 16 live births; 1 family of every 10; statistical factors responsible: race, maternal age, sex

C. Prevention

  1. Early recognition of all birth defects

  2. Professional genetic counseling

  3. Research—new methods of testing genetic carriers

  4. Early prenatal care and supervision

  5. National Foundation (March of Dimes) research and study of congenital defects, educational programs and materials, treatment centers

D. Birth defects of digestive system

  1. Cleft lip and palate

  2. Galactosemia and phenylketonuria

  3. Atresia of esophagus

  4. Obstructions of duodenum and small intestine

  5. Imperforate anus

E. Birth defects of circulatory system

  1. Hemolytic disease—destruction of red cells, with anemia (a result of ABO incompatibility blood grouping or Rh blood systems of parents)

    a. Etiology—transfer of incompatible blood from fetal to maternal circulation with antibody formation, transfer of antibodies through placental barrier to fetus, with resulting agglutination and destruction of red cells

    b. Symptoms—jaundice at birth or within the first 24 hours, anemia, edema in varying degrees, enlargement of liver and spleen, lethargy, feedings taken poorly, vomiting, tremors and convulsions indicative of kernicterus

c. Treatment—prompt reporting of early jaundice; blood from umbilical cord at delivery affords prompt diagnosis and treatment; positive Coombs' test indicates presence of antibodies, bilirubin concentration of 4 mg. or more warrants immediate transfusion, exchange with Rh-negative blood

d. Prevention—amniocentesis; amniotic fluid evaluation with increase in antibody titer in mother followed by intrauterine transfusion after 25 weeks' gestation; RhoGAM to mother not sensitized first 72 hours postpartum, repeated after each subsequent pregnancy

2. Patent ductus arteriosus—tetralogy of Fallot (p. 348)

F. Birth defects of musculoskeletal system
1. Clubbed foot
2. Congenital hip dislocation (p. 541)

G. Birth defects of central nervous system
1. Spina bifida
2. Hydrocephalus (p. 407)

H. Birth defects of urinary system
1. Hypospadias—epispadias
2. Exstrophy of bladder (p. 540)

I. Chromosomal aberrations
1. Down's syndrome
2. Turner's and Klinefelter's syndromes
3. Phocomelia—improper development of body limbs

J. Support of family of infant with birth defect

7. **Infections of female reproductive organs**

A. Health supervision—routine yearly examination for women 30 years of age or over (include physical, pelvic examination, and Papanicolaou smear)

B. Organisms invade reproductive system
1. Fungus (Candida albicans)
   a. Vagina—wet dark environment optimum for growth of bacteria
   b. Symptoms—pruritus, redness, thick cheesy discharge
   c. Treatment—local application 5% gentian violet, nightly insertion propion gel, Mycostatin, oral broad-spectrum antibiotic
2. Protozoa (Trichomonas vaginalis) thrive in alkaline environment
   a. Symptoms—increased vaginal discharge, pruritus, burning, redness
   b. Treatment—change pH to acid with vinegar douches; Flagyl (anti-

protozoal medication) given to husband and wife to eliminate reinfection (contraindicated during pregnancy)

3. Streptococcal infection
   a. Prevention of tissue breakdown, strict aseptic technique during maternity cycle, gynecologic examination, maintenance of optimum health
   b. Signs and symptoms—elevated BMR, elevated pulse and respirations, elevated WBC, abdominal pain, distention, nausea and vomiting, and peritoneal invasion
   c. Treatment and nursing care—bed rest, alleviation of pain with sedation, parenteral fluids, antibiotics specific for Streptococcus, surgical intervention with localization

4. Gonococcus infection (gram-negative diplococci)
   a. Signs and symptoms—profuse purulent vaginal discharge, redness, irritation, pruritus, burning on urination; symptoms may be absent

5. Spirochete (syphilis) Treponema pallidum (p. 364); syphilis during pregnancy
   a. Prevention—serologic examination early and late in pregnancy, immediate treatment to protect growing fetus
   b. Treatment—large doses of penicillin; observe infant at birth for symptoms

C. Nursing care
1. Feelings of women associated with female reproductive organs, womanliness, reproduction, sexual competency
2. Follow through on treatment of all contacts by public health nursing service
3. Hand washing and prevention of reinfection through health teaching
4. Referral to public health department for community control of venereal diseases

8. **Childbirth injuries**

A. Injuries to birth canal and perineum
1. Hematoma
   a. Broad ligament, spontaneous rupture of vein, pain lateral to uterus following delivery, abdominal dis-

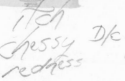

tention, pain on palpation, absence of vaginal bleeding
  (1) Treatment—supracervical hysterectomy
 b. Labia or blood vessel following episiotomy repair; observation of perineum for edema, ecchymosis; painful to touch
  (1) Immediate treatment—cold applications, with evacuation under aseptic technique
2. Episiotomy—incision into perineum prior to delivery
 a. Purposes—facilitates delivery, prevents lacerations and overstretching of pelvic floor, prevents undue pressure and trauma to head of newborn, prematurity, forceps application, breech delivery, fetal distress
 b. Types—median, left or right mediolateral
3. Lacerations
 a. Indications—bleeding from cervix, vagina, or perineum with firm uterus
 b. Types—first: vaginal mucosa, skin; second: skin, levator ani muscle and perineal body; third: entire perineum, external sphincter, partial or complete; fourth: entire perineum, rectal sphincter, and mucous membrane of rectum
4. Nursing care
 a. Area clean and dry
 b. Perineal exercise to increase circulation and reduce swelling
 c. Heat lamp
 d. Commercial sprays for anesthetic effect
 e. Lubricant cathartics to soften stool
B. Relaxations of vaginal outlet
1. Etiology—overstretching of perineal tissues during childbirth
2. Types
 a. Cystocele—defect of tissues supporting bladder
 b. Rectocele—defect of tissues supporting rectum
 c. Prolapse—cervix visible or entire uterus protrudes through vagina
3. Signs and symptoms
 a. Looseness, heaviness in vaginal region
 b. Backache (bearing down) feeling
 c. Urinary and fecal incontinency

4. Treatment
 a. Conservative—Kegal's exercises
 b. Surgical repair
5. Nursing care
 a. Preoperative—perineal preparation, cleansing of lower bowel, insertion of Foley catheter, explanation and support of patient, spiritual attendance
 b. Postoperative—vital signs, intake and output, clean dry perineum, early ambulation when indicated, leg motion and deep breathing, lubricating cathartics
C. Displacements of uterus
1. Retroflexion—bending backward of fundus with normal placement of cervix
2. Retroversion—tilting backward in varying degrees
3. Anteflexion—bending forward upon itself, cervix displaced toward posterior pelvis
4. Signs and symptoms—backache, menstrual disorders, infertility and abortions during pregnancy
5. Treatment—pessaries (mild displacements during pregnancy), surgical intervention
D. Rupture of uterus
1. Prevention
 a. Repeat cesarean section with disproportion
 b. Determining cause of prolonged labor
 c. Adequate anesthesia in operative obstetrics
 d. Cautious use of oxytocins for induction
2. Types
 a. Rupture of a previous cesarean scar
 b. Spontaneous rupture of intact uterus
 c. Traumatic rupture of uterus
3. Causes
 a. Grandmultiparity
 b. Cephalopelvic disproportion
 c. Injudicious induction
 d. Version, extraction, injudicious use of fundal pressure
4. Nursing care—same as in bleeding
9. **Abnormal uterine bleeding**
A. Anatomic—lesions, growths of uterus, tubes, or ovaries
1. Cervical erosions—replacement of squamous epithelium with columnar

a. Symptoms—increased vaginal secretions and bleeding
b. Treatment—cauterizations, vinegar douches, biopsy to rule out cancer
2. Cervical polyps—small growths at external os
  a. Symptoms—slight intermenstrual bleeding, bleeding during coitus and defecation (same as in cervical carcinoma)
  b. Treatment—surgical removal; dilatation and curettage (D and C) to rule out malignancy, follow-up exam every 6 months during premenopause and menopause
3. Myomas—fibroids—growths of uterus; originate in muscle cells (common in fundus)
  a. Signs and symptoms—asymptomatic, diagnosed on vaginal examination; hypermenorrhea or metrorrhagia; pain, sensation of bearing down; frequency, dysuria, constipation with large growths
  b. Myomas and pregnancy—may be responsible for infertility, abortions, premature labor
    (1) Symptoms—usually asymptomatic; myoma may cause pain, fever, tenderness, leukocytosis second trimester; last trimester and at delivery fibroids cause premature bleeding, uterine inertia, mechanical blocking of birth canal
    (2) Treatment—conservative, pelvic examination every 6 months, surgical intervention, radiotherapy if surgical risk, preceded by diagnostic D and C
4. Malignant growths (most frequent sites breast and cervix)
  a. Cancer of cervix
    (1) Etiology—unknown, incidence high in married women, early marriage, first coitus early age
    (2) Pathology—common site at squamous columnar junction
    (3) Symptoms — intermenstrual bleeding; may be bleeding after coitus or with severe straining on defecation, pain in late stages
    (4) Diagnosis — Papanicolaou smear, Schiller test, biopsy, conization

    (5) Treatment—depends upon extent of invasion; either surgical or irradiation therapy
  b. Cancer of uterus
    (1) Incidence—higher in white women, past menopausal age
    (2) Symptoms—same as above
    (3) Diagnosis—D and C, microscopic examination
    (4) Treatment—individual consideration given to age, health, stage of disease
  c. Cancer of ovary
    (1) Types—cystic, benign; or solid, malignant; quickly invade lymphatics and metastasize
    (2) Symptoms—obscure until late in disease; menorrhagia and metrorrhagia, ascites, enlarged mass in lower abdomen
    (3) Treatment—surgical intervention, postoperative irradiation; prognosis grave with malignancy
  d. Cancer of vulva
    (1) Symptoms—early: slight soreness and pruritus, patchy, grayish thickening of skin, leukoplakia (predisposing factor)
    (2) Treatment—early: vulvectomy; late: lymphadenectomy
  e. Nursing care with irradiation therapy
    (1) Radium—destroys tissue, careful handling; careful inspection of bed linens; report any elevation in temperature; avoid displacement of implanted radium
    (2) X-ray—skin erythema; keep skin dry and clean; avoid excessive water; use no soap
      (a) Contraindicated: creams, ointments, alcohols, tub baths, showers
      (b) Light, soft, nonconstricting clothing; low-residue diet prevents bowel evacuation that might displace radium; Foley catheter keeps bladder empty
      (c) Anorexia, nausea, vomiting, diarrhea frequent
      (d) Flat in bed and in single room, if possible; avoid contact with nurse who is

of childbearing age and during pregnancy

B. Dysfunctional uterine bleeding—not associated with tumors, inflammation, or pregnancy
   1. Diagnosis by
      a. Pelvic examination
      b. D and C during postovulatory or secretory phase of menstrual cycle
   2. Treatment—determined by cause and by age of woman

C. Nursing care following surgery of reproductive organs
   1. Psychological implications—feelings associated with sexual incompetency, loss of womanliness, feelings associated with deprivation related to motherhood
   2. Physiologic implications—sudden disturbance of hormones, metabolic, urinary, and digestive changes, all greatly related to psychological
   3. Preoperative preparations
      a. Skin preparation, enemas and douches in selected women, dependent on surgical procedure
      b. Extensive surgery, indwelling catheter
      c. Spiritual attendance
      d. Psychological preparation by doctor and nurse
   4. Postoperative nursing care
      a. Vital signs
      b. Restoration of normal body functions of digestion, circulation, excretion; comfort measures
      c. Frequent checking operative site
      d. Parenteral fluids
      e. Changing position, early ambulation
      f. Vaginal repair, tub baths
      g. Antibiotics, prevent infection

10. Infertility and sterility

A. Definition
   1. Sterility, absolute factor preventing procreation
   2. Infertility, inability to initiate the reproductive process after a desired or a 1-year period
      a. Primary (absolute)—pregnancy never occurs, causative factors cannot be corrected, absence of genital organs
      b. Secondary (relative)—one pregnancy has occurred, causative factor can be corrected

B. Causes
   1. Female
      a. Cervical factors 20%
      b. Tubal factors 30% to 35%
   2. Male 30% to 35%
   3. Hormonal 15%

C. Diagnosis
   1. Both partners involved
   2. Male examined first, less expensive, history and physical, semen analysis, and examination
   3. Female—serology for CBC, sedimentation rate, and syphilis, urinalysis, serum protein-bound iodine, chest x-ray film, BMR, Sims-Huhner test, endometrial biopsy, tubal insufflation, hysterosalpingography, culdoscopy

D. Male genital factors
   1. Disturbance in spermatogenesis
   2. Obstruction of seminiferous tubules
   3. Changes in amount and quality of seminal fluid
   4. Anomalies of ejaculatory process

E. Female genital factors
   1. Congenital anomalies of vagina and vulva
   2. Bacterial invasion of vagina
   3. Violent orgasm during coitus, in highly erotic
   4. Developmental anomalies of reproductive organs
   5. Blockage of cervical os or fallopian tubes
   6. Endocrine dysfunction
   7. Emotional factors
   8. Cervical factors—position, patency of external os, quality and quantity of cervical secretions

F. Treatment in male and female depends on causative factor

11. Menopause

Period of menstrual cycle in which there is gradual cessation of ovarian function with cessation of menstruation (climacteric or change of life)

A. Symptoms
   1. Somatic
      a. Atrophy of reproductive organs due to decrease in hormonal action
      b. Vasomotor symptoms, hot flashes, upper part of body with diaphoresis
      c. Weight gain, facial hair growth, skin texture changes
      d. Anatomic changes, increased susceptibility to infection and dyspareunia

2. Psychic
   a. Anxiety and irritability
   b. Decrease in sexual feelings
   c. Loss of feelings of womanliness
   d. Economic insecurities

B. Treatment
   1. Mild symptoms—mild sedative
   2. Severe symptoms—estrogen therapy
   3. Dyspareunia—vaginal creams

12. **Unmarried parents**

A. Incidence
   1. Highest percentage in 20- to 30-year age groups
   2. Higher in poor, nonwhite population

B. Needs of unmarried parents
   1. Importance of early prenatal care, toxemia prevalent, higher in young
   2. Maternity shelter when indicated
   3. Social caseworker, to help mother plan for baby (father also gets help)
   4. Education of both parents
   5. Added support by medical personnel, during childbearing crisis and following delivery, by referral to appropriate agencies

C. Long-term goals
   1. Community efforts to provide adequate housing, education, job, and social opportunities
   2. Provision for adequate social services to unmarried parents
   3. Provisions for continuing education during childbearing

13. **Trends in maternal child health (MCH) services**

A. Vital statistics
   1. Births recorded on local, state, and national levels
   2. Birth record for right to citizenship, inheritance, proof of age, Social Security
   3. 1968—3.46 million births
   4. 1970—expected 5.5 million births
   5. Causes of maternal deaths
      a. Hemorrhage 26.5%
      b. Infection 23.4%
      c. Other—anesthesia and embolism 30.6%, etc.
      d. Toxemia 19.5%
   6. Causes of neonatal deaths (infants 20 weeks' gestation to 1 month of age)
      a. Prematurity
      b. Respiratory distress syndrome
      c. Birth defects

B. Government agencies involved in providing MCH services

   1. World Health Organization—founded in 1948 by United Nations; 100 or more countries exchange knowledge and collaborate on achieving highest level of health throughout world
   2. Children's Bureau—founded in 1912, under Dept. of HEW in Washington, D. C.; purpose: improve services for maintenance of health in children through research, care, and teaching; 1921—monies provided for improving health services to mothers and babies; 1935—under Social Security Act, federal aid through Crippled Children's Commission and for orthopedic and muscular problems with rehabilitative services; White House Conferences held every 10 years to identify and improve health services to mothers and children
   3. Department of Family and Children Services, HEW—federal monies for food, shelter, and medical services for dependent children, so mother is at home during early important months
   4. Women's Bureau—under Department of Labor provides supervision of conditions existing in industry where pregnant women are employed
   5. National Institutes of Health—monies provided for research on child health and human development

C. Lay organizations providing MCH services
   1. La Lèche League Internationale—organized in 1956, interested in fostering and encouraging mothers desiring to breast-feed; referral by hospital and public health nurses
   2. International Childbirth Education Association—a federation of groups and individuals interested in fostering family-centered maternity and infant care; main objective—create an interest for education for childbirth, emotional support during labor, delivery, and breast-feeding; fosters closeness of father, mother, and baby during the early moments surrounding birth
   3. Pre-Cana Conferences—held under Roman Catholic auspices providing subject matter related to preparation for a Christian marriage; discussions conducted by priests, doctors, and lay couples

D. Nurse midwife—a registered nurse with

neonatal—20 wks gestation to 1 month of age

added knowledge and skill who manages the care of mother and baby throughout the maternity cycle when the childbearing process is normal

REVIEW QUESTIONS FOR OBSTETRIC AND GYNECOLOGIC NURSING
Multiple choice

Read each question carefully and consider all possible answers. When you have decided which answer is best, blacken the corresponding space on the answer sheet. There is only *one* best answer in each question (or implied question).

1. One of the objectives of maternity nursing is to provide for
   1. Early medical supervision
   2. Safe care of mother during maternity cycle
   3. Total care of mother, infant, and family
   4. Physical, emotional, and spiritual welfare of mother and infant
2. Statistics in relation to marriages show that
   1. Marriages now occur less frequently in younger age groups (17 to 25 years) than previously
   2. Young people are generally better prepared for marriage and parenthood than previously
   3. Marriages between people of varying cultural, social, and racial backgrounds occur less frequently than previously
   4. Marriages now occur more frequently in the older age groups (27 to 35 years) than previously
3. Human reproduction is accomplished by
   1. Fission
   2. Budding
   3. Fragmentation
   4. Sexual union
4. The period before birth is known as the
   1. Intrapartum period
   2. Postpartum period
   3. Perinatal period
   4. Prenatal period
5. Embryonic development of the reproductive organs begins during the
   1. Second to third week of pregnancy
   2. Fifth to sixth week of pregnancy
   3. Tenth to twelfth week of pregnancy
   4. Eighteenth to twentieth week of pregnancy
6. Spermatogenesis in the male occurs
   1. During embryonic development
   2. Immediately following birth
   3. At the time of puberty
   4. At any time following birth
7. The testes are suspended in the scrotum to
   1. Facilitate the passage of sperm through the urethra
   2. Protect the sperm from the acidity of urine
   3. Protect the sperm from high abdominal temperatures
   4. Facilitate their maturation during embryonic development
8. The two functions of the penis are
   1. To act as organ of copulation, to transport urine from the bladder
   2. To act as organ of copulation, to protect sperm during spermatogenesis
   3. To act as reservoir for sperm, to transport urine from the bladder
   4. To act as organ of copulation, to secrete urine
9. The vagina in the female has the following function(s)
   1. It is the canal through which the menstrual flow escapes
   2. It is the female organ of copulation
   3. It is the birth canal at time of delivery
   4. It is all of these
10. The vaginal canal normally has
    1. An acid environment
    2. An alkaline environment
    3. A neutral environment
    4. An environment difficult to determine
11. The internal genitalia in the female are
    1. Uterus, ovaries, fallopian tubes, clitoris
    2. Uterus, ovaries, clitoris, vagina
    3. Uterus, fallopian tubes, vagina, labia minora
    4. Uterus, ovaries, fallopian tubes, vagina
12. The muscles in the uterus are
    1. Entirely nonstriated
    2. Partially striated and partially nonstriated
    3. Striated in the fundus and nonstriated in lower segment
    4. Nonstriated in the fundus and striated in lower segment
13. The main blood supply to the uterus is *directly* from the
    1. Uterine and ovarian arteries
    2. Uterine and hypogastric arteries
    3. Ovarian arteries and the aorta
    4. Aorta and the hypogastric arteries
14. The primordial follicles are usually found in the
    1. Medulla of the ovary
    2. Fallopian tubes
    3. Cortex of the ovary
    4. Fundus of the uterus
15. The following hormones are responsible for the menstrual cycle
    1. Estrogen and progesterone
    2. Gonadotropins
    3. Gonadotropins and estrogen
    4. Gonadotropins, estrogen, and progesterone
16. The hormone(s) responsible for maturation of the graafian follicle is (are)
    1. Follicle-stimulating hormone—FSH
    2. Luteinizing hormone
    3. Follicle-stimulating hormone and estrogen
    4. Follicle-stimulating hormone and progesterone
17. Ovulation may be defined as rupture of graafian follicle, followed by
    1. Discharge of a mature ovum
    2. Discharge of an immature ovum
    3. Secretion of estrogen
    4. Secretion of luteinizing hormone
18. The time of ovulation may be determined by taking the basal temperature. During ovulation the basal temperature
    1. Drops markedly
    2. Drops slightly and then rises
    3. Drops markedly and remains low
    4. Rises suddenly and then falls

19. Maturation of ovum and sperm is a process whereby the number of chromosomes in the ovum and sperm is established at
    1. 22 + X or Y
    2. 23 + X or Y
    3. 23 − X or Y
    4. 22 − X or Y

20. The product of the first cell division following union of a mature ovum and sperm is known as a
    1. Zygote
    2. Germ cell
    3. Morula
    4. Blastocyte

21. While the fertilized ovum is traveling through the fallopian tube toward the uterus, it is in the
    1. Trophoblastic phase
    2. Morula phase
    3. Blastocytic phase
    4. Meiotic phase

22. Penetration of the chorionic villi into the maternal surface is called
    1. Fertilization
    2. Impregnation
    3. Fecundation
    4. Implantation

23. A rudimentary circulatory system is formed by the end of which lunar month?
    1. Fourth
    2. Third
    3. Second
    4. First

24. During pregnancy the uterine lining is known as
    1. Endometrium
    2. Perimetrium
    3. Decidua
    4. Chorion

25. First fetal movements felt by the mother are known as
    1. Ballottement
    2. Engagement
    3. Lightening
    4. Quickening

26. Growth is most rapid during which phase of prenatal development?
    1. Implantation
    2. First trimester
    3. Second trimester
    4. Third trimester

27. By which week of pregnancy is the placenta usually formed?
    1. Second
    2. Sixth
    3. Tenth
    4. Sixteenth

28. The blood vessels in the umbilical cord consist of
    1. Two arteries and one vein
    2. Two arteries and two veins
    3. One artery and two veins
    4. One artery and one vein

29. In which of the fetal blood vessels is the oxygen content highest?
    1. Umbilical artery
    2. Ductus arteriosus
    3. Ductus venosus
    4. Pulmonary artery

Situation: Mr. and Mrs. J are a young married couple. John J is 24, Mary J is 21. John is a veteran and is studying accounting under the G.I. bill. Mary is working as a keypunch operator at a large insurance company. They have been married six months and have just purchased a small house in the suburbs. In order to meet the expenses entailed in establishing the new home, John J has accepted a part-time job in an accountant firm, where he works two or three nights a week and most weekends. They both want children, but have decided to postpone having a family until John finishes his education in two years. Mary has therefore taken an oral contraceptive since shortly before the marriage. Mary has always had a very regular menstrual cycle. She therefore becomes very concerned when she misses her regular menstrual period. After three weeks pass and the period does not occur, she decides to go to a physician for a checkup. She tells the nurse interviewing her that she suspects she may be pregnant, because she missed taking her contraceptive pills for more than a week when she had the flu. Questions 30 to 47 refer to Mrs. J's situation.

30. In relation to the patient's statement about her possible pregnancy, the best response for the nurse to make would be
    1. "Contraceptive pills are very unpredictable anyhow. You probably would have become pregnant even if you had taken them regularly as prescribed."
    2. "You may well be correct; one of the reasons for prescribing an exact specific schedule is that the effect of contraceptive drugs depends on the regularity with which they are taken."
    3. "Don't think about that now. It's too late to worry anyhow. First find out whether or not you really are pregnant. If you are, you may want to decide to have an abortion. That will solve your problems."
    4. "That's the trouble with using contraceptive pills. People become too careless and don't use proper restraint. If you had used the rhythm method, this would not have happened and you would not be here worrying now."

31. While Mrs. J is being prepared for the examination, she complains of feeling very tired and of being "sick to her stomach," particularly in the morning. The best response for the nurse to make would be
    1. "This is a common occurrence during the early part of pregnancy and you need not worry."
    2. "This is a common occurrence due to all the changes going on in your body."
    3. "These are common occurrences; you say your sick feelings bother you most often in the morning?"
    4. "Perhaps you might discuss this with the doctor when he arrives."

32. Mrs. J asks, "Is it true the doctor will do an internal examination today?" The nurse would answer
    1. "Yes, an internal is done on all mothers on the first visit."

2. "Yes, an internal is done on all mothers, but it is only slightly uncomfortable."
3. "Are you fearful of having an internal examination done?"
4. "Yes, he will; have you ever had an internal examination done before?"

After a thorough examination, the physician determines that Mrs. J is about 6 weeks pregnant.

33. All of the following findings contributed to his diagnosis except
    1. Cervix soft and compressible
    2. Breasts slightly tender
    3. Slight bluish discoloration of vagina
    4. Elevated blood pressure

34. Mrs. J asks when she may expect her baby. She states that her last menstrual period was April 14, 1972. Her expected date of delivery most likely will be
    1. December 21, 1972
    2. January 7, 1973
    3. January 21, 1973
    4. February 1, 1973

35. Following the pelvic examination the doctor indicates Mrs. J has a normal gynecoid pelvis. A normal gynecoid pelvis has
    1. Well-hollowed sacrum, movable coccyx, blunt spines, and wide pubic arch
    2. Flat sacrum, a movable coccyx, prominent spines, and a wide pubic arch
    3. Deeply hollowed sacrum, immovable coccyx, narrow pubic arch, and blunt spines
    4. Flat sacrum, movable coccyx, narrow pubic arch, and prominent spines

36. Mrs. J is concerned, since she has read that nutrition during pregnancy is important for proper growth and development of the baby. She wants to know something about the foods she should be eating. The nurse would best proceed by
    1. Giving her a list of foods to refer to in planning meals
    2. Asking her what she usually eats at each meal
    3. Emphasizing the importance of limiting salt and highly seasoned foods
    4. Instructing her to continue eating a normal diet

37. Mrs. J's work as a keypunch operator would of necessity have implications for her plan of care during pregnancy. The nurse most likely would recommend that Mrs. J
    1. Ask for time in the morning and afternoon to elevate her legs
    2. Tell her employer she cannot work beyond the second trimester
    3. Ask for time in the morning and afternoon to obtain nourishment
    4. Try to walk about every few hours during the workday

38. For the next few months Mrs. J will be asked to return to the physician's office at regular intervals. For the next few months if everything goes well she can expect to go for a checkup every
    1. Week
    2. Other week
    3. 3 to 4 weeks
    4. 6 to 8 weeks

39. At each visit the following will be done
    1. C.B.C., check of blood pressure, weight taken
    2. Vaginal examination, urine test for albumin, weight taken
    3. Check of blood pressure, urine test for albumin, C.B.C.
    4. Check of blood pressure, weight taken, urine test for albumin

40. During one of the visits, the nurse notices that Mrs. J wears round garters. The best action for the nurse to take, since she observes that Mrs. J has no sign of varicose veins, is to
    1. Do nothing
    2. Tell the physician about it and ask him what she should do
    3. Ask Mrs. J if she knows that round garters are prohibited during pregnancy
    4. Explain to Mrs. J that round garters are constricting and predispose to the development of varicose veins

41. Mrs. J returns to the physician's office regularly and is now in her eighth month. When the nurse asks "how are things going?" she answers: "I am sick and tired of wearing these same old clothes. How I wish all this would be done and over with." The best response for the nurse to make at this time would be
    1. "Is there something bothering you; you appear so discouraged?"
    2. "You are kind of weary at this point and feel that time is dragging?"
    3. "I went through this myself."
    4. "I can understand how you feel right now; what do you know about labor?"

42. In the previous comment, the nurse's reply would be based on the nurse's assumption that Mrs. J was
    1. Weary of pregnancy
    2. Rejecting her baby
    3. Fearful of oncoming labor
    4. Upset about something

43. Mrs. J asks what her baby would look like at this time (approximately 34 to 36 weeks). The most appropriate response would be that the baby
    1. Is still incompletely developed and would not be viable if born now
    2. Is exactly like a full-term baby, only weighs less, but has a good chance of survival
    3. Is exactly like a full-term baby in every respect and has the same chances for survival
    4. Looks the same as a full-term infant, only is extremely small, and has a very slim chance for survival if born

44. The nurse asks Mrs. J what she has ready for the baby, and Mrs. J tells her "Oh, I don't believe in buying anything until after the baby is born; there's really no sense in buying anything now, is there?" The best response would be
    1. "Many mothers feel the way you do; but it is easier for you after delivery to have things ready."
    2. "You would rather wait than buy anything now?"
    3. "Many mothers tell me the very same

thing; I suppose you have some superstitious beliefs."

4. "Many mothers feel the way you do; can you tell me why you would rather wait?"

45. Since Mrs. J is a primigravida, she would be told to come to the hospital when
1. Contractions are 2 to 3 minutes apart and she cannot walk about
2. Contractions are every 10 to 15 minutes apart
3. She has a bloody show
4. Membranes rupture, or contractions are 5 to 8 minutes apart

46. During the examination the nurse asks Mrs. J if she would like to listen to her baby's heartbeat. She is delighted and after listening comments on how rapid it is. She appears frightened and asks if this is normal. The nurse would respond
1. "The baby's heart rate is usually twice the mother's pulse rate."
2. "The baby's heartbeat is rapid to accommodate his nutritional needs."
3. "The baby's heart rate is normally rapid, so you needn't worry."
4. "It is far better that the heart rate is rapid; when it is slow, there is need to worry."

47. Since Mrs. J is in her last trimester, consideration of her diet is essential. In the last trimester the diet should include an increase in minerals and
1. Fats
2. Vitamins
3. Carbohydrates
4. Proteins

Situation: Mrs. K is a primigravida at term and is admitted to the labor room. Her prenatal record reveals that she has had an uneventful pregnancy. She has attended education for childbirth classes together with her husband. Both Mr. and Mrs. K have decided that Mr. K will remain in the labor room and, if possible, will go to the delivery room with his wife. The physician and the nursing staff of the unit are very supportive of this arrangement. When Mrs. K is admitted, she is experiencing contractions every 5 to 8 minutes, which last approximately 30 seconds. She also has a slight bloody discharge. The physician's examination reveals that the cervix is about 3 cm. dilated and almost fully effaced. The vertex is presenting at a +1 station, with the occiput toward the left side of the symphysis pubis. The vital signs are recorded as follows: F.H. 144, L.L.Q.; B.P. 118/74; T.P.R. 98.8-82-22. Mrs. K is quite cheerful and at ease. Questions 48 to 61 refer to this situation.

48. The term vertex refers to which kind of presentation?
1. Shoulder
2. Breech
3. Cephalic
4. Transverse

49. The findings in relation to Mrs. K's contraction and cervical dilatation indicate that Mrs. K is most likely in which stage of labor?
1. Early first stage
2. Transition phase of first stage

3. Second stage
4. Not in labor yet

50. Mrs. K asks the nurse if it is all right for her to get up and walk around. Based on her observation of Mrs. K's contractions and her knowledge of the physiology and mechanism of labor, the best action for the nurse to take would be to tell Mrs. K
1. "Please stay in bed, because walking may interfere with proper uterine contractions."
2. "I can't make a decision on that, you will have to ask the doctor."
3. "You will have to stay in bed, because otherwise your contractions cannot be timed and no one can listen to the fetal heart."
4. "It is quite all right for you to be up and about as long as you feel comfortable and your bag of waters is intact."

51. An enema is ordered for Mrs. K. Reasons for giving enemas to patients in labor include all of the following except
1. Expulsion of feces during labor predispose the patient to infection
2. A full rectum tends to hinder the progress of labor
3. It is a routine procedure carried out for every patient in labor
4. A full lower bowel predisposes to postpartum discomfort

52. Mrs. K's contractions gradually increase in strength and become more frequent and last longer. Her membranes rupture. The *first* action for the nurse to take after putting Mrs. K to bed is to
1. Listen to the fetal heart
2. Call the physician
3. Time the contractions
4. Check B.P. and pulse

The nurse observes the amniotic fluid.

53. Normal amniotic fluid is
1. Clear, dark amber-colored
2. Milky, greenish yellow, containing shreds of mucus
3. Clear, almost colorless, containing little white specks
4. Cloudy, greenish yellow, containing little white specks

54. An examination reveals that Mrs. K is 7 to 8 cm. dilated and that the vertex is low in the midpelvis. To alleviate discomfort during contractions, the nurse would instruct Mr. K to encourage his wife in
1. Panting
2. Abdominal breathing
3. Pelvic rocking
4. Athletic chest breathing

55. Mrs. K becomes very tense with contractions and quite irritable. She frequently states "I cannot stand this a minute longer." This kind of behavior is indicative of the fact that she
1. Is entering the transition phase of labor
2. Needs immediate administration of an analgesic or anesthetic
3. Developing some abnormality in terms of uterine contractions
4. Has been very poorly prepared for labor in the parents' classes

56. Mr. K is becoming very tense at this time.

He asks: "Do you think it is best for me to leave, since I don't seem to do my wife much good?" The most appropriate answer to this statement would be:
1. "If you feel that way, you'd best go out and sit in the father's waiting room with all the others."
2. "I know this is hard for you. Why don't you go have a cup of coffee and relax and come back later if you feel like it?"
3. "This is the time your wife needs you. Don't run out on her now."
4. "This is hard for you. Let me try to help you coach her during this difficult phase."

57. The beginning of the second stage of labor can be recognized by the patient's desire to
1. Relax during contractions
2. Push during contractions
3. Pant during contractions
4. Blow during contractions

58. Mrs. K delivers a baby boy spontaneously under saddle block anesthesia. Since she is awake, she asks to hold her baby. After the nurse places him in Mrs. K's arm, Mrs. K asks; "Is he normal?" The most appropriate response for the nurse would be
1. "Of course he is, why shouldn't he be? You had a fine pregnancy."
2. "If you worry that way, I'll have to take him back."
3. "He must be all right, he has such a strong healthy cry."
4. "Maybe you would like me to unwrap him, so that you can look him over yourself."

59. The baby is given an Apgar score of 9. This indicates that he is
1. In imminent danger of asphyxia
2. Having a considerable amount of mucus
3. In excellent condition
4. Pale and lethargic

60. Shortly following delivery Mrs. K tells the nurse that she feels as if she is bleeding. On checking, the nurse finds a steady trickling of blood from the vagina. The first action of the nurse would be to
1. Go out and call the physician
2. Check the fundus, hold it, and have someone call the physician
3. Check the patient's pulse and blood pressure and call the physician
4. Check the patient's pulse and blood pressure and prepare for transfusion

61. A newborn must be observed carefully for the first 24 hours particularly for
1. Respiratory distress
2. Change in body temperature
3. Desire for feeding
4. Frequency in voiding

Situation: Mrs. E is a primipara. She delivered a 6½-pound baby girl about 1 hour ago. She tells the nurse admitting her to the room that she planned to breast-feed her baby but that she is afraid she won't be able to do so because she has very small breasts. She also says that she hopes breast-feeding won't make her fat and change her figure because her husband is very proud of her petite figure. Questions 62 to 69 refer to the above situation.

62. In terms of Mrs. E's statements, the best response for the nurse to make is
1. "The size of the breast is completely irrelevant in the production of milk."
2. "The amount of glandular tissue rather than the size of the breast determines the amount of milk produced."
3. "The amount of glandular tissue coupled with the stimulation of suckling determines the amount of milk produced."
4. "The amount of fat and connective tissue together with the glandular tissue determines the amount of milk produced."

63. The most appropriate response to Mrs. E's concern in relation to retaining her petite figure is
1. "This is a difficult decision to make. If your primary concern is with maintaining your slim figure, you should not try to breast-feed, since this invariably causes sagging of the breasts."
2. "You really have to make up your mind what is important to you. If you really care about your baby's future welfare, you will breast-feed her regardless of what happens to your figure."
3. "The actual process of breast-feeding does not affect your figure. Nursing mothers who gain weight do so because they eat and drink too many high-caloric foods and fluids and don't take care of themselves."
4. "The breasts enlarge during pregnancy in preparation for breast-feeding. You can avoid sagging breasts and spoiling your figure by eating a well-balanced diet sufficient in calories for both you and the baby and by wearing a proper uplift support."

64. Mrs. E decides to breast-feed her infant. She asks the nurse what to do about cleansing the nipples. The best response for the nurse to make is that it is important to
1. Thoroughly scrub the nipples with soap and water prior to each feeding
2. Wipe the nipples with sterile water prior to each feeding
3. Wash breasts and nipples with a mild soap and water
4. Cleanse the nipples with an alcohol sponge prior to and following each feeding

65. Factors that influence lactation are
(a) Increased protein and calories in the mother's diet
(b) Rest and relaxation
(c) Increased intake of fluids
(d) Adequate breast size to support milk production
1. a, b, and c
2. a, b, and d
3. a and c only
4. b, c, and d

66. On the third day, Mrs. E states that she has a great deal of pain in her breasts and that she is afraid that the baby will hurt her when she tries to grasp the nipple. The most appropriate action for the nurse to take is to explain the reasons for the patient's discomfort and to
1. Call the physician to obtain his advice
2. Administer a medication for pain

3. Express some of the milk manually before putting the baby to breast
4. Suggest that the patient limit fluids and not try to nurse the baby for the next 2 days

67. Mrs. E is concerned about what will happen when she goes home. Her neighbor told her that the minute she got home her breasts dried up and she had to discontinue breast-feeding. The most appropriate comment for the nurse to make is
   1. "This is a common problem. The best thing to overcome this is to try to relax and put the baby to breast more frequently for a short time in order to stimulate the breasts."
   2. "This is a very common problem. We therefore provide you with formula and directions to make formula so that the baby does not go hungry until your milk returns."
   3. "I don't know who gave you this information, but there is absolutely no basis for it. Once the milk supply has been established, it does not diminish."
   4. "Don't worry unnecessarily. You have plenty of milk now, so there is a good chance that this will not happen to you."

68. Mrs. E tells the nurse that she has heard about "demand" feeding and wonders how anyone ever finds time to do anything but feed the baby. The best response for the nurse to make is
   1. "Most mothers find babies on breast do better on demand feeding, since the amount of milk ingested varies at each feeding."
   2. "Perhaps a schedule might be better, since the baby is already used to hospital routine."
   3. "Although the baby is on demand, he will eventually set his own schedule, so there will be time for your household chores."
   4. "Most mothers find that feeding the baby whenever he cries works out fine."

69. Mrs. E wants to know whether or not it is true that she will not have to use contraceptives while nursing. The most appropriate response is
   1. "Since lactation suppresses ovulation, you don't have to worry about becoming pregnant."
   2. "As long as you have no menstrual period you won't have to worry about using contraceptives."
   3. "It is best to use contraceptive measures, since ovulation is likely to occur without initiation of a menstrual period."
   4. "It is best to delay any sexual relations until the occurrence of the first menstrual period and then to practice the rhythm method of birth control."

Situation: Mrs. A is a primipara. She is 18 years old. At this time, she is 7 months pregnant. She has had an uneventful pregnancy to date and has had prenatal care since the beginning of her third month. On her first visit, she weighed 124 pounds, her B.P. was 112/78, and the physical examination showed

her to be in excellent health. She was working as a secretary. She made plans to work as long as she could and to return to work after six to eight weeks, since her mother lived in the same house and was able to care for the baby. The physician told her that she could work until about three weeks before her due date. Mrs. A is of Italian descent and loves her mother's cooking—pasta, sauces, etc. Two weeks ago she weighed 133 pounds, her B.P. was 110/72, and the F.H. was 146 and regular. On this visit, her B.P. was 138/96, her weight 140 pounds, and the F.H. 152 and regular. The physician advised her to stay home and rest for a few days and placed her on a low-calorie diet. On examination, he found no edema. The urine was negative for albumin. He made the diagnosis of mild preeclampsia. Questions 70 to 76 refer to the above situation.

70. On which of the following findings was the diagnosis of mild preeclampsia most likely based? Excessive weight gain and
   1. Marked increase in diastolic B.P.
   2. Marked increase in fetal heart rate
   3. Absence of edema
   4. Absence of albumin in the urine

71. Which of the following is a most likely contributor to Mrs. A's weight gain?
   1. Kidney dysfunction
   2. Stress on the job
   3. Improper diet
   4. Hypertension

72. Mrs. A has gained a total of 16 pounds during her pregnancy. What action should the nurse take to support Mrs. A's prenatal nutritional needs?
   (a) Caution her about any further weight gain, as it will cause complications
   (b) Explore her diet with her to be sure it is optimum in needed nutrients, especially extra protein, vitamins, and minerals
   (c) Encourage sufficient caloric intake to spare protein and to meet added energy demands
   (d) Encourage limitation of weight gain to about 25 pounds, to ensure proper growth and development of the baby and meet maternal needs
      1. a and c
      2. a only
      3. b, c, and d
      4. b only

73. A general physiologic edema is normal during pregnancy because
   (a) The total body fluid circulating through blood vessels and interstitial tissues increases
   (b) There is a subsequent diluting of blood constituents with a lowering of plasma protein
   (c) The lowered plasma albumin contributes to slowed return of interstitial fluid to capillaries due to reduced colloidal osmotic pressure (COP)
   (d) There is reduced fluid output by the kidneys
      1. a and d
      2. b and c
      3. b and d
      4. a, b, and c

74. The nurse explains to Mrs. A that she needs added amounts of protein of high biologic value during her pregnancy to
    (a) Synthesize additional plasma proteins, especially albumin, necessary to maintain COP and normal circulation of tissue fluid
    (b) Build tissue required for the rapid fetal growth and development
    (c) Help control her appetite and avoid weight gain
    (d) Lessen the tendency to nausea, as protein is easier to digest
        1. a and b
        2. a and d
        3. b and c
        4. c and d

75. Adequate intake of salt, rather than its restriction, during pregnancy is advisable because
    (a) Fetal needs for Na require sufficient amounts in the maternal diet
    (b) Food without salt tends to be less tasteful and curtails adequate intake of needed nutrients and calories
    (c) The physiologic edema of pregnancy is related more to plasma protein levels, not sodium, and hence is not responsive to sodium restriction
    (d) Low sodium diets during pregnancy, especially combined with use of potent diuretics, pose dangers of fluid and electrolyte imbalances
        1. a, b, and c
        2. b, c, and d
        3. a, c, and d
        4. All of these

76. Mrs. A was told to report any headache or visual disturbance immediately to the physician. The reason for this is that headaches and visual disturbances frequently
    1. Are forerunners of severe preeclampsia
    2. Are side effects of diuril
    3. Are side effects of low-sodium diets
    4. Are indicative of kidney dysfunction

Situation: Mrs. F brought her 16-year-old daughter Lois to the emergency room because, Mrs. F said, "She has had a fit, foaming at the mouth and all. She has not been right for a few days and yesterday complained about a bad stomachache and had spots before her eyes. She is about 8 months pregnant, I think. I have been taking care of her and she has been fine until now." Physical examination showed Lois to be about 32 weeks pregnant with B.P. 198/112, T. 100°, P. 98, R. 26, F.H. 156 and regular. There was edema present over entire body, especially marked facial edema. Lois was drowsy and responded poorly. The physician's orders read nothing by mouth, bed rest, morphine sulfate 0.015 Gm. stat., 50 ml. of 50% glucose in distilled water stat., by intravenous infusion, vital signs q. ½ hr., and observe for signs of labor. Patient's diagnosis was eclampsia. (See questions 77 to 85.)

77. The diagnosis of eclampsia was most likely based on which of the following findings?
    1. Pain in epigastric region
    2. Hypertension
    3. Facial edema
    4. Convulsions

78. Morphine sulfate 0.015 Gm. is equal to
    1. 150 mg.
    2. 1.5 mg.
    3. ¼ gr.
    4. ½ gr.

79. Morphine sulfate is given to
    1. Relax the cervix
    2. Increase the pain threshold
    3. Stimulate the central nervous system
    4. Depress the central nervous system

80. Tests of BUN, blood uric acid, and CO_2 combining power were ordered. These blood tests are commonly done in severe preeclampsia and eclampsia. Which of the following are found in severe preeclampsia?
    1. Decrease in urea nitrogen and uric acid and increase in carbon dioxide combining power
    2. Increase in urea nitrogen and uric acid and decrease in carbon dioxide combining power
    3. Decreases in all of the above
    4. Increases in all of the above

81. Which of the following is frequently a complication of preeclampsia or eclampsia?
    1. Abruptio placentae
    2. Placenta praevia
    3. Dystocia
    4. Malpresentation

82. Hypertonic glucose was ordered for Lois to
    1. Decrease body toxins
    2. Decrease cerebral edema
    3. Lower blood pressure
    4. Provide nourishment

83. Since Lois was semiconscious, the best position for her was
    1. On her side with foot of bed elevated
    2. On her side with bed flat
    3. On her back with head of bed elevated
    4. On her abdomen with pillow under her chest

84. Lois has had a severe "stomachache." This type of epigastric pain is usually indicative of which of the following in pregnant women?
    1. Ruptured gastric ulcer
    2. Sudden onset of labor
    3. Impending convulsion
    4. Severe gastrointestinal infection

85. As soon as Miss F was able to eat, a high-protein, high-calorie diet with added vitamins and minerals was ordered for her. The nurse explained that
    (a) She need not try to eat if she had no appetite
    (b) The food contained important minerals she needed to build up the protein and red cells in her blood
    (c) Not getting enough of the foods needed during pregnancy contributes to problems like this
    (d) A number of small meals would be provided for her if need be to help her get in the food she needed
        1. a and c
        2. b, c, and d
        3. a and d
        4. b and d

Situation: Mr. and Mrs. Q had been married almost 7 years when Mrs. Q experienced symptoms that led her to believe that she was pregnant. She went to her obstetrician who, after a thorough examination including laboratory tests, confirmed that she was 10 to 12 weeks pregnant and that everything was progressing normally. Both Mr. and Mrs. Q were overjoyed, since they wanted children and Mrs. Q had tried for a number of years to become pregnant. About 10 days after her visit to the physician, at the time of her normal menstrual period, Mrs. Q started to stain. The physician told her to go to bed immediately and remain on complete bed rest for at least 72 hours. Since Mr. Q could not stay at home and Mrs. Q had no one else to care for her, she was admitted to the hospital. Questions 86 to 89 refer to the above situation.

86. Mrs. Q was admitted because of
 1. Threatened abortion
 2. Inevitable abortion
 3. Ectopic pregnancy
 4. Missed abortion
87. After a few hours Mrs. Q began to experience "bearing-down" sensations and suddenly expelled the fetus in bed. In order to give safe nursing care the nurse would *first*
 1. Take her immediately to the delivery room
 2. Check the fundus for firmness
 3. Give her the sedation ordered
 4. Immediately notify the doctor
88. Following delivery Mrs. Q should be observed for
 1. Dehydration and hemorrhage
 2. Hemorrhage and infection
 3. Subinvolution and dehydration
 4. Signs of toxemia
89. When Mrs. Q returns to her room, both she and her husband are visibly upset. The nurse notices that Mr. Q has tears in his eyes and that Mrs. Q has her face turned to the wall and is sobbing quietly. The best approach for the nurse to take is to go over to Mrs. Q and say
 1. "I know how you feel, but you must not be so upset now, it will make it more difficult for you to get well quickly."
 2. "I can understand that you are upset, but be glad it happened at this time in your pregnancy and not after you carried the baby for the full time."
 3. "I know that you are upset now, but hopefully you will become pregnant again very soon and then everything will be fine."
 4. "I see that both of you are very upset. I brought you some hot coffee and hot tea and will be right here if you want to talk about it."

Situation: Mrs. H, a Cuban gravida iii para ii, was admitted to the hospital at 32 weeks gestation because of moderate vaginal bleeding. On admission, the bleeding had stopped, her B.P. was 114/72, P. 92, R. 24, and F.H. 128 and regular. She had no contractions and membranes were intact. The diagnosis on admission was "possible placenta praevia." In taking the history, the nurse observed that Mrs. H had some difficulty expressing herself in the English language, but that she was able to understand and follow instructions if the nurse spoke

slowly. Another observation was that Mrs. H was pale and restless, wringing her hands, and generally showed signs of being upset. The physician's orders read complete bed rest, blood type and crossmatch, C.B.C., vital signs q.2.h., and watch for signs of labor. Have 2 pints of whole blood available for immediate administration, if needed. (See questions 90 to 104.)

90. Complete bed rest was ordered to prevent
 1. Premature rupture of the membranes
 2. Onset of labor
 3. Further bleeding
 4. Precipitous drop in blood pressure
91. No enema was ordered on admission. The primary reason for this was that an enema would likely cause
 1. Bleeding
 2. Infection
 3. Onset of labor
 4. Rupture of the membranes
92. Vital signs were checked frequently in order to detect early signs of
 1. Anemia
 2. Hemorrhage
 3. Labor
 4. Toxemia

Placenta praevia and abruptio placentae are two complications occurring mostly in late pregnancy or during labor. The statements in 93 to 99 refer to these conditions. Please respond to each statement as follows: blacken space No.
 1. If the statement refers to placenta praevia only
 2. If the statement refers to abruptio placentae only
 3. If the statement is applicable to both conditions
 4. If the statement is not specifically applicable to either condition
93. Separation of normally implanted placenta, prior to delivery of baby
94. Necessitates immediate induction of labor
95. Implantation of placenta over or near the internal cervical os
96. Signs of shock with or without visible bleeding
97. Excruciating abdominal pain accompanied by boardlike rigidity of abdomen
98. Frequently a complication of preeclampsia
99. Often characterized by intermittent vaginal bleeding
100. After several hours, Mrs. H. experienced uterine contractions, which rapidly and progressively grew stronger, more regular, and more frequent. There was a moderate amount of vaginal bleeding. The fetal heart was strong, regular, 144 L.L.Q., B.P. 112/78, P. 98, R. 24. The physician ordered Mrs. H to be prepared for vaginal examination. Based on her knowledge of the condition, the nurse would
 1. Tell the physician that a vaginal examination was contraindicated
 2. Set up for a sterile vaginal examination in the delivery room with preparation for an immediate cesarean section if needed
 3. Set up for a vaginal examination in bed and notify the operating room that there

was the possibility of an eventual cesarean section

4. Suggest to the physician to delay the examination until the patient showed signs of nearing the second stage of labor

101. Mrs. H became progressively more distressed and murmured "my baby," "my baby." The nurse would recognize that her anxiety was most likely due to all of the following *except*
1. Unfamiliarity with surroundings
2. Inability to fully comprehend what was happening
3. Desire to be up and about
4. Fear for her own and the baby's safety

102. In order to reassure Mrs. H the most appropriate comment for the nurse to make would be to assure her of understanding, and add
1. "You must relax, then your baby will be fine."
2. "I'll stay here with you. We are doing everything possible for you and the baby."
3. "Try not to worry. The doctor is doing everything he can. Call me when you want me."
4. "Worrying makes things so much harder for you. You are in labor now and things will progress just fine."

Mrs. H delivered a baby girl by elective low forceps. A midline episiotomy was done under saddle block anesthesia. The baby was small, but had good color and cried spontaneously. The baby was immediately transferred to the premature nursery in an Isolette.

103. A low forceps delivery was done in order to
1. Hasten delivery
2. Prevent exhaustion of the mother
3. Prevent laceration of the perineum
4. Minimize trauma to the infant

104. The infant was placed into an Isolette in order to
1. Maintain body temperature for survival
2. Provide oxygen that the infant needed
3. Provide stimulation for adequate respirations
4. Maintain body fluids by supplying humidity

Situation: Mrs. L is a gravida iv para ii. She has been admitted to the labor room at term. Her contractions are occurring every 4 minutes and lasting 45 to 50 seconds. She has a heavy bloody show. Her B.P. is 194/106, her pulse 88, her respirations 24. The fetal heart rate is 156. On rectal examination, Mrs. L is found to be 5 cm. dilated. The cervix is almost 50% effaced. During her last pregnancy she had a mild preeclampsia that readily responded to treatment. This pregnancy has been uneventful. Both of her previous deliveries have been normal. She has had one abortion, at 12 weeks, between the last and this present pregnancy. At the present time, the fetus is found to be abnormal. Suddenly, after about 1 hour of regular gradually increasing contractions, Mrs. L complains of severe abdominal pain. The pain is accompanied by abdominal rigidity and a trickle of dark red blood from the vagina. Her abdomen is so sensitive to touch that the nurse is unable to place the stethoscope in order to listen to the fetal heart. Mrs. L's pulse increases to 104, and her skin becomes cold

and clammy. All this occurs within the space of approximately 5 minutes. Questions 105 to 109 relate to this patient.

105. Mrs. L's symptoms are indicative of possible
1. Imminent delivery
2. Abruptio placentae
3. Placenta praevia
4. Dystocia

106. The immediate action for the nurse to take would be to
1. Have someone call the physician
2. Prepare for immediate delivery
3. Place the patient in Trendelenburg position
4. Check the vital signs

107. In a patient with ruptured membranes all of the following are signs of fetal distress *except*
1. Increase in F.H. rate from 130 to 158 beats per minute
2. Decrease in F.H. rate from 150 to 120 beats per minute
3. Any change in rate of more than 2 beats per minute
4. Passage of meconium in a vertex presentation

108. Mrs. L was delivered of a living baby boy by emergency cesarean section, but the baby was in evident severe respiratory distress. The most important immediate measure in the care of this infant was to
1. Stimulate the infant vigorously to initiate respirations
2. Aspirate the mucus quickly to maintain an open airway
3. Stimulate respirations immediately with positive pressure oxygen
4. Give the infant a respiratory stimulant intramuscularly stat.

109. In addition to hemorrhage, for which of the following complications must Mrs. L be watched closely for the first 24 to 48 hours?
1. Infection
2. Convulsions
3. Peritonitis
4. Thrombophlebitis

Situation: Mrs. V had missed two menstrual periods when she came to the obstetrician for examination. During the course of the examination, she stated that she had had rheumatic fever when she was 12 years old and that she had had some cardiac involvement at that time, which caused her to curtail all strenuous activities. However, she felt that she actually had been able to lead a normal life. She was presently working as a secretary. The obstetrician diagnosed her as pregnant and referred her to a cardiologist for evaluation. She was diagnosed as having a Class I functional lesion. The cardiologist placed Mrs. V on a low-sodium diet and suggested that she change her schedule to include a morning and an afternoon rest period. He also suggested that she stop working as soon as she became fatigued and that she be checked biweekly by the obstetrician until the 24th week and, after that, weekly. (See questions 110 to 116.)

110. According to the American Heart Association Classification, Class I cardiac disease signifies that

1. Ordinary physical activity does not cause undue fatigue, palpitation, dyspnea, or anginal pain
2. Less than ordinary activity results in exhaustion, palpitation, dyspnea, or anginal pain
3. Symptoms of congestive failure occur as soon as activity is increased
4. Palpitation, dyspnea, or anginal pain is present at all times

111. Rest is an important factor in the management of a pregnant woman with heart disease because
    1. There is a decrease in blood volume during pregnancy
    2. Heart disease predisposes to premature delivery
    3. Pregnancy normally places added stress on the cardiovascular system
    4. Pregnant women are normally more easily fatigued than nonpregnant women

112. Consultation with the nutritionist is requested. A careful diet history reveals that, because of her anxiety and inadequate nutrition education at the beginning of her pregnancy, Mrs. V had been following an extremely rigid diet of only 500 mg. Na and 1,000 calories. In case conference with the obstetrician, cardiologist, and the nurse, the nutritionist recommended a diet only mildly restricted in Na (2 to 3 gm.) and sufficient calories to meet the nutritional needs of both her pregnancy and of her heart condition. The nurse explained to Mrs. V that
    (a) She needed increased amounts of protein during pregnancy
    (b) More calories were needed during pregnancy to spare protein for building and to supply needed energy
    (c) More vitamins and minerals were needed to strengthen heart muscle action, especially proper amounts of iron and potassium
    (d) Dividing her food into six small meals during the day would help avoid a heavy work load on the heart
       1. a and b
       2. c and d
       3. a and d
       4. All of these

Mrs. V's pregnancy continued uneventful until at about 28 weeks gestation she suddenly experienced dyspnea accompanied by a nonproductive cough and an elevation of temperature. The cardiologist as well as the obstetrician advised immediate admission to the hospital.

113. Mrs. V was admitted at this time because her symptoms were indicative of
    1. Early signs of pneumonia
    2. Impending cardiac failure
    3. Exhaustion
    4. Myocardial infarction

Mrs. V was discharged after 2 weeks, with instructions to remain at home, come for regular checkups every week, and return to the hospital for admission a week prior to her due-date.

114. The reason for admitting Mrs. V a week ahead of her expected date of delivery is that

1. Extensive laboratory tests have to be done prior to delivery
2. She will be placed on a monitor in the I.C.U. prior to delivery
3. Antibiotic therapy will be started to prevent subacute bacterial endocarditis
4. A period of bed rest and close supervision will increase her chances for an uncomplicated labor

115. When Mrs. V is in active labor, the best position for her to assume is
    1. Dorsal recumbent
    2. Lithotomy
    3. Sims
    4. Semi-Fowler

116. Mrs. V's labor progressed normally and fairly rapidly. When she reached the second stage, the most appropriate action for the nurse to take was to immediately notify the physician and to
    1. Encourage Mrs. V to push with each contraction
    2. Have Mrs. V pant vigorously during contraction
    3. Encourage Mrs. V to relax as much as possible between contractions
    4. Keep her in semi-Fowler position, with knees flexed, and allow her to push without straining

Situation: Mr. and Mrs. E. (questions 117 to 121) are both diabetic. Mr. E's condition had been diagnosed during a routine physical examination shortly after their marriage. Mrs. E has been a diabetic since early childhood. They have sought genetic counseling and are well aware of the implications that the disease has on their own future and on that of their potential offspring. After 5 years of marriage Mrs. E suspects that she is pregnant because she is experiencing breast changes, some early-morning nausea, and excessive fatigue. She also has missed two menstrual periods. Despite the nausea and fatigue her urine tests are consistently negative for sugar. Mrs. E seeks the advice of an obstetrician, who confirms the diagnosis of pregnancy. Mrs. E is taking 30 units of NPH insulin daily at this time.

117. Both Mr. and Mrs. E are very apprehensive about the outcome of the pregnancy for Mrs. E as well as for the baby. During one of the early visits, Mr. E asks the nurse if it is true, as he has heard, that most babies of diabetic parents are either aborted early, born dead, or born with malformations. The best response for the nurse to make would be
    1. "I suppose you have heard many stories that are old wives' tales, which you must try to forget."
    2. "Yes, it is true; however, we will have Mrs. E checked quite often during pregnancy to prevent such a catastrophe."
    3. "This was a common occurrence in past years, but with our new knowledge more women who are diabetics are having uneventful pregnancies."
    4. "This is really not true in all women; it depends on many factors."

118. Mrs. E is referred to the clinic nutritionist for

nutrition assessment and counseling. The dietary program worked out for her is
(a) A low-carbohydrate, low-calorie diet to stay within her present insulin coverage and avoid hyperglycemia
(b) A diet high in protein of good biologic value, and increased calories
(c) Adequate balance of carbohydrate and fat to meet energy demands and avoid ketosis
(d) Insulin adjusted as needed to balance increased dietary needs
1. a and c
2. b and d
3. b, c, and d
4. a and b

119. Which of the following would be most likely to contribute to the development of acidosis in Mrs. E?
1. Constipation
2. Urinary frequency
3. Vomiting
4. Chloasma

120. Pregnancy is usually terminated several weeks before term in moderately severe diabetics because
1. Diabetics have very large babies
2. Intrauterine fetal death occurs more often during the last weeks of pregnancy
3. Early termination of pregnancy helps in preventing diabetes in the infant
4. Diabetes is impossible to control during the last weeks of pregnancy

121. Babies of diabetic mothers are more likely than average to have which of the following characteristics?
1. Hyperbilirubinemia
2. Respiratory distress during neonatal period
3. Hypoglycemia during neonatal period
4. All of these

Situation: After an uneventful pregnancy and labor, Mrs. H (questions 122 to 126) was delivered of a 7-pound boy with bilateral cleft lip and palate. After 10 years of marriage, during which both had undergone extensive tests, this was Mrs. H's first pregnancy. Both were very happy at the prospect of having a baby. Mrs. H had received a general anesthetic and had not seen the baby before he was brought to the nursery. Mr. H had been told of the defect and also had seen the baby. After seeing the baby, he became very upset. His major concern was what reaction Mrs. H would have. The physician indicates that he will explain the baby's condition to Mrs. H. Mr. H is relieved but states that he will be present, since he feels she needs his support at this time. While looking at the baby, he says to the nursery nurse: "Oh, what am I going to do, how could this happen to us, what is my wife going to do? It would have been better if she had never become pregnant."

122. The most appropriate response for the nurse to make is
1. "How can you say that? You have a lovely healthy baby; the cleft lip can be fixed and then the baby will be fine."
2. "I know how hard this must be for you. But believe me, you will love the baby so

much, you won't even notice that he is disfigured."
3. "This must be very hard on you. Would it help if I went with you when the doctor talks to your wife?"
4. "I know that this is very difficult for you. But you can't think of yourself now. Your wife needs you. You must be strong."

123. After the physician talks to Mrs. H she seems quite composed and asks to see the baby. In order to assess Mrs. H's reaction, the nurse would
1. Bring the baby to her immediately
2. Tell her exactly what the baby looks like before bringing him to her
3. Encourage her to express and explore her feelings; bring the baby to her and stay with her during this time
4. Show her some pictures and give her some literature on harelip and cleft palate and discuss the treatment with her before bringing the baby to her

124. When Mrs. H sees the baby she becomes very disturbed, pushes him away, and says: "Oh, take him away, I never want to see him again." This reaction would indicate that
1. Mrs. H is unable to cope with the situation and that arrangements will have to be made to place the baby into a foster home, at least for the first few months
2. Mrs. H responds as most normal new mothers do, who find it difficult to accept that their baby is less than perfect
3. Mrs. H is severely emotionally disturbed and is in immediate need of psychiatric help
4. Mrs. H is rejecting the baby and he will have to be placed for adoption

125. Mr. and Mrs. H decide to take the baby home as soon as feasible. The nurse has many concerns relating to the baby's welfare and the ability of the mother to care for him. The most important of these is
1. Mother-infant relationship
2. Feeding of the infant
3. General physical care for the infant
4. Long-range plans for repair of the defects

126. Afterward Mrs. H asks how she is going to feed the baby if his mouth is deformed and he cannot suck properly. The nurse teaches her carefully and gently how feedings are to be given
(a) Try using a soft nipple with an enlarged opening so that he can get the milk through a chewing motion
(b) Since he tires easily, it is best to have him lying in bed while he is being fed
(c) He should be held in an upright position and fed slowly to avoid aspiration
(d) Give him brief rest periods and frequent burpings during feedings to expel swallowed air
1. a, c, and d
2. b and d
3. a and c
4. a, b, and d

Situation: Baby P (questions 127 to 131) was admitted to the nursery after a very difficult labor and a forceps delivery. His original Apgar score was 5. After 15 minutes the Apgar score was 7.

127. An Apgar score of 5 indicates that the baby is
   1. In excellent condition and no special care is necessary
   2. In fair condition and needs to be watched
   3. In severe distress and drastic measures have to be taken
   4. Immature and needs to be placed into an incubator

128. Which of the following complications may result from a difficult forceps delivery?
   1. Facial paralysis
   2. Brachial nerve paralysis (Erb's palsy)
   3. Torticollis
   4. Cephalohematoma

129. After Baby P was admitted, the nurse observed suddenly that he was gagging on some mucus. Her first action should be to
   1. Call the physician
   2. Place the baby into Trendelenburg position and aspirate him
   3. Hold the baby by its feet and slap him between the shoulder blades to dislodge the mucus
   4. Administer oxygen

130. Which of the following symptoms would indicate that Baby P has possible brain damage?
   1. High shrill cry
   2. Poor or no sucking reflex
   3. Absence of Moro reflex
   4. All of the above

131. The Apgar scoring is done to appraise the infant in terms of
   1. Respiratory effort
   2. Rh sensitization
   3. Evidence of brain damage
   4. Evidence of birth defects

Situation: Miss C teaches parents' classes at the local hospital in a predominantly Puerto Rican neighborhood. Part of the classes are devoted to a discussion of fetal development, antepartum care including nutrition, preparation for labor and delivery, care of the infant, and postpartum care. The last 15 minutes of each class is devoted to a discussion of concerns or problems raised by any of the class participants. Questions 132 to 143 deal with such concerns.

132. One of the parents wants an explanation of family-centered care. The best statement by the nurse would be that family-centered care implies that
   1. Both parents participate in the childbearing process, supported by the nurse and physician
   2. The husband takes over the nurse's role during labor
   3. The husband must remain with his wife throughout labor and delivery
   4. The mother must be delivered by the psychoprophylactic method

133. One of the mothers asks if it is true that she should not climb or stretch because the baby's cord will wrap itself around the baby's neck and strangle him. Based on her knowledge of pregnancy and fetal development, the best response for the nurse to make is
   1. "That's nonsense. You can do anything you want to do."
   2. "Climbing and stretching may throw you off balance and that is a reason why it should be avoided."
   3. "This is a question only the doctor can answer. Why don't you ask him the next time you see him?"
   4. "You are quite correct. Stretching, in particular, causes strain on the uterine muscles and this tends to lift the cord up and around the baby's neck."

134. To the question "What is the most important reason for rooming-in?" the best response would be that rooming-in is designed to
   1. Alleviate the nursing shortage by placing the baby in the care of the mother from the start
   2. Strengthen family relationships from the start by bringing mother, father, and baby together in a supportive environment
   3. Have the mother learn to bathe, change, and feed the baby properly
   4. Teach the mother to develop a proper schedule for herself and the baby

135. One of the mothers asks why she can't take a tub bath during the last month of pregnancy; the best response would be
   1. "At that time you lose your balance easily and may slip and fall."
   2. "There is no reason why you can't take a tub bath."
   3. "A tub bath is dangerous all during pregnancy because of the chance of infection."
   4. "Soaking in the tub may stimulate contractions and start labor prematurely."

136. "You say that I need to increase the protein in my diet while I am pregnant. What are some ways I can do that?"
   (a) "Add more meat such as chicken to rice dishes—*arroz con pollo.*"
   (b) "Add cheese to beans and sofrito dishes."
   (c) "Use added eggs and codfish with the cooked viandas."
   (d) "Increase milk intake by adding more boiled milk to coffee."
      1. a and b   3. a and d
      2. c and d   4. All of these

137. "Why do I need more iron?"
   (a) "To help you avoid anemia due to the increased blood volume during pregnancy."
   (b) "Iron is necessary to build red blood cells and you need more of them since the amount of blood is increased."
   (c) "Red blood cells carry the oxygen to your cells, which need an extra amount of oxygen to carry on their extra work during pregnancy."
   (d) "Your baby needs to have iron stored in his liver while he is developing, because his first food—milk—is low in iron."
      1. b and c   3. a, b, and c
      2. a and d   4. All of these

138. "How can I get enough iron in my diet?"
   1. "Use 2 eggs every day."

2. "Increase your daily portions of rice and beans."

3. "Add generous amounts of dried skim milk to your coffee."

4. "It is difficult to get sufficient iron from food sources alone, so be sure that you take the daily iron supplement ordered for you."

139. "I'm worried about gaining too much weight because I've heard it's bad for me."
    (a) "Yes, weight gain causes complications during pregnancy."
    (b) "Don't worry primarily about gaining weight. We are more concerned if you don't gain enough weight to ensure proper growth of your baby."
    (c) "The quality of the weight gain is more important than the amount, that it is gained from eating enough of the foods you need."
    (d) "If you gain over 15 pounds, you'll have to follow a low-calorie diet."
    1. a and d   3. c and d
    2. b and c   4. a and c

140. "What is the best way to get the extra calcium I need?"
    (a) "Try to increase the amount of meat in your rice and bean dishes."
    (b) "You need to include more fruit in your diet."
    (c) "Try to increase the amount of milk in your diet and use dried skim milk if you need a cheaper form."
    (d) "Add more cheese to your rice and bean dishes."
    1. a and b   3. c and d
    2. a and c   4. b and d

141. "Is it all right for me to use salt? My girl friend said she was told not to use salt when she was pregnant."
    (a) "There is usually no need to cut out salt. An adequate amount of salt is needed during pregnancy."
    (b) "It is usually best to use salt to taste so that you can get in the added amounts of key foods you need by having them seasoned as you like them."
    (c) "It is best not to go by instructions given someone else, because her situation may have been different from yours."
    (d) "You should not use salt in your food because it is harmful to you and your baby."
    1. a, b, and c   3. c and d
    2. b and c   4. d only

142. "Will milk give my baby all the things he needs?"
    (a) "It will supply all his needs for about the first 3 months but after that he'll need additional solid foods."
    (b) "Milk is not a 'perfect' food because it doesn't contain iron and vitamin C."
    (c) "The amount of iron stored in your baby's liver during your pregnancy usually lasts only about 3 months or so."
    (d) "If you continue indefinitely giving him only milk he will develop 'milk anemia' eventually."

1. b and c   3. c and d
2. a and d   4. All of these

143. "What solid foods should I begin giving him then that will add iron?"
    (a) "Fruit juices, especially citrus."
    (b) "Enriched cereals."
    (c) "Egg yolk."
    (d) "Strained yellow vegetables."
    1. a and d   3. b and d
    2. b and c   4. a and c

Situation: Miss B, the nursery nurse, responds to the call of Mrs. Q (questions 144 and 145), who is very upset and says: "Look nurse, I am sure my baby is sick; she sneezes a lot and look how she breathes. Her breathing is so rapid and shallow and not regular. My neighbor's baby had to return to the hospital after she was home a week because she had pneumonia. I hope this does not happen to my baby."

144. The best action for the nurse to take is to
    1. Pick up the baby and tell the mother that she will watch her closely
    2. Look the baby over and tell the mother that the baby is fine, there is nothing wrong with her
    3. Look the baby over and explain to the mother that sneezing is normal and helps the baby to get rid of mucus and that a baby normally has rapid, shallow, irregular respirations
    4. Look the baby over, take her to the nursery immediately, and return to the mother to tell her that the physician has been called, since the baby is obviously in respiratory distress

145. Miss B's action is based on her knowledge that a normal infant's respirations are
    1. Regular, initiated by the chest wall, 40 to 60 per minute, shallow
    2. Irregular, abdominal, 30 to 40 per minute, shallow
    3. Regular, abdominal, 30 to 40 per minute, deep
    4. Irregular, initiated by chest wall, 30 to 60 per minute, deep

146. Mrs. R, who has three children under 5 years of age at home, comments to the nursery nurse that she cannot hold the baby for feedings once she gets home. She has just too much to do, and anyhow it spoils the baby. The best response for the nurse to make is
    1. "That's entirely up to you, you are the mother."
    2. "Holding the baby is an absolute must, you will just have to find a way."
    3. "It is most unsafe to prop a bottle. If anything happens, you alone are responsible."
    4. "You seem concerned about time. Let's talk about it."

Situation: Baby S (questions 147 to 150) has been delivered at 29 weeks' gestation. He weighs 3 pounds 9 ounces. His mother is 15 years old, unmarried, and had no antepartum care. On admission her B.P. was 196/112, her urine showed 3+ albumin, and she had marked edema of her face and hands.

She delivered spontaneously after a short labor (4½ hours).

147. Baby S was considered to be in critical condition. According to his size and length of gestation, Baby S would be classified as
1. Premature
2. Immature
3. Nonviable
4. Low birthweight infant
148. Which of the following factors is (are) likely to have contributed to Baby S's condition?
1. Age of the mother
2. Presence of preeclampsia
3. Lack of antepartum care
4. All of the above
149. Baby S is being fed by gavage. This type of feeding is indicated in prematures because
1. The feeding can be given quickly, so that handling is minimized
2. Vomiting is prevented
3. It conserves the baby's strength and does not depend on the swallowing reflex
4. The amount of food given can be more accurately regulated
150. Baby S is placed in an incubator to maintain his body temperature at a constant level, because the heat regulation mechanism in prematures is one of the least-developed functions. Which of the following conditions is responsible for this?
1. The surface area of the premature is smaller than that of the normal newborn
2. The premature lacks subcutaneous fat, which would furnish some insulation
3. The premature perspires a great deal, thus losing heat almost constantly
4. The premature has a limited ability to produce antibodies against infections
151. In caring for a premature, which of the following precautions should be taken against retrolental fibroplasia?
1. Oxygen should be kept at less than 40% concentration and be discontinued as soon as feasible
2. Temperature and humidity should be controlled very carefully
3. A high concentration of oxygen (above 75%) should be maintained together with high humidity
4. Phototherapy should be used to prevent jaundice and retinopathy
152. The temperature of the incubator should be regulated so that the baby's temperature is maintained
1. Between 93° and 95° F.
2. Between 97° and 98° F.
3. Between 99° and 100° F.
4. At 100.4° F.

Option type questions

This section of the test consists of questions in a form that is likely to be new to you. In each question, you are presented with two statements, A and B, and you are to choose your answer from the following list of four options:

1. Both A and B are true, and A helps to explain or confirm B.
2. Both A and B are true, and A does not help to explain or confirm B.
3. A is false, B is true.
4. Both A and B are false.

In answering these questions, the *first* step is to make judgments concerning the truth or falsity of the two statements: is A true or false; is B true or false? If you decide that the A statement is false, your answer to the item will be either 3 or 4, depending upon whether B is true or false. Make your choice, fill in the proper space on the answer sheet and go to the next item. If, however, you decide that A is true and B is true, you must make a judgment concerning the relationship of A to B: does A help to explain or confirm B? Here is an example:

A. The time of ovulation may be determined by taking the basal temperature.
B. The temperature drops with a sudden rise at the time of ovulation.
   1 2 3 4

Since both A and B are true statements, ignore answers 3 and 4, since the correct option would be either 1 or 2. You can now focus on the relationship part of this question: that is, does A help to confirm or explain B? Since ovulation is determined by taking the basal temperature and there is a drop with sudden rise during ovulation, A helps to explain B; therefore, option 1 is correct.

The following questions relate to the interpregnancy period. Using the option type questions and associated guide, encircle your choice.
153. A. Routine gynecologic examination done yearly on all women of childbearing and menopausal age is essential for maintenance of optimum health.
B. Obstetrics and gynecology are so closely related that often good obstetrics is preventive gynecology.
   1 2 3 4
154. A. *Candida albicans* is a rodlike bacillus causing vaginitis in women.
B. Fungi thrive well in a dry dark environment.
   1 2 3 4
155. A. *Candida albicans* found in the infant's mouth immediately following birth is usually a secondary infection from the mother.
B. Mycostatin is a broad-spectrum antibiotic used for fungal infections.
   1 2 3 4
156. A. Any change in vaginal pH from acid to alkaline may favor invasion of organisms.
B. In treating vaginal infections, medications

of an acid nature are used to clear up the infection.
1 2 3 4

157. A. The gonococcus is a gram-negative diplococcus.
B. The gonococcus has an affinity for Skene ducts and Bartholin glands.
1 2 3 4

158. A. Lacerations of the perineum heal more readily than do episiotomies.
B. An episiotomy is an incision into the perineum, which facilitates delivery and prevents lacerations.
1 2 3 4

159. A. Healing of perineal incisions and lacerations is facilitated by keeping the area clean and dry.
B. Perineal cleansing from the vagina toward the rectum is considered safe technique.
1 2 3 4

160. A. The most common site of cancer of the uterus is the corpus.
B. The most common site of cancer of the uterus is the cervix.
1 2 3 4

161. A. Pessaries are devices used to correct malpositions of the uterus.
B. Removal of tissue for diagnosis is known as a biopsy.
1 2 3 4

162. A. Culdoscopic examinations are usually done for diagnosis in infertility studies.
B. Pain during sexual intercourse is known as dysmenorrhea.
1 2 3 4

Multiple choice

Situation: Mrs. P, 35 years of age, had her third baby 6 months ago and is returning for a routine gynecologic examination. The doctor finds a small erosion of the cervix. He cauterizes the area with silver nitrate and tells her to douche once daily with 3 tablespoons of vinegar to 2 quarts of water. Questions 163 to 167 relate to this situation.

163. Erosions of the cervix
1. Are not common unless there has been a long labor
2. Are common when the cervix stretches during delivery and there is an unhealed laceration
3. Are common when the cervix is not dilated completely and delivery occurs
4. Are common when the normal acidity of the vagina is altered

164. Douches are ordered for Mrs. P to
1. Keep the vaginal canal clean and free of bacteria
2. Promote healing by heat and elimination of sloughed tissue
3. Promote healing by altering the pH of the vagina
4. Make her comfortable

165. In taking a douche the best position to use for beneficial results would be
1. Knee-chest   3. Dorsal
2. Sims'   4. Fowler's

166. Mrs. P should be instructed to direct the douche nozzle
1. Downward
2. Upward
3. Downward and backward
4. Backward and upward

167. Early treatment of cervical erosions prevents
1. Infections of the reproductive system
2. Cancer of the cervix
3. Metrorrhagia
4. Further erosions from occurring

Situation: Mrs. G, a 56-year-old woman, is admitted for repair of a cystocele and rectocele. She has nine children, three of whom are married, two are away at college, and four are still at home. The youngest child is 17 years old. Her husband is a Civil Service worker. Questions 168 to 171 relate to this situation.

168. Which of the following symptoms have most likely been experienced by Mrs. G?
1. Sporadic bleeding accompanied by abdominal pain
2. Stress incontinence, feeling of low abdominal pressure
3. Heavy leukorrhea, pruritus
4. Change in acidity level of vagina, leukorrhea, spotting

169. Rectocele and cystocele
1. Are usually due to relaxation of musculature of the pelvic floor
2. Are usually due to injury during childbirth
3. Are usually due to infection of the bladder and rectum
4. Are usually due to trauma in repair of an episiotomy or laceration

170. Based on Mrs. G's age and parity status, the surgery done will *most* likely be
1. Insertion of a pessary
2. Abdominal hysterectomy
3. Vaginal hysterectomy
4. Vaginoplasty

171. Mrs. G returned from the operating room with a Foley catheter in place. The reason for this procedure was to prevent all of the following *except*
1. Retention with overflow
2. Bleeding following surgery
3. Discomfort due to bladder distention
4. Loss of bladder tone

Situation: Mrs. U is 45 years old. She has three children—ages 12, 9, and 5 years, respectively. She was admitted to the hospital with the diagnosis of severe metrorrhagia and menorrhagia of 1 year's duration. She was found to have a submucous myoma 6 months ago and has been carefully examined monthly. On the last examination, a week ago, the myoma was found to have grown appreciably and she was told that a hysterectomy was necessary. See questions 172 to 175.

172. The term metrorrhagia refers to
1. Periods of severe bleeding in between menstrual periods
2. Severe bleeding during each menstrual period
3. Presence of occult blood in vaginal discharge
4. Spotting or staining at time of ovulation

173. Mrs. U expressed concern about having a hysterectomy done at her age, because she had heard from friends that she would undergo severe symptoms of menopause after surgery. Based on her knowledge, the most appropriate response for the nurse to make would be
1. "This is something that does occur in older women on occasion, but you don't have to worry about it."
2. "It's too bad you did not discuss this with your doctor. I really can't give you any kind of information about this."
3. "You were misinformed. This never happens following this type of surgery. Your friend probably had a different diagnosis."
4. "Some women occasionally experience exaggerated symptoms of menopause. This is usually transitory, since the ovaries are mainly responsible for maintenance for the hormone balance."

174. Mrs. U wants to know if it would be wise for her to take hormones right away in order to prevent symptoms. The most appropriate response would be
1. "It is best to wait; you may not have any symptoms at all."
2. "You have to wait until symptoms are severe; otherwise, hormones will have no effect."
3. "This is something you should discuss with your physician, since it is important for him to know how you feel and what your concerns are."
4. "Isn't it comforting to know that hormones are available if you should need them?"

175. Mrs. U, when being prepared for the night, starts to sob a little and says: "I told my husband today that, after this operation, I will only be half a woman. He reassured me, but I know that was just a front." The most appropriate response would be
1. "You feel this operation will have an effect on how your husband feels about you as his wife?"
2. "You know of course that this is complete and utter nonsense. I wish you would not worry about such irrelevant things. The main thing is that you have to get well quickly."
3. "It must be frightening to know that your husband rejects you as a woman."
4. "I think I'll call your physician. He might want to postpone the operation until you and your husband have adjusted better to the outcomes of a hysterectomy."

Situation: Mrs. P has been married for 6 years and has been unable to become pregnant. Mr. and Mrs. P have decided to discuss this problem with a physician, who suggests that some studies be done. (See questions 176 to 181.)

176. The physician explains that the studies will involve both Mr. and Mrs. P (and Mr. P first) because
1. 50% to 55% of all infertility is due to female factors
2. Each partner provides support for the other when both undergo testing

3. The largest majority of infertility problems are due to male factors
4. If the male partner is azoospermic, it is useless to do expensive and time-consuming studies on the woman

177. In couples with no demonstrated physical cause for infertility all of the following will help to increase chance of pregnancy except
1. Sexual intercourse only between days 13 and 15 of the menstrual cycle
2. Removal of emotional tensions
3. A general improvement in health and nutrition of both partners
4. Increasing frequency of sexual intercourse

178. After ovulation has occurred, the ovum is believed to remain viable for
1. 1 to 6 hours
2. 12 to 18 hours
3. 24 to 36 hours
4. 48 to 72 hours

179. A test commonly used to determine number, motility, and activity of sperm is the
1. Rubin test
2. Huhner test
3. Papanicolaou test
4. Friedman test

180. In the female, evaluation of all the pelvic organs of reproduction is accomplished by
1. Cystoscopy
2. Biopsy
3. Culdoscopy
4. Hysterosalpingogram

181. A factor in sterility may be related to the pH of the vaginal canal. A frequent medication that is ordered to alter the pH would be
1. Sulfur insufflations
2. Sodium bicarbonate douches
3. Lactic acid douches
4. Estrogen therapy

Situation: Mrs. W, age 24, complains of menstrual irregularity and infertility. See questions 182 to 185.

182. A drug which the physician may prescribe to treat both of Mrs. W's complaints is known as
1. Methallenestril (Vallestril)
2. Ergonovine (Ergotrate)
3. Norethynodrel with mestranol (Enovid)
4. Relaxin (Releasin)

183. After this medication is discontinued, Mrs. W becomes pregnant. When Mrs. W complains of spotting, which of the following groups of drugs might be used to maintain the pregnancy
1. Oxytocics
2. Gonadotropins
3. Androgens
4. Luteal hormones

184. Mrs. W is hospitalized when her membranes rupture during the 38th week of pregnancy. If the obstetrician decides to induce labor, he is likely to request which of the following drugs?
1. Ergonovine maleate
2. Progesterone
3. Oxytocin (Pitocin)
4. Lututrin (Lutrexin)

185. During the period of induction, Mrs. W should be observed carefully for signs of which of the following?
1. Uterine tetany
2. Severe pain
3. Prolapse of the umbilical cord
4. Hypoglycemia

Situation: Mrs. R is seen at the gynecology clinic because of profuse vaginal discharge, pruritus, and burning. A smear for microscopic examination was done and revealed presence of *Trichomonas vaginalis.* (See questions 186 to 188.)

186. A trichomonal infection is caused by which organism?
   1. Fungus
   2. Yeast
   3. Spirochete
   4. Protozoa
187. Mrs. R would be treated by medication and
   1. Douches with sodium bicarbonate to decrease the pH of the vagina
   2. Douches of acetic acid to decrease the pH of the vagina
   3. Douches with sodium bicarbonate to increase the pH of the vagina
   4. Douches with acetic acid to increase the pH of the vagina
188. It is most likely that which drug will be prescribed orally for treatment of *Trichomonas vaginalis?*
   1. Gentian violet
   2. Condicidin
   3. Metronidazole (Flagyl)
   4. Nystatin

Situation: Mrs. V is 42 years old and mother of two children, ages 3 and 7. She is admitted to the hospital because of spotting between menstrual periods. The bleeding increased during intercourse and when straining on defecation. Her admission diagnosis read "possible cervical polyps." She was scheduled for a D and C and polypectomy. The nurse admitting her noted that she was pale, wringing her hands, and unable to sit still but not speaking unless asked a direct question. From these observations, the nurse deduced that Mrs. V was very anxious. Questions 189 to 196 apply to this situation.

189. All of the following factors *except which one* are most likely to be contributory to Mrs. V's anxiety?
   1. Worry about the children
   2. Fear of surgery
   3. Relief that something is finally being done
   4. Worry about the outcome of the laboratory tests
190. In order to get Mrs. V to express her anxieties, the best approach for the nurse to use would be to
   1. Tell Mrs. V that there is no need to worry; a polypectomy and a D and C are considered minor surgery
   2. Say "I can tell that something is troubling you. It might help you to talk about it. I might be able to help you."
   3. Tell Mrs. V that it is normal for her to be anxious; everybody coming to the hospital is fearful, even when there is no reason.
   4. Ask "Why are you so upset?"
191. Mrs. V finally tells the nurse that she believes she has cancer, because the doctor told her that he would have to remove the polyps and wait for laboratory reports. The best response of the nurse would be
   1. "No operation is done without specimens being sent to the laboratory."

   2. "Of course you don't have cancer; polyps are always benign. The laboratory report is simply routine."
   3. "Worrying today is not going to help you at all. It will only interfere with your rest; and you need to be relaxed for the surgery."
   4. "It is very upsetting to have to wait for a laboratory report. It might help you to know that most of the time polyps are not cancerous. I'll be with you and try to help you as much as I can."
192. The nurse knows that
   1. Cervical polyps are usually benign but curettage of the uterus is always done to rule out malignancy
   2. Cervical polyps are usually malignant and curettage is always done
   3. Cervical polyps do not cause bleeding until they are malignant
   4. Cervical polyps are never malignant and do not necessitate further study
193. Following surgery, the laboratory reports revealed a stage 0 lesion. According to the International Federation of Gynecology and Obstetrics, stage 0 is indicative of
   1. Carcinoma in situ
   2. Carcinoma strictly confined to cervix
   3. Early stromal invasion
   4. Parametrial involvement
194. The most common site for cancer cell growth in the cervix is
   1. At the internal os
   2. At the external os
   3. At the junction of the columnar and squamous epithelium of the internal and external os
   4. At the junction of the cervix and lower uterine segment
195. Following discharge, Mrs. V was asked to return in 3 months for a Papanicolaou smear. This was done because
   1. Mrs. V had suspicious cells in the report following the D and C
   2. Mrs. V is being followed carefully because of the findings on the laboratory test
   3. Mrs. V is very anxious about her condition and needs a great deal of reassurance
   4. It is a routine practice on all women under 50 years of age
196. The Papanicolaou smear on Mrs. V was reported to be class I. Class I indicates that
   1. The smear contains only normal cells
   2. The smear contains atypical cells (none suggestive of malignancy)
   3. The smear contains cells suggestive of, but not diagnostic of, cancer
   4. The smear contains malignant cells

Situation: Mrs. E is a 52-year-old woman admitted to the hospital with the diagnosis of cancer of the cervix. She is scheduled for a hysterectomy and insertion of radium. She returns to the floor from the recovery room with a Foley catheter in place, and vaginal packing. The packing is to be removed in 24 hours. (See questions 197 to 200.)

197. The nurse checking the perineum found the packing protruding from the vagina. The im-

mediate action to take would be to report this situation to the physician at once because
1. The packing is radioactive
2. The purpose of the packing is to increase the distance between the insert and the rectum and/or bladder
3. The packing must be removed
4. The purpose of the packing is to prevent bleeding

198. In caring for Mrs. E the nurse would do all of the following except
1. Plan the care to limit the time spent at or close to the bedside
2. Keep Mrs. E as quiet as possible so as not to dislodge the radium insert
3. Check all bed linen carefully before discarding
4. Spend as much time as possible in close contact with Mrs. E to alleviate her anxiety

199. Following radium insertion, which of the following symptoms is (are) significant as reaction to the radium?
1. Nausea and vomiting
2. Pain and elevation of temperature
3. Restlessness and irritability
4. Vaginal discharge

200. Which of the following are important procedures to follow when assisting with radium removal?
1. Radium must be handled carefully, with long forceps
2. Radium must be cleansed carefully in ether or alcohol, using long forceps
3. Date and hour of removal and total time of treatment must be charted
4. All of these must be carried out

Situation: Joan Y, 16 years of age, comes to the clinic because of severe burning on urination, persistent vaginal discharge, and irritation of the vulva. On examination, the vulva and vagina appear red and irritated and there is profuse greenish yellow discharge. A cervical culture and smear are taken. The smear reveals a gonorrheal infection. (See questions 201 to 206.)

201. The causative organism of gonorrhea is
1. *Treponema pallidum*
2. Gonococcus
3. *Staphylococcus*
4. Döderlein's bacillus

202. In relation to gonorrhea, the nurse understands that it is a highly infectious disease and also that
1. It is easily cured
2. It can produce sterility
3. It occurs very rarely
4. It is limited to the external genitalia

203. In relation to the public health implications of this condition, the nurse would be *most* interested in
1. The reasons for Joan's promiscuity
2. Interviewing Joan's parents to find out how she got this infection
3. Finding Joan's contacts
4. Instructing Joan in birth control measures

204. If a woman with untreated gonorrhea is allowed to deliver, the infant is in danger of being born with
1. Ophthalmia neonatorum
2. Congenital syphilis
3. Thrush
4. Pneumonia

205. The drug of choice for the treatment of gonorrhea is
1. Penicillin
2. Actinomycin
3. Chloromycetin
4. Colistin

206. Appropriate drug therapy for treatment of gonorrhea can be expected to
1. Cure the infection
2. Prevent complications
3. Control its transmission
4. Reverse pathologic changes

Additional questions:

207. Which of the following does *not* contribute to the diagnosis of syphilis in the newborn?
1. Blebs on soles of feet and palms of hands
2. Snuffles
3. Mongolian spots
4. General skin eruption of rose spots

208. Ectopic pregnancy refers to any pregnancy outside of the uterus, the most common site being
1. Abdominal cavity
2. Cervix
3. Fallopian tube
4. Ovary

209. Symptoms of an ectopic pregnancy *usually* occur
1. Before the first missed period
2. During the first trimester
3. During the second trimester
4. During the third trimester

SCORES

NAME ______________ (LAST) ______________ (FIRST) ______________ (MIDDLE) DATE ______________

SCHOOL ______________ CITY ______________

1 ______________ 2 ______________

1 ______	5 ______	
2 ______	6 ______	
3 ______	7 ______	
4 ______	8 ______	

DATE OF BIRTH ______________ AGE ______ SEX ______ (M OR F)

GRADE OR CLASS ______ INSTRUCTOR ______________

NAME OF TEST ______________ PART ______

DIRECTIONS: Read each question and its numbered answers. When you have decided which answer is correct, blacken the corresponding space on this sheet with the special pencil. Make your mark as long as the pair of lines, and move the pencil point up and down firmly to make a heavy black line. If you change your mind, erase your first mark completely. Make no stray marks; they may count against you.

SAMPLE:

1. Chicago is

1—1 a country
1—2 a mountain
1—3 an island
1—4 a city
1—5 a state

1 ▯1 ▯2 ▯3 ▮4 ▯5

1 — 1 2 3 4 5	31 — 1 2 3 4 5	61 — 1 2 3 4 5	91 — 1 2 3 4 5	121 — 1 2 3 4 5
2 — 1 2 3 4 5	32 — 1 2 3 4 5	62 — 1 2 3 4 5	92 — 1 2 3 4 5	122 — 1 2 3 4 5
3 — 1 2 3 4 5	33 — 1 2 3 4 5	63 — 1 2 3 4 5	93 — 1 2 3 4 5	123 — 1 2 3 4 5
4 — 1 2 3 4 5	34 — 1 2 3 4 5	64 — 1 2 3 4 5	94 — 1 2 3 4 5	124 — 1 2 3 4 5
5 — 1 2 3 4 5	35 — 1 2 3 4 5	65 — 1 2 3 4 5	95 — 1 2 3 4 5	125 — 1 2 3 4 5
6 — 1 2 3 4 5	36 — 1 2 3 4 5	66 — 1 2 3 4 5	96 — 1 2 3 4 5	126 — 1 2 3 4 5
7 — 1 2 3 4 5	37 — 1 2 3 4 5	67 — 1 2 3 4 5	97 — 1 2 3 4 5	127 — 1 2 3 4 5
8 — 1 2 3 4 5	38 — 1 2 3 4 5	68 — 1 2 3 4 5	98 — 1 2 3 4 5	128 — 1 2 3 4 5
9 — 1 2 3 4 5	39 — 1 2 3 4 5	69 — 1 2 3 4 5	99 — 1 2 3 4 5	129 — 1 2 3 4 5
10 — 1 2 3 4 5	40 — 1 2 3 4 5	70 — 1 2 3 4 5	100 — 1 2 3 4 5	130 — 1 2 3 4 5
11 — 1 2 3 4 5	41 — 1 2 3 4 5	71 — 1 2 3 4 5	101 — 1 2 3 4 5	131 — 1 2 3 4 5
12 — 1 2 3 4 5	42 — 1 2 3 4 5	72 — 1 2 3 4 5	102 — 1 2 3 4 5	132 — 1 2 3 4 5
13 — 1 2 3 4 5	43 — 1 2 3 4 5	73 — 1 2 3 4 5	103 — 1 2 3 4 5	133 — 1 2 3 4 5
14 — 1 2 3 4 5	44 — 1 2 3 4 5	74 — 1 2 3 4 5	104 — 1 2 3 4 5	134 — 1 2 3 4 5
15 — 1 2 3 4 5	45 — 1 2 3 4 5	75 — 1 2 3 4 5	105 — 1 2 3 4 5	135 — 1 2 3 4 5

BE SURE YOUR MARKS ARE HEAVY AND BLACK.
ERASE COMPLETELY ANY ANSWER YOU WISH TO CHANGE.

16 — 1 2 3 4 5	46 — 1 2 3 4 5	76 — 1 2 3 4 5	106 — 1 2 3 4 5	136 — 1 2 3 4 5
17 — 1 2 3 4 5	47 — 1 2 3 4 5	77 — 1 2 3 4 5	107 — 1 2 3 4 5	137 — 1 2 3 4 5
18 — 1 2 3 4 5	48 — 1 2 3 4 5	78 — 1 2 3 4 5	108 — 1 2 3 4 5	138 — 1 2 3 4 5
19 — 1 2 3 4 5	49 — 1 2 3 4 5	79 — 1 2 3 4 5	109 — 1 2 3 4 5	139 — 1 2 3 4 5
20 — 1 2 3 4 5	50 — 1 2 3 4 5	80 — 1 2 3 4 5	110 — 1 2 3 4 5	140 — 1 2 3 4 5
21 — 1 2 3 4 5	51 — 1 2 3 4 5	81 — 1 2 3 4 5	111 — 1 2 3 4 5	141 — 1 2 3 4 5
22 — 1 2 3 4 5	52 — 1 2 3 4 5	82 — 1 2 3 4 5	112 — 1 2 3 4 5	142 — 1 2 3 4 5
23 — 1 2 3 4 5	53 — 1 2 3 4 5	83 — 1 2 3 4 5	113 — 1 2 3 4 5	143 — 1 2 3 4 5
24 — 1 2 3 4 5	54 — 1 2 3 4 5	84 — 1 2 3 4 5	114 — 1 2 3 4 5	144 — 1 2 3 4 5
25 — 1 2 3 4 5	55 — 1 2 3 4 5	85 — 1 2 3 4 5	115 — 1 2 3 4 5	145 — 1 2 3 4 5
26 — 1 2 3 4 5	56 — 1 2 3 4 5	86 — 1 2 3 4 5	116 — 1 2 3 4 5	146 — 1 2 3 4 5
27 — 1 2 3 4 5	57 — 1 2 3 4 5	87 — 1 2 3 4 5	117 — 1 2 3 4 5	147 — 1 2 3 4 5
28 — 1 2 3 4 5	58 — 1 2 3 4 5	88 — 1 2 3 4 5	118 — 1 2 3 4 5	148 — 1 2 3 4 5
29 — 1 2 3 4 5	59 — 1 2 3 4 5	89 — 1 2 3 4 5	119 — 1 2 3 4 5	149 — 1 2 3 4 5
30 — 1 2 3 4 5	60 — 1 2 3 4 5	90 — 1 2 3 4 5	120 — 1 2 3 4 5	150 — 1 2 3 4 5

Printed by the International Business Machines Corporation, Endicott, N. Y., U. S. A.
IBM FORM I.T.S. 1000 B 108

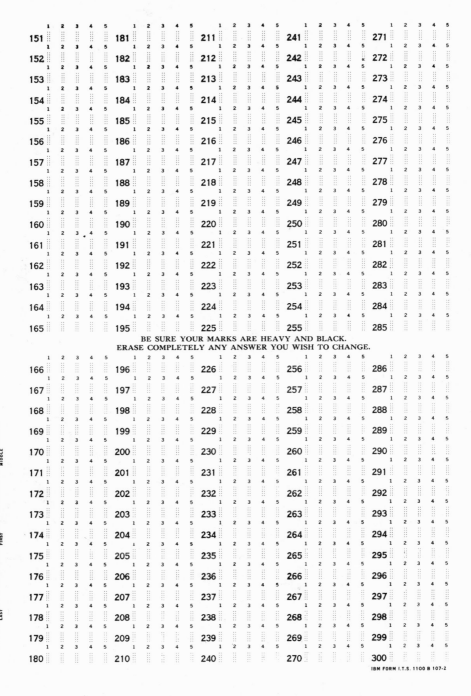

BE SURE YOUR MARKS ARE HEAVY AND BLACK.
ERASE COMPLETELY ANY ANSWER YOU WISH TO CHANGE.

SCORES

5
6
7
8

1
2
3
4

NAME

LAST

FIRST

MIDDLE

IBM FORM I.T.S. 1100 B 107-2

11

PEDIATRIC NURSING

American Academy of Pediatrics: Report of the Committee on Infectious Diseases 1970, Evanston, Ill., 1970, The Academy.

Anderson, G., Arnstein, M. G., and Lester, M. R.: Communicable disease control, ed. 4, New York, 1962, The Macmillan Co.

Benenson, A. S., editor: Control of communicable diseases in man, ed. 11, New York, 1970, The American Public Health Association.

Bergmann, T., and Freud, A.: Children in the hospital, New York, 1965, International Universities Press.

Blake, F. G., Wright, F. H., and Waechter, E. H.: Nursing care of children, ed. 8, Philadelphia, 1970, J. B. Lippincott Co.

Bossard, J. H. S., and Boll, E. S.: The sociology of child development, ed. 3, New York, 1960, Harper & Brothers.

Brechenridge, M. E., and Murphy, M. N.: Growth and development of the young child, ed. 7, Philadelphia, 1963, W. B. Saunders Co.

Brechenridge, M. E., and Vincent, E. L.: Child development, ed. 5, Philadelphia, 1965, W. B. Saunders Co.

Duvall, E. M.: Family development, ed. 4, Philadelphia, 1971, J. B. Lippincott Co.

Erickson, F.: Reactions of children to hospital experience, Nursing Outlook 6:501, Sept., 1958.

Erickson, F.: When 6 to 12 year olds are ill, Nursing Outlook 13:48, July, 1965.

Geist, H.: A child goes to the hospital, Springfield, Ill., 1965, Charles C Thomas, Publisher.

Gesell, A., and Ilg, F. L.: Child development, New York, 1949, Harper & Brothers.

Government documents available from the United States Government Printing Office, Division of Public Documents, Washington, D. C. 20402.

Harper, P. A.: Preventive pediatrics: child health and development, New York, 1962, Appleton-Century-Crofts.

Hurlock, F. B.: Child development, ed. 4, New York, 1964, McGraw-Hill Book Co.

Johnston, D. F.: Essentials of communicable disease: with nursing principles, St. Louis, 1968, The C. V. Mosby Co.

Kagan, J., and Moss, H. A.: Birth to maturity. A study in psychological development, New York, 1962, John Wiley & Sons, Inc.

Krugman, S., and Ward, R.: Infectious diseases of children, ed. 5, St. Louis, 1973, The C. V. Mosby Co.

Landreth, C.: Early childhood, behavior and learning, ed. 2, New York, 1967, Alfred A. Knopf, Inc.

Latham, H. C., and Heckel, R. V.: Pediatric nursing, ed. 2, St. Louis, 1972, The C. V. Mosby Co.

Leifer, G.: Principles and techniques in pediatric nursing, ed. 2, Philadelphia, 1972, W. B. Saunders Co.

Marlow, D. R.: Textbook of pediatric nursing, ed. 3, Philadelphia, 1969, W. B. Saunders Co.

Moore, M. L.: The newborn and the nurse, Philadelphia, 1972, W. B. Saunders Co.

Murphy, L. B.: The widening world of children. Paths toward mastery, New York, 1962, Basic Books, Inc., Publishers.

National Communicable Disease Center, U. S. Public Health Service: Morbidity and Mortality Weekly Reports, Atlanta, Ga.

Nelson, W. E., Vaughan, V. C., and McKay, R. J.: Textbook of pediatrics, ed. 9, Philadelphia, 1969, W. B. Saunders Co.

Plank, E. N.: Working with children in hospitals, Cleveland, 1962, The Press of Case Western Reserve University.

Prugh, D. G., Staub, E. M., Sands, H. H., Kirschbaum, R. M., and Leniham, E. A.: A study of the emotional reactions of children and families to hospitalization and illness, American Journal of Orthopsychiatry 23:70, Jan., 1953.

Robertson, J.: Hospitals and children: a parent's eye view, New York, 1962, International Universities Press.

Robertson, J.: Young children in hospitals, New York, 1962, Basic Books, Inc., Publishers.

Roe, R. L., editor: Developmental psychology today, California, 1971, Communication Research Machines.

Stone, L. J., and Church, J.: Childhood and adolescence, ed. 2, New York, 1968, Random House, Inc.

Stuart, H. C., and Prugh, D. G.: The healthy child: his physical, psychological, and social development, Cambridge, Mass., 1964, Harvard University Press.

Top, F. H., and Wehrle, P. F., editors: Communicable and infectious diseases, ed. 7, St. Louis, 1972, The C. V. Mosby Co.

Vernon, D., Foley, J., Sipowicz, R., and Schulman, J.: The psychological responses of children to hospitalization and illness, Springfield, Ill., 1965, Charles C Thomas, Publisher.

Ziai, M., editor: Pediatrics, Boston, 1969, Little, Brown & Co.

CHALLENGE AND SCOPE OF PEDIATRIC NURSING

1. **Public documents expressing philosophy of human concern**
A. Constitution of United States
B. The Children's Charter
C. Children's Bill of Rights
D. Pledge to Children
E. United Nations Universal Declaration of Human Rights
2. **Health services—a promise to the child for his way of life**
A. Vast expansion of many kinds of health services for the child
B. Official—the federal, state, and local services extended to all children
C. Children and Youth Projects, comprehensive health care programs for children (federal funding support)
D. Maternal and Infant Projects, comprehensive health care for mothers and their unborn and new infants (federal funding support)
E. Health insurance plans favorably influence total family health
F. Family-centered child health care
G. Hospitalization—stay for acute illnesses decreased, while there is little change in hospital stay for illnesses requiring long-term care
H. Increased availability of ambulatory health services for the child and his family
I. Ever-growing body of knowledge in the health and social sciences
J. New and improved methods of medical diagnosis
K. Rapid development of drug therapies for specific illnesses
L. Widespread immunization programs
M. Improved surgical techniques for congenital handicaps
N. Public documents, such as the United Nations Universal Declaration of Human Rights

3. **Concerns and responsibilities of pediatric nursing**
A. It is concerned with
1. Growth and development of the child from embryonic life up through adolescence
2. Genetic factors that influence the child's potential for development
3. Environment that helps determine the present and the future life of the child
4. Health and illnesses of the child
5. Family that assumes responsibility for the love and care of the child
6. Health services for the child in which nursing plays a vital role
B. It deals with changes in size or complexity of function of the child's
1. Various organ systems
2. Emotional responses
3. Motor and mental abilities
4. Ability to respond to disease
C. It assumes responsibility for
1. Giving needed care to both the healthy and the sick child
2. Helping the child stay well
3. Helping the child help himself to overcome many aspects of illness or disability
4. Teaching the child about his health and his illness
5. Making careful and systematic observations of the child
6. Teaching parents how to care for the healthy and the sick child
7. Working with the physician to achieve the health goals of the child
8. Contributing as member of a multidisciplinary professional team for the health care of the child
9. Promoting and participating in preventive aspects of illness
10. Contributing to total health furtherance for the child
11. Encouraging research for the improvement of nursing care to the infant and child
12. Planning for the improvement of nursing care to all children, in the many varieties of institutions and agencies that provide health care for the child

THE CHILD AND HIS ENVIRONMENT

1. **Needs of the child**
A. Physical needs

1. Food, shelter, warmth, comfort, rest, and exercise
2. Play, companionship, growth, communication

B. Social, emotional, and spiritual needs—to
1. Feel safe and unafraid
2. Feel that people care about him
3. Have approval and acceptance
4. Develop trust
5. Be trusted by others
6. Think well of himself
7. Express his feelings
8. Make some choices
9. Have opportunity to play and be imaginative
10. Love and be loved
11. Grow, through experience
12. Maintain self-integrity
13. Be understood
14. Be recognized as a person of worth

C. Health provisions
1. Maintenance of health
2. Prevention of illnesses and accidents
3. Ambulatory and acute care for illnesses
4. Healthy environment in which to live
5. Adequate nutrition for health

2. **Conditions essential to development of sense of security and autonomy in the child**
A. Assurance that he is wanted, loved, and enjoyed by his parents
B. Stable home where his needs are met
C. Assurance of protection
D. Sense of being allowed and encouraged to grow, learn, and achieve
E. Faith in information received from parents
F. Assurance that he will be treated as individual with own unique worth
G. Schooling that provides for optimal development of the child and in turn enhances his family and community life

3. **Behaviors that require understanding by parents and by nurses**
A. Hostility and aggression
1. Urgent need to be aggressive and self-indulgent
2. Recognition of behavior limits consistent with developmental level
3. Limitations set should be consistent
4. Impulsive behavior may promote drastic response in parent
   a. Temper tantrum
      (1) Child needs assurance and love
      (2) Precipitating factors prior to tantrum

(3) Standards too high for child
(4) Child overexcited or tired
   b. Provision of channels for release of hostility in play

B. Sex interests
1. Part of normal development
2. Sometimes a cause of feelings of guilt and shame
3. Conflict between natural impulses and their moral evaluation by adults

C. Fears
1. Some fear reaction normal and desirable
2. Understanding of fear-provoking object or situation also desirable

4. **Symptomatic behavior of the child**
A. Emotional tension often symptomatic of underlying problem
1. Symptoms of emotional tension
   a. Nail-biting
   b. Thumb-sucking beyond period of infancy
   c. Bed-wetting or soiling clothing after learning elimination control
   d. Refusal of foods
   e. Temper tantrums
   f. Masturbation
   g. Crying
   h. Withdrawal from usual activities
2. Possible causes of tension
   a. Unhappy environmental conditions
   b. Rejection
   c. Sibling jealousy
   d. Overprotection
   e. Goals too high for comfortable accomplishment

5. **The child's play and recreation**
A. Value of play—an aid in
1. Learning physical coordination
2. Social and emotional development
3. Personality development
4. Cognitive development
5. Learning to get along with others
6. Developing imagination
7. Encouraging freedom of movement
8. Providing pleasure for the child

B. Criteria for judging suitability of toy
1. Safety
2. Attraction and appeal
3. Compatibility with child's need, age, and experience
4. Usefulness in variety of ways
5. Enhances sensory-motor development
6. Enhances personal and social development
7. Challenges the development of the child

8. Provides outlet for some strains to his emotions

C. Types of toys to avoid—those which
1. Are beyond range of experience
2. Encourage destructiveness
3. Are unsafe
4. Are of transient value
5. Overstimulate
6. Have limited uses

D. Care of toys
1. Storage space accessible to child
2. Encouragement in care

E. Books for children—principles of selection in general are the same as for adults
1. Good print
2. Good illustrations
3. Eye appeal
4. Content suitable to stage of development
5. Lasting value
6. Nursery rhymes
7. Poetry
8. Easily cleansed (washable)—for very young child

F. Other cultural materials
1. Excerpts from world's collection of good music
2. Finger paints
3. Crayons
4. Water-solvent paints

G. Play in the hospital
1. Director of recreational programs
2. Play space (outdoor and indoor)
3. Prevention of overstimulation
4. Responsibility of nurse for child's play
5. Storage of toys and play equipment
6. Cooperation and participation in child life program

6. **Home in life of the child**

A. Influence of family
1. Importance of good parent-child relationship
2. Home as community force
   a. Migrant versus stable
   b. Poverty versus affluence
3. Need for consistency in developing patterns of conduct

B. Changes in function of home and influence on child rearing
1. Homemaker services
2. Foster homes
3. Care of children of working mothers
   a. Day care services
   b. Child rearing problems of care
4. Care of handicapped child
   a. Special day care services
   b. Special day schooling

C. Development of security
1. Parental acceptance of child as he is
   a. Approval of progression at his own rate in friendly atmosphere without rigid standards
   b. Encouragement of self-reliance and independence
2. Avoidance of both excessive indulgence and overprotection

D. Child's need for satisfaction
1. "Mothering" vs. mechanical handling
2. Success vs. persistent frustration

E. Child's need for exercise
1. Activities suitable to age and degree of development
2. Prevention of overfatigue and overstimulation

F. Parental attitudes
1. Some parents show loving acceptance of infant
2. Others seem unable to assume parental roles because of their own immaturity
3. In some cases the infant apparently interferes with mother's career
4. Infant may not be of the sex preferred by the parents
5. Economic factors may cause some rejection of infant
6. Infant may be neglected because of parents' lack of knowledge about infant and child care
7. Infant or child may be outlet for hostilities of parents and be victim of battered-child syndrome
8. Infant born out of wedlock is particularly subject to rejection and neglect

G. Nature of relationship of infant to adult who assumes responsibility for his care
1. Infant's responses depend upon
   a. Nurturing pattern and, particularly, the regularity in pattern
   b. Time lapse between need arousal of the infant and his receiving of care
   c. Kinds and amount of physical contact
   d. Separation from the adult figure, which produces anxiety
   e. Amount and kind of vocalization between infant and adult
2. Infant learns or feels
   a. Satisfactions gained by having his physiologic needs cared for
   b. Some of the pleasures to be gained from the parental figure in the nurturing process

c. Anticipation of attentions from parents
d. Some anxiety when the anticipated nurturing needs are not met
e. Close one-to-one relationship with the mother or person who provides the nurturing
f. Enjoyment of the presence and vocalizations of siblings who also provide him with nurturing needs
g. Some anxiety in the presence of strangers after he has established the one-to-one relationship with the mother figure

3. Infant and mother both are disturbed by some problems of the infant
a. Crying without apparent reason
b. Poor sleeping patterns
c. Vomiting
d. Irregular feeding patterns and variations in desire for food

4. Infant's relationship to parents leads to his development of trust and then of some autonomy

GROWTH AND DEVELOPMENT (HUMAN DEVELOPMENT)

1. **Children are constantly changing**
A. Traditional definitions
   1. Growth—physical maturation
   2. Development—functional maturation
B. Current concepts
   1. Human development—interacting processes of growth and development to achieve maturation
   2. Patterns of human development (growth and development) are
   a. Described in terms of norms and normal range
   b. Noted for a child over a lengthy period of time
   c. Evaluated in relation to other parameters, such as health, genetic inheritance, and specific abnormalities due to disease

2. **Periods readily identified in growth**
A. Infancy—rapid growth
B. Slow and uniform growth from preschool age to puberty
C. Growth spurt of pubertal period
D. Decline in growth rate until it ceases

3. **Human development is viewed in the context of**
A. Perinatal history of the child (including genetic factors)
B. Family history
C. Health history of the child

D. Socioeconomic factors
E. Cultural factors
F. Physical and mental development (findings)
G. Rate of development and growth
H. Environmental factors

4. **Development**
A. Is a continuous process from embryonic age to maturity
B. Follows a sequence, but the rate varies from child to child
C. Is a change from mass and undifferentiated activity to that of specific responses
D. Is closely related to the maturation of the nervous system
E. Changes from some reflexes, such as the grasp, which disappears for a period of time, and is then replaced by voluntary activity
F. Is in the cephalocaudal direction, or head-to-foot, and the proximodistal, or center-to-periphery

5. **Characteristics of biologic growth**
A. Hemoglobin
   1. 17 grams at birth, then decreases to 11.5 to 12 grams per 100 ml. at 1 year
   2. At ages 1 to 12 years there is a gradual increase in hemoglobin to 14.5
   3. Red blood cells in children contain less hemoglobin than in adults
   4. Hemoglobin in children has a greater affinity for oxygen than in adults
   5. Fetal hemoglobin (60% to 90%) gradually decreases in first year of life, to less than 5% of total hemoglobin
B. Blood sugar
   1. Blood sugar levels gradually rise from 75 to 80 mg. per 100 ml. in infancy to 95 to 100 during adolescence
   2. Premature infants have lower blood sugar levels than do full-term infants
C. Basal metabolism
   1. Highest rate is found in the newborn
   2. Males have slightly higher rates than females
D. Vital capacity
   1. Boys' capacity exceeds girls'
   2. Gradual increase in capacity throughout childhood and adolescence
E. Heart rate
   1. Rate decreases with increase in age (from 100 to 110 at 1 year to 60 to 70+ at 18 years)
   2. After age 10, girls' rates are slightly higher than boys'
F. Blood pressure (base 60 to 90 mm. systolic, 20 to 60 mm. diastolic)

1. Gradual increase in pressure with age, 2 to 3 mm. per year
2. Systolic higher in adolescent boy than in girl

G. Kidney
   1. Premature and full-term newborn have some inability to concentrate urine
   2. Glomerular filtration rate greatly increased by 6 months of age

6. **Developmental concepts**
A. Erikson: personality and childhood

Stages	Characteristics
Infancy—oral, sensory	Basic trust vs. mistrust
Toddler—muscular, anal	Autonomy vs. shame, doubt
Preschooler—locomotor, genital	Initiative vs. guilt
Childhood—latency	Industry vs. inferiority
Puberty and adolescence	Identity vs. role confusion
Young adulthood	Intimacy vs. isolation

B. Piaget: cognitive development

Ages	Phase
Infancy, toddler	Sensorimotor
Years 3 to 4	Preconceptual, beginning language
5 to 7	Intuitive thought
8 to 12	Concrete operations
13	Formal operations

INFANCY

1. **Terminology**
A. Embryonic stage—first 8 weeks of intrauterine life
B. Fetal age—that period of time between beginning of embryonic life and birth
C. Neonatal period—first 4 weeks of extrauterine life
D. Perinatal—fetal and neonatal periods of life
E. Dysmature infant—one small at birth in relation to gestational age
F. Premature infant—newborn infant whose gestational age is less than 37 weeks
G. Low birth weight infant—infant whose weight at birth is 2,500 grams or less
H. High-risk infant—infant born of a high-risk mother, a teen-ager, an elderly (36 to 40's) mother, an unwed mother, one who has special health problems, or one from low socioeconomic level

2. **Behaviors of infants**
A. The 28-week gestational age infant
   1. Body limp, and grasp difficult to obtain
   2. Almost constant spontaneous activity
   3. Suck and swallow weak, infant lacking persistence in these
   4. Reflexes, if present, feeble

B. The 32-week gestational age infant
   1. Some abduction and flexion of limbs
   2. Almost constant spontaneous activity
   3. Improved suck and swallow
   4. Reflexes still weak

C. The 36-week gestational age infant
   1. Improved flexion but still froglike position of legs
   2. Some occasional spontaneous activity
   3. Suck and swallow fair to good
   4. Most reflexes present

D. The 40-week or full-term infant
   1. Limbs strongly flexed
   2. Frequent spontaneous activity
   3. Reflexes present and easily elicited, particularly the
      a. Moro reflex—abduction and extension of the arms followed by adduction and flexion of the arms when the head is suddenly released from firm support, or as a response to a bang or other loud noise
      b. Tonic neck reflex—flexion of the right arm and leg and extension of the left arm and leg when the head is turned toward the left
   4. Almost complete head lag

3. **Newborn's adjustments**
A. Assessment of immediate adjustment (Apgar)
   1. Measured at 60 seconds of life: heart rate, respiratory effort, muscle tone, reflex irritability, color
   2. Maximum score of 2 for each of above: 2 for heart rate over 100, 1 for less than 100; 2 for well-flexed, 1 for some flexion; 2 for cry as response to stimulation, 1 for only motion as a response; 2 if body is completely pink, 1 if body pink and extremities blue; score of 0 for absence of these behaviors
   3. Score of 8 to 10 shows a good adaptation; score of 5 to 7 is only fair; and infant with a score of 4 or less is depressed

B. Transition period (Desmond has identified these periods, and transition nurseries are now in existence because of her)
   1. Six steps
      a. Stimulation from the contracting uterus
      b. New stimuli at birth—light, temperature, sound
      c. Initiation of air breathing
      d. Changes in function of organ systems—e.g., the lungs

e. Reorganization of metabolic processes

f. Achievement of level of steady state—i.e., normal pH

2. First period of reactivity
   a. Outburst of diffuse and purposeless movements occurs
   b. Respiratory rate may reach 80
   c. Heart rate may be as high as 180 and then fall to 120 to 140 during period of intense purposeless movement activities
   d. Infant becomes quiet and may have a sleep period up to 2 hours

3. Second period of reactivity
   a. Awakening, the infant becomes hyperresponsive to stimuli
   b. Heart rate increases
   c. Excessive oral mucus appears

4. Period of stabilization
   a. Begins after completion of the second reactivity period
   b. Actual time span of first and second periods may be 12 hours

4. **First 3 months of life**
A. Gains 5 to 7 ounces per week
B. Grows an inch in length per month
C. Learns to raise head to 90° angle in prone position
D. At about 3 months Moro and tonic neck reflexes are less pronounced
E. Usually smiles at 2 months and laughs at 3 months
F. Learns to follow objects with eyes
G. Is taking orange juice, has added cereals, and is beginning to add fruits and vegetables to diet
H. May have fussy periods
I. Gradually has longer periods of being awake
J. Discussion and teaching of parents
   1. Space is required for crib
   2. Infant may reject a rigid schedule of feeding
   3. Parent should talk to infant, who will soon learn to regard face of mother; infant likes this
   4. Infant gradually learns to enjoy play period with mother and/or father
   5. Infant requires protection from
      a. Other young children
      b. Persons with infections
      c. High places, from which he may roll and fall (table, bed)
      d. Continuous, strong sunlight
   6. Needs for attendance at clinic or seeing pediatrician for beginning of immunizations and/or health supervision
   7. Gradual orderly growth and development of the infant

5. **3 to 6 months of age**
A. Grows about an inch in height per month, and by 6 months has doubled birth weight
B. Around the fifth or sixth month, rolls from abdomen to back or vice versa
C. Central lower incisors begin erupting at around 6 months
D. Sits well with assistance and learns to sit alone momentarily
E. Reaches for objects and likes favorite toy
F. Vocalizes socially and does some cooing and babbling
G. Begins to recognize strangers as different persons
H. Diet is being increased to include egg yolk and some meats
I. May transfer toy from one hand to the other at 6 months

6. **6 months to 1 year**
A. Grows about ½ inch in stature each month and gains about 3 to 5 ounces per week
B. At 9 months has good hand-to-mouth coordination and then learns good pincer grasp
C. Around 9 months creeps; then learns to pull self up and stand and walk with support at 1 year
D. Has learned to like pat-a-cake and peek-aboo
E. May try to help with his dressing
F. Still takes long naps
G. May have one or two words at a year
H. Meals include all basic foods; child enjoys table foods

7. **1 year to 18 months**
A. Gains only ½ pound per month and gets about 2½ inches taller in this time period
B. Walks unassisted and learns to climb
C. Increases his independence and may learn to use a few more words
D. Is aware of other persons and some of his own feelings
E. May begin toilet training
F. Enjoys foods from the family table
G. Number of teeth increases to 16 by the end of this period

8. **Nurse and the newborn infant**
A. Changes that occur at birth
   1. Respiration—placental exchange of oxygen and carbon dioxide cut off at birth; infant must breathe to survive

a. Immediate recognition of need for resuscitation (Apgar assessment)
b. Abandonment of drastic measures of resuscitation
c. Adoption of conservative methods of resuscitation
d. Pulmonary inflation a gradual process during neonatal period
e. Some causes of failure of newborn to breathe spontaneously
  (1) Aspiration of fluid or mucus
  (2) Premature separation of placenta
  (3) Umbilical cord wrapped around neck
  (4) Anomalies
  (5) Drugs and anesthetics administered to mother during labor and delivery
  (6) Trauma of labor
  (7) Prematurity
  (8) General weakness or debility
  (9) Disease in mother
  (10) Hyaline membrane disease
  (11) Central nervous system damage
  (12) Glottic edema
  (13) Atelectasis
  (14) Anoxia
f. Responsibilities of nurse
  (1) Accurate observation and reporting
  (2) Thorough understanding of physician's orders
  (3) Always having lifesaving equipment in readiness
  (4) Certainty of her responsibilities and exactitude in carrying out orders

2. Circulation
a. Changes in circulation of newborn more gradual than was once supposed
b. Obliteration of fetal circulatory system
  (1) More oxygen in postnatal than in fetal circulation
  (2) High hemoglobin and red blood count aid in compensating for smaller amount of oxygen in fetal blood

B. Immediate care of newborn
1. Mouth and throat—clear of secretions
2. Resuscitation if necessary
3. Provision for warmth
4. Eyes
a. Instill drug into eyes as prophylactic against ophthalmia neonatorum
b. Use care in administration of eye drops
  (1) Lids should be gently separated without pressure on eyeball
  (2) Drops should not fall from height
  (3) Drops should not fall directly onto cornea
  (4) Drops should enter eye and spread over entire surface
c. Report any sign of discharge from eyes so that smears may be obtained before secretions washed away

5. Identification of newborn
a. Immediate and accurate—methods
  (1) Necklace or bracelet of lettered beads
  (2) Identical identification tags for mother and infant
  (3) Permanent record made by taking prints of palm and foot of infant, and index finger of mother

6. Reporting of birth
a. Time of birth
b. Sex of infant
c. Surname and given names of parents

7. Care of skin
a. Customs regarding first bath
b. Variation in present practices

C. Appraisal of newborn—clinically first 2 weeks
1. Appearance and characteristics
a. Initially, purplish red
b. After vernix has worn off, skin firm, pink, elastic
c. Poor nutrition of pregnant woman may result in flabby tissues and inelastic skin in newborn
d. Varying amounts of lanugo present
e. Nails extend at least to tips of fingers and toes
f. Amount of hair varies
g. Small hips, narrow chest, and protruding abdomen
h. Head large in proportion to rest of body (25% of total length in infancy, 11% in adulthood)
i. Relatively short legs and long arms
j. Abnormalities may not be notice-

able at birth but may be detected on reexamination

k. Tongue may be furred; coating disappears as food and fluid taken

l. Initial weight loss due to low intake and to loss through urine, stool, skin, and respiration

2. Response of newborn
   a. Lies in position of flexion, fingers clenched, legs flexed, soles of feet often together
   b. Complexity and variety of responses indicate he is not inert mass; can sneeze, cough, yawn, grasp, suck, swallow, and respond to sound and dermal stimuli
   c. Infant may roll over; this may be accidental rather than result of a definite effort to move
   d. Moro reflex
   e. Flexion response to sudden stimulation
   f. Absence of Moro reflex or startle pattern may indicate presence of intracranial lesion

3. Weight and length of newborn
   a. Comparison with tables of averages may give erroneous impression for judging normality of size for particular infant
   b. Variations influenced by
      (1) Race
      (2) Size and age of parents
      (3) Number of pregnancies
      (4) Interval since last pregnancy
      (5) Health of mother
      (6) Sex of infant
      (7) Socioeconomic status of family
   c. Criteria of intrauterine age
      (1) Length of period of gestation
      (2) Length of infant
      (3) Weight

4. Stools of newborn
   a. First stool called meconium
   b. Notation of time and description of all stools important (type more important than number); absence of stools in newborn may indicate
      (1) Obstruction due to hardened meconium
      (2) Rectal or intestinal anomalies
   c. Change in character of normal stools—may be result of food
   d. Stools usually soft in breast-fed baby; may be somewhat drier in artificially fed infant

5. Urinary output
   a. Output may be small in first few days
   b. First voiding always to be noted and reported
   c. Variations in time and amount great
   d. By tenth day, infant will void about 10 times a day with total 24-hour output varying from 100 to 300 ml.; urinary output may approximate 2/3 of fluid intake

6. Conditions of blood
   a. Bleeding, external or internal
      (1) Greater tendency to bleeding in prematures; due to immaturity of vascular walls, delayed clotting time in first few days of life
      (2) Value of vitamin K variable
      (3) Cerebral hemorrhage
   b. Jaundice
      (1) Due to retention of excess bilirubin released through destruction of red blood cells after birth
      (2) Often appears second or third day of life; normally disappears spontaneously in about 2 weeks

D. Birth injuries
   1. Shock (not specific injury but occurrence in varying degrees in newborn may be serious)
      a. Avoid chilling and excessive handling
      b. Treat each newborn as one with marginal case of shock
      c. Shock said to be more common in infants with grossly abnormal blood chemistry at birth
      d. Shock one factor affecting amount of weight loss in newborns
   2. Caput succedaneum—swelling of scalp due to pressure during delivery
   3. Cephalhematoma
      a. Result of subperiosteal hemorrhage during delivery causing tumorlike mass over some part of head (usually over parietal bones)
      b. Blood in tumor slowly absorbs; no treatment necessary unless mass becomes infected
      c. Head should be carefully handled and infant's position changed frequently

d. Parental fears should be allayed through discussion with physician and nurse

e. Hematomas may occur in muscle tissue due to pressure during delivery

4. Fractures

a. Clavicle fracture one of most common; may be detected by absence of Moro reflex

b. Fracture of ribs, arm, leg, or skull less common, but may occur

5. Paralysis (face or upper arm most commonly involved)

a. Result of injury to nerve supplying part

(1) Abnormal intrauterine position

(2) Pressure during birth process

E. Infection

1. Skin infections

a. Furunculosis

b. Impetigo

2. Respiratory tract infections

a. Newborn very susceptible

b. Atelectasis and aspiration of food and fluid may predispose to development of infection or a viral infectious disease

3. Septicemia

4. Infectious diarrhea

a. Characteristics

(1) Speed of attack and prostration

(2) Watery stools with resulting dehydration

b. Treatment

(1) Restoration of fluid balance in body by use of parenteral fluids

(2) Gradual reestablishment of oral fluids and foods

c. Prevention

(1) Safe preparation and storage of formulas

(2) Immediate separation of infected infants from well newborns with separate staff for each nursery

(3) Elimination of overcrowding in nursery

(4) Provision of sufficient small nurseries rather than one large one

(5) Suitable health inspection of any ill staff member before return to work in nursery

(6) Periodic inspection of sewerage and water systems in hospital

(7) Safe disposal of waste, handling of linen and supplies

(8) Cooperation between administration, medical, and nursing staff

(9) Individual technique in care of newborn

F. Providing emotional satisfaction for child and for mother

1. Sense of touch well established at birth

a. Tactile stimulation about lips evokes suckling response

b. Satisfaction achieved by gratification of suckling and rooting reflex

2. Variability in rhythm of hunger contractions

a. From infant to infant

b. From day to day in same infant

c. Regularity of feeding may not satisfy child

d. Physiologic tension may be produced by hunger contractions

(1) Crying in response to need for gratification

(2) Studies indicate decrease in number and duration of crying spells in own home after discharge from hospital nursery

3. Infant and mother sharing same room in hospital

a. Provides early practice in infant care

b. Gives infant feeling of security; needs can be immediately met

4. Experimental programs have demonstrated that crying in nursery can be reduced greatly if personnel detect and remedy first signs of distress in each infant

5. Teaching parents

a. Begin early in pregnancy

b. Encourage parents to discuss problems and fears

c. Refrain from passing judgment on mother who does not wish to nurse her infant

d. Give assurance that attention to infant's needs is not "spoiling" him

e. Teach when parents indicate need to learn; do not force instruction; adapt plan to meet their requirements

f. Provide practice in handling and caring for newborn infant

g. Provide many opportunities and encourage discussion of minor details of care, and any other problems confronting parents

6. Learnings of the infant
   a. What his immediate world is like
   b. How people affect each other and how they affect him
   c. That there is world beyond himself which he must learn to trust
   d. How he can recognize differences between affection and rejection, indulgence and force
   e. That he can find self-expression through cooing, crying, gurgling, and other elementary speech
      (1) Infancy is often called "oral" period
         (a) Exploration through sucking and putting objects into mouth
         (b) Satisfaction of oral needs develops feelings toward outer world; infant needs love, "belonging," opportunity to explore and learn at his own rate

9. **Infant feeding**
A. Self-regulation schedule
   1. Studies indicate healthy infant is good judge of his intake needs
   2. Each infant born with different degree of maturity and rhythm of needs
   3. Feeding behavior key to understanding infant personality
   4. Denial of satisfaction may be cause of tension in mother and child
   5. Assurance of satisfaction has been found to cause less rather than more crying
   6. Periods of nursing vary greatly in number and length
   7. Good hygienic care of child necessary to successful operation of self-regulation schedule
B. Self-selection of food
   1. Studies show infants can select suitable intake to maintain good nutrition if offered proper foods
   2. Definite preferences for food change from time to time and unpredictable
   3. Maximum amount taken at given age exceeds that usually prescribed
C. Nutritional requirements

1. Nutrition as it affects growth
   a. Difference in opinion regarding desirability of giving oral feedings to prevent or lessen weight loss immediately after birth
   b. Initial weight loss normally regained by tenth day of life
   c. Birth weight usually doubled in fifth to sixth month, and tripled in year
      (1) Small babies may gain more rapidly
      (2) Normally, baby need not be weighed daily in home
   d. Healthy, well-nourished baby active and happy when awake, sleeps well, takes and digests food well
   e. Satisfactory or unsatisfactory progress judged by
      (1) Weight
      (2) Muscular development
      (3) Tissue tone and turgor
      (4) General appearance and activity
      (5) Presence or absence of symptoms of illness
      (6) Amount of crying
2. Proper feeding essential to good infant care
   a. Good general nutrition
   b. Prevention of nutritional deficiencies
   c. Prevention of gastrointestinal disturbances
   d. Establishment of good eating habits
3. Factors to consider in providing adequate diet
   a. Bacteriologic safety
   b. Easy digestibility
   c. Content and proper proportion of food elements—amounts adequate for optimal growth and development
      (1) Protein
      (2) Fats—caloric value higher than an equal amount of protein or carbohydrate
      (3) Carbohydrate
      (4) Vitamins and minerals
      (5) Fluid
D. Breast-feeding
   1. Preparation for breast-feeding
      a. Psychological readiness a factor in successful nursing
      b. Attitude during pregnancy toward breast-feeding

  c. Mother who does not breast-feed infant should not be made to feel guilty

  d. Adequate diet, prenatal and post-natal

  e. Sufficient rest for mother

  f. Suitable exercise

  g. Prevention of tension in mother and infant

 2. Advantages of breast-feeding

  a. Greater immunity to infection

  b. Lower death rate

  c. Aid to ensuring normal healthy babyhood

 3. Length of nursing period

  a. Self-demand studies recommend nursing baby as long as he desires

  b. Healthy baby said to consume ½ to ¾ of total feeding in first 5 minutes

  c. Some recommend that if baby is unable to obtain sufficient food in 20 minutes of nursing another method of feeding should be considered

 4. Nursing baby

  a. Mother and infant in comfortable position, usually with baby semi-erect

  b. During feeding, and at end of feeding, hold baby over shoulder to allow escape of air from stomach

   (1) Gently pat or rub the back

   (2) Avoid jarring

  c. Range of breast milk intake

   (1) From 1/7 to 1/6 of baby's weight per day

   (2) 2½ to 3 ounces of milk per pound of body weight per day

 5. Contraindications to breast-feeding

  a. In mother

   (1) Active tuberculosis

   (2) Acute contagious disease

   (3) Chronic disease, such as cancer, advanced nephritis, cardiac disease

   (4) Extensive surgery

   (5) Temporary cessation if mastitis develops

  b. In infant

   (1) Prematurity

   (2) Cleft lip or palate preventing grasp of nipple

E. Artificial feeding

 1. Factors influencing success of artificial feeding

  a. Pasteurization of milk

  b. Tuberculin testing of cows

  c. Sanitation in milk handling

  d. Adequate refrigeration

  e. Understanding of infant's nutritional needs

 2. Fresh milk

 3. Evaporated milk

  a. Removal of half of water content from whole milk

  b. Resterilization after canning

 4. Dried milks (whole or skimmed)

 5. Diluents

 6. Proprietary milks

 7. Calculation of formula

  a. Based on facts regarding requirements in calories, proteins, minerals, vitamins, and fluids

  b. Relatively more food required by infants to provide material for growth

  c. Number of calories needed influenced by age, weight, size, and activity of infant

  d. 1½ to 2 ounces of whole milk per day per pound expected body weight for given age; add carbohydrate up to 5% of amount milk used; dilute with water to amount child will take

  e. Standards for formula construction only estimates of baby's needs

  f. Infant should regulate artificial formula intake as he does in breast-feeding

  g. Little danger of overfeeding if formula properly constructed; each baby must be individually considered

  h. All formulas and feeding equipment should be free from harmful bacteria

  i. Formula should be readily digestible

F. Warm feedings

 1. Remove required formula bottles from refrigerator with clean hands

 2. Warm to body temperature in water bath; keep level of water in warmer below cap

 3. Wash and sterilize warmer at least daily; constant warm temperature in warmer conducive to bacterial growth

G. Giving feedings

 1. Have infant warm, clean, dry

2. See that hands and clothing of nurse are clean
3. Hold infant in semierect position unless specifically contraindicated; holding him provides body warmth and gives him feeling of security
4. Hold bottle so nipple always filled with milk
5. After feeding completed, and during feeding if necessary, hold infant over shoulder to allow for expulsion of air from stomach
6. Place infant on abdomen or on right side

H. Preparation of formula in home
  1. Directions should be simple and easy to follow
  2. Equipment should be simple and readily available in usual home
  3. Mother should observe demonstration of formula preparation and then practice under supervision until she feels secure in procedure

10. Summary of care of newborn
A. Establishment of respiration
B. Care of eyes
C. Adequate and accurate identification of infant
D. Maintenance of suitable environment with optimum temperature, humidity, and circulation of air free from dust
E. Maintenance of personal health of all personnel
F. Prevention of development of infection
G. Sterilization of feedings and feeding equipment; safe administration of feeding
H. Vigilant observation
I. In infants born by cesarean section, watch for symptoms of delayed shock
  1. Grunting
  2. Shallow respirations
  3. Accelerated weak pulse
  4. Air hunger
  5. Cyanosis
  6. Dyspnea
  7. Vomiting
  8. Convulsions

11. Premature infant
A. Contributing factors in prematurity
  1. In mother
    a. Accidents and injuries
    b. Emotional shock
    c. Multiple pregnancy
    d. Previous miscarriage
    e. Syphilis
    f. Toxemias
    g. Abdominal operations
    h. Disease of heart or kidneys
    i. Acute infections
    j. Premature separation of the placenta
    k. Placenta praevia
  2. In infant
    a. Faulty nutrition
    b. Syphilis
    c. Congenital malformations
B. Prevention of prematurity
  1. Improvement and extension of prenatal care
  2. Education of pregnant woman regarding prevention of factors contributing to premature labor
  3. Institution of antisyphilitic treatment, if necessary
  4. Assurance of suitable dietary regimen for mother
C. Appearance of premature infant
  1. Lack of subcutaneous fat, with skin hanging in folds
    a. Pinched appearance
    b. Ribs easily visible
    c. Greater loss of body heat
  2. Skin thin, delicate, and relatively transparent
    a. Underlying blood vessels readily visible
    b. Usually profuse lanugo
  3. Nails may not extend to ends of fingers and toes
D. Muscular activity
  1. Little activity
  2. Cries little, and then as whine rather than lusty cry
  3. Lacks muscular tonus
    a. Weak swallowing reflex
    b. May be unable to suck
E. Development of body systems
  1. Respiratory and circulatory systems
    a. Slow pulmonary inflation
    b. Often, diminished excitability of respiratory system
    c. Pulmonary circulation impeded by atelectasis
    d. Respiratory movements inhibited by weak musculature
  2. Osseous system
    a. Softer bones than in full-term infant
  3. Other systems
    a. All systems may function less satisfactorily than in full-term infant

b. Icterus neonatorum often more severe and persistent than in full-
term infant
c. Kidney function may be inadequate
F. Disease conditions of premature infant
1. Subject to all diseases of newborn
2. Unable to cope with them
3. Prone to develop deficiency diseases
G. Nursing care of premature infant
1. Compensate as effectively as possible
for shortened period of intrauterine
life
2. Adapt skills used in care of normal
newborn, for care of premature infant
3. Protect against hazards of extrauterine
life
a. Inability to maintain optimum body
temperature
(1) Lack of subcutaneous fat
(2) Greater body surface in relation to cubical contents of
body; thus more heat loss
(3) Temperature tends to fluctuate
with environment, due to muscular inactivity and to immaturity of heat-regulating center
(4) Overheating or chilling may
have harmful effects
b. Tendency toward asphyxiation
(1) Respiratory muscles weak and
system defective
(2) Areas of atelectasis
(3) Soft, pliable bony cage of chest
c. Predisposition to feeding problems
and to gastrointestinal upsets
(1) Incomplete development of
cardiac sphincter permits easy
regurgitation
(2) Weak suck and swallow reflex
(3) Absence or impairment of
cough or gag reflex may result in choking
(4) Absorption of food may be
hampered
d. Inability to combat infection; immunity not fully developed
e. Tendency to hemorrhage
f. Unstable pulse
g. Unstable respiration
(1) Rapid, shallow, irregular
(2) May show prolonged periods
of apnea
4. Establish rapport with parents; encourage their questions and expression of feelings

5. Understand community program for
premature care
a. Adequate preparation for hospital
discharge
(1) Ability to maintain satisfactory
body temperature in environment of 70° to 75° F.
(2) Evidence of steady weight
gain
(3) Favorable home environment
(4) Preparation of parents in home
care of infant
b. Home follow-up
c. Special preparation in nursing care
of prematures
d. Maternal and child welfare services
12. **Health problems and nursing in infancy
—congenital problems, acute illnesses,
long-term illnesses, and health supervision**
A. Prematurity—about 8% of infants are
classified as premature and the percent-
ages are higher in some cities
1. Infant requires intensive nursing care
—adequate warmth, special feedings,
prevention of infection, special handling
2. Respiratory difficulties are common
and are due to
a. Immaturity of lungs; capillary net-
work and alveolar cells are not at
a stage in development to permit
an adequate exchange of gases, and
atelectasis results
b. Aspirations causing atelectasis and
pneumonias
c. Hyaline membrane disease, insufficiency of surface tension material
on surface of lungs (surfactin) to
facilitate expansion of terminal air
sacs and prevent their closure
3. Increased amounts of oxygen
a. Concentrations over 40% may
cause retrolental fibroplasia, retinal
neovascularization, retinal detachment, and resultant blindness
b. When positive pressure is used to
administer oxygen, a minimal pressure should be used to prevent
damage to the alveoli of the lungs
4. Body temperature maintenance
a. Small infants require incubator to
maintain body temperature of
36.2° to 37° C.
b. Desired humidity for body comfort

and temperature control is usually
60%
5. Nutritional needs
   a. Require nasogastric or gavage when
      suck and swallow reflexes are weak
   b. Require low-fat diet because of
      milk-fat absorption problems
   c. Require frequent small feedings
6. Additional problems of premature infants
   a. The lower the birth weight, the
      higher the incidence of mental re-
      tardation
   b. Incidence of neurologic handicaps
      is high
   c. Morbidity and mortality rates are
      high for the first year of life
B. Other high-risk infants who present problems similar to those of prematurity
   1. Infant of diabetic mother
   2. Infant with rubella syndrome
   3. Infant with chromosomal aberration
   4. Very small full-term infant
   5. Postmature infant
C. Health team essential for care of premature infant
   1. Pediatricians (particularly, neonatol-
      ogist and physicians in clinics)
   2. Nurses—in nursery, in postpartal unit
      or clinic, and public health (home
      evaluation and care)
   3. Social workers
D. Infant's parents
   1. Require teaching in care of infant be-
      fore discharge from hospital
   2. Frequently require financial assistance
E. Tax-supported programs
   1. Aimed at prevention of prematurity
   2. Directed toward preparation of pro-
      fessional and other persons in the care
      of the infant, through special educa-
      tional programs
   3. May provide for a total care program
      for the infant

Congenital problems

1. **Chromosomal abnormalities**
A. Autosomal (23 pairs, or 46 chromosomes)
   1. Down's syndrome, with trisome or
      triplicate rather than normal pair of
      chromosome 21, is known as mongol-
      ism; person may have other anoma-
      lies—such as cardiac defects, hernia,
      or duodenal atresia—and will be men-
      tally retarded
   2. Trisome 18 infant is small at birth,

fails to thrive, usually has cardiac defects, and dies within the first year of
life
   3. Aberrations may be due to differing
      lengths of chromosomes, or there may
      be a partial deletion of a portion of
      a chromosome
B. Sex chromosome (1 pair, or 2 chromosomes)—combinations other than XX or
   XY result in abnormalities of endocrine
   and metabolic functioning (Turner's syndrome, Klinefelter's syndrome, etc.)
2. **Inborn errors of metabolism and other
   genetic and familial problems**
A. PKU or phenylketonuria—a lack of the
   enzyme phenylalanine hydroxylase, which
   changes phenylalanine into tyrosine; can
   be detected early in life and many state
   laws require that newborns be tested for
   this condition; treatment is a low-phenyl-
   alanine diet; failure to treat infant or
   child results in mental retardation; tests
   for PKU known as Guthrie test and the
   ferric chloride test
B. Other inborn errors include galactosemia,
   which is usually first detected as a feeding problem in infancy; dietary measures
   are the treatment used; mental retardation may result if treatment is not instituted
C. Other inherited genetic problems include
   hemophilia (from mother to son), sickle
   cell anemia, and thalassemia; each of
   these presents a major health and nursing problem; treatment consists of transfusions and prevention of injuries
D. Rh factor and other incompatibilities
   such as the ABO; maternal antibodies
   enter fetal circulation, cause erythrocyte
   destruction, resulting in hemolytic disease in infant; treatment of infant consists of transfusions; hyperbilirubinemia
   may be a cause of kernicterus and child
   may later have neurologic damage and
   mental retardation; a new therapy (as
   of June, 1968) is to give RhoGAM, gamma globulin containing antiRh antibody,
   to the mother almost immediately after
   delivery and thus prevent erythroblasto-
   sis in future infants
E. Congenital malformations (structural
   anomalies present at birth) frequently
   require both intensive and long-term
   nursing and medical care
   1. Cleft lip and/or cleft palate—failure
      of fusion of maxillary and premaxil-

lary processes (defect usually occurs about fifth week of intrauterine life)

2. Congenital laryngeal stridor—a crowing sound noted on inspiration; is usually caused by flabbiness of the epiglottis; treatment may be unnecessary in mild cases, but severe ones may require tracheotomy and laryngoplasty

3. Choanal atresia—an obstruction of the posterior nares; the infant breathes through his mouth and may become cyanotic at feedings; surgery may be indicated

4. Atresia of the esophagus—the esophagus is closed at some point; also there may be a fistula; surgery is imperative; at birth, infant has excessive mucus that is readily detected by the nurse

5. Diaphragmatic hernia—a protrusion of the abdominal viscera through an opening into the thoracic cavity; the infant has a small abdomen, severe respiratory difficulty, and a large chest in which the affected side does not expand with respirations; immediate surgery is essential to the life of this infant

6. Intestinal obstruction—usually characterized by abdominal distention, vomiting of bile, and absence of stools; symptoms are frequently first noted by the nurse; surgery is imperative

7. Imperforate anus—noted when nurse is unable to insert rectal thermometer; there is no meconium stain or infant does not pass meconium; surgery is indicated, depending upon the type and degree of the anomaly

8. Hypospadias—the urethra opens on the lower surface of the penis or into the vagina; plastic surgery is required

9. Exstrophy of the bladder—the entire lower urinary tract is exposed; kidneys may be damaged because of urine back pressure; long-term treatment with surgery is essential; possible infections present a problem

10. Amelia—absence of one or more limbs

11. Clubfoot
   a. Talipes equinovarus—most common type of clubfoot; foot turns inward and downward; cannot be held in normal position

b. Purpose of treatment—correction of condition, with maintenance of correction until normal muscle balance attained

c. Treatment used in infancy
   (1) Gentle repeated manipulations, or forcible manipulation under anesthesia, followed by cast; either with frequent changes of cast or with cast wedgings for gradual correction
      (a) Watch for signs of circulatory impairment; make sure it is possible to see all toes beneath cast
      (b) Observe cast for signs of weakness and wear; cast on which child has been allowed to stand or walk, or cast that has been repeatedly dampened, may lose all power of support; protect top of cast with waterproof material
   (2) Denis Browne splint
      (a) Success of apparatus depends on alternate kicking and extension of baby's legs; encourage activity
      (b) Watch for circulatory impairment due to swelling around tape; watch skin around tape for signs of irritation
      (c) Clean child's skin very gently when tape is removed; avoid harsh cleansers such as benzine
      (d) Pick child up frequently; respiratory infections common with this type of treatment

d. Treatment of older child
   (1) Surgery usually necessary: wedge resection, plantar fascia stripping, posterior capsulotomy of ankle joint, etc.
   (2) Usually immobilized in long leg cast; keep leg elevated on rubber-covered pillows, groin to heel; canvas hammock attached to overhead bar may be used to elevate leg
   (3) Watch for hemorrhage; may

be noticed at thigh level because blood runs back along thigh under cast; mark bleeding area on cast with pencil and check frequently

(4) Observe for circulatory impairment

e. Follow-up care of patient with clubfoot

(1) Great tendency to recurrence; patient should be under care of physician for long time after correction; child cannot be considered cured until he is able to wear normal shoe and walk normally

(2) Follow-up treatment emphasizes muscle reeducation and walking

(3) Braces or shoes prescribed after clubfoot treatment must be kept in repair; shoes must not be allowed to become worn and run-down, either at heel or at sole; night splints may be ordered

(4) Corrective clubfoot shoes may have sole and heel lifts on lateral border

12. Congenital dislocation of hip (three different clinical and roentgenologic syndromes)

a. First group—hip unstable, slight tightening of adductors, Ortolani sign positive, shallow acetabular roof, upper end of femur and femoral head normal, hip dislocated but easily reduced in infant

(1) Treatment—pillow splint (Frejka splint) or abduction brace

(a) Keeps thigh in flexion and abduction

(b) Worn continuously for several months; then worn at night as prescribed

(c) Apparatus worn until roentgenograms show a normally developed hip joint

(2) Instruction of mother very necessary part of care

(a) Hold pillow in place by romperlike garment

(b) Protect with plastic pants

(c) Position with each diaper change

b. Second group—tight adductors, asymmetry of thigh folds, Ortolani sign negative; roentgenograms show hip not dislocated, but acetabular roof slanting; these hips may develop normally, or subluxation may occur

(1) Treatment—pillow splint, worn till sloping acetabulum corrected

c. Third group—hip dislocated at birth, adductors tight, femoral head lodged in a secondary acetabulum, Ortolani sign negative, thigh on involved side appears shorter, anteversion of femoral neck may be present

(1) Treatment—closed or open reduction

(a) Open reduction necessary with older child

(b) In closed reduction that is difficult—to avoid trauma to femoral head —traction is applied for several weeks to stretch thigh muscles and to pull head of femur down; also Putti splint, or other type of abduction splint, may be used before reduction to stretch soft structures

(2) Reduction maintained with hip spica plaster cast

(a) Position of 90° to 100° of hip flexion and 70° of abduction

(b) Plaster cast extended to knee, if hip stable; if unstable, cast extended below knee

(c) Plaster cast—well molded posteriorly over greater trochanter to prevent redislocation

(d) Subcutaneous tenotomy of adductor tendon prevents excessive pressure on femoral head

(e) Protect cast about perineum with small strips of waterproof material; secure outer edge with plaster or tape; tuck inner edge of Pliofilm under cast edge; use diaper as perineal pad; change frequently

(f) Instruct parents in all phases of cast care; written instructions desirable

(g) Child wears cast several months as prescribed by physician; cast cut above knee to permit crawling

(h) Abduction brace may be applied when cast is removed; keeps legs in same position as cast; worn continuously for 2 or 3 months; parents instructed about care of child and wearing of brace; later, brace may be removed several hours daily as prescribed by physician

(i) If roentgenograms satisfactory, use of brace gradually decreased; brace continued at nighttime for several years; acetabulum then well developed

d. Clinical signs of congenital dislocated hip

(1) In infant, hips seem unusually movable in all directions except abduction, which is limited

(2) A palpable or audible click when hip being abducted—Ortolani sign

(3) Perineum may seem somewhat wider than normal

(4) Extra folds may be apparent in buttock or thigh; unequal leg lengths

(5) In older child, walking with waddling gait (bilateral dislocation) or marked limp (unilateral dislocation) common; increased lumbar curve, protruding abdomen, and broadened buttocks may be noticed

e. Treatment of older child

(1) Skeletal traction may be used to bring head down as near acetabulum as possible; usually pin or wire inserted through condyles of femur

(2) Shelving operation, arthroplasty, bifurcation operation, or subtrochanteric osteotomy may be done, followed by hip spica cast or traction

Surgical problems and accidents of infancy

1. **Acute—most surgery necessary because of congenital abnormalities**

A. Anomalies interfere with normal development of organ systems

B. Small size of infant presents problems
   1. Body warmth and temperature control
   2. Maintenance of fluids; infant has a high percentage of extracellular fluid that can be quickly excreted
   3. Susceptibility to respiratory diseases and other infections
   4. Toxic reactions to many drugs because of immaturity of organs

C. Goals in nursing care
   1. Minimal interruption in voluntary and involuntary physical motion
   2. An uninterrupted relationship of adult and infant or child
   3. Minimal restraints in an effort to keep suture lines clean, dry, and free from damage by the infant

D. Surgical procedures include cleft lip repair, later the palate repair, release of tight bands in pyloric stenosis, hernia repairs, and other minor repairs essential in the infancy period

2. **Problems requiring long-term care and, frequently, long hospitalization**

   Mostly these are associated with major handicaps due to congenital anomalies

A. Infants with problems of acute care also have problems in long-term care

B. Special consideration is given to provision for continued physical and personal relationships that enhance total development

C. The problems are an acute burden on the family and may become a chronic burden

D. Many health agencies may assume some responsibility for the care of the infant and child

E. Mental retardation is frequently associated with handicaps of a neurologic nature

3. **Accidents in infancy and toddler periods**
Accidents have a high incidence, and mortality rates due to this cause are also high
A. Design of all health facilities and equipment must be geared to accident prevention
B. Preventive aspects are essential in teaching and working with parents
4. **Many problems in caring for the infant and small child are related to other factors**
A. Renal functioning—the newborn and premature do not concentrate their urine
B. Interstitial tissues contain a large amount of fluid—water, and this small being is prone to edema
C. Electrolyte balance is a problem because of the above two factors
D. Blood vessels are still developing structurally; therefore there is an increased probability of cell fragility with hemorrhage
E. Newborn is still developing some essential enzymes, such as glucuronyl transferase, which is essential for the conjugation of bilirubin; hence increased jaundice and concomitant neurologic problems may result
F. Primary defense mechanisms, antibodies, are just being developed; and the loss of antibodies from fetal life increases the infant's susceptibility to diseases and infections of different kinds
   1. Antibody is low at 6 weeks to 2 months; then infant begins to develop his own
   2. At the age of 1 year this problem recedes
5. **Nursing care of tracheotomized child**
A. Symptoms indicating need for tracheotomy
B. Special factors in postoperative care
   1. Good general nursing care
   2. Increased humidity of inspired air
   3. Use of suction machine
   4. Anticipate needs; child has no voice
   5. Clean and change tube
   6. Drugs contraindicated
   7. Precautions
      a. Maintenance of patent airway
      b. Accurate observation and reporting
      c. Ensuring plenty of rest
   8. Allaying fears—explanation of procedures to parent and to child if old enough

C. Teaching child to eat, drink, talk without choking
D. Complications
E. Decannulation
F. Rehabilitation

Health supervision

1. **Nurse's role**
A. Working closely with the physician and reporting to him on observations relating to all aspects of growth and development—physical, social, personal, and intellectual
B. Teaching parents about nutrition and other needs of the infant and small child
C. Participating and developing immunization programs
D. Teaching parents some health care, the preventive aspects of illness, and means of staying well
2. **Immunization schedule (approved by Committee on Infectious Diseases, American Academy of Pediatrics, October, 1971)**

2 months	DTP	TOPV
4 months	DTP	TOPV
6 months	DTP	TOPV
1 year	Measles	Tuberculin test
1 to 12 years	Rubella	Mumps
1½ years	DTP	TOPV
4 to 6 years	DTP	TOPV
14 to 16 years	Td	And thereafter every 10 years

(DTP = diphtheria and tetanus toxoids combined with pertussis vaccine
TOPV = trivalent oral poliovirus vaccine
Td = combined tetanus and diphtheria toxoids)
Routine smallpox vaccination no longer recommended

Maternal nutrition, the infant and child

1. **Some requirements and results in nutrition**
A. Placenta has great ability to concentrate nutrients for the fetus
B. Anemia in mother may result in low iron storage in infant with resultant anemia in infancy
C. Undernourished mother may produce breast milk of thiamin deficiency, resulting in
   1. Fulminant heart failure
   2. Encephalopathy
D. Inadequate supplies of dietary requirements result in
   1. Slowing of growth
   2. Reduction of cellular multiplication
   3. Providing only maintenance needs

4. Severely lessened activity
5. Tissues consumed to preserve life
E. Average daily total requirement for first year of life is 100 cal. per kilogram body weight
F. Protein, in the form of amino acids, is required for both growth and repair (yields 4 cal. per gram)
   1. Over 50% of amino acids required for absorption are endogenous in origin (e.g., pancreatic enzymes)
   2. Some amino acids play a vital role outside of protein synthesis; e.g., tyrosine is the precursor of thyroxine, epinephrine
   3. Amount required by the body depends on the rate of growth—the infant having the highest requirement, at least 2.5 gm. per kilogram weight per day, and by 1 year requiring at least 1 gm. per kilogram of weight
   4. Milk is the essential source of protein for the infant
   5. Infections, particularly viral, inhibit protein synthesis
G. Carbohydrate (yields 4 cal. per gram)
   1. Provides most of the energy in human diets
   2. Provides 50% of calories in human breast milk
   3. May provide 90% of calories in lower socioeconomic group
   4. Consumed mostly in the form of
      a. Starches—the polysaccharides, absorbed in the stomach and small bowel
      b. Lactose and sucrose—the disaccharides, intestinal mucosa
      c. Glucose—the monosaccharides, mucosal cells
H. Fat (yields 9 cal. per gram)
   1. Provides essential fatty acids
   2. Carrier of fat-soluble vitamins
   3. High-caloric density (9 cal. per gram)
   4. Lends palatability to food
   5. 95% of dietary fat is absorbed
   6. Lipids are stored in the liver
   7. For periods of rapid growth, 30% to 40% of calories should be fat
   8. Premature infant is unable to absorb animal fat
I. Minerals
   1. Calcium
      a. Breast milk provides 30 mg. per 100 ml.; cow's milk provides four times as much calcium
      b. 99% of calcium in body is present in the bony skeleton
      c. Levels in body fluids kept constant by parathyroid and thyroid hormonal control
   2. Phosphorus
      a. 80% is located in bone
      b. Remainder is in essential nucleic acids
      c. Is essential for metabolism
   3. Iron
      a. Iron deficiency is the most common disorder in man and particularly the child
      b. Only around 10% of food iron is absorbed
      c. Copper is essential for the absorption of iron
   4. Fluorine (in drinking water)
      a. Lowers incidence of dental caries
      b. Reduces incidence of osteoporosis (in the adult)
J. Vitamins, essential biochemical catalysts
   1. Fat-soluble A (1,500 IU for infants to 5,000 IU for adults)
      a. Essential for growth (may be stored in body)
      b. Poor absorption of this vitamin in celiac disease, cystic fibrosis, congenital biliary atresia
      c. Average balanced diet contains sufficient amounts of this vitamin
      d. Hypervitaminosis—anorexia, fretfulness, headaches, and prolonged condition of tenderness over long bones
   2. Fat-soluble D (400 IU per day; may be stored in body)
      a. Adequate amounts in fortified milk
      b. Exposure to sunlight essential
      c. Deficiency disease symptoms—restlessness, irritability, constipation
      d. Overt deficiency disease
   3. Fat-soluble vitamins E and K
      a. Found in foods
      b. Vitamin K, fat-soluble form, prevents hemorrhage in newborn
   4. Vitamins B, water-soluble (not stored in the body)
      a. 11 vitamins comprise the B complex
      b. Concerned with metabolism of carbohydrates and the release of energy
      c. Thiamin, riboflavin, and niacin deficiencies produce health problems

d. Thiamin—cerals high in this vitamin

TODDLER PERIOD OF LIFE

1. Development is characterized by
A. Completion of some skills, such as walking
B. Greater skill in performance of motor activities
C. Acquiring a sense of autonomy
D. Acquiring and using language skills
E. Using play to express himself
F. Strong maternal relationship
G. Use of self play rather than group play
H. Accepting some responsibilities for self, such as feeding
I. Proneness to accidents, due to cognitive immaturity
2. Acute conditions
A. High incidence of nasopharyngeal and respiratory infections
B. Accidents such as ingestion of poisons
C. Gastrointestinal problems such as parasites
3. Chronic conditions or long-term care needs
A. Burns and some poisonings that require long-term care
B. Long-term problems of infancy such as celiac disease, cerebral palsy
C. Sensory problems such as deafness or blindness

PRESCHOOL CHILD

1. Development is characterized by
A. Refinement of some motor skills
B. Imitating behavior of adults and others
C. Imagination and creativity
D. Liking to perform many tasks for mother
E. Learning self-care, such as dressing, toileting
F. Playing with one or two other children
G. Enjoying organized group activities for his age group
H. Little girl's possibly becoming possessive of her father, and a little boy possessive of his mother
I. Having a high incidence of accidents
2. Acute or short-term care
A. Communicable diseases (many can be prevented by immunizations)
B. Acute glomerulonephritis (highest incidence is in this age group)
C. Respiratory illnesses and nasopharynx diseases
D. Accidents, such as fractures

3. Long-term care and chronic conditions
A. Cardiac surgery for congenital problems such as tetralogy of Fallot
B. Leukemia
C. Emotional problems
D. Allergies and asthma

SCHOOL-AGE CHILD

1. Development is characterized by
A. Play away from home
B. Cooperating with others
C. Acquires great amount of knowledge and skills
D. Is very industrious
E. Imitates the parent of his sex
F. Period of refinement of many skills
2. Acute conditions
A. Those acquired at school, pediculosis or scabies
B. Appendicitis, osteomyelitis, and other acute conditions that require surgery or drug therapy
3. Long-term care
A. Rheumatic fever (incidence appears to be decreasing)
B. Diabetes mellitus
C. Emotional problems

PUBERTY AND THE ADOLESCENT

1. Development is characterized by
A. Growth spurt
B. Personality growth
C. Development of secondary sex characteristics
D. Emphasis on sense of identity
E. Importance of friends
F. Interest in the opposite sex, and beginning of intimate relationships
G. Consideration of adult vocation
H. Preparation for adult vocation
2. Health problems
A. Acne
B. Diabetes
C. Tuberculosis
D. Poor nutrition
E. Emotional problems, incidence of suicides is high
F. Chronic inherited and acquired health problems of childhood

UNDERSTANDING AND TREATING THE CHILD AS AN INDIVIDUAL

1. Means used and the child's reactions
A. Observation
B. Listening
C. Establishing child's confidence

D. Giving of self
E. Anticipating child's needs and behaviors
F. Consideration of the child
   1. Accept child as he is
   2. Deleterious effects of fear, threats, punishment, separation, trauma
   3. Tensions to be overcome
   4. Explain procedures and allow child to handle equipment whenever feasible
   5. Avoid taking child by surprise
      a. Frightening sensation of sudden awakening, glare of lights, voices, appearance of a strange face
      b. Encourage expression of fears
   6. Relief of discomfort and anticipation of needs appreciated by child
   7. Importance of consistency in handling child
   8. Harmonious relationships among personnel—essential
G. Emotional response to illness
   1. Unpredictable
   2. Possible sequelae
      a. Mental disturbances
      b. Fears
      c. Night terrors
      d. Aggressive behavior
      e. Regressive behavior
   3. Hospital experience may be first separation from home
H. Discipline
   1. As a destructive force
      a. Threats and withdrawal of love
      b. Isolation
      c. Goals too high
      d. Failure to use praise and reward
      e. Unjust punishment
   2. As a cooperative venture
I. Effect of child care practices
   1. Effect of deprivation
   2. Role of "mothering"
   3. Influence of relationships between parents
   4. Reaction to stress in environment influenced by child's degree of emotional maturity
   5. Influence of nurse
      a. To help child overcome fears and worries
      b. To be aware of disturbing elements in daily life
      c. To relieve tensions
   6. Providing opportunity for happy, spontaneous relationships with other children
   7. Developing climate conducive to recovery of ill child and to maintenance of positive health
   8. Reducing child's feelings of insecurity
   9. Learning to read behavior cues
J. Food, the infant, the child
   1. Preparation for mealtime
      a. Happy pleasant association necessary
      b. Physical comfort and cleanliness
      c. Respect of child's needs for food, likes and dislikes
   2. Transition from breast or bottle to cup
      a. Gradual, without force
      b. Begin early
   3. Feeding schedule
      a. Infant can help to establish own rhythm
      b. Develop good habits of eating in infancy
      c. Occasional decreased intake not important
      d. Persistent poor eating requires investigation
   4. Introducing new foods
      a. Gradual, just taste at first
      b. Do not start new foods when
         (1) Child overly fatigued
         (2) Child not feeling well
         (3) Child fed in strange surroundings
      c. Beginning at 6 to 8 weeks, cereals; then other solids gradually added
      d. Chopped foods introduced when child has enough teeth to chew
   5. Feeding self
      a. When he demonstrates desire
      b. In comfortable environment with equipment suitable to age
   6. Nutrition of sick child
      a. Means of encouraging oral fluids
      b. Means of allaying thirst if fluids restricted
      c. Other than oral route for administration of fluids
         (1) Rectal
         (2) Subcutaneous
         (3) Intravenous, including continuous drip
      d. Meal hour for child in hospital
         (1) Means of tempting flagging appetite
            (a) Attractive dishes and servings
            (b) Proper preparation of child
            (c) Feeding helpless child

(d) Preparation of food so child can handle it

(2) Adapting special diet from general diet

(3) Care of child after meals

HOSPITAL CARE

1. Genuine interest in obtaining facts necessary in nursing care

A. Is more than one language spoken?
B. What language does child speak?
C. Does child have nickname that he likes?
D. How are toilet needs made known?
E. What are child's favorite toys? stories?
F. What are child's food likes or dislikes?
G. Is this first experience away from home?
H. Does child sleep in room by himself?
I. Has he any fears?
J. Does he play with other children?
K. Eating and sleeping habits
L. Other hospital experiences? illnesses?

2. Making child feel comfortable in hospital

A. Introduce to nearby children
B. Inform child how to make his wants known
C. Inform about daily ward activity
D. Supply place for personal belongings and equipment
E. Give name of nurse caring for him
F. Listen to child

3. Reactions to maternal separation

A. Protest
  1. Prolonged loud crying
  2. Continual asking to go home
  3. Rejection of nurse
  4. Excessive preoccupation with strangers
B. Despair
  1. Poor sleep
  2. Decreased appetite
  3. Diminished interest and reactivity (listlessness)
  4. Relative immobility
  5. Blandness of facial expression
  6. Failure to smile
  7. Quietness
  8. Withdrawal from environment
  9. Weight loss
  10. Unresponsiveness to stimuli
C. Detachment
  1. Excessive preoccupation with strangers
  2. Cheerful undiscriminating friendliness
  3. Lack of interest in parents when they visit

4. Mother as overnight guest

A. Make provision for her comfort
B. Familiarize with any regulations

5. Anticipation (and explanation whenever possible)

Unfamiliar and possibly frightening factors—sounds, equipment, etc.

A. Buzz of voices
B. Noise of elevator
C. Lights and shadows
D. Equipment
E. Different clothing
F. Height of bed, side rails
G. Method of serving food
H. Toilet equipment
I. Physical examination
J. Treatment and drugs

6. Recognition and relief of symptoms of apprehension, insecurity, anxiety

7. Factors in providing comfort

A. Position, good alignment
B. Provision for rest
  1. Suitable temperature, humidity, and ventilation
  2. Treatments and medications timed to minimize interference with rest
  3. Exclusion of external stimuli of light and noise
  4. Relief of pain and thirst
  5. Care of toilet needs
  6. Suitable covering and clothing
  7. Allaying fears
  8. Something familiar in his surroundings
C. Care of skin
D. Proper food
E. Recreation and play
F. Respect for privacy

8. Maintenance of comfort during procedure

A. Equipment suitable to situation
B. Explanation of procedure within child's range of comprehension
C. Comfortable position
D. Sufficient warmth
E. Inspection of person after treatment finished
F. Reassurance
G. Skill in performance

9. Operative care

A. Mental
  1. Elimination, as far as possible, of worry, apprehension, fear
  2. Truthful explanation in line with child's ability to understand
  3. Familiarity with possible emotional sequelae
B. Physical

1. According to individual orders and type of operation
2. Means of allaying thirst
3. Identification
4. Report any untoward symptoms

C. Postoperative
1. Preparation of bed, room, and equipment
2. Caution in lifting unconscious child
3. Vital functions may be depressed under anesthesia
4. Sensitivity to trauma, exposure, chilling
5. Anticipation of symptoms of shock
6. Expert nursing care to minimize surgical risks
7. Continued emotional support
8. Early ambulation
   a. Advantages
   b. Contraindications
   c. Precautions

DISEASES AND ANOMALIES AFFECTING BODY SYSTEMS

1. Health problems of childhood

A. Hearing problems
1. Congenital anomalies
2. Otitis media (acute or chronic)
   a. Symptoms
      (1) Infant frets and rubs his ear and is prone to infection because of short, wide, and horizontal eustachian tube
      (2) Older child complains of popping noises in the ear or may have dull throbbing ache or acute pain
   b. Streptococci and pneumococci most frequently found organisms
   c. Frequently occurs in child with diseased tonsils and adenoids
   d. Antibiotics are given, usually penicillin
   e. Ear canal must be kept clean with use of sterilized cotton pledgets
3. Mastoiditis
   a. Symptoms
      (1) Pain
      (2) Chills and fever
      (3) Swelling of mastoid area
   b. Treatment
      (1) Chemotherapy
      (2) Surgery
   c. Complications
      (1) Septicemia
      (2) Sinus thrombosis

4. Foreign body
5. Deafness
6. Conservation of hearing

B. Throat infections
1. Enlargement of tissues
2. Infections
   a. Pharyngitis
   b. Tonsillitis
   c. Peritonsillar abscess
   d. Retropharyngeal abscess (may follow acute upper respiratory infection)
      (1) Symptoms
         (a) High fever
         (b) Difficulty in swallowing
         (c) Refusal of feedings
         (d) Noisy respiration
         (e) Retraction of head
         (f) Prostration
      (2) Treatment and nursing care
         (a) Nursing care of acutely ill infant
         (b) Use of antibiotics
         (c) Incision and drainage of abscess
      (3) Complications
         (a) Septicemia
         (b) Erosion of blood vessels
   e. Laryngitis
      (1) Spasmodic (false croup), acute, self-limited inflammation of larynx
      (2) Acute

C. Pyopneumothorax and lung abscess
1. Cause
   a. Infection
   b. Foreign body
   c. Trauma
2. Treatment
   a. Aspiration
   b. Surgical drainage
   c. Chemotherapy
3. Complications
   a. Atelectasis
   b. Gangrene

D. Bronchitis
1. Symptoms may include
   a. High temperature
   b. Dry cough, hoarseness, dryness of throat, sore chest
   c. Thick, tenacious secretions; later may have loose cough and purulent sputum
   d. Obstruction of bronchi due to secretions
   e. Swollen membranes

    f. Noisy and embarrassed, rapid respiration

  2. Treatment may include

    a. Rest

    b. Increased humidity of inspired air

    c. Drugs to allay discomfort

    d. Bronchoscopy

    e. Tracheotomy

  3. Complications

    a. Chronic bronchitis

    b. Bronchiectasis

    c. Atelectasis

E. Acute laryngotracheobronchitis (acute infection of larynx, trachea, and bronchi)

  1. Cause

    a. Virus

    b. Bacteria

  2. Characteristics

    a. Onset abrupt and prostrating

    b. Edema of larynx

    c. High temperature

    d. Cough and hoarseness

    e. Thick, viscid exudate of tracheobronchial tree

    f. Change in respiration

    g. Toxemia

  3. Treatment and nursing care

    a. Warm, moist air

    b. Oxygen

    c. Rest (by well-planned nursing care)

    d. Liberal fluids

    e. Soft, nourishing diet

    f. Close observation

    g. Ensure patent airway

    h. Detect signs of cardiac failure

    i. Tracheotomy if necessary

    j. Avoid opiates (tendency to inhibit cough reflex and to dry secretions)

  4. Complications

    a. Pneumonia

    b. Asphyxia

    c. Bronchiectasis

    d. Cardiac failure

F. Pneumonia

  1. Causes

    a. Bacteria

    b. Virus

    c. Aspirated material or foreign body

    d. Chemicals

  2. Predisposing factors

    a. Lowered resistance, allowing invasion of virus or bacteria

    b. Excessive fatigue

  3. Symptoms (great variation, dependent somewhat upon cause, age of child, area of lung involved) may include

    a. Sudden high temperature in previously well child

    b. Vomiting, diarrhea, distention

    c. Toxemia and prostration

    d. Cough, dyspnea, cyanosis

    e. Restlessness

    f. Muscular and chest pains

    g. Chills

    h. Respiratory distress

      (1) Shallow respiration

      (2) Movement of ala nasi

    i. Signs of meningeal irritation

    j. Signs of cardiac or respiratory failure

  4. Treatment and nursing care

    a. Good physical and mental care (according to age and degree of illness)

    b. Adequate rest (nurse and doctor plan for care to avoid frequent disturbances)

    c. Adequate fluid intake (parenteral if necessary)

    d. Easily digestible, nourishing diet (constituents depend upon age)

    e. Provision for fresh, moist, comfortably warm air

    f. Oxygen, if needed

    g. Relief of persistent distention

    h. Early detection and reporting of symptoms of respiratory or cardiac failure

G. Diaphragmatic hernia

  1. Function of diaphragm

  2. Type of hernia

    a. Congenital

    b. Acquired (traumatic)

  3. Symptoms may include

    a. Cyanosis

    b. Dyspnea

    c. Rapid respiration

    d. Vomiting

    e. Evidence of intestinal obstruction if viscera are greatly displaced

H. Foreign bodies aspirated

  1. Cause (almost any object capable of being aspirated)

  2. Prevention

    a. Keep small dangerous objects out of child's reach

    b. Teach child not to run or laugh with food or drink in his mouth

    c. Avoid giving young children foods easily aspirated

d. Teach child to masticate food well before swallowing
3. Symptoms
  a. Respiratory and pulse rate increased
  b. Retraction, substernal
  c. Restlessness
  d. Cough
  e. Cyanosis (late symptom)
4. Treatment
  a. Location by
    (1) Fluoroscopy
    (2) X-ray
  b. Removal by
    (1) Oral bronchoscopy
    (2) Tracheotomy
I. Infections of mouth
  1. Thrush (moniliasis)
    a. Cause
      (1) Spore-bearing organisms, may occur in healthy newborn
      (2) Lack of cleanliness may predispose to development
      (3) Positive correlation between maternal vaginal and infantile oral moniliasis
    b. Prevention
      (1) Prevention of abrasions of oral mucous membrane
      (2) Maintenance of good physical condition
      (3) Cleanliness of feeding equipment
      (4) Identification and treatment of vaginal moniliasis during pregnancy
      (5) Isolation of infected persons
    c. Treatment
      (1) Individual care of feeding equipment
      (2) Gentle application of antiseptics
  2. Stomatitis (Vincent's infection, Vincent's angina, or trench mouth)
    a. Location
      (1) Gingival margins; may spread to tongue, cheeks, and pharynx
    b. Symptoms
      (1) Headache
      (2) Malaise
      (3) Symptoms of toxemia
      (4) Lesions in mouth
    c. Treatment (varies with severity of condition)
      (1) Therapeutic doses of vitamin B complex and nicotinic acid
      (2) Cleansing of mouth with hy-

drogen peroxide or solution of sodium perborate
      (3) Local application of mild antiseptics
    d. Complications
      (1) Gingivitis due to traumatic lesions or infectious agents; may occur in vitamin C and B complex deficiencies, heavy metal poisoning, leukemia, and in poorly controlled diabetes
J. Esophageal disorders
  1. Traumatic stricture due to caustic poisons
    a. Amount of scarring depends upon amount and strength of solution (lye, acids, various caustics)
    b. Stenosis may be sudden and severe or increase gradually
    c. Treatment
      (1) Administration of dilute antidote (lavage may be contraindicated)
      (2) Dilatation
      (3) Analgesics to relieve pain
      (4) Gastrostomy (if food cannot pass through stricture)
      (5) Parenteral feedings if necessary
    d. Special attention to psychological needs of child
  2. Congenital atresia
  3. Tracheoesophageal fistula
    a. Type
    b. Diagnosis
      (1) Immediate regurgitation of feedings
      (2) Inability to pass catheter more than few centimeters
      (3) X-ray findings
    c. Correction—surgical repair of fistula (gastrostomy may be necessary for feedings)
    d. Preoperative care
      (1) Prevention of aspiration of fluids from blind pouch
      (2) Parenteral feedings
    e. Postoperative care
      (1) Careful aspiration of mouth and pharynx
      (2) Parenteral feedings
      (3) Oral feedings begun gradually when ordered
      (4) Good nursing care of newborn not yet well adjusted to ex-

trauterine life and now under effects of anesthetic
    (5) Continuous gentle suction of chest
    (6) Chemotherapy
    (7) X-ray to test competency of anastomosis
    (8) Dilatation after healing takes place

K. Congenital pyloric stenosis
1. Cause—overgrowth of muscular tissue about pyloric opening of stomach
2. Symptoms—usually manifested in third or fourth week of life
    a. Vomiting (usually projectile)
    b. Dehydration and weight loss
    c. Constipation and diminished urinary output
    d. Peristaltic waves over abdomen
3. Preoperative care
    a. Parenteral fluids
    b. Gastric lavage
4. Postoperative care
    a. Influenced by type of anesthesia
    b. General care as for any child of same age
    c. General care as for any unconscious child of same age
    d. Parenteral fluids
    e. Time and interval of feedings will vary with individual situation

L. Intussusception (invagination of one segment of bowel into another)
1. Symptoms
    a. Sudden sharp pain
    b. Vomiting
    c. Prostration
    d. Constipation
    e. Small amounts of bloody mucus passed by rectum
    f. Free blood encountered on rectal examination
2. Treatment
    a. May subside spontaneously
    b. Surgical correction
3. Prognosis—good if disease corrected immediately; poor if correction delayed 24 hours or more

M. Megacolon (Hirschsprung's disease)
1. Symptoms
    a. Dilatation of colon (may have chronic obstruction of lower bowel)
    b. Retention of gas and feces, obstinate constipation
    c. Enlargement of abdomen
    d. Faulty nutrition

2. Treatment
    a. Search for obstruction
    b. Induce evacuation
    c. Surgical removal of distal segment
    d. Care of chronically ill child
    e. Dietary

N. Anal anomalies
1. Partial or complete occlusion at birth, requires immediate surgery
2. Fistula, surgical correction necessary
    a. Between rectum and vagina
    b. Between rectum and urethra
3. Fissure, caused by trauma or disease
4. Rectal prolapse, often self-corrective after replacement
    a. Relieve local irritation
    b. Prevent straining at stool
    c. Low residue diet

O. Hemophilia (factor VIII)
1. Transmission
2. Characteristics—delayed clotting time of blood, resulting in prolonged bleeding
3. Treatment
    a. Pressure to bleeding area if possible
    b. Transfusion
    c. Application of thromboplastic preparations

P. Leukemia
1. Cause—malignant neoplasm of unknown cause
2. Manifestations
    a. Anemia
    b. Spongy gums with necrosis of tissues of mouth
    c. Weakness, fatigue, and irritability
    d. Anorexia
    e. Vomiting and abdominal pain
    f. Dyspnea and palpitation
    g. Tenderness and swelling of joints
    h. Tendency to hemorrhage in mucous membranes, skin, and organs of body
    i. Lymphadenopathy and enlarged liver and spleen
    j. Presence of abnormal white blood count important in the diagnosis
3. Treatment—palliative (certain treatments may be contraindicated in some forms of disease)
    a. Irradiation by x-ray, radium, or administration of radioactive substances
    b. Folic acid antagonists
    c. Steroids
    d. 6-Mercaptopurine

e. Blood transfusions

f. Bone marrow extracts

4. Nursing care

    a. Very gentle oral hygiene because of sore, bleeding gums

    b. Careful handling because of tendency to hemorrhage and because of painful joints

    c. Infinite patience because of child's irritability and pain

    d. Plan for chronic condition as it may last years with periodic remissions

5. Prognosis—may become rapidly fatal or become subacute with periodic remissions

Q. Rheumatic fever

1. Predisposing factors (no universal agreement); found in all socioeconomic levels; cause cannot be solely attributed to poor living conditions

    a. Damp, crowded living quarters

    b. Poor nutrition

    c. Frequent respiratory infections of streptococcal origin

    d. Sensitization to protein antigens

    e. Virus infection

    f. Sudden wide temperature range of environment and exposure to chilling

2. Incidence

    a. Exact incidence not known, since not reportable in all areas

    b. Essentially disease of childhood and early adolescence

    c. Leading cause of death of school-age children

    d. Possible reasons for increased incidence

        (1) Migration of rural population to cities

        (2) Greater recognition of subclinical and borderline cases

        (3) Establishment of state programs of control including case finding

3. Signs and symptoms—often insidious with vague and transient symptoms, which include

    a. Loss of appetite

    b. Failure to gain weight and actual weight loss

    c. Carditis

    d. Increased pulse rate

    e. Some fever

    f. Arthritis

    g. Tendency to fatigue

    h. Increased sedimentation rate during active infection

    i. Presence of rheumatic nodules

    j. Tendency to nasal bleeding

    k. Symptoms of heart failure in some instances

4. Duration

    a. Acute phase may last weeks or several months

    b. Always possibility of recurrence

5. Treatment and nursing care

    a. Bed rest to reduce work load of heart; child may not be aware of significance of rest

    b. Gentle handling of tender, aching joints

    c. Chemotherapy

    d. Protection from overfatigue

    e. Nutritious diet stimulating to appetite

    f. Anticipation of his needs

    g. Team planning

    h. Diversions and hobbies suitable to age and degree of illness

    i. Emotional support, may rebel at long convalescence, may develop fear of death

    j. Good skin care, may perspire profusely in acute stage

    k. Adequate plan for convalescence

        (1) To prevent recurrences

        (2) Continue general hygienic measures

        (3) Resume activity gradually

        (4) Prevent "invalidism"

        (5) Continue with school activities, under special plan if necessary

        (6) Maintain child's status in home and community

    l. Vocational preparation

    m. Counseling program

6. Complications—some of most common

    a. Recurrence of acute phase

    b. Subacute bacterial endocarditis

    c. Congestive heart failure

    d. Rheumatic heart disease

    e. Polyarthritis

    f. Chorea

7. Public health aspects of disease include need for

    a. Unified community program of control, case finding, and prevention

    b. Long-range programs

c. Adequate care during acute illness and convalescence

d. Improvement of housing conditions in lower economic levels

e. Encouragement of suspects to seek physical examination and counseling

f. Better health programs in public schools

g. Wise planning for use of federal and state funds

h. Coordination of services

R. Chorea, Sydenham's chorea
  1. Symptoms—onset often gradual
     a. Emotional instability
     b. Lack of fine muscle coordination
     c. Exaggerated muscular movements, often with facial grimacing
     d. Restless and unable to maintain one position
  2. Treatment and nursing care (see also care of child with rheumatic fever)
     a. Symptomatic
     b. Conserve child's strength; it may be necessary to do everything for him during acute stage
     c. Protect from injury
     d. Calm environment

S. Congenital heart disease
  1. Circulatory changes after birth
     a. Pulmonary circulation rapidly increases
     b. Foramen ovale, ductus arteriosus, and ductus venosus closure
  2. Diagnosis
     a. History
     b. Clinical observation
     c. X-ray and fluoroscopic examinations
     d. Cardiac catheterization, electrocardiography, and angiocardiography
  3. Types of defects, great variety (only 2 types considered here)
     a. Acyanotic group—patent ductus arteriosus the principal example for which remedial surgery available
        (1) Persistence of deformity may lead to
            (a) Cardiac decompensation
            (b) Development of fatal bacterial infection
        (2) Correction—surgical
     b. Cyanotic group—e.g., tetralogy of Fallot
        (1) Defects
            (a) Stenosis or atresia of pulmonary artery
            (b) High interventricular septal defect
            (c) Dextroposition of aorta
            (d) Hypertrophy of right ventricle
        (2) Signs and symptoms, number and severity depend upon extent of defects
            (a) Cyanosis and dyspnea on exertion
            (b) Clubbing of ends of fingers, toes
            (c) Undernutrition
            (d) Possibility of some retardation of physical and mental growth and development
        (3) Preoperative preparation
            (a) Continuous competent medical supervision
            (b) Protection from overfatigue and infections
            (c) Provision for all reasonable opportunity for normal growth and development
            (d) Frequent rest periods for runabout child—squatting position often diagnostic sign
            (e) Adequate plan of care so other children in family not neglected
            (f) Attention to emotional needs
            (g) Possible restricted school attendance, avoid infections, provide immunizations, good nutrition, and general health care
            (h) Immediate preoperative care—skillful hospital admission; adjustment to hospital without long anxious anticipation of surgery; adequate fluid intake (parenteral fluids and plasma if necessary); chemotherapy to prevent infection; familiarity with oxygen apparatus
        (4) Surgical correction—aim to increase blood supply to lungs by connecting systemic artery (usually subclavian) to pulmonary artery (age at which

performed varies with individual child)
    (a) Postoperative care
T. Burns and scalds
  1. Prevention
  2. Type
    a. Thermal
    b. Radiation
    c. Chemical
    d. Electrical
  3. Treatment
    a. Local—may or may not include cleansing and debridement; variety of types of dressings; many now favor pressure dressings
      (1) Provide rest for tissues
      (2) Daily dressing may be eliminated
      (3) Relieve pain
      (4) Prevent loss of serum
      (5) Prevent infection
      (6) Prevent contractures
    b. Daily soaks
    c. Systemic
      (1) Control of shock
      (2) Chemotherapy
      (3) Parenteral fluids and plasma
      (4) Abundance of oral fluids
      (5) High-vitamin, high-caloric diet
    d. Early skin grafting
    e. Control of infection
  4. Nursing care
    a. Attention to emotional needs, allay fears, give encouragement and support
    b. Good general care of helpless individual
    c. Adequate intake of foods and fluids
    d. Accurate record of urinary output
    e. Prompt reporting of any change in condition
    f. Protection of dressings to prevent soiling
    g. Friendly, understanding contact with parents
    h. Care after skin grafts or other plastic operations will vary with individual surgeon; long-range rehabilitation plans
U. Skin infections
  1. Prevention
    a. Cleanliness
    b. Prevent development of breaks in skin
    c. Prevent wound contamination
  2. Types

    a. Impetigo—infectious skin disease
      (1) Isolation
      (2) Local application of gentian violet, ammoniated mercury, or penicillin ointments
      (3) Chemotherapy
      (4) Prevention of scratching infected areas
    b. Furunculosis—infection of sebaceous glands or hair follicles
      (1) Chemotherapy
      (2) Surgical drainage if necessary
      (3) Local application of antiseptics
      (4) Prevention of scratching infected areas
      (5) Measures for comfort
    c. Ringworm (tinea) fungous disease
      (1) Scalp (tinea capitis)
        (a) Shave head so lesions readily observed
        (b) Ointments, ultraviolet light, and epilation have been used in treatment
      (2) Feet (athlete's foot)
        (a) Symptoms—scaly fissures between toes; vesicles on sides of feet; chronically thickened skin
        (b) Treatment—treated with antiseptic soaks, ointment, powders
    d. Miliaria rubra (prickly heat)
      (1) Manifestation
      (2) Treatment
        (a) Local application of soothing lotions may be helpful
        (b) Cleanliness of skin and exposure to air usually produce prompt healing
    e. Intertrigo and diaper rash, excoriation due to moisture and chafing
      (1) Keep area clean and dry
      (2) Expose to air and light
      (3) Apply bland ointment at night
      (4) Avoid strong alkalies in diaper washing
    f. Scabies—produced by itch mite
      (1) Sulfur ointment effective remedy, although several other drugs are useful also
      (2) Prevent spread to others
      (3) Prevent scratching, as secondary skin infection may develop if skin is broken
    g. Pediculosis—infestation with lice

(1) Lice may infest hair and scalp, pubic region, or entire body

(2) Head louse most common in children

(3) Generalized dermatitis may develop due to scratching

(4) Admission procedure should include thorough inspection of hair and scalp

(5) Institute immediate treatment (number of remedies available); inspect hair and scalp daily and continue treatment until cured

V. Genitourinary conditions
 1. Infections
  a. Pyelitis and pyelonephritis
   (1) Colon bacillus common invader; other organisms may be present
   (2) More common in female infants
   (3) Infection frequently ascends through urethra
   (4) Diagnosis made by presence of pus in urine
   (5) Symptoms vary with age of child; may include
    (a) Sudden high fever
    (b) Vomiting
    (c) Increased frequency of urination
    (d) Varying degrees of prostration
    (e) Irritability of central nervous system
    (f) Convulsions
   (6) Treatment and nursing care
    (a) Chemotherapy, depending upon causative organism
    (b) Drugs to acidify urine may be indicated
    (c) Build up general health of child
    (d) Bed rest during acute stage
    (e) Search for possible malformation of urinary tract
    (f) Nursing care similar to that provided for any acutely ill child
   (7) Complications
    (a) Chronic infection resulting in kidney damage
    (b) Hypertension
  b. Acute glomerulonephritis

   (1) Incidence—often follows focal or systemic infection in 3- to 7-year age group
   (2) Frequent causative organism hemolytic *Streptococcus*
   (3) Classification—several; acute hemorrhagic nephritis the only acute glomerulonephritis considered here, because of many similar characteristics
   (4) Symptoms vary in severity
    (a) May appear acutely ill
    (b) Hematuria
    (c) Possible initial high temperature
    (d) Low-grade temperature may persist
    (e) Edema may or may not be visible
    (f) Urinary output often decreased
    (g) Anorexia
    (h) Vomiting, constipation, headache (not constant symptoms but may occur)
   (5) Complications
    (a) Hypertension and cardiac involvement
    (b) Chronic nephritis
   (6) Treatment and nursing care—specific treatment depends upon individual child
    (a) Antibiotic therapy to control infection
    (b) Drugs to lower blood pressure and edema
    (c) Digitalis
    (d) Sedatives
    (e) Good nursing care
     (1) If fluids restricted, spread wisely through 24 hours
     (2) Use methods of allaying thirst
     (3) Meticulous oral hygiene
     (4) Frequent skin care with attention to pressure points
     (5) Comfortable clothing and covering to prevent chilling
     (6) Comfortably warm room without direct drafts
     (7) Coax lagging appetite

(8) Recreation, hobbies, etc., suitable to age and condition of child

(9) Suitable change of position

(10) Provision for maximum rest and protection from upper respiratory infection

(11) Assist child and family to adjust to child's chronic illness

(12) Measures to relieve strain on heart

(13) Parenteral fluids, such as blood, plasma, glucose, amino acids

2. Nephrosis
   a. Incidence—essentially disease of early childhood
   b. Symptoms
      (1) Generalized edema
      (2) Free fluid may be found in chest and abdomen
      (3) Listlessness
      (4) Pallor
      (5) Poor appetite and poor state of nutrition
   c. Treatment and nursing care
      (1) Adequate rest
      (2) Directed toward achieving normal body fluid balance, control of infection, establishment of good nutrition
      (3) Parenteral fluids, such as amino acids and plasma
      (4) Drainage of fluids from chest and abdomen if necessary
      (5) Administration of diuretics if indicated
      (6) Chemotherapy to control infection
      (7) Change of position frequently because of dependent edema
      (8) Special care of tender, edematous, easily abraded skin
      (9) Relief of discomfort due to edema of genitals, keep skin clean and dry, support genitals if necessary
      (10) Special care of eyes, conjunctiva may be irritated and eyelids very swollen
      (11) Planning with child and parents for home convalescence

W. Malformations of urinary tract
   1. Congenital cystic kidneys
      a. May occur in one or both kidneys
      b. Cysts may be numerous and small, very large, or even single one
      c. Surgical removal of single cyst may be advisable; no known cure for multiple, bilateral cysts
      d. Renal insufficiency possible complication if
         (1) Lesions are extensive
         (2) Child survives to adulthood
   2. Exstrophy of bladder, partial or complete; exposure of bladder mucosa through abdominal wall (penis or vagina may also be malformed)
      a. Exposed mucosa very sensitive, ulceration may occur if not protected
      b. Skin may become irritated because of incontinence of urine
      c. Treatment and nursing care
         (1) Implantation of ureters into sigmoid or other urinary diversion
         (2) Plastic repair of bladder and external genitals
         (3) Attention to emotional needs of child and parents; older child may suffer embarrassment, fear, shame, guilt
   3. Other anomalies of genitourinary tract
      a. Absence of organ
      b. Duplication of organ
      c. Kinks in urinary tract
      d. Stenosis or atresia
      e. Fistulas
      f. Hypospadias, urethral opening behind glans penis, treat surgically
   4. Methods of diversion of urine
      a. Indwelling urethral catheter
      b. Suprapubic cystotomy
      c. Ureteral catheter in kidney
      d. Nephrostomy
      e. Surgical transplant of ureters
      f. Ureteroileocutaneous anastomosis
         (1) Ileum has rich blood supply and strong peristaltic quality
         (2) Eliminates fecal contamination
         (3) Continuity of intestinal tract maintained
   5. Other conditions of genitourinary tract
      a. Adherent prepuce, foreskin adherent to glans

b. Phimosis, narrowing of preputial opening
   (1) May not require treatment
   (2) Retraction may be indicated
   (3) Circumcision may be necessary
c. Hydrocele, collection of fluid in scrotum, spontaneous recovery usually takes place
d. Undescended testes

X. Neuromuscular disorders
   1. Rheumatoid arthritis (Still's disease)
      a. Characteristics
         (1) Slowly progressive, painful swelling, stiffness, and limited motion of joints
         (2) Shifting type of pain
         (3) Usually insidious onset with weight loss, fatigue, low-grade fever, tachycardia, weakness, and paresthesia of fingers and toes
         (4) Mental depression
         (5) Possible enlargement of liver, spleen, and lymph nodes
         (6) Frequently, increased sedimentation rate
      b. Treatment
         (1) Eradicate foci of infection
         (2) High-vitamin, nutritious diet
         (3) Bed rest during active phase
         (4) Local heat for comfort
         (5) Drugs (many drugs, vaccines, foreign proteins, etc. have been tried)
            (a) Gold therapy
            (b) Analgesics may be necessary
            (c) Cortisone and ACTH have been tried but further evaluation is necessary
         (6) Consider child and family to help them to maintain courage and continue treatment
   2. Hydrocephalus
      a. Cause
         (1) Congenital malformation in spinal column
         (2) Acute infection such as meningitis or syphilis
         (3) Subdural hematoma or tumor
      b. Symptoms
         (1) Enlarged head due to accumulation of spinal fluid in ventricles
            (a) Stretching of scalp pulls eyelids up, exposing sclera
            (b) Veins of scalp become prominent
         (2) Widely separated sutures
         (3) Variable degree of mental impairment
         (4) Communicating hydrocephalus: normal communication between ventricles and subarachnoid space, with enlarged head
         (5) Noncommunicating: block between ventricles and subarachnoid space; enlarged head results, and problem is usually more serious than communicating type, which also requires surgery
      c. Nursing care
         (1) Because of large head, careful handling to prevent injury of neck
         (2) Position for greatest comfort, may be unable to lie on back or abdomen
         (3) Turning and special skin care to prevent breakdown, skin is thin and veins prominent
         (4) Special care of eyes, they may be pulled open because skin over head is stretched
         (5) Careful feeding to prevent choking, may not be possible to hold child for feedings
   3. Cerebral palsies
      a. Some causes thought to be
         (1) Developmental malformations of cerebrum which occur in utero
         (2) Intracranial injury at birth
         (3) Postnatal damage to cerebrum as result of head injury or infection
      b. Main types
         (1) Athetoid, in which motion involuntary
         (2) Spastic, characterized by tension of certain muscles, especially under strain
         (3) Ataxic, with disturbance of balance and sense of posture
      c. Frequency
         (1) Largest single cause of crippling
         (2) Estimate of 7 children with

cerebral palsy born each year in population of 100,000
d. Treatment and nursing care must include team approach
(1) Early diagnosis
(2) Teaching plan for motor co-ordination, education, play, speech, etc.
(3) Special educational programs
(4) Special equipment often nec-essary
(a) Patience in all care giv-en
(b) Clothing simple with large buttons
(c) Chair, table, etc., adjusted to individual needs
(d) Special training chairs and tables for posture, bal-ance, exercise
(e) Special handles on feed-ing equipment, toothbrush, etc.
(5) Encouragement of parents to continue care and assistance with remedial program
(6) Good general care with proper food, protection against infec-tions, ample rest, avoidance of overstimulation
(7) Goals of performance fixed at levels so that child can experi-ence joy of achievement, praise for effort and achievement
(8) Trained therapist to guide pro-gram of care
(9) Periodic evaluation of program and achievement
(10) Love, affection, emotional sup-port
4. Epilepsy
a. Cause somewhat obscure
b. Manifestations—paroxysmal tonic or clonic seizures of varying de-grees of intensity and regularity
(1) Petit mal, very little muscular spasm
(2) Grand mal, severe generalized spasm
c. Treatment and nursing care di-rected toward
(1) Provision for normal physical, mental, and emotional growth and development
(2) Prevention of seizures
(a) Gentle handling in calm quiet atmosphere

(b) Avoid sudden and exces-sive stimulation
(3) Attention to measures for safe-ty in all activities and during seizures
(4) Anticipation of seizure when-ever possible
(5) Emotional support, may shun playmates
(6) Encourage parental participa-tion in making and executing plans for care
(7) Adequate supervision during and after seizure
(a) Safety
(b) Accurate description of areas involved, duration, severity, position of child, position and movement of eyes, in what part of body attack began, sequence, incontinence, etc.
(c) Reaction of child after at-tack
(d) After seizure leave child clean, dry, comfortable, and allow him to sleep
(8) Encouragement in eating spe-cial diet
(a) Ketogenic diet tends to create mild acidosis and prevent seizures
(b) Alkalinity of body fluids encourages seizures
(9) Anticonvulsant drugs
(10) Continued care at home
(a) Assist in readjustment to school and community
(b) Do not press child beyond ability to achieve
(c) Encourage parents to con-tinue medical supervision
5. Spina bifida, meningocele, and me-ningomyelocele
a. Cause—defect in closure of bony structure of spinal cord, may or may not be externally visible
b. Characteristics of visible defect
(1) Herniation of meninges through opening
(2) Lesion may or may not be covered with skin
(3) Infection may occur if mem-brane ruptures
c. Treatment and nursing care
(1) Surgical correction, effective-

ness depends upon type and extent of lesions and presence or absence of infection

 (2) Chance of infections from urine, stool, and other sources should be decreased before and after surgery

 (3) Good nursing care suitable for any child of that age

 (4) Keep off back until wound heals

 (5) Understanding approach to parents

Y. Nutritional, metabolic, and endocrine disturbances

 1. Celiac disease, chronic disturbance of nutrition

  a. Age group—any age child (most common 1 to 5 years)

  b. Characteristics

   (1) Defective absorption of fat

   (2) Passage of large, pale, offensive smelling stools

   (3) Malnutrition and growth failure

  c. Treatment and nursing care (need long-range planning)

   (1) Dietary regulation

   (2) Liver extract

   (3) Vitamin B complex

   (4) Good general care

   (5) Stimulation of appetite

   (6) Prevention of infection

   (7) Encouragement of parents to continue treatment

 2. Rickets

  a. Prevention

   (1) Sufficient exposure to ultraviolet rays

   (2) Sufficient intake of vitamin D

   (3) Good health habits

  b. Symptoms

   (1) Irritability

   (2) Constipation

   (3) Perspiration of head

   (4) Increase in head size

   (5) Delayed dentition

   (6) Rachitic rosary enlarged wrists and ankles, leg deformities

  c. Complications prone to develop

   (1) Respiratory infections

   (2) Chronic gastrointestinal disturbance

  d. Treatment

   (1) Adequate amounts of vitamin D

   (2) Exposure to ultraviolet radiation

   (3) General hygienic measures and building up good nutrition

 3. Allergy—sometimes called "great imitator"

  a. Area affected—almost any part of body

  b. Some manifestations

   (1) Asthma

   (2) Hay fever

   (3) Angioneurotic edema

   (4) Eczema

   (5) Vasomotor rhinitis

   (6) Diarrhea and other gastrointestinal upsets

   (7) Conjunctivitis

  c. Treatment—general

   (1) Comprehensive study of child and his surroundings

   (2) Enlistment of child and parental cooperation in long-range program of attack

    (a) Avoid offending allergens in food, inhalants, contact

    (b) Immunization to the offending allergen

    (c) Symptomatic treatment

  d. Asthma

   (1) Manifestations

    (a) Swelling or secretions in bronchioles cause wheezing

    (b) Spasm of smooth muscle and edema prevent expectoration of bronchial secretions causing dyspnea

   (2) Treatment symptomatic

    (a) Drugs to relieve spasm and promote expectoration

    (b) Supply moist air

    (c) Administration of oxygen or oxygen and helium

    (d) Sedation if necessary

    (e) Long-range program to find cause and build up child's general condition

  e. Eczema may occur in infant or in older child

   (1) Manifestation

    (a) Red, inflamed, itching skin

    (b) Circumscribed or general lesions

    (c) Oozing or crusting of broken skin

(2) Treatment and nursing care
   (a) Bathe skin with mineral oil to remove loose crusts
   (b) Provide adequate restraint to prevent scratching, remove restraints one at a time and change position often to rest child
   (c) Provide smooth surface under child to minimize irritation
   (d) Keep perspiration from collecting
   (e) Apply ordered ointment often enough to keep area covered
   (f) Expose area to light (protect eyes from glare, control temperature for comfort)
   (g) Measures to prevent upper respiratory infection
   (h) Diet as prescribed

4. Cystic fibrosis of pancreas
   a. Cause
      (1) Genetic origin
      (2) Probably inborn error of metabolism
   b. Symptoms
      (1) Vary in number, severity, and age of onset
      (2) Some resemble celiac disease
      (3) Poor weight gain
      (4) Repeated and persistent upper respiratory infection
      (5) Thick, tenacious pulmonary secretions
      (6) Enlarged liver
      (7) Peripheral edema
      (8) Retinal hemorrhages
      (9) Right ventricular hypertrophy may develop
      (10) Obstructive emphysema
      (11) Large foul-smelling stools
   c. Diagnosis
      (1) Absence of trypsin in pancreatic secretions
      (2) Elevated chloride content of sweat (normal is 1 to 60 mEq. per liter)
      (3) Large amount of fat in stools
   d. Treatment and nursing care
      (1) Alleviate and control symptoms
      (2) Protect against respiratory infections

(3) Provide adequate rest, nutrition, and health supervision
(4) Repair and prevent electrolyte depletion
(5) Guard against cardiac failure

5. Thyroid disorders
   a. Hypothyroidism
      (1) Congenital
         (a) Cause—absence or underdevelopment of gland causes cretinism
         (b) Symptoms — stunted growth; short thick neck; broad hands, short fingers; tongue thick and protruding; skin dry and scaly; mental retardation may be marked
         (c) Treatment—early recognition; administration of desiccated thyroid
      (2) Acquired hypothyroidism (myxedema)
         (a) Cause—trauma; disease; removal of thyroid
         (b) Symptoms — impaired growth and development
         (c) Treatment — desiccated thyroid
   b. Hyperthyroidism (exophthalmic goiter)
      (1) Symptoms—caused by excess of thyroxine
         (a) Emotional disturbance
         (b) Overactive
         (c) Excitable and irritable
         (d) Metabolism increased and weight loss occurs
         (e) Easily fatigued
         (f) Fine tremor of outstretched hands
         (g) Dyspnea
         (h) Palpitation
         (i) Tachycardia
         (j) Possible development of symptoms of cardiac enlargement
      (2) Treatment
         (a) Prolonged bed rest
         (b) Iodine by mouth, often in form of Lugol's solution
         (c) May inhibit formation of thyroid hormone with thiouracil

(d) Digitalis may be needed for cardiac symptoms

(e) Surgical removal may be necessary

(3) Nursing care

  (a) Develop plan to minimize symptoms

  (b) Eliminate hurry and competition

  (c) Reassurance of child

  (d) Quiet diversions according to age and condition

  (e) Have child assist with plan whenever possible

6. Diabetes mellitus

  a. Symptoms—juvenile diabetes may be more severe and variable than disease in adults

    (1) Increased thirst and fluid intake

    (2) Increased hunger and food intake

    (3) Increased urinary output

    (4) Malnutrition, metabolism balance upset

  b. Tests for diabetes

    (1) Sugar in urine not always indicative; may be present in other conditions

    (2) Sugar and acetone in urine, plus elevated fasting blood sugar strongly indicative

    (3) Glucose tolerance test

  c. Complications

    (1) Diabetic acidosis or coma

      (a) Abdominal and/or generalized body pain

      (b) Drowsiness

      (c) Cherry red lips

      (d) Deep respirations

      (e) Acetone on breath

      (f) Acetone in urine

  d. Treatment and nursing care

    (1) Treat as normal child in home, school, community

    (2) Nutritionally adequate diet and fluids

    (3) Good hygienic care

    (4) Prevention of infections

    (5) Care of child in diabetic coma similar to that for any comatose child

    (6) Insulin

    (7) Teach child how to care for self and contribute to control of disease

      (a) Administration of insulin

      (b) Testing urine

      (c) Preparation and variation of diet

      (d) Recognition of symptoms of hypoglycemia and appropriate treatment

      (e) Recognition of hyperinsulinism and appropriate treatment

    (8) Help child and parents with psychological acceptance of condition

      (a) May rebel against insulin injections

      (b) Testing urine may become boring

      (c) May object to rest periods

      (d) May find difficulty in resisting candy and family desserts

      (e) Chronicity of disease

2. Poisonings

A. Possible sources

  1. Household drugs, insecticides, cleaning agents, chemicals

  2. Accidental administration of excess dosage of drug

  3. Lead paint of toys or furniture

  4. Eating poisonous paints or crayons

  5. Eating unwashed fruit or vegetables treated with poisonous insecticide sprays

  6. Use of well water in which nitrate compounds exist; converted to nitrites that change hemoglobin to methemoglobin

B. Prevention

  1. Eliminate sources of lead available to child; make parents aware of sources

  2. Legislation to control ingredients in nostrums and to assure accurate labeling

  3. Keep all drugs and household poisons out of reach of children

  4. Administer only prescribed drugs and in correct amounts

  5. Use safe paints on toys and equipment

  6. Teach older children methods of preventing poisoning

  7. Thoroughly wash fresh fruits and vegetables

C. Diagnosis

  1. Parent may know what child has swallowed

2. May produce local lesion
3. Oral ingestion may produce irritation of gastrointestinal tract and central nervous system
4. Examination of stomach contents
5. X-ray—especially in lead poisoning
D. Treatment and nursing care
   1. Removal of source of poison
   2. Administration of antidote
   3. Gastric lavage using appropriate solvent, absorbent, or neutralizing agent (lavage may be contraindicated in some instances)
   4. Supportive treatment
      a. Parenteral fluids to combat dehydration
      b. Oxygen
      c. Stimulants if necessary
      d. Artificial respiration
      e. Prevention and treatment of shock
      f. Sedation if necessary
   5. Save vomitus and excretions for analysis
   6. Withhold food by mouth if necessary to rest gastrointestinal tract
E. Education of public
F. Function of poison centers

3. Mental retardation

A. Definition
   1. Symptom rather than disease
   2. Definition adopted by American Association on Mental Deficiency
B. Current concerns
   1. Contribution of research
   2. Preparation of personnel
   3. Program development
      a. Finding children early
      b. Complete evaluation
      c. Role of parents
      d. Continuity of care and guidance
C. Highlights of progress
   1. Mobilization of resources
   2. Shift in philosophy of care
   3. Development of special education
   4. Expansion of program for training specialists
   5. Organization of National Association for Retarded Children
   6. Appointment of
      a. President's Panel on Mental Retardation
      b. Technical Committee on Clinical Programs
   7. First worldwide Congress on Mental Deficiency—London, 1960; second Congress—Poland, 1970

8. Development of study centers
D. Possible causes of retardation
   1. Prenatal
      a. Blood incompatibilities
      b. Deficient maternal diet
      c. Genetic factors
      d. Infections
      e. Toxic agents
   2. Trauma of labor and delivery
   3. Postnatal conditions
   4. Unknown causes
E. Prevention
   1. Adequate supervision of every woman during pregnancy
   2. Guaranteeing right of every child to be "well born"
   3. Improving depressed environments
   4. Control of infectious diseases
   5. Recognition of right of every person to achieve maximum potential
F. Care of retarded child; recognition that needs similar for all children
   1. Love and affection
   2. To feel wanted
   3. Opportunity to respond to others
   4. Support to cope with anxiety, fear, anger, frustration, etc.
   5. Acceptance of self
   6. Health needs
   7. To be family member
   8. Education appropriate to him
G. Role of nurse enhanced by working knowledge of
   1. Normal growth and development
   2. Objectives of program
   3. Interlocking roles of various disciplines
   4. How to cooperate with families
   5. Existing community resources
   6. Gaps in resources
   7. Contribution of research
H. Role of National Institute of Neurological Diseases and Blindness
I. Long-term and short-term goals
J. Phenylketonuria (PKU)—example of cause of mental retardation
   1. Discovery
   2. Genetic and biochemical pattern
   3. Incidence
   4. Clinical manifestations
   5. Screening programs
   6. Treatment—team approach

4. Rehabilitation

A. Chief causes of crippling
   1. Result of infection
   2. Group of palsies
   3. Congenital anomalies and genetic factors

4. Traumatic conditions due to burns and other accidents
B. Reasons for increase in number of persons known to need rehabilitative services
   1. Lower mortality rates
   2. Adequacy of case finding
   3. Advances in knowledge about rehabilitation
C. Through eyes of child
   1. Same basic needs as any child
   2. Needs recognition of being able to do things for himself and others
   3. Security
   4. Moral support in accepting things that set child apart from others, such as braces, crutches, prostheses, special equipment
   5. Affection and encouragement in learning process
   6. Handicaps not to be excuse for overindulgence
   7. Practice principles of good mental health
   8. Look for compensatory qualities to cultivate in child
D. Understand factors in prolonged convalescence; child may
   1. Be excessively irritable and emotionally unstable
   2. Have temper tantrums and nightmares
   3. Have intensified behavior problems
   4. Be easily overfatigued
   5. Withdraw from social contacts
   6. Be shocked if part of his body is paralyzed or missing
   7. Resist any pressure to achieve
E. Understanding siblings
F. Through eyes of parents
   1. Cost of care
   2. Special plans for education of child
   3. Adjustment in social life
   4. Plans for other family members
   5. Danger of overanxiety and overprotection
   6. Guilt feelings and conflicting attitudes of parents
   7. Permit child to give of himself
   8. Familiarity with suitable games, crafts, toys
   9. Encouragement to continue rehabilitation measures
G. Assisting child to
   1. Achieve good health to limit of capacity
   2. Live with his handicap
   3. Achieve security within himself, in home and community

4. Participate in all possible activities of normal child
5. Receive education (academic, cultural, and vocational in accord with abilities and desires)
6. Receive guidance in preparing for employment
7. Process of rehabilitation centers around
   a. Activities of daily living (ADL)
   b. Satisfaction of basic creative urges
   c. Making best use of functions and abilities he possesses
   d. Retraining lost functions
   e. Developing new skills
   f. Care of prostheses and other equipment
   g. Synthesis of services
   h. Good interpersonal relationships

5. Drug therapy
A. Infants and children have
   1. Increased toxicity to some drugs
   2. Greater numbers of untoward reactions to drugs
B. Medication chests; and all medicines should be made inaccessible to child, by use of locked cupboards and other safety measures
C. Medications may be given in syrup to help child accept oral drug
D. Second nurse or person may be needed to help hold child, lend ego support, when some medications are given, such as parenteral ones
E. Determination of dosage by physician according to rules
   1. Surface area

$$\text{Child dose} = \frac{\text{Surface area of child in sq. M} \times \text{Adult dose}}{1.75}$$

   2. Clark's rule (most frequently used)

$$\text{Child dose} = \frac{\text{Adult dose} \times \text{Weight in pounds}}{150 \text{ (weight of average adult)}}$$

   3. Young's rule

$$\text{Child dose} = \frac{\text{Age} \times \text{Adult dose}}{\text{Age in years} + 12}$$

6. Drug abuse—taking of drugs, or drug-producing agents that are not needed for treatment of disease
A. Organs of body that are targets of greatest toxicity
   1. Brain
   2. Liver

B. Smoking
   1. Increased use of cigarettes by youth (nicotine and irritants)
   2. Possible increase of lung cancer is great
C. Alcohol
   1. Brain damage, interference with glucose oxidation
   2. Malnutrition
   3. Eventually liver damage results
D. Barbiturates, sedatives
   1. Symptoms are irritability, compromise of judgment, slurred speech, staggering gait
   2. Goofballs
      a. Luminal—"purple hearts"
      b. Seconal—"pinks," "redbirds"
      c. Tuinal—"rainbows," "tuies"
      d. Nembutal—"yellow jackets"
      e. Sodium Amytal—"bluebirds," "blue heaven"
E. Amphetamines, stimulants
   1. Symptoms are irritability, being agitated, loud, unable to sleep, and delusions of persecution
      a. Pep pills
         (1) Methamphetamine—"speed"
         (2) Dexedrine—"capilots," "dexis"
         (3) Benzedrine—"bennies," "bambitos"
         (4) Biphetamine—"goofballs"
F. Tranquilizers
   1. Same symptoms as barbiturate abuses
   2. Deaths have been reported from abuse
   3. Common drugs
      a. Librium
      b. Meprobamate (Equanil, Miltown)
      c. Valmid
G. Aspirin—constant use
   1. Bleeding, particularly stomach and upper intestinal tract
   2. Overdose is particularly toxic to young child—drowsiness, stupor
H. Vapor sniffing, thrill-seeking experience of glue sniffers
   1. Bodily damage related to substance
      a. Gasoline and naptha—cause sudden death
      b. Toluene—kidney and neurologic damage
   2. Many effects similar to acute alcoholism
I. LSD (lysergic acid diethylamide)
   1. Growing evidence that it produces irreversible changes in life style and personality
   2. Fantasy replaces reality
J. Marijuana
   1. Controversy over its reactions in the human being
   2. Associated with changes in life style of the youth

COMMUNICABLE DISEASES IN CHILDREN

For definitions and principles of communicable disease control, see chapter on medical-surgical nursing, pp. 427 and 435.

1. **Immunizing agents**
A. Vaccines—consist of active agent of disease or closely related organism
   1. Live attenuated—modified so not to cause disease
   2. Killed noninfective—inactivated by heat or chemicals
   3. Toxoid—exotoxin, detoxified
   4. Vaccines produce active, artificially acquired immunity
   5. Administered prior to exposure
   6. Primary antigenic stimulus after initial series of vaccine or toxoid
   7. Secondary antigenic stimulus follows booster of same preparation—produces long-lasting immunity
   8. Reinforcing injections may be delayed several years
   9. Some vaccines available from National Communicable Disease Center, for medical investigation
B. Antisera-antitoxins
   1. Neutralize toxins produced by certain organisms
   2. Produce passive, artificially acquired immunity lasting 2 to 3 weeks
   3. Produced in body of animals, usually horses
   4. Human gamma globulin
      a. Made from serum of person recovered from specific disease, or from human placenta
      b. Administered to prevent or modify some diseases
      c. Given with Edmonston B strain of measles vaccine to modify side effects of vaccine
   5. Sensitization tests done prior to administering antitoxins
C. Antimicrobial drugs
   1. May be given to prevent infection
   2. Given to check infection during incubation period
   3. Given to control disease and prevent complications

D. Skin tests—many tests developed; most have limited use
1. Allergic reaction to infection
   a. Tuberculin test
   b. Histoplasmin test
   c. Blastomycin test
   d. Coccidioidin test
2. Bacterial infections
   a. Schick test
   b. Lepromin test
   c. Dick test—little used today
   d. Test for tularemia
3. Viral infections
   a. Mumps antigen
   b. Rubella—field trials in progress
4. Fungus infections
   a. Trichophytons—all 3 genera that cause cutaneous dermatomycosis
5. Parasitic infections
   a. *Trichinella* skin test most widely used
6. Allergy
2. **Diphtheria**
Incidence in the United States low due to immunization; endemic in some parts of world
A. Etiology—*Corynebacterium diphtheriae* (diphtheria bacillus) produces powerful soluble toxin
B. Transmission—direct or indirect contact, droplet infection or droplet nuclei, asymptomatic carriers
C. Incubation period—2 to 5 days
D. Symptoms—onset insidious, fatigue, malaise, fever 100° to 102° F., slight sore throat, prostration; later necrotic tissue over tonsils and uvula, grayish membrane turning dull white and possibly extending into trachea; cervical adenitis
E. Diagnosis—clinical and bacteriologic, cultures from nose and throat
F. Treatment—diphtheria antitoxin, penicillin may be given, analgesics
G. Complications—myocarditis; paralysis of soft palate, pharynx, larynx, ciliary muscles of eye, extremities, respiratory muscles
H. Nursing—isolation minimum 14 days, with bacteriologic release following 3 negative nose and throat cultures; medical asepsis; frequent pulse, respiratory rates, and blood pressure; absolute rest, flat in bed; observe for complications, cyanosis, vomiting, pallor, abdominal pain, palatal paralysis, stertorous breathing, restlessness

I. Prevention—immunization; diphtheria toxoid usually combined with pertussis and tetanus vaccines as DPT: three injections, interval 4 to 6 weeks, beginning at 1 to 2 months of age; booster doses at 3- to 5-year intervals until 12 years of age; patient after age 12 given adult diphtheria tetanus toxoid; mandatory reporting, information exchange with World Health Organization
3. **Pertussis (whooping cough)**
Incidence declining in the United States due to immunization; mortality rate about 0.2 per 100,000 population
A. Etiology—*Bordetella pertussis*
B. Transmission—direct contact, droplet infection; carriers not important
C. Incubation period—7 to 10 days; may be 21 days
D. Symptoms—3 stages, duration about 6 weeks
   1. Catarrhal stage—coryza, sneezing, lacrimation, dry cough, leukocytosis; most contagious
   2. Paroxysmal stage—paroxysms of coughing with whoop, cyanosis, eyes red, vomiting; epistaxis or hemorrhage possible during paroxysm of coughing
   3. Convalescent stage—gradual decrease of all symptoms
E. Complication—interstitial pneumonia, atelectasis, umbilical hernia, central nervous system involvement, otitis media
F. Diagnosis—stage 1, bacteriologic study from cough plate, nasal swabs; clinical signs and history of exposure; paroxysmal stage, characteristic whoop
G. Treatment—hyperimmune convalescent serum or gamma globulin, light sedation; chemotherapy of little value
H. Nursing—if in hospital, isolate, observe medical asepsis, maintain airway, keep warm, record food eaten and retained
I. Prevention—exclude nonimmune children from school for 14 days after last contact; immunize with pertussis vaccine (DPT) 3 injections, beginning at 1 to 2 months of age, and booster doses each 3 to 5 years until 12 years of age; pertussis vaccine alone may cause cerebral pathology
4. **Scarlet fever (streptococcal tonsillitis or pharyngitis)**
Epidemic in most countries, including the United States
A. Etiology—*Streptococcus pyogenes* (group A hemolytic *Streptococcus*)

1. Scarlet fever, skin rash
2. Streptococcal tonsillitis, no skin rash

B. Transmission—direct or indirect contact, droplet infection or droplet nuclei, possible transmission through milk
C. Incubation period—24 hours to 10 days
D. Symptoms—abrupt onset, fever 101° to 104° F., sore throat, vomiting, headache, chill may occur, increase in pulse rate, skin rash after 48 hours, "circumoral pallor" about mouth, "strawberry tongue"—later becoming red, dry, cracked "raspberry tongue," after 10 days' desquamation of skin
E. Complications—otitis media, mastoiditis or cervical adenitis, meningitis, septic arthritis
F. Diagnosis—clinical signs, throat cultures, tests; Schültz-Charlton and Dick tests of questionable value, Schilling hemogram of some value
G. Treatment—penicillin, tetracycline drugs, supportive care
H. Nursing—isolation, medical asepsis, warm olive oil to relieve pruritus, intake-output records; observe for complications
I. Prevention—active immunization not recommended; passive immunity with hyperimmune human gamma globulin or prophylactic penicillin

5. **Congenital syphilis**
Infection in utero occurs between 4 and 5 months; if mother in secondary stage, abortion likely and if term completed, stillbirth likely; if fetus infected, symptoms of early congenital syphilis develop between 3 weeks and 3 months
A. Anogenital skin rash may be mistaken for diaper rash; rash on palms of hands and soles of feet
B. Snuffles—stuffiness of nose and mucopurulent discharge
C. Fissures about mouth
D. Splenomegaly, pseudoparalysis, osteochondritis; symptoms of late congenital syphilis begin between 6 and 9 years of age
   1. Hutchinson's teeth
   2. Saber shin
   3. Interstitial keratitis
   4. Eighth nerve deafness
   5. Juvenile paresis
6. **Cytomegalovirus (CMV)**
Also known as cytomegalic inclusion disease (CID)
A. Congenital infection due to virus crossing the placental barrier

1. Virus may be present in oropharyngeal secretions and urine of mother who appears to be asymptomatic
2. May range from mild manifestation of disease to those resulting in fatality
   a. Enlarged liver
   b. Enlarged spleen
   c. Microcephaly
   d. Mental retardation
   e. Motor disability
   f. Jaundice
   g. Petechiae
   h. Chorioretinitis
   i. Cerebral calcification
3. No known specific treatment
4. Infants may be isolated while in nursery
5. Care for infant should not be given by pregnant personnel
B. Acquired
   1. Associated with debilitating diseases
      a. Pneumonia
      b. Infectious mononucleosis
      c. Kidney transplant
      d. Need for transfusions
   2. Other disease condition receives usual therapy
7. **Measles (rubeola)**
Worldwide distribution; endemic and epidemic; incidence in the United States decreased due to immunization
A. Etiology—a filtrable virus whose precise classification is undetermined
B. Transmission—respiratory route, direct contact
C. Incubation period—10 to 14 days
D. Symptoms—coryza, conjunctivitis, lacrimation, sneezing, fever 104° to 105° F., dyspnea, photophobia, Koplik's spots in mouth, skin rash followed by fine desquamation
E. Diagnosis—clinical signs, history of exposure; laboratory tests that may be used include examination for leukopenia, hemagglutination inhibition antibody test; differential diagnosis important
F. Complications—rare; usually due to bacterial invasion
   1. Otitis media
   2. Bronchopneumonia
   3. Bronchitis
   4. Encephalitis
G. Treatment—none in uncomplicated cases; symptomatic and supportive measures may include
   1. Sedative cough mixture

2. Nonimmunized children may be given immune human gamma globulin within 1 week following exposure; not effective after onset of disease

H. Nursing
1. Isolation for 5 to 7 days after appearance of skin rash
2. Medical asepsis
3. No bright lights
4. Avoiding use of soap and water during exanthem stage
5. Tepid sponges for fever (no alcohol)
6. Diet liquid during febrile period
7. Observing for increase in temperature, cyanosis, dyspnea, croup, or convulsions

I. Prevention—young infants have passive immunity
1. Measles vaccine given to newborn infants extends period of passive immunity
2. Active acquired immunity at 9 to 12 months; one injection of live attenuated measles vaccine of Edmonson B strain is used with gamma globulin, or Schwarz strain without gamma globulin; may last for life

8. **Mumps (epidemic parotitis)**
Worldwide occurrence

A. Etiology—filtrable virus of myxovirus group
B. Transmission—by respiratory system, direct or indirect contact, spread by droplet infection, possibly droplet nuclei and urine from infected persons
C. Incubation period 12 to 26 days, usually 14 to 21 days
D. Symptoms
1. Headache
2. Anorexia
3. Fever may reach 104° F.
4. Swelling of parotid gland; salivary glands may be involved
5. Pain
E. Diagnosis—clinical signs; laboratory tests may include complement-fixation and hemagglutination inhibition antibody tests; tissue culture methods use oral secretions, urine, cerebrospinal fluid; skin test not diagnostic
F. Complications
1. Orchitis and oophoritis most common; other glands may be affected
2. Disease implicated in abortion and birth defects
G. Treatment—none; complete bed rest; other treatment symptomatic and supportive
H. Nursing—isolation until swelling subsides, concurrent disinfection, liquid or soft diet
I. Prevention—active acquired immunity with mumps virus vaccine, live
1. Military forces
2. Other adults
3. All children over 1 year of age
4. Should not be given during pregnancy
5. Should not be given to persons sensitive to egg protein or neomycin
6. Mumps skin test not reliable indication of immunity

9. **Poliomyelitis (infantile paralysis)**
Endemic worldwide; decline in the United States, with about 50 cases reported annually

A. Etiology—one of 3 serotypes of poliovirus classified as types 1, 2, and 3; type 1 causes most epidemics
B. Transmission—not completely resolved; believed to be by oral route by direct and indirect contact
C. Incubation period—unknown; believed to be 3 to 35 days with an average of 7 to 12 days
D. Symptoms and forms of disease
1. Abortive—cannot support diagnosis; onset abrupt, headache, fever, nausea, vomiting, anorexia; may recover in 24 hours
2. Nonparalytic—all of above symptoms with stiffness of neck, back, and pain
3. Paralytic—above symptoms with paralysis
   a. Spinal and bulbar forms; involvement depends upon part of nervous system affected
   b. Spinobulbar—combination of spinal and bulbar
E. Diagnosis—clinical diagnosis difficult; stool specimens during first 10 days, spinal fluid examination, complement-fixation tests
F. Complications
1. Respiratory failure
2. Circulatory collapse
3. Bacterial infection
4. Electrolyte imbalance
5. Paralysis of bladder plus retention of urine
6. Abdominal distention
G. Treatment—no specific therapy; symptomatic and supportive care based on

individual patient needs; team of specialists required

H. Nursing—isolation for 7 days with medical asepsis (p. 567)
1. Firm mattress, fracture boards, no pillow
2. Personal hygiene
3. Proper positioning
4. Hot packing
5. Nutritious diet
6. Care may include respirator care
7. Convalescence and restorative care may be prolonged

I. Prevention—epidemiologic investigation; immunization
1. Inactivated poliovaccine (Salk)—is begun at 1 to 2 months, 3 injections of 1 ml. each at 4- to 6-week intervals; patient may be given quadruple vaccine (DPT and polio); reinforcing dose required at 7 months and at 2- to 3-year intervals
2. Live attenuated poliovirus vaccine (Sabin oral)—given at 1 to 2 months or between 4 and 5 months, dropped on tongue of infant; 2 feedings of trivalent vaccine or 3 feedings of monovalent vaccine at 4- to 6-week intervals
3. Vaccine may be administered to adults who are at risk, military personnel, and overseas travelers; also given in epidemics

10. **Rabies (hydrophobia)**
Worldwide incidence; about 5 cases in the United States annually
A. Etiology—disease of wild and domestic animals transmitted to humans; unclassified neurotropic viral agent
B. Transmission—inoculation by bite of infected animal; airborne transmission believed possible
C. Incubation period—variable, 4 weeks to 1 year; in dogs, 3 to 8 weeks
D. Symptoms—virus attacks brain; three phases of disease
1. Prodromal period with headache, malaise, nausea, sore throat, fever 100° to 103° F., rapid pulse rate, mental depression, numbness and tingling about site of wound, photophobia, sensitiveness to exteroceptive stimuli
2. Excitation period—irritability, restlessness, anxiety, apprehension, spasm of muscles of swallowing and respiration, drooling, spitting, manic behavior,

convulsions, dyspnea, apnea, cyanosis, death due to cardiac failure
3. Paralytic phase—stupor, coma, progressive paralysis, death
E. Diagnosis—clinical signs, history, fluorescent antibody test for antibodies in blood serum
F. Treatment—none; always fatal; therapy symptomatic, heavy sedation, antispasmodic and analgesic drugs
G. Nursing—isolate to control environment; wear gown, gloves, and mask; preserve medical asepsis; protect from self-injury; give continuous care; no running water, bathing; I.V. fluids should not be visible to the patient
H. Prevention
1. Control disease in animals
2. Preexposure immunization with duck embryo rabies vaccine for high-risk groups: weekly injection of 1 ml. for 3 weeks, and 1 ml. 5 to 6 months later; some variation in schedules
3. If person exposed, 1 ml. of vaccine given; if exposure is severe, injections are given for 10 to 20 days
4. Postexposure Semple killed virus vaccine (Pasteur treatment) may cause encephalomyelitis; rabies hyperimmune serum given with rabies vaccine; sensitization tests made prior to administration; duck embryo vaccine being used more extensively for postexposure treatment; contraindications in allergy

11. **Rubella (German measles)**
Usually very mild; occurs in epidemics, worldwide; in 1964, 1.8 million cases in the United States
A. Etiology—filtrable pseudoparamyxovirus related to virus causing measles
B. Transmission—direct contact with droplet infection
C. Incubation period—14 to 21 days
D. Symptoms—variable; malaise, coryza, headache, sore throat, fever 101° to 104° F., conjunctivitis, tender lymph nodes, pale pink macular skin rash
E. Diagnosis—may be difficult; hemagglutination-inhibition antibody test to evaluate immunity
F. Treatment—none; therapy symptomatic; gamma globulin being advised against, but is used by some physicians
G. Complications—self-limiting arthritis; disease occurring in first 14 weeks of preg-

nancy causes serious defects in 15% to 20% of offspring, and in 50% if during first 4 weeks of pregnancy; increased incidence of abortion and stillbirth

H. Nursing—isolation for 7 days after rash; concurrent disinfection; isolation for newborn with congenital rubella

I. Prevention—immune human gamma globulin may be given to children first 4 or 5 days after exposure to modify disease

   1. Live rubella virus vaccine may be administered to children between the ages of 1 year and puberty—first priority

   2. Adolescent boys and adult males—lower priority

   3. Vaccine should not be given to pregnant women or to adolescent girls because of danger of undiagnosed pregnancy

   4. If vaccine given to women of childbearing age, pregnancy must be avoided for following 2 months

12. Smallpox (variola)
Distribution worldwide; last cases in the United States, 1953

A. Etiology—filtrable virus of poxvirus group; disease classified as variola major, variola minor (alastrium), and varioloid

B. Transmission—direct contact; possibility of insect vectors

C. Incubation period—average 10 to 12 days

D. Symptoms—sudden onset, aching of head, back, and extremities, malaise, chills, vomiting, fever 105° F., prostration, delirium, sore throat, skin rash that progresses through stages of macule, papule, vesicle, pustule, crust

E. Diagnosis—based on clinical signs, characteristics and distribution of skin lesions; difficult during preeruptive stage; differential diagnosis may be problem in some patients

F. Complications—pulmonary edema, heart failure, pneumonia, septicemia; abortion and hemorrhage complicate pregnancy

G. Treatment—none; therapy symptomatic and supportive, with analgesics, narcotics, electrolyte replacement, antibiotics to prevent complications

H. Nursing—isolation until all crusts are off; strict medical asepsis, autoclaving of linens; extra care of skin, mouth, and eyes; avoid soap-and-water bathing during eruptive stage, use warm oil on crusts to relieve pruritus; observe pregnant

women for onset of labor; no danger to nurse who is successfully vaccinated

I. Prevention [elective]—vaccination after 12 months of age and booster every 5 years; required for foreign travel; oral prophylactic agent 33T57, Marboran, under investigation and said to be highly effective; vaccination and quarantine of all contacts for 16 days

13. Varicella (chickenpox)
Worldwide distribution

A. Etiology—herpesvirus varicella

B. Transmission—direct contact with droplet infection

C. Incubation period—14 to 21 days

D. Symptoms—malaise, headache, fever, aching, skin rash that appears in crops and goes through progressive stages of macule, papule, vesicle, crust; vesicles on mucous membrane of mouth, pruritus; disease may be mild or severe

E. Complications—rare; secondary infection due to *Staphylococcus* or *Streptococcus*

F. Diagnosis—clinical signs, history of exposure, laboratory examination of vesicular fluid by tissue culture technique

G. Treatment—palliative: antipruritic lotion; antipyretics for fever

H. Nursing—isolation not required; no special care

I. Prevention—no immunologic agent; avoid exposure; children may be excluded from school; policy varies among states

14. Toxoplasmosis (parasitic disease)

A. *Toxoplasma gondii*, a protozoan parasite found in all mammals and in many birds and reptiles is cause

B. Transmission

   1. Excreta of animals most common source

   2. Sometimes associated with immunosuppressive therapy, Hodgkin's disease, or neoplasms

C. Incubation period

   1. Uncertain

   2. May be several months

D. Congenital symptoms

   1. Chorioretinitis

   2. Jaundice

   3. Anemia

   4. Seizures

   5. Hydrocephaly or microcephaly

   6. Lymphadenopathy

E. Acquired

   1. Mononucleosis-like syndrome

   2. Fever

3. Rash
4. Pneumonia
5. Encephalitis
6. Myocarditis
F. Prognosis
1. Acquired—severe cases may be fatal
2. Congenital—fatal, or person may be permanently handicapped
15. **Staphylococcal infections** (p. 323)
16. **Brucellosis** (p. 324)
17. **Tuberculosis** (p. 341)
18. **Hepatitis** (p. 379)
19. **Encephalitis** (p. 408)
20. **For other communicable diseases** that affect both adults and children see Chapter 9 on medical-surgical nursing

REVIEW QUESTIONS FOR PEDIATRIC NURSING
Multiple choice

Read each question carefully and consider all possible answers. When you have decided which answer is best, blacken in the corresponding space on the answer sheet. There is only one best answer for each question (or implied question).

Situation: Baby Star, newly admitted to the newborn nursery, had an initial Apgar score of 4. Questions 1 through 10 relate to this infant.

1. The nurse interprets this score to indicate
   (a) Vigorous infant
   (b) Depressed infant
   (c) Respiration readily established
   (d) Respiration rate at least 20
   1. a and c   3. a, c, and d
   2. b and d   4. b only
2. Immediate critical observations for Apgar scoring include
   (a) Respiratory effort
   (b) Heart rate
   (c) Voiding and passing meconium
   (d) Moro reflex
   1. a and b   3. a, b, and d
   2. a, b, and c   4. All of above
3. Within 3 minutes after birth the normal range of heart rate for this infant may be
   1. 100 to 180   3. 120 to 140
   2. 120 to 160   4. 100 to 120
4. Within this same period the normal respiratory rate may soar to
   1. 100   3. 60
   2. 80   4. 50
5. The nurse may obtain a Moro reflex by
   (a) Creating a bang noise
   (b) Lessening support of infant's head when it is raised
   (c) Stimulating the feet
   (d) Grasping a hand of the infant
   1. a and b   3. a and d
   2. a and c   4. All of above

6. Moro reflex is marked by
   1. Extension of arms
   2. Extension of legs
   3. Adduction of arms
   4. Abduction and then adduction of the arms
7. At 10 hours of life Baby Star has a large amount of mucus and becomes slightly cyanotic. The nurse
   (a) Gives infant oxygen
   (b) Inserts Levin tube
   (c) Notes it may be a period of reactivity
   (d) Suctions the mucus as needed
   1. a only   3. c and d
   2. a and c   4. All of above
8. During his initial feeding Baby Star will probably
   (a) Reject the feeding
   (b) Have some gagging and choking
   (c) Have good rooting reflex
   (d) Have some regurgitation
   1. a and b   3. b and d
   2. a, b, and c   4. b, c, and d
9. When Baby Star's mother removed his blanket and started to examine her infant, she became concerned because he assumed a fencing position as she turned his head; the mother suspected neurologic damage. The nurse would discuss with the mother that
   (a) This is normal response
   (b) The doctor had been notified of this suspicious response
   (c) Reflex disappears around 6 months of age
   (d) Tonic neck reflex rarely indicates neurologic damage in the newborn
   1. a only   3. b and d
   2. a and c   4. a, c, and d
10. On his discharge from the hospital Baby Star's mother asks again about cord base care. The nurse would explain that the
    (a) Cord band helps prevent hernias
    (b) Cord will be detached before 2 weeks of age
    (c) Cleanliness of cord base is advised
    (d) Cord base area should be kept dry
    1. a and b   3. b, c, and d
    2. a, b, and c   4. All of above

Situation: The nurse brought the summary sheet of information about little newborn Nelda and presented it to the staff on the pediatric unit. It is noted that Nelda seems to breathe through her mouth most of the time and occasionally appears to be cyanotic. Questions 11 through 15 relate to this infant on the pediatric unit.

11. Which of the following may give the nurse some clue as to Nelda's problem and a possible plan of nursing care?
    (a) Vaginal delivery, ROA
    (b) Membranes ruptured 15 hours prior to delivery
    (c) Mother had some analgesia during early labor
    (d) Gestational period of 248 days
    1. a, b, and c   3. d only
    2. a, c, and d   4. All of above
12. Which of the following may give some clues as to the possible problem that would necessitate intensive care for this infant?

(a) Birth weight of 3,500 grams
(b) Apgar score of 3
(c) 20 ml. of milky-colored fluid in stomach at time of birth
(d) Umbilical cord having two vessels
1. a, b, and c 3. a, b, and d
2. b and c 4. b and d

13. Among known causes related to cyanosis in the newborn for which the nurse observes and notes the color are
(a) High levels of hemoglobin
(b) Bronchial obstruction
(c) Wilms' tumor
(d) Nasopharyngeal obstruction
1. a, b, and c 3. b and d
2. a and d 4. a, b, and d

14. The physician diagnoses the problem as bilateral choanal atresia, an anomaly located in the
(a) Nasopharynx
(b) Intestinal tract
(c) Pharynx and larynx
(d) Anal area
1. a only 3. b and d
2. a and c 4. d only

15. While feeding little Nelda, the nurse notices that she
(a) Chokes on her feedings
(b) Requires frequent rest periods
(c) Lacks a swallow reflex
(d) Does not appear to be hungry
1. a, b, and d 3. a, b, and c
2. a and b 4. All of above

Situation: Another newborn in this infant unit is very jaundiced and the diagnosis is an Rh incompatibility problem. Questions 16 through 18 relate to this infant.

16. While caring for this infant the nurse may notice that
(a) He appears to be slightly edematous
(b) He refuses glucose water as an initial feeding
(c) He sleeps quietly
(d) His abdomen is slightly distended
1. a and c 3. a, c, and d
2. a, b, and c 4. b, c, and d

17. The high bilirubin level that necessitated immediate medical and nursing consideration was
(a) Unconjugated by the glucuronyl transferase enzyme
(b) Accompanied by anemia
(c) A neurologic threat
(d) Indirect Coombs-positive in infant
1. a and b 3. a, c, and d
2. a, b, and c 4. b, c, and d

18. Nursing care during the critical period is directed toward
(a) Maintaining a warm body temperature
(b) Preventing infection
(c) Lowering bilirubin levels
(d) Keeping the cord base and cord stump moist with sterile solution and gauze
1. a and c 3. a, b, and d
2. a, b, and c 4. All of above

19. When clinically manifest, ABO incompatibilities are more frequently mild than are Rh incompatibilities. ABO disease may be a threat to

1. Life and cerebral functioning
2. Life only
3. Cerebral function only
4. Normal physical growth

Situation: Another baby on this unit has Down's syndrome. Questions 20 to 22 relate to this situation.

20. Which of the following are known to be expected in this infant?
(a) Slow development
(b) Trisomy 21 (chromosome)
(c) Increased incidence of cardiac problems
(d) Proneness to respiratory infections
1. a and b 3. a, c, and d
2. a and c 4. All of above

21. Nursing of this infant presents the following requirements
(a) Frequent handling and rocking to keep him from crying
(b) Helping parents to learn about their child
(c) Teaching infant to nipple-feed
(d) Preventing aspiration of formula, by frequent bubbling
1. a and b 3. a, c, and d
2. a, b, and c 4. b, c, and d

22. Which of the following possibly presents least concern to this infant's parents?
(a) Their other children's reaction to the infant
(b) Their ability to give physical care to this infant
(c) Their decision on the present and future life of this child
(d) Their possible total rejection of this infant
1. b only 3. a and b
2. d only 4. b and c

23. A month-old infant on this unit appears to be lethargic and to be having some problem in digesting his formula feeding. These problems lead the nurse to look for
(a) Jaundice and convulsion, which may accompany phenylketonuria (PKU)
(b) Maple sugar odor of urine of PKU
(c) Drowsiness and jaundice of galactosemia
(d) Diarrhea and convulsions associated with galactosemia
1. a and c 3. c and d
2. a and b 4. c only

24. Galactosemia is similar to phenylketonuria in which of the following ways?
(a) Metabolism error is involved
(b) Diet must exclude cereals
(c) Mental retardation may occur if diet is not prescribed
(d) Transmission occurs by autosomal recessive genes
1. a, b, and c 3. b, c, and d
2. a, c, and d 4. All of above

25. Primary treatment of an infant who has an inherited inborn error problem consists mostly of
(a) Hormonal control
(b) Dietary control
(c) Controlled activities
(d) Sensory stimulation
1. a and b 3. b and c
2. b only 4. a and d

26. Which of the following can be associated with PKU (phenylketonuria)?
    (a) Mental retardation
    (b) Guthrie test
    (c) Transmission by an autosomal recessive gene
    (d) Possible detection in the first month of life
    1. a and b   3. b and c
    2. a and c   4. All of above

27. In working with a mother of an infant or child who has phenylketonuria the nurse should know
    (a) A low-phenylalanine diet is required
    (b) A phenylalanine-free diet is required
    (c) Phenylalanine can have another amino acid substitute for growth
    (d) Phenylalanine is necessary for growth
    1. a only   3. a and d
    2. a and c   4. b and c

28. Amounts of phenylalanine in equal amounts of foods vary in which ways?
    (a) Cereals are higher than fruits
    (b) Vegetables are usually lower than fruits
    (c) Soups are higher than fruits
    (d) Milk substitutes contain a balance of fats, carbohydrates, vitamins, and minerals
    1. a, b, and c   3. a, c, and d
    2. a, b, and d   4. All of above

29. A nurse can readily test urine for PKU with ferric chloride 5%
    (a) By use on fresh wet diaper
    (b) By noting that red gives a positive indication
    (c) By noting that green gives a positive indication
    (d) When the child is at least 6 weeks of age
    1. a and b   3. a, b, and d
    2. a and c   4. a, c, and d

30. Fat absorption and utilization is a problem noted in feeding
    (a) Premature infant
    (b) Infant and child with cystic fibrosis
    (c) Child who has been on hypoallergic, milk-free diet for eczema
    (d) In a teen-ager who has jaundice due to hepatitis
    1. a, b, and c   3. b, c, and d
    2. a, c, and d   4. All of above

31. When vomiting is uncontrolled in an infant, the nurse should observe for signs of
    1. Tetany
    2. Alkalosis
    3. Acidosis
    4. Hyperactivity

32. In talking with mother about vitamins, several points should be stressed
    (a) Balanced diet contains most essential vitamins
    (b) Vitamin D is produced through a chemical action when the skin is exposed to sunlight
    (c) Excess vitamin D intake may slow down linear growth
    (d) Vitamin C is found in cabbage as well as in orange juice

    (e) Breast milk contains large amounts of vitamin D
    1. a, b, c, and d   4. b, d, and e
    2. a, b, d, and e   5. All of above
    3. b, c, d, and e

33. A newborn of a few hours appears to be less cyanotic when he cries. The nurse should observe for
    1. Twitchings of the body for neural damage
    2. Equality of chest expansion for an atelectasis problem
    3. Heart rate for an atrioventricular septal defect
    4. Sternal retractions of respiratory distress syndrome

34. A mother talks to the nurse about her sick infant and she is disturbed because she did not realize the baby was ill. Which of the following is frequently the only sign of illness that her infant may have?
    1. Longer periods of sleep
    2. Grunting and rapid respirations
    3. Perspiring profusely
    4. Desire for increased fluids during the feedings

35. A small toddler is admitted to the hospital because of sudden hoarseness and an insistence on a continuous pattern of his somewhat unintelligible talking. In talking with the mother, the nurse will be particularly concerned about
    (a) Acute respiratory infection
    (b) Undetected laryngeal abnormality
    (c) Respiratory tract obstruction due to a foreign body
    (d) Retropharyngeal abscess
    1. a and b   3. c
    2. b and c   4. b and d

36. Febrile convulsions in children are not uncommon and
    (a) Frequently accompany an acute infection
    (b) Rarely occur after 4 years of age
    (c) May occur in minor illnesses
    (d) Cause is usually readily identified
    1. a and b   3. a, c, and d
    2. a, b, and c   4. b, c, and d

Situation: Loren E, age 14, is admitted to the hospital and is scheduled to have orthopedic surgery the following day. Questions 37 through 39 apply to this situation.

37. At the conclusion of visiting hours, Loren's mother hands the nurse a bottle of capsules and says, "These are for Loren's allergy. Will you be sure he takes one about 9 o'clock?" The nurse might best respond with which of the following statements?
    1. "One capsule at 9 P.M.? Of course, I will give it to him."
    2. "Did you ask the doctor if he should have this tonight?"
    3. "I am certain the doctor knows about Loren's allergy."
    4. "We will ask Loren's doctor to write an order so we can give this medication to him."

38. Postoperatively, Loren is to be given codeine

sulfate 1 gr. every 3 to 4 hours when necessary for relief of pain. An hour after he is given this medication, he complains of severe pain. Which of the following actions would the nurse best initiate?

1. Administer another dose of codeine, since it is a relatively safe drug
2. Tell Loren he cannot have any additional medication for 2 more hours
3. Report that Loren has an apparent idiosyncrasy to codeine
4. Request the physician to evaluate Loren's need for additional medication

39. About 8 hours later, Loren complains of itching. Antihistaminic drugs that may be ordered to relieve this symptom include which of the following?
    (a) Chlorpheniramine (Chlor-Trimeton)
    (b) Diphenhydramine (Benadryl)
    (c) Tripelennamine (Pyribenzamine)
    (d) Promethazine (Phenergan)
    1. a and c   3. a, b and c
    2. b and d   4. All of above

40. A young mother has been reading several books about the development and behavior of the newborn. The mother is concerned about an occasional twitching and some tremors of the baby. In order to discuss the matter intelligently with the mother, the nurse should know that tremors and twitching
    (a) Occur without obvious cause
    (b) Are a normal reflex
    (c) Accompany hypoglycemia
    (d) Are seen more frequently in premature infants
    1. a, b and c   3. a, c, and d
    2. a, b, and d   4. a and d

41. In talking with a mother about tremors and twitchings the nurse will no doubt discuss
    (a) Feeding patterns of the baby
    (b) Formula preparation
    (c) Some expected normal responses of the baby
    (d) Disease conditions that may be related to tremors or twitching
    1. a, b, and c   3. b, c, and d
    2. a, c, and d   4. All of above

42. A mother brings her week-old newborn to clinic because he continually regurgitates. Chalasia is suspected, and the nurse instructs the mother about
    (a) The value of frequent, small feedings
    (b) Keeping the infant in a sitting or semi-sitting position, particularly after feeding
    (c) Not permitting the child to cry
    (d) The possibility that the sphincter at the cardiac end of the stomach will probably function properly long before the baby learns to walk
    1. a, b, and c   3. b, c, and d
    2. a, b, and d   4. All of above

43. It is expected that, after some surgical intervention for atelectasis, lung expansion will occur within
    1. An hour   3. 4 hours
    2. 3 hours   4. 12 to 48 hours

44. Normal expected responses of the infant,

which are noticed by the nurse following the surgical procedure for atelectasis, include
    (a) Tachypnea
    (b) Hyperpnea
    (c) Dyspnea
    (d) Cyanosis
    1. a and c   3. b, c, and d
    2. b and c   4. None of above

45. An infant scheduled for surgery is diagnosed as having a diaphragmatic hernia. Some emergency measures that are omitted at this time include
    (a) Positive pressure oxygen by mask
    (b) Positive pressure oxygen by intratracheal tube
    (c) Increased oxygen concentration by any method
    (d) Humidity of 40%
    1. a and b   3. a, c, and d
    2. a, b, and d   4. a, b, and c

46. A young mother has become concerned about her 9-month-old infant's development. The baby no longer has the same strong grasp that he had shortly after birth; nor does he have a similar response to startle that he had at an early age. The nurse should discuss with the mother that
    (a) Neurologic examination is desirable
    (b) Failure of these responses may be related to mental retardation
    (c) These responses are usually replaced by a voluntary activity at 5 to 6 months of age
    (d) The infant needs additional sensory stimulation to aid in the return of these responses
    1. a and b   3. c only
    2. a and c   4. a, b, and d

47. When picked up by either the mother or the nurse, a 9-month-old infant screams. The scream seems to be that of pain. At his clinic visit the nurse will note and talk particularly to the mother about
    (a) The infant's food and specific vitamins given to him, including vitamins C and D
    (b) Accidents and injuries and the importance of their prevention
    (c) Any other behavior of the infant, such as tremors or convulsions, that may have been noticed by the mother
    (d) Limiting the play time and activities that this infant has with other children in the family
    1. a and b   3. a, c, and d
    2. a, b, and c   4. b, c, and d

48. The physician asked a mother in a well baby clinic to stay in a cubicle area. This mother became upset, for she thought that disinterest in foods and formula by the infant was a normal phase and that her infant was not ill, as was stated by the physician. The nurse would explain to the mother that
    (a) Lack of appetite may precede fever in the infant
    (b) Infants and small children often vomit at the onset of an infection
    (c) After several months of age the baby will respond more severely to respira-

tory infections than will older children in the family

(d) Usually when the baby is not feeling well or is ill there should be no plan to change feeding patterns by the introduction of new foods
  1. a and b
  2. a, b, and c
  3. a, b, and d
  4. All of above

Situation: At the time of his birth the tube passed into Baby Thomas' stomach for routine aspiration of fluid met with some obstruction, and an atresia was suspected. Questions 49 to 51 apply to Baby Thomas.

49. In view of the situation, the nurse was careful to note
  (a) Abdominal distention
  (b) Excessive salivation and drooling
  (c) Cyanosis, if any
  (d) Coughing and gagging
  1. a, b, and c
  2. a, b, and d
  3. a, c, and d
  4. b, c, and d

50. Inasmuch as his weight was only 1,600 grams and his condition did not warrant primary repair, Baby Thomas was scheduled for two-stage surgery. His 2 post-surgery tubes were primarily to
  (a) Remove secretions from the trachea and bronchi
  (b) Prevent aspiration pneumonia
  (c) Prevent distention, by use of gastrostomy tube
  (d) Provide feeding, by a gastrostomy tube
  1. a and b
  2. b and c
  3. b and d
  4. a and d

51. Nursing care for him at this time is directed toward
  (a) Keeping Baby Thomas as quiet as possible
  (b) Providing high humidity, at least 80%
  (c) Preventing infection
  (d) Providing some normal sensory stimulation
  1. a and c
  2. b and c
  3. a, b, and d
  4. b, c, and d

Situation: At 2 weeks of age Baby Williams began to vomit after his feedings and was admitted to the hospital for observation with a tentative diagnosis of pyloric stenosis. Questions 52 and 53 relate to this situation.

52. The nurse was careful to note
  (a) Signs of dehydration
  (b) Coughing and gagging after feeding
  (c) Force with which undigested formula was vomited
  (d) Quality of cry
  1. a, b, and c
  2. a and c
  3. a and d
  4. a, c, and d

53. Surgery was performed and Baby Williams' condition was good. The nurse caring for him noticed that his postoperative orders were similar to those for other infants having such surgery and included
  (a) Withholding of all feedings for the first 24 hours
  (b) Frequent small feedings of glucose water
  (c) Additional glucose feedings after the first 24 hours
  (d) Diluted formula feeding 4 to 6 hours after surgery
  1. a and b
  2. a, b, and c
  3. a and c
  4. b and d

54. Results of deprivation studies on infants in institutions indicate that the major depriving factor in the situation is
  1. Absence of interaction with a mother figure
  2. Lack of multisensory inputs
  3. Care provided only by mother substitute
  4. Lack of play objects

55. Which of the following aspects of development have been repeatedly found to be most seriously affected by continuing deprivation in the environment?
  (a) Language development
  (b) Physical growth
  (c) Emotional response
  (d) Social development
  1. a and b
  2. a, b, and c
  3. b, c, and d
  4. All of above

56. A significant development in the past quarter century concerns the steady growth of evidence that the quality of parental care which a child receives in his earliest years is of vital importance for his future mental health. Absence of the warm, continuous relationship is called maternal deprivation. It has been found that
  (a) A child may suffer from maternal deprivation in his natural home
  (b) Most children in institutions suffer maternal deprivation
  (c) Most children respond alike to maternal deprivation
  (d) Maternal deprivation is inevitable if mother and child are separated
  1. a and b
  2. a, b, and c
  3. b, c, and d
  4. All of above

57. Literature on the effects of maternal deprivation describes infants who have been in an institution for some time as
  1. Extremely active
  2. Prone to illnesses
  3. Very responsive to stimuli
  4. Obese

58. Studies of young children institutionalized for some time indicate that they show signs of retarded development. Not all aspects of development are equally affected. The *least* affected is
  1. Neuromuscular development
  2. Hearing
  3. Ability to understand
  4. Ability to express himself

59. The immediate effect of return of a young child to his mother after long separation has been observed as
  1. Hostile reaction toward mother
  2. Excessive demands
  3. Cheerful but shallow attachment to any adult
  4. Apathetic withdrawal from all emotional ties to mother

60. Conclusions drawn as a result of studying the histories of children who early in life have suffered prolonged maternal deprivation indicate that these children

1. Are unable to love
2. Establish warm relationships quickly with mother substitute
3. Recall past experiences vividly
4. Are particularly conscious of time

61. What is the outstanding characteristic of growth and development?
    1. It occurs in a uniform manner
    2. Each individual follows a unique pattern
    3. It is a simple process
    4. It rarely influences behavior

62. What significance does understanding growth and development have for the nurse?
    1. It has little significance in an ill child
    2. Most children of the same age can be treated alike
    3. A keen appreciation of human variability is essential
    4. It has little effect on nursing care plans

63. Learnings associated with a particular stage of development often are referred to as "developmental tasks." What is characteristic about these tasks?
    1. There is no uniform time for learning a task
    2. Tasks are learned at the same age in children
    3. Tasks occur with predictable rhythm
    4. Most developmental tasks are learned by school age

64. When is toilet training best accomplished?
    1. When sphincter control is sufficiently mature
    2. Before 1 year when the child enjoys sitting still
    3. As soon as the child can communicate
    4. Whenever the mother has sufficient time

65. Parents of a newborn with a cleft lip and palate are usually very disturbed about the appearance of their infant. Modern treatment provides excellent corrective care and may include
    (a) Prosthesis for palate until repair can be made
    (b) Lip repair early, frequently at 1 month of age
    (c) Palate repair after the child has some teeth
    (d) Speech therapy until at least 5 years of age
    1. a and b   3. b, c, and d
    2. a, b, and c   4. All of above

66. Nursing care for the infant with a surgical lip repair includes
    (a) Keeping the suture area clean and dry
    (b) Placing the infant in a semisitting position
    (c) Keeping the infant from crying
    (d) Spoon-feeding the first 2 days after surgery
    1. a and b   3. a and c
    2. a, b, and c   4. a, b, and d

Situation: Mr. and Mrs. B were emotionally upset when their baby girl Sue was born with a cleft palate and double cleft lip. Questions 67 to 72 apply to this infant.

67. How could the nurse give the most support to the parents?

1. Discourage them from talking about the baby
2. Encourage them to express their worries and fears
3. Tell them not to worry, because the defect could be repaired
4. Show them postoperative photographs of babies who had similar defects

68. What is the most critical factor in the immediate care of Sue after repair of the lip?
    1. Maintenance of a patent airway
    2. Administration of drugs to reduce oral secretions
    3. Administration of parenteral fluids
    4. Prevention of vomiting

69. During Sue's hospitalization the parents had several talks with the doctor, social worker, and nurse. How would the parents be encouraged to cooperate?
    1. Limit their questions to Sue's care
    2. Discuss any problem that bothers them
    3. Plan for special education for Sue
    4. Refrain from discussing Sue's condition with her brothers

70. At 2 years of age Sue returned for palate surgery. What was the most important factor in preparing her for this experience?
    1. Her previous hospital visits
    2. Gratification of all her wishes
    3. Never being left with strangers
    4. Assurance of affection and security

71. A toothbrush was not used on Sue immediately after palate surgery because
    1. The suture line might be injured
    2. She was not accustomed to a brush at home
    3. Her mouth was too small after palate closure
    4. It might be frightening to her

72. The nurse, in her attempt to provide assurance for the patient and parents, may increase their fears. Which is the best response to parents?
    1. "There seems to be little wrong with your child."
    2. "Don't worry about the child."
    3. "Tell me why you feel worried."
    4. "You should ask the doctor."

73. What does make-believe play in the hospital provide for a child?
    1. Opportunity to accept a mother substitute
    2. Opportunity to reject the reality of the hospital
    3. Opportunity to learn to know other children more quickly
    4. Opportunity to cope with his fears

74. The maintenance of fluid and electrolyte balance is more critical in children than in adults because
    1. Renal function is immature in children
    2. Cellular metabolism is less stable than in adults
    3. The proportion of water in the body is less than in adults
    4. The daily fluid requirement per unit of body weight is greater than in adults

75. What is the most critical factor confronting the nurse in the administration of intravenous fluids to a small, dehydrated infant?

1. Maintenance of the prescribed rate of flow
2. Maintenance of the fluid at body temperature
3. Calculation of the total intake
4. Maintenance of the height of the column of fluid

76. If a drug is to be given by intravenous injection, which of the following is recommended?
    1. Using the antecubital vein
    2. Replacing the needle used to withdraw the drug from the vial
    3. Being honest with the child
    4. Injecting the dose over a 15-minute period

77. Studies of children's responses to hospitalization indicate that much of the resulting trauma can be attributed to
    1. Anxiety and fear of mutilation
    2. Fear of hospital personnel
    3. The illness itself
    4. Strange surroundings

78. During nursing care to the small child in the hospital, home, or clinic, the child should
    (a) Be asked to cooperate with all procedures
    (b) Be told firmly what he is to do
    (c) Be told what is expected of him
    (d) Have recognition for his cooperative behavior
    1. a and b   3. b, c, and d
    2. a and c   4. All of above

79. The mother's participation in the care of the sick infant or child requires
    (a) Telling her when procedures will be painful
    (b) Daily conference with the physician
    (c) Letting her hold the child at crucial times, thus lending ego support
    (d) Including her in implementing the plan of nursing care
    1. a and b   3. a, b, and c
    2. a, c, and d   4. All of above

80. Nursing observations of the infant as well as those reported by the mother may be some of the first clues of a genitourinary tract problem. These observations include
    (a) His diaper appears to be always wet
    (b) He voids only small amounts of urine
    (c) He appears to have some difficulty in voiding
    (d) His bladder appears to be distended
    1. a, b, and c   3. b, c, and d
    2. a, b, and d   4. All of above

81. In the care of the child with cystic fibrosis much of the nursing is directed toward
    (a) Promoting postural drainage
    (b) Controlling humidity
    (c) Helping the child conserve his energy
    (d) Preventing any coughing
    1. a and b   3. b and c
    2. a, b, and c   4. b, c, and d

82. The problem of cystic fibrosis is sometimes first noted by the newborn nursery nurse because of
    (a) Increased heart rate
    (b) Feeding problems
    (c) Abdominal distention
    (d) Excessive crying
    1. a and b   3. a, c, and d
    2. b and c   4. b, c, and d

83. A sad-looking little boy of 3 years has been readmitted to the hospital because of celiac disease. His inability to absorb some foods and his foul-smelling stools present problems to the nursing staff and to his mother. Most of the nursing problems arise because he
    (a) Is irritable
    (b) Sleeps poorly
    (c) Lacks appetite
    (d) Has apparent mental retardation
    1. a and b   3. b, c, and d
    2. a, b, and c   4. All of above

84. The nurse works with others on the health team to help the mother of the child in question 83 understand that
    (a) Her son is prone to infections
    (b) He should have moderate amounts of protein foods
    (c) He should be given foods that he seems to tolerate
    (d) New foods should be introduced slowly
    1. a and b   3. a, c, and d
    2. a, b, and c   4. All of above

85. Nursing of a small child with megacolon (Hirschsprung's disease) consists primarily of
    (a) Giving relief by use of enemas and rectal irrigations (tap water)
    (b) Giving relief by use of enemas and rectal irrigations (isotonic solutions)
    (c) Keeping him in a semisitting to a sitting position (relief of respiratory distress)
    (d) Giving frequent and smaller feedings
    1. a, c, and d   3. b, c, and d
    2. a and c   4. b and d

86. Malignancies in children ages 1 to 14 are not uncommon, and recent reports show that
    (a) The mortality rate is 7.8 per 100,000
    (b) The mortality rate has shown a sharp decrease in the past few years
    (c) They account for approximately 20% of deaths in this age group
    (d) Malignancy is one of the top three causes of death in the United States in this age group
    1. a and b   3. b, c, and d
    2. a and d   4. All of above

87. Many of the nursing problems that must be met in caring for the leukemic child are focused on
    (a) Relieving the irritability of the child through patience and consistent behavior by the nurse
    (b) Accepting parents' manner of expressing their grief
    (c) Relieving the boredom of hospitalization by changing his routine pattern of care
    (d) Permitting usual play activities that include those which rely on use of the larger muscles
    1. a and b   3. b and d
    2. b and c   4. a, b, and d

88. The child with leukemia has many of the same problems as the child with almost any kind of anemia, and nursing measures include
    (a) Helping the child avoid bumps that cause bruises
    (b) Protecting the child from infection
    (c) Providing extra-large servings of foods at regular mealtimes

(d) Providing rest periods for the child
    1. a and b   3. a, b, and d
    2. a and c   4. All of above

89. The primary reason for using prednisone in the treatment of acute leukemia in children is that is it able to
    1. Suppress mitoses in lymphocytes
    2. Reduce irradiation edema
    3. Decrease inflammation
    4. Increase appetite and sense of well-being

90. A combination of drugs, which includes Vincristine (Oncovin) and prednisone, is prescribed. The toxic symptoms that are most likely to occur are
    1. Neurologic
    2. Irreversible alopecia
    3. Anemia and fever
    4. Gastrointestinal

91. In teaching a mother about the quality of milk for her infant the nurse would emphasize
  (a) Evaporated milk contains all food constituents except vitamin D
  (b) Cow's milk contains more protein than human milk
  (c) Human milk contains more iron than cow's milk
  (d) Dried milk is lacking in vitamins A and D
  (e) Human milk produces small fine curds
    1. a, b, and c   4. b, c, d, and e
    2. a, c, and d   5. All of above
    3. b, d, and e

92. Mothers will need to know that the quantity of intake for the infant
  (a) Will be determined to a great extent by the baby himself
  (b) Usually is 3½ to 4 ounces fluid per pound baby weight
  (c) Usually is 2½ to 3 ounces fluid per pound baby weight
  (d) Should provide for a weight gain of about 4 ounces per week in his first 3 months of life
    1. a and b   3. b and c
    2. a and c   4. b and d

93. Supplemental iron given to an infant or child
  (a) May be stored
  (b) Should be mixed with fruit juices
  (c) Should be given in small doses
  (d) Is more irritating to intestinal than to gastric mucosa
    1. a, b, and c   4. b and c
    2. a, b, and d   5. b, c, and d
    3. a and c

94. John, age 4, and Jim, age 7, may have which of the following as common experiences to hospitalization?
  (a) Fear of pain
  (b) Fear of body mutilation
  (c) Punishment fantasy
  (d) Separation anxiety
    1. a, b, and c   4. b, c, and d
    2. a, b, and d   5. All of above
    3. a, c, and d

95. Jean and Bill, both toddlers, will have long-term hospitalizations. Nursing for these would include
  (a) Social play with each other
  (b) Placement of cribs so they may have their own kind of communications with each other
  (c) Assignment of the same nurse to provide care each day
  (d) Provision of TV as one means of simulating normal home environment
    1. a, b, and c   3. b and c
    2. a, b, and d   4. a, c, and d

96. Which of the following would the nurse systematically observe for, in the growth and development of the child?
  (a) Trust, autonomy, industry, intimacy, identity
  (b) Trust, autonomy, initiative, industry, identity
  (c) Fine and gross motor activities
  (d) Language
  (e) Intelligence level
    1. a, b, and d   3. b, c, and d
    2. a, c, d, and e   4. b, c, d, and e

97. Carol Ann (questions 97 to 99), who looks to be about 2 years old, wears an anxious look; one arm hangs limp; she has multiple bruises, some of which appear to be old; and, with her noncrying and nonwhimpering behavior, she sits by her father in the emergency room. The nurse would
  (a) Observe her silent reaction to injuries
  (b) Observe her reaction to her father
  (c) Talk about the injury, as a possible abuse, to the father
  (d) Look for discrepancies in history given by father
    1. a, b, and c   3. a, b, and d
    2. a, c, and d   4. b, c, and d

98. Her father says she has shown evidence of retardation because she did not walk until almost 14 months of age, is not completely toilet trained, and uses only a small number of words when speaking. The nurse screens her development on the Denver (Denver Developmental Screening Tool) tool for
  (a) Fine motor
  (b) Language
  (c) Personal-social
  (d) Gross motor
    1. a, b, and c   3. a, c, and d
    2. a, b, and d   4. All of above

99. The nurse learns from the screening that Carol Ann is within the normal range for three of the four categories. With this as a clue, the nurse might suspect child abuse and would further observe and seek information regarding
  (a) Fear of parent by child
  (b) Clinics or physicians where child received care
  (c) Social play with another toddler in the ER
  (d) Her pattern of weight gain
    1. a, b, and c   3. a, c, and d
    2. a, b, and d   4. b, c, and d

100. Rodney (questions 100 and 101) is a healthy muscular toddler of 14 months who cried as though he had severe pains in his belly and his mother wondered if he had eaten some-

thing that would upset him, because his stools had mucus and a little blood. The nurse suspects he has intussusception as she screens him for care in the pediatric emergency room. Clues for this were

(a) Healthy state of appearance other than pain
(b) Sex and age of the patient
(c) Character of the stool
(d) Apparent pain
    1. a, b, and c   3. b, c, and d
    2. a, b, and d   4. All of above

101. She makes a decision, based on these clues, as to immediacy and kind of treatment for his problem
(a) Refer to physician for immediate care
(b) Place ice bag on abdomen while waiting for physician
(c) Have mother rock infant while waiting for physician
(d) Recognize this as an emergency
    1. a, b, and d   3. a and d
    2. a, c, and d   4. All of above

102. One of the most frequent problems encountered by a child is that of an infection of his respiratory tract. Many of these problems require
(a) Warm moist air
(b) Cool moist air
(c) Forcing of fluids
(d) Antibiotics
    1. a and c   3. a or b, c, and d
    2. b, c, and d   4. a, c, and d

Questions 103 to 105 relate to the problem identified in 103.

103. One of the most bothersome health problems of the teen-ager is that of scoliosis. It is
(a) Usually associated with rotation of the spine
(b) Found most frequently in girls
(c) Occurs at the end of the period of this rapid growth
(d) Found any time in this period of rapid growth, 12 to 16 years
    1. a, b, and c   3. b and c
    2. a, b, and d   4. b and d

104. Types are known as
(a) Correctable or functional
(b) Fixed or structural
(c) Congenital or acquired
(d) Traumatic or injury-born
    1. a only   3. b only
    2. a and b   4. c and d

105. Treatment usually consists of
(a) High-protein, mineral and vitamin diet
(b) Braces
(c) Cast with turnbuckle
(d) Posture exercises
    1. a, b, and d   3. b, c, and d
    2. a, c, and d   4. All of above

106. Coxa plana, Legg-Perthes disease, is known for
(a) Attacking school-age child
(b) Hip involvement
(c) Requiring long-term care
(d) Frequently resulting in permanent injury to bone
    1. a, b, and c   3. b and c
    2. a, b, and d   4. c and d

107. Congenital dislocation of the hip may be suspected by the nurse, on her first visit to the home of the newborn, because of
(a) Increased number of gluteal folds
(b) Decreased number of gluteal folds
(c) Limitation in abduction of affected limb
(d) Limitation in adduction of affected limb
    1. a only   3. b and c
    2. a and c   4. b and d

108. Burns of the child continue to present a problem to the child, his family, society at large, and to both nurses and physicians. Some important facts about burns are that
(a) They are one of the two most frequently occurring injuries of childhood
(b) Highest incidence is in the preschool child
(c) Matches are often a source of this problem in the home during winter months
(d) The smaller the child, the greater is the problem encountered in maintaining fluid and electrolyte balance
    1. a, b, and d   3. b, c, and d
    2. a, c, and d   4. All of above

109. The open technique of treatment provides several aspects of care in which there is
(a) No dressing   1. a and b
(b) No eschar   2. a, b, and c
(c) Little fever   3. a and c
(d) Little odor   4. b, c, and d

110. Some nursing measures that are essential, whether the open technique or the closed or pressure bandage method is used, include
(a) Protection from infection of any kind
(b) Body alignment to prevent contractures
(c) Keeping careful records on intake and output
(d) Permitting the child to see other children through a window if at all possible
    1. a and c   3. a, c, and d
    2. a, b, and c   4. All of above

Situation: A small, thin but alert infant about 1 year of age in the well baby clinic is reported to be slightly cyanotic at times; otherwise, his mother states, he seems quite good. Questions 111 through 117 relate to this patient.

111. In talking with this mother the nurse hopes to learn
(a) What real concern the mother has about the cyanosis
(b) Whether the cyanosis decreases or increases when the baby cries
(c) If the baby has frequent fevers and chills
(d) If the baby has been unconscious
    1. a and b   3. a, b, and d
    2. a, b, and c   4. a, c, and d

112. The mother is eager to talk about the baby and, in addition to his health problem, the fact that he is a good baby. Additional things the nurse may consider pertinent for discussion are
(a) Whether the baby is always as alert as he seems today
(b) When the mother first noticed this problem
(c) Why the mother did not bring the baby to a clinic or doctor at an earlier date
(d) The mother's concept of the baby's problem

1. a and b   3. a and d
2. a, b, and c   4. All of above

113. Discussion reveals that the mother is a working mother and a relative cares for her boy most of the time. Other things the nurse should talk about with the mother are
   (a) Amount of rest that can be afforded the baby in the relative's home
   (b) Presence of preschoolers and school-age children in this other home
   (c) Financial arrangements for care of child
   (d) Place of employment of the father and the mother
      1. a and b   3. a, b, and d
      2. a, b, and c   4. a, c, and d

114. The physician, after his examination of the infant, gives a tentative diagnosis of tetralogy of Fallot. Hospitalization is advised for specific examinations, and a date for this is scheduled. The nurse now talks to the mother about
   (a) Smaller and more frequent feedings that should be given to the baby
   (b) Crawling and walking, which should be discouraged
   (c) Reporting of illnesses of the other children where the baby stays
   (d) Teaching the baby to spoon-feed
      1. a and b   3. a, b, and c
      2. a and c   4. a, c, and d

115. A cardiac catheterization was ordered for the baby after his admission to the hospital. The nurse is aware that this procedure will give information about
   (a) Pressures of the different heart chambers
   (b) Sizes of the valves
   (c) Blood samplings, used for blood gas determinations
   (d) Pathway of the blood flow
      1. a and b   3. a, c, and d
      2. a and c   4. All of above

116. The mother asks the purpose of the examinations and if the procedures will harm her baby. The nurse knows that the importance of these procedures has been explained to the mother by the physician. In view of the fact that the mother still has questions, the nurse would
   (a) Explain the procedures in some detail
   (b) Reiterate the need for the study procedures
   (c) Answer questions in simple language
   (d) Stress the fact that no child could be harmed by the procedures
      1. a, b, and c   3. c and d
      2. b and c   4. b, c, and d

117. The physician is hopeful that surgery can be delayed until the child is older. The present problem is working with the mother so that good care is given to the child until surgery is scheduled. Plans are focused on
   (a) Public health nurse, clinic nurse, and social worker conferring with the nurse and physician on planning care
   (b) Limiting all physical activities
   (c) Providing toys that are light and easily handled
   (d) Close health supervision of the child
      1. a and b   3. a, c, and d
      2. a, b, and c   4. b, c, and d

118. The heart rate is also a cardinal sign that must be observed and reported, in caring for children. This rate varies, and *upper* limits of so-called normal rates are
   (a) At birth, 180
   (b) Newborn period, 140
   (c) At 1 year, 130
   (d) At 4 years, 110
      1. a and b   3. c and d
      2. b and c   4. a and d

119. Electrocardiograms are done on infants and children for various diagnostic purposes
   (a) To determine congenital heart problems
   (b) To determine needed dosage of digitalis preparation
   (c) To determine size of heart chambers and valves
   (d) To detect electrolyte metabolic problems in the premature
      1. a and b   3. a, b, and c
      2. a and c   4. a, b, and d

120. Among the last signs of heart failure in the infant and child is (are)
   (a) Rapid respiratory rate in the supine position
   (b) Some orthopnea
   (c) Tachypnea
   (d) Peripheral edema
      1. a and b   3. c only
      2. a only   4. d only

121. Blood pressure readings in children give important data on the health of the child. Which of the following are important for the nurse to know in obtaining these measurements?
   (a) Crying may double the systolic blood pressure in children
   (b) Children with septicemia usually have elevated blood pressure readings
   (c) Blood pressure at birth usually ranges between 60 and 90
   (d) Unequal blood pressure readings in the arms of children may be related to a congenital heart problem
      1. a, b, and c   3. b, c, and d
      2. a, b, and d   4. All of above

122. The method and techniques used in taking blood pressures on infants and children have a direct bearing on the measurements obtained. Which of the following are true?
   (a) A cuff that is smaller than ½ the length of the upper arm may give a reading that is too low
   (b) Systolic pressures in the legs are higher than those of the arms after 1 year of age
   (c) The first pulsation felt (by palpation) when the cuff is deflated is lower than that obtained by auscultation
   (d) The first flushing noted when the flush method is used gives a fairly accurate reading
      1. a and b   3. b, c, and d
      2. b and c   4. a, b, and d

123. Several things are important in caring for the infant or child who has an ear problem of some kind. These include
   (a) Pulling the auricle down for a treatment in the infant

(b) Pulling the auricle up and back for a treatment in the older child

(c) When bleeding occurs, noting whether there are foreign bodies that have been pushed into the canal by the infant or child

(d) Noting swelling around and behind the ears

1. a and b   3. c and d
2. b, c, and d   4. All of above

124. Some of the first signs observed by the mother that may alert her to a health problem of diabetes in her child are

(a) Bed wetting   1. a and b
(b) Extreme thirst   2. a, b, and c
(c) Sunken eyeballs   3. a, b, and d
(d) Refusal to play   4. b, c, and d

125. In work with the mother in the care of a diabetic child several things should receive due consideration

(a) Oral hypoglycemic agents are usually effective in children

(b) Cooperation of the child is paramount to treatment

(c) Minimal exercise helps maintain blood sugar levels

(d) Omission of insulin results in severe problems such as coma

1. a and b   3. b and d
2. b and c   4. b, c, and d

126. Before Jane, who has diabetes, is discharged from the hospital she should be taught to regulate her dosage of insulin by

1. Injection of glucagon every morning
2. Decreasing intake of carbohydrates
3. Increasing the protein content of her diet
4. Regular testing of samples of urine

127. In working with a child who has diabetes and with his parents the matter of diet should be discussed in terms of

(a) Normal nutritional needs of the child

(b) Protein requirement, although roughly only 5% of total calories, is the first food considered in planning the diet (1 gm. per kg.)

(c) Food requirements for carbohydrates and fat may be equal in number of calories

(d) Refined or free sugars should be avoided

(e) Regular and routine eating habits are desirable

1. a, b, c, and e   3. b, c, d, and e
2. a, c, d, and e   4. All of above

128. A "free" diet for the diabetic child means

(a) Food as the child desires

(b) Appetite guides choice of foods

(c) Sugar spillage in the urine is allowed

(d) Insulin does not have to be adjusted

1. a and b   3. b, c, and d
2. a, b, and c   4. All of above

129. Hernias are not too uncommon in infants and children. In working with the mother of a child who has a hernia it is well to mention that

(a) These require medical supervision

(b) Incarceration may occur unless surgery is performed

(c) Umbilical hernia may disappear as the infant grows

(d) Femoral hernias are common in young children

1. a and b   3. a, c, and d
2. a, b, and c   4. All of abbve

130. A small boy has acute glomerulonephritis with edema of the face and hemorrhage due to glomerular damage. His mother is staying with him in the hospital and she needs to understand that

(a) He must have bed rest

(b) She should be free of colds and infections

(c) His chances of cure are slim

(d) He will require special diets for many years

1. a and b   3. a, b, and c
2. a and c   4. a, b, and d

131. In care of the infant or child with pyelonephritis the usual nursing measures include

(a) Careful recording of intake and output

(b) Encouraging the child to empty his bladder when voiding

(c) Supervising his limited fluid intake

(d) Obtaining necessary clean specimens for laboratory study

1. a and b   3. a, c, and d
2. a, b, and d   4. All of above

132. In working with parents in the preventive aspects of rheumatic fever the nurse would stress primarily

(a) The prevention of childhood diseases

(b) Early treatment of upper respiratory infections

(c) Rheumatic fever itself is infectious

(d) Most children who have had this disease have a permanent handicap

1. a and b   3. b only
2. b and d   4. b and c

133. Nursing of children with congenital anomalies of the meninges or cord requires long-term planning because of the handicaps that accompany these anomalies. Nursing is planned to assure

(a) Mental development—human contacts and toys

(b) Neuromuscular development—handling, music, opportunity for exercise

(c) Acceptance by parents of the child

(d) Preparation for school activities

1. a and b   3. a, b, and c
2. a and c   4. All of above

134. The drug that is likely to be used in the treatment of Wilms' tumor is

1. Achromycin
2. Dactinomycin
3. Vincristine
4. Iododeoxyuridine

135. The after-hospitalization effects that have been identified for the young child include

(a) Sleep disturbances

(b) Refusal to eat

(c) Regression of toilet habits

(d) Hostility toward parents

1. a, b, and c   3. b, c, and d
2. a, c, and d   4. All of above

136. Separation from the mother is interpreted to have, for the young child, some behavioral meanings, such as

(a) Fear of abandonment

(b) Loss of need for maternal love
(c) New feelings of revenge and guilt
(d) Positive effects on developing autonomy in the child
  1. a and b   3. a, c, and d
  2. a and c   4. All of above

137. Which of the following factors must be considered on an individual basis—that is, according to age and health problem—for each child who is hospitalized? The mother's presence may
(a) Give ego support
(b) Contribute to anxiety of child
(c) Damage a trusting relationship
(d) Not be desired by the mother
  1. a only   3. a, b, and c
  2. a and b   4. All of above

138. Some of the more important aspects of development of the 1- to 5-year-old child include
(a) Control of gross movements in walking, running, and bicycling
(b) Use of language as a tool
(c) Self-concept in motor development
(d) Finer coordination in using tools
  1. a and b   3. a, b, and d
  2. a, b, and c   4. All of above

Situation: Cara L has rheumatic fever. Drug therapy includes the administration of sodium salicylate and sodium bicarbonate, gr. 10 of each given four times daily. Questions 139 to 141 apply to this situation.

139. During the salicylate therapy, the nurse should observe Cara for which of the following groups of symptoms?
1. Nausea, dizziness, edema, headache
2. Gastric distress, nausea, vomiting, tinnitus
3. Constipation, deafness, nausea, headache
4. Diarrhea, gastric distress, edema of the face

140. Sodium salicylate is classified as an
1. Antibiotic and antipyretic
2. Analgesic and antipyretic
3. Analgesic and sedative
4. Antipyretic and hypnotic

141. Which of the following actions is sodium bicarbonate expected to produce?
1. Increase the absorption of sodium salicylate
2. Reduce undesirable side effects from sodium salicylate
3. Potentiate the action of sodium salicylate
4. Prevent excessive excretion of sodium salicylate

142. In discussing diet with mother of a child who has tuberculosis and is receiving isonicotinic acid hydrazide the nurse would
(a) Stress importance of vitamins A and D supplements
(b) Stress importance of vitamin B₆
(c) Ask mother to note neurologic signs or complaints from the child
(d) Stress importance of high-caloric diet
  1. a and b   3. b and c
  2. a and c   4. c and d

143. Hospital care of the child has been changing to include knowledge learned in the behavioral sciences. Nursing care is planned so that
(a) Child can continue to express himself in play activities
(b) Interruption in daily living activities with the family can be minimized
(c) Play can be used to reduce fears of intrusive procedures
(d) All school activities can be continued
  1. a and b   3. a, b, and c
  2. a and c   4. All of above

144. A sense of trust is developed at a definite time period in the life of the child. This period is primarily during
(a) Infancy
(b) Preschool years
(c) Elementary school years
(d) Adolescence
  1. a and b   3. b and c
  2. a only   4. c and d

145. When the quality of the infant's food intake of protein is inadequate, he
(a) Has flabby musculature
(b) Has slow weight gain
(c) Has little resistance to infection
(d) Has retention of some body fluids
  1. a, b, and c   3. b, c, and d
  2. a, b, and d   4. All of above

146. One of the minerals that may be eaten by the toddler is lead. Lead is
(a) Laid down in bones
(b) Not released from bone
(c) Known to severely affect the central nervous system if taken in large amounts
(d) Also found in some polluted city air
  1. a, b, and c   3. b, c, and d
  2. a, c, and d   4. All of above

147. Nutritional anemia is prevalent among children
(a) Mostly from lower middle class socioeconomic groups
(b) Who drink an insufficient amount of milk
(c) Who have a high intake of cereal grain in their diet
(d) Who eat large amounts of solid foods
  1. a and b   4. b and d
  2. a and c   5. None of above
  3. b and c

148. The antifibrinolytic agent that is most useful in the treatment of hemophilia is
1. Vitamin K (menadione)
2. Aminocaproic acid
3. AHG
4. Whole blood

149. Selection of drugs of choice for the treatment of pneumonia depends primarily upon
1. Selectivity of the organism
2. Tolerance of the patient
3. Preference of the physician
4. Sensitivity of the organism

150. Using live virus vaccines against measles is contraindicated in children receiving corticosteroids or antineoplastic or irradiation therapy, because these children may
1. Have had the disease or have been immunized previously
2. Be unlikely to need this protection during their shortened life-span
3. Be allergic to rabbit serum, which is used as a base for these vaccines
4. Be susceptible to infection due to their depressed immune response

151. Abuse of narcotic drug may cause
   1. Viral hepatitis–like syndrome
   2. Dilated pupils and tremors
   3. Disconnected, free-flowing ideas and deviations in memory
   4. Exaggerated spatial perception
152. Drug abuse can in its broadest sense be defined as
   1. Compulsive use of drugs to maintain a feeling of well-being
   2. Self-administration of a drug, which varies from culturally approved medical and social behavior
   3. Psychological dependence or habituation
   4. Physiologic dependence
153. Some of the major health problems of the adolescent are
   (a) Eye and visual difficulties
   (b) Dental problems
   (c) Allergies
   (d) Gastrointestinal difficulties
1. a and b	3. a and d
2. a and c	4. b and d
154. The incidence of malnutrition is highest in
   1. Male school child
   2. Female school child
   3. Male teen-ager
   4. Female teen-ager
155. One of the gravest types of health problem in the high school youth is
   1. Neuromuscular
   2. Emotional and behavioral
   3. Infectious and parasitic
   4. Cardiovascular
156. In implementing the concept of habilitation for the handicapped child, the nurse plans his care to
   (a) Help him attain independence
   (b) Help him with his developmental tasks
   (c) Provide for interaction with his peers
   (d) Make hospitalization a maturing experience
1. a, b, and c	3. b, c, and d
2. a, b, and d	4. All of above
157. When the United Nations came into being, it established a Commission on Human Rights whose first main task was to draft a bill of human rights. That document declares that the rights described in the Declaration pertain to
   1. All human beings in countries that belong to the United Nations
   2. All human beings in all countries and territories
   3. All human beings in democratic countries
   4. All human beings in countries that pay money to support the United Nations
158. The need for protecting young children from economic exploitation and premature employment is well known. The principle of a minimum age for employment of youth has been universally recognized in
   1. National legislation
   2. Employer statements of responsibility
   3. The Declaration of the Rights of the Child
   4. Social Security regulations
159. Child neglect and abuse are not new phenomena in society. What is new is the increase and violence in attacks on infants and young children by parents or other caretakers, as reported by medical personnel. Results of such abuse produce what physicians call "the battered-child syndrome." The task of assembling information and starting action regarding child abuse and neglect was undertaken in 1961 by the
   1. American Medical Association
   2. American Academy of Pediatrics
   3. Children's Bureau
   4. National Institutes of Health
160. Recently the agency recognized as foremost among forces committed to improving the lot of children in economically underdeveloped countries was the
   1. United Nations International Children's Emergency Fund
   2. World Health Organization
   3. Children's Bureau
   4. Food and Agricultural Organization
161. Under what authority does the World Health Organization operate?
   1. As an independent American agency under its own board
   2. Under the United States Public Health Service
   3. As a specialized agency of the United Nations
   4. As an international agency under an international board
162. During a preemployment examination Mr. Johns was found to have pulmonary tuberculosis. The disease was diagnosed as active and moderately advanced, with a small cavity in the right apex. His family consists of his wife Mary and children, Jerry, age 10, Nida, age 6, and Joe, age 3. The physician has advised Mr. Johns to enter the tuberculosis hospital for further study and adjustment on therapy. Immediate services to be rendered to the family will include which of the following?
   1. Tuberculin tests for family contacts
   2. X-ray examination for all members of the family
   3. BCG vaccine for all of the children
   4. Contacting the Welfare Department for financial help
163. Mrs. Johns and Jerry were found to have negative tuberculin tests. According to the present eradication program which of the following would be in order?
   1. Administer BCG vaccine
   2. Consider that no further care is required
   3. Place on prophylactic isoniazid
   4. Repeat tuberculin test in 6 months
164. Nida and Joe had positive tuberculin tests; therefore, which of the following would be indicated?
   1. Admission to the hospital
   2. Exclusion of Nida from school
   3. Sputum examination for each
   4. X-ray examination of the chest
165. A positive tuberculin test indicates the following:
   1. Active primary tuberculosis
   2. A delayed allergic reaction
   3. Extrapulmonary infection
   4. Active acquired immunity

166. Before Mr. Johns is placed on a regular schedule of drug therapy which of the following will be done?
    1. Provision for economic assistance
    2. Report of the disease to the Public Health Department
    3. Drug sensitivity tests
    4. Referral of patient back to private physician

167. The following communicable diseases are causing considerable attention because of their ability to cause abortion, stillbirth, and congenital defects:
    (a) Rubella
    (b) Cytomegalic disease
    (c) Mumps
    (d) Toxoplasmosis
    (e) Influenza
        1. b, c, and e   3. a, d, and e
        2. a, c, and e   4. All of above

168. Malaria has become an important disease in the United States because of the following conditions:
    (a) Its worldwide distribution
    (b) Travel into and out of the United States
    (c) Failure to secure malaria vaccine
    (d) Drug resistance of the etiologic agent
    (e) Failure to control the vector
        1. All but e   3. Only b
        2. a and b   4. a, b, and d

169. The most common form of malaria is caused by which species of *Plasmodium?*
    1. *P. ovale*   3. *P. vivax*
    2. *P. malariae*   4. *P. falciparum*

170. Hepatitis occurs as sporadic cases and in isolated outbreaks. Exposure to virus B homologous serum hepatitis (SH) may be expected to occur in hospitals because of the following:
    1. Increased use of blood and blood products
    2. Careless handling of excreta
    3. Asymptomatic carriers
    4. Increasing use of aerosols

171. The following applies to both virus A and virus B hepatitis:
    (a) No isolation for virus B hepatitis
    (b) Both A and B may be transmitted parenterally
    (c) Isolation of patient with virus A for 7 days
    (d) Symptoms of viruses A and B indistinguishable
    (e) Viruses A and B cause different forms of the same disease
        1. d and e   3. a, b, and d
        2. b and c   4. b, d, and e

172. In nursing patients with virus A hepatitis, the nurse should include which of the following?
    (a) Wear gloves for venipunctures and dressings
    (b) Wear gloves for giving enemas and rectal temperatures
    (c) Autoclave linens and nondisposable equipment
    (d) Fumigate room on recovery
    (e) Destroy thermometer on recovery
        1. All of these   3. All but d
        2. All but c   4. a, b, and c

173. Diseases for which a bacteriologic release from isolation is required include

    (a) Typhoid fever
    (b) Pertussis
    (c) Shigellosis
    (d) Diphtheria
    (e) Staphylococcal infection
        1. a and d   3. a, b, c, and d
        2. All but b   4. a, c, and d

174. The administration of a series of injections of a vaccine may be expected to produce a
    1. Primary antigenic stimulus
    2. Passive immunity
    3. Secondary antigenic stimulus
    4. Lifelong immunity

175. Which of the following is DPT a combination of?
    1. Serum and toxoid
    2. Antitoxin and a vaccine
    3. Toxoids and a vaccine
    4. Vaccine and sera

176. For which of the following diseases is immunization unavailable?
    (a) Tetanus
    (b) Varicella
    (c) Poliomyelitis
    (d) Rubella
    (e) Typhoid fever
        1. a, c, and e   3. b, c, and e
        2. b only   4. a, b, c, and e

177. Mrs. Amos is a patient on the maternity service where she has just delivered a baby. There are 2 other children of preschool age in the family. The nurse learns that the children have never received any immunizations. This is an opportunity for the nurse to advise Mrs. Amos about the protection for her children. The diseases that the children should be immunized for are
    (a) Diphtheria
    (b) Poliomyelitis
    (c) Pertussis
    (d) Rubeola
    (e) Tetanus
        1. All but d   3. All but e
        2. All of these   4. a, c, and e only

178. Children in the family who have been exposed to but show no evidence of tuberculosis
    1. Can be considered to be immune
    2. Should be treated with INH and PAS
    3. Given massive doses of penicillin
    4. X-rayed every 6 months and observed for evidence of tuberculosis

179. If a person has been exposed to tuberculosis but shows no signs or symptoms except a positive tuberculin test, prophylactic drug therapy is usually continued after his last exposure for a time period of
    1. 3 weeks   3. 1 year
    2. 6 months   4. 5 years

180. Members of the family who have developed a positive tuberculin test are candidates for treatment with
    1. Old tuberculin
    2. BCG vaccine
    3. INH and PAS
    4. Purified protein derivative of tuberculin

181. The drugs that are most effective against tuberculosis and cause fewest toxic effects are
    1. Streptomycin, isoniazid, and aminosalicylic acid

2. Penicillin, dihydrostreptomycin, and erythromycin
3. Cycloserine, viomycin, and kanamycin
4. Streptomycin, acetylsalicylic acid, and pyrazinamide

182. Mrs. Amos asks the nurse when immunizations for the new baby should be started. The nurse's reply would be
   1. At 4 months
   2. At 6 months
   3. Between 1 and 2 months
   4. Anytime after birth

183. The first immunizations given to an infant are for the following diseases:
   (a) Rubella
   (b) Tetanus
   (c) Diphtheria
   (d) Poliomyelitis
   (e) Pertussis
      1. All but a   3. c, d, and e
      2. b, c, and e   4. c only

184. Vaccine for measles should be administered during the first year. The recommended age is
   1. 6 months   3. Give with DPT
   2. 4 to 6 months   4. 12 months

185. Pertussis vaccine is not recommended for children over 12 years of age for the following reason:
   1. They have a passive immunity
   2. Severe reactions may occur
   3. They are not likely to contract the disease
   4. They would fail to develop antibodies

186. The Joint Committee of the American Academy of Pediatrics and the American College of Physicians as recommended that all infants be tested for tuberculosis at
   1. 6 to 12 months of age
   2. Birth
   3. 2 to 4 months of age
   4. Before 6 months of age

187. Chemotherapeutic drugs are not effective in the treatment of viral diseases. Which of the following diseases is an exception to this?
   1. Varicella   3. Psittacosis
   2. Parotitis   4. Rubella

188. The nursing care of patients with enteric communicable diseases requires that particular attention be given to the following:
   (a) Early ambulation
   (b) Hand washing
   (c) Using pasteurized milk
   (d) Handling and disposal of excreta
   (e) Wearing a gown
      1. All of these   3. All but a
      2. b, d, and e   4. All but c

189. Of which of the following diseases may the etiologic agent be isolated from the stools?
   (a) Typhoid fever
   (b) Brucellosis
   (c) Cholera
   (d) Virus A hepatitis
   (e) Poliomyelitis
      1. a, c, and d   3. All but e
      2. a and d   4. All of these

190. Which of the following communicable diseases are most important and are endemic in the United States at the present time?
   (a) Rubella
   (b) Tuberculosis
   (c) Yellow fever
   (d) Syphilis and gonorrhea
   (e) Malaria
      1. All but c   3. b and d
      2. All of these   4. b, d, and e

191. The incidence of hospital-acquired infection has increased since the development of antibiotics and their extensive use. Although several pathogenic organisms are involved, one of the most important is *Staphylococcus aureus*. According to the best evidence at the present time, the exact method of transmission is unknown, but is believed to be the following:
   1. Asymptomatic carriers
   2. Direct contact with infected patient
   3. Airborne infection
   4. Contaminated fomites

192. Certain groups of patients in the hospital are considered to be at high risk and should be protected from nosocomial infections. These groups include the following:
   (a) Newborn infants
   (b) Outpatients
   (c) All surgical patients
   (d) Maternity patients
   (e) Elderly debilitated patients
      1. a, c, and d   3. All but b
      2. a and d   4. All of these

193. Rubella, usually a mild afebrile disease, occurs in cyclic epidemics. In 1964 in the United States 1,800,000 cases occurred. If the disease occurred during the first 4 weeks of pregnancy, it may be expected that the risk to the pregnancy and to the fetus would be
   1. 10%   3. 5%
   2. 25%   4. 50%

194. Malaria, once considered to be eradicated in the United States, has become a present-day problem. The primary source of infection is among the following:
   (a) Servicemen returning from Vietnam
   (b) Returning missionaries
   (c) Peace Corps volunteers
   (d) Foreign travelers in the United States
   (e) United States citizens traveling abroad
      1. All of these   3. a, b, and c
      2. Only a   4. a and d

195. A certain area of the southeastern United States has been declared a yellow fever–receptive area. This means which of the following?
   1. Yellow fever exists in the area
   2. The area is infested with *Aedes aegypti*
   3. There has been a breakdown in control measures
   4. Carriers exist in the area

196. John was admitted to the hospital because of minor injuries suffered in an automobile accident. During the examination the physician noticed a rash on the skin and found that John had suffered from a sore throat for several days. Based on the clinical examination the physician made a tentative diagnosis of secondary syphilis, pending a report on the serologic test. Secondary syphilis is classified as which of the following?
   1. Primary syphilis   3. Infectious syphilis
   2. Latent syphilis   4. Late syphilis

197. The report of the serologic test was reactive.

In view of the clinical examination and history of exposure the physician confirmed the diagnosis of secondary syphilis. The nursing care of the patient should include the following:
1. Thorough hand washing after patient care
2. Isolation for 7 days
3. Autoclaving linens
4. Boiling dishes

198. Many serologic tests for syphilis have been developed, but many are no longer used. The test most widely used at present is
1. Wassermann   3. VDRL
2. Kahn   4. TPI

199. John was exposed to syphilis through sexual contact with an infected person. It is important to locate the source of his infection and also persons whom he may have infected. Therefore, all sexual contacts should be located and examined for the past
1. 3 months   3. 30 days
2. 6 months   4. 3 weeks

200. The treatment prescribed for John consisted of which of the following?
(a) Methacycline 1,200 mg. orally
(b) Bicillin 2.4 million units I.M.
(c) Bicillin 2.4 million units weekly for 10 weeks
(d) PAM
(e) Sensitivity tests for penicillin
    1. a and b   3. c and e
    2. b and e   4. Only e

201. At the present time the incidence of infectious syphilis is highest among which of the following age groups?
1. 25 to 35 years   3. Past 40 years
2. Under 14 years   4. Under 25 years

202. The control of syphilis and gonorrhea in the United States involves a variety of economic, cultural, and personality problems. Some of the problems include the following:
(a) Premarital and extramarital sex contact
(b) The ease and availability of treatment
(c) Deprivation
(d) Promiscuity
(e) Conformity among teen-age population
    1. Only d   3. All of these
    2. All but e   4. a and b

203. In January, 1968, a live virus vaccine for active immunization against mumps was released. The vaccine is advised for high-risk groups that include which of the following?
(a) Military personnel
(b) Elderly persons
(c) Nonimmune pregnant women
(d) Infants under 1 year
(e) All children over 1 year of age
    1. a and e   3. a, b, and c
    2. a, c, and e   4. All but d

204. Rabies is a disease of wild and domestic animals that may be transmitted to humans by the bite of a rabid animal. Although few cases occur in humans in the United States, they are almost 100% fatal. The disease is endemic to epidemic among wild animals in many parts of the United States. Recently a new preexposure vaccine for immunization became available. This vaccine is known as
1. Semple killed virus vaccine
2. Rabies hyperimmune serum

3. Pasteur treatment
4. Duck embryo vaccine

205. During recent years a number of serious epidemics of arthropod-borne viral encephalitis has occurred. The disease is transmitted to humans by the bite of an infected mosquito. The reservoir of infection is among
1. Domestic and wild birds
2. Culex mosquitoes
3. Asymptomatic carriers
4. Wood ticks

206. Viral encephalitis may affect persons of all ages. The eastern form results in greater mortality among the young and elderly persons. The nurse caring for a child with eastern encephalitis may expect the following to occur:
(a) Convulsions
(b) Diarrhea
(c) Progressive neurologic symptoms
(d) Leukopenia
(e) Fever 104° to 105° F.
    1. c, d, and e   3. d and e
    2. a, c, and e   4. All but b

207. The nursing care of most communicable diseases is essentially the same as
1. Good medical-surgical nursing care
2. Required in special communicable disease hospitals
3. Outlined by the U. S. Public Health Service
4. Outlined in hospital policies

208. The nurse who is assigned the care of communicable diseases must be knowledgeable about which of the following:
(a) The etiologic agent
(b) Methods for its destruction
(c) Route of escape from the body
(d) Medical asepsis
(e) Clean versus contaminated
    1. All but a   3. All of these
    2. d and e   4. b, d, and e

209. Ringworm of the scalp frequently seen in children is
(a) Caused by tinea
(b) May be treated with griseofulvin
(c) A superficial fungus infection
(d) Noninfectious
(e) Transmitted by direct contact
    1. All of these   3. a, b, and c
    2. All but d   4. d and e

210. The nurse caring for communicable diseases must be a teacher and be capable of instructing patients and their families in the following:
(a) Importance of hand washing
(b) Symptoms of communicable diseases
(c) Need for immunization against preventable diseases
(d) Covering nose and mouth when coughing and sneezing
(e) Using bacteriocidal soap
    1. All but e   3. a, b, and d
    2. All but b   4. a, c, and d

211. The following skin test(s) may be administered to a person with suspected histoplasmosis:
(a) Lepromin test
(b) Tuberculin test

(c) Histoplasmin test
(d) Schick test
(e) Blastomycin test
    1. a and c   3. b only
    2. c and e   4. b and c

212. Prevention of infections caused by helminths requires which of the following?
(a) Personal hygiene
(b) Control of pollution of streams
(c) Sanitary disposal of excreta
(d) Thorough cooking of beef, pork, and fish
(e) Public education
    1. All of these   3. a and d
    2. a, c, and e   4. All but c

213. Every professional nurse should be familiar with the community facilities where immunizations for communicable diseases may be obtained. In some communities the following may be available:
(a) Public Health Department clinics
(b) Veterans Administration Hospitals
(c) Rehabilitation centers
(d) Private physicians
(e) Hospital outpatient clinics
    1. a and e   3. a, d, and e
    2. d only   4. All of these

214. The prevention and control of communicable diseases is the responsibility of
1. The National Communicable Disease Center
2. The State Health Department
3. The Public Health Laboratory
4. Every citizen

215. Agencies that have legal responsibility for the control of communicable diseases include
(a) State Department of Agriculture
(b) City-County Health Department
(c) National Tuberculosis Association
(d) W. K. Kellogg Foundation
(e) City Health Officer
    1. b, c, and e   3. a, b, and c
    2. a, b, and e   4. Only e

SCORES

SCORES

1 _____ 5 _____
2 _____ 6 _____
3 _____ 7 _____
4 _____ 8 _____

DIRECTIONS: Read each question and its numbered answers. When you have decided which answer is correct, blacken the corresponding space on this sheet with the special pencil. Make your mark as long as the pair of lines, and move the pencil point up and down firmly to make a heavy black line. If you change your mind, erase your first mark completely. Make no stray marks; they may count against you.

SAMPLE:
1—1 a country
1—2 a mountain
1—3 an island
1—4 a city
1—5 a state

1. Chicago is

BE SURE YOUR MARKS ARE HEAVY AND BLACK.
ERASE COMPLETELY ANY ANSWER YOU WISH TO CHANGE.

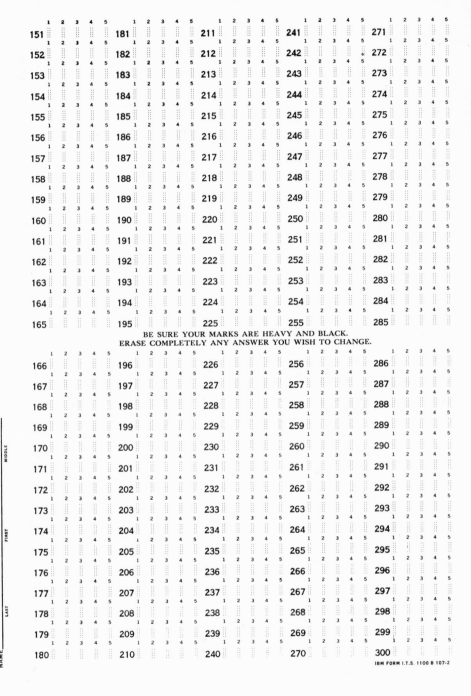

BE SURE YOUR MARKS ARE HEAVY AND BLACK.
ERASE COMPLETELY ANY ANSWER YOU WISH TO CHANGE.

SCORES

5
6
7
8

1
2
3
4

NAME

LAST   FIRST   MIDDLE

IBM FORM I.T.S. 1100 B 107-2

12

PSYCHIATRIC NURSING

Aguilera, D. C., Messick, J. M., and Farrell, M. S.: Crisis intervention—theory and methodology, St. Louis, 1970, The C. V. Mosby Co.

Blum, R. H., and others: Society and drugs. Drugs I, Social and cultural observations; Drugs II, College and high school observations, San Francisco, 1970, Jossey-Bass, Inc., Publishers.

Bodie, M. K.: When a patient threatens suicide, Perspectives in Psychiatric Care 6:76, 1968.

Fenichel, O.: Psychoanalytic theory of neurosis, New York, 1945, W. W. Norton & Co., Inc.

Freedman, A. M., and Kaplan, H. I.: Interpreting personality; a survey of twentieth century views, New York, 1972, Athenium Press.

Glasser, W.: Reality therapy, New York, 1965, Harper & Row, Publishers.

Goode, E.: The marijuana smokers, New York, 1970, Basic Books, Inc., Publishers.

Green, H.: I never promised you a rose garden, New York, 1964, Signet Books, The New American Library, Inc.

Greenblatt, M., Levinson, D. J., and Williams, R. H.: The patient and the mental hospital, New York, 1957, The Free Press of Glencoe.

Grinspoon, L.: Marijuana reconsidered, Cambridge, Mass., 1971, Harvard University Press.

Hays, J. S., and Larson, K. H.: Interacting with patients, New York, 1963, The Macmillan Co.

Jones, M.: The therapeutic community, New York, 1953, Basic Books, Inc., Publishers.

Jones, M.: Beyond the therapeutic community; social learning and social psychiatry, New Haven, 1968, Yale University Press.

Kolb, L. C.: Noyes modern clinical psychiatry, ed. 7, Philadelphia, 1968, W. B. Saunders Co.

Maloney, E. M.: The fears and feelings of the patient on electro-convulsive therapy, American Journal of Nursing 58:560, 1958.

Matheney, R. V., and Topalis, M.: Psychiatric nursing, ed. 5, St. Louis, 1970, The C. V. Mosby Co.

Mereness, D.: Essentials of psychiatric nursing, ed. 8, St. Louis, 1970, The C. V. Mosby Co.

Parad, H. J.: Crisis intervention: selected readings, New York, 1965, Family Service Association of America.

Peplau, H. E.: Interpersonal relations in nursing, New York, 1952, G. P. Putnam's Sons.

Peplau, H. E.: Interpersonal techniques: the crux of psychiatric nursing, American Journal of Nursing 60:50, 1962.

Roche Laboratories: Aspects of alcoholism, vols. 1 and 2, Philadelphia, 1966, J. B. Lippincott Co.

Roche Laboratories: Aspects of anxiety, Philadelphia, 1966, J. B. Lippincott Co.

Schwartz, M. S., and Shockley, E. L.: The nurse and the mental hospital, New York, 1956, Russell Sage Foundation.

Singer, R. G., and Blumenthal, I. J.: Suicide clues in psychotic patients, Mental Hygiene 53:346, 1969.

Small, L.: The briefer psychotherapies, New York, 1971, Brunner/Mazel Publishers, Inc.

Stanton, A. H., and Schwartz, M. S.: The mental hospital, New York, 1954, Basic Books, Inc.

Toward therapeutic care, Topeka, Kansas, 1961, Group for Advancement of Psychiatry, Committee on Psychiatric Nursing.

Wallace, M. A.: The nurse in suicide prevention, Nursing Outlook 15:55, 1967.

The Child Study Association of America: You, your child, and drugs, New York, 1971, The Child Study Press.

UNDERSTANDING THE DEVELOPING PERSONALITY

1. **Meaning of personality**
   The sum total of an individual's physical, intellectual, emotional, and social formation in conjunction with the hopes, fears, needs, drives, prejudices, and capabilities that are part of the total life's experience

2. **Historical contributions to psychiatry and the understanding of mental health and the treatment of mental illness**

A. Adler, Alfred (1870-1937)—defined the basic concepts of the individual as related to his social environment and the interrelatedness of body and mind (the holistic approach)

B. Alexander, Franz (1891-1964)—emphasized the importance of the total personality in disease processes (the interdepending of the "psyche" and the "soma")

C. Beers, Clifford (1876-1943)—founded mental hygiene movement in 1908

D. Binet, Alfred (1857-1911)—developed first intelligence test in 1904

E. Bini, Lucio (1908-1964)—developed electroshock therapy in 1937 with Ugo Cerletti

F. Bleuler, Eugen (1857-1939)—contributed to understanding of schizophrenia and evolved notion of schizoid and syntonic personalities; contributed notion of autistic thinking and evolved concept of ambivalence

G. Cerletti, Ugo (1877-1963)—developed electroshock therapy in 1937 with Lucio Bini

H. Charcot, Jean (1825-1893)—French neurologist who inspired research into cause and nature of hysteria and effects of hypnosis

I. Dix, Dorothea Lynde (1802-1887)—instrumental in humanizing care and improving conditions for mental patients in United States

J. Ehrlich, Paul (1854-1915)—introduced salvarsan for treatment of syphilis in 1910

K. Freeman, Walter (1895-   )—prefrontal lobotomy in 1936 with Egas A. Moniz

L. Freud, Sigmund (1856-1939)—father of psychoanalysis; introduced revolutionary contributions to the understanding of personality; described an unconscious area of the mind, which is a realm of wishes and pleasures that form the motivational force behind human action

M. Juaregg, von, Julius Wagner (1857-1940)—treated syphilis with malaria in 1917

N. Jung, Carl (1875-1961)—student of Freud; developed analytical psychology and the concept of "the collective unconscious" or "objective psyche"

O. Korsakoff, Sergei (1853-1900)—in 1887 described alcoholic psychosis characterized by personality change and blunting of intellectual capacity

P. Kraeplin, Emil (1856-1926)—described dementia praecox and manic-depressive psychoses; developed classification of mental illness

Q. Meduna, von, Ladislas (1896-1964)—developed Metrazol (pentylenetetrazol) therapy in 1935

R. Meyer, Adolph (1856-1950)—father of psychobiology; considered mental illness to be a regression to infantile behavior as a means of self-cure or defense

S. Moniz, Egas A. (1874-1955)—prefrontal lobotomy operation in 1936 with Walter Freeman

T. Noguchi, Hideyo (1876-1928)—verified presence of *Treponema pallidum* in brain tissue of paretics

U. Pinel, Philippe (1745-1826)—humanized care and treatment of mental patients in France by having chains and restraints removed

V. Quincke, Heinrich (1842-1922)—performed first lumbar puncture in 1890

W. Rank, Otto (1884-1939)—proposed theory of birth trauma as origin of anxiety

X. Sakel, Manfred (1900-1957)—developed insulin therapy in 1933

Y. Sullivan, Harry Stack (1892-1949)—proposed theory that all behavior derives from conditioning in the interpersonal realm

Z. Wassermann, von, August Paul (1866-1925)—demonstrated antibodies in cerebrospinal fluid and blood serum of known syphilitics

3. **Theoretical structure of psyche**

A. Id—the reservoir of instinctual drives and the source of psychic energies

B. Ego—the tool by which a person organizes outside information, tests perception, selects memories, governs actions adaptively, and integrates the capacities of orientation and planning

C. Superego—portion that has the function of deciding which impulses are acceptable and which are not

4. **Levels of consciousness**

A. Conscious—taking in of the external world (perception); mastery of the motor apparatus (motility); ability to bind tension (countercathexis) for later effective energy discharge

B. Preconscious—memory traces, which can be made conscious by a simple act of attention; one function of the preconscious is to maintain censorship (repression of unconscious wishes and desires)

C. Unconscious—realm of repressed wishes and desires that form the motivational force behind human action

5. **Contributions of prenatal and natal period to developing personality**
A. Hereditary: genetic influence
B. Constitutional endowment
C. Intrauterine environment
6. **Contributions of infancy period to developing personality**
A. Oral sensory stage of life—the first year —trust vs. mistrust
   1. Develops basic feeling that his wants will be satisfied
   2. Experiences through mouth as most sensitive and pleasurable zone of body
   3. Mother or "other" acts as reality agent through which infant's needs are gratified and societal expectations are formed
   4. Learns process of getting, through which he can learn to give
   5. If basic trust is strong, an inbuilt and lifelong sense of hope is established
B. Influence of experience in oral period on adult behavior
   1. Interdependence and moderation vs. dependency and excessive indulgence (a feeling of never being satiated)
   2. Hopefulness vs. feelings of doom, frustration, and bitterness
   3. Alcoholism and addiction are residuals of unresolved experiences in oral period
   4. Eating, drinking, and merrymaking continue to be vital throughout life; in excess, these normal functions become problematic
7. **Mechanisms of adjustment originating in oral period**
A. Compensation—defense with which one unconsciously disguises undesirable trait by developing and emphasizing a desirable one
B. Substitution—defense mechanism by which an acceptable object is unconsciously selected in place of the unacceptable wish or desire
C. Fixation—situation in which psychic energy remains attached to one level of psychosexual development and impedes maturational progression
8. **Contributions of early childhood period to developing personality**
A. Muscular-anal stage—1 to 3 years—autonomy vs. shame and doubt
   1. Child learns to walk, talk, feed himself, and control the anal sphincter muscles; he can choose to retain or release

   2. Through testing out the mastery of his new accomplishments he gains confidence in his autonomy; begins important individuation
   3. Feels a balance of love over hate, cooperation over willfulness, self-expression over suppression
   4. Anus and urethra become erotic zones
B. Residuals of anal period in adult life
   1. Orderliness, perseverance, and independence are some of the positive acquisitions of personality development; if child is overly controlled and given to believe that his feces are "bad," he comes to feel enraged at his impotence; once shamed, he mistrusts his own rightness and comes to doubt himself
   2. Can learn to control and relate to others by withholding of emotion, as he had retained or released his feces as a sign of pleasure and approval or of anger and defiance
9. **Development of personality—3 to 6 years of age**
A. Awakening of sexual awareness—phallic-genital stage
   1. Interest in differences between male and female
   2. Penis and clitoris are primary areas of erotic pleasure
   3. Attraction to and identification with parent of opposite sex; comparison to and competition with parent of same sex; oedipal situation develops
B. Continued development and testing of ego and superego
C. Struggle for parental affection with siblings
   1. Introduction into social-political structure of nursery school, street, playground, etc.
   2. Initiation of masculine and feminine identification
D. Potential residuals of adjustments originating in phallic-genital period
   1. Unresolved oedipal situation
   2. Castration fear in male, penis envy in female
E. Mechanisms of basic and complex defenses and adjustments originating in phallic-genital period
   1. Displacement—unconscious shifting of emotion from one idea or object to another that resembles the original in some aspect or quality

2. Rationalization—pseudoreasonable explanations, which may not be valid, are used in an attempt to hide the actual motives from self and others
3. Regression—return to an earlier stage of functioning, in which gratification was assured, as means of avoiding tension and conflict evoked at the present
4. Repression—unconscious wishes, impulses, and affects are forgotten in an attempt to inhibit unacceptable sexual impulses

10. **Development of personality—ages 6 to 12 years**
A. Latency or normal homosexual period
   1. Social formation of personality outside of home
   2. Identification stronger with someone of same sex
   3. Models of experiment and experience are peer group–centered, in school, clubs, gangs, cliques
   4. Using adult tools—language, deduction, the written word, machines, etc.—child seeks confidence in self
   5. Reservoir of useful achievement and identity is stored up to develop sense of value
B. Homosexuality—may be considered an incomplete resolution of the oedipal conflict; the child has identified with the parent of the opposite sex and chosen the parent of the same sex as a love object; this choice of an object is based, in part, on its sexual resemblance to the individual himself
C. Mechanisms of basic and complex adjustment originating in latency period
   1. Projection—individual attributes his own feelings and wishes to another person because his own ego is unable to assume the responsibility for these feelings or tolerate the painful affects they evoke; associated with ego immaturity and vulnerability

11. **Puberty-adolescence and ego identification versus role confusion**
A. Heterosexual period
   1. Group identity becomes important and necessary as youth initiates process of separation from family
   2. Suspension between the learned morality of the child and the developing ethic of the adolescent
   3. Great deal of attention paid to how

one looks, since exterior presence helps commit one to a concept of "selfness"; falls in love with heroes, ideologies, and members of opposite sex
   4. Reflects image of others to get a clearer picture of self
   5. Biologic maturation of sexual development

12. **Young adulthood and intimacy versus isolation**
A. Once identity is secured, individual can invest in caring about others without losing own identity
B. In true intimacy there is a mutuality of love, trust, ability, and willingness to regulate life's work, play, and procreation and to accept responsibility for the healthy development of offspring; potential for sharing of self in intense and long-term relationships
C. Sense of isolation is evidenced by self-interest and self-indulgence

13. **Adulthood—middle years of life**
A. Generativity versus stagnation
   1. Vital interest outside the home in establishing and guiding the oncoming generation or in bettering society
   2. The new generation depends upon the adults, and the adults upon the young—an interdependency that gives a sense of connection and purpose between past and future
   3. The alternative—stagnation—is to satisfy personal needs and engage in self-absorption

14. **Maturity—later years of life**
A. Ego integrity versus despair
   1. Strong sense of self and the value of life, his own and every other life
   2. Realistic understanding and acceptance of limited or uncertain future
   3. Strength comes from looking back to a life that has produced satisfaction
   4. Without that sense of satisfaction, there are both fear of death and despair

15. **Contributions of psychology**
A. Administering and interpreting projective techniques
   1. Tests that employ projective techniques include Rorschach, Murray Thematic Apperception, Szondi, etc.
   2. Purpose of projective techniques—to objectively evaluate personality structure and deviations and to measure nonintellectual traits of personality

B. Evaluating intellectual abilities
1. Tests that evaluate intellectual abilities include Binet-Simon, Otis, and Bellevue-Wechsler
2. Other tests, which discover areas of special impairment and/or vocational aptitude, aid in treatment and in planning for discharge

16. **Factors that may contribute to mental illness**
No single set of factors may be considered separately when seeking to identify the causes of mental illness; the individual must be considered in totality

A. Genetic factors—insufficient evidence, to date, prevents any definitive conclusion of genetic factors having primary influences in the development of mental illness; studies of identical twins and the exceptionally high incidence of parallel psychosis evidenced, however, indicate that heredity plays a role

B. Organic factors
1. Trauma—damage to brain tissue may result in degeneration with accompanying psychopathology
2. Infectious disease—syphilis, encephalitis, etc. can frequently produce brain tissue pathology resulting in psychic disorders with accompanying physical disabilities
3. Brain tumor—an organic condition, which may be accompanied by a variety of mental and physical symptoms
4. Alcohol—may result in progressive personality and social disintegration; a major health problem in United States
5. Drug abuse—becoming a major social, psychiatric, and medical health problem in United States
   a. Casual and indiscriminate usage can precipitate psychotic state
   b. Excessive and prolonged usage can cause irreversible organic brain damage
   c. Strong evidence indicates genetic chromosomal defects, mutations, and changes as a result of habitual usage
6. Age
   a. Sharp rise in incidences of psychosis and "psychotic-like" disorders in adolescence
   b. Sharp rise in incidence of psychosis during involutional period is caused

by continued social, emotional, and physical factors

C. Psychogenic factors—most significant causative factors in mental illness
1. Involve individual's subjective and emotional feelings of self (self-esteem, security, well-being, personal value, guilt, and inadequacies)
2. Collapse of defense mechanisms due to acute or prolonged stresses and anxiety
3. Breakdown of significant interpersonal relationships

D. Cultural factors—the culture into which one is born superimposes many ideas and values
1. Rigid sex roles, although once clearly defined, are now being challenged
2. Culture imposes problems and restrictions upon minority groups, which are limiting and stressful
3. Cultural conflict can lead to adjustment problems resulting in such high levels of anxiety that individuals are forced to utilize abnormal or exaggerated defense mechanisms

UNDERSTANDING THE INDIVIDUAL WITH IMPAIRED FUNCTIONAL-ADAPTATIONAL DEVELOPMENT

1. **Definitions**
A. Psychoneurosis—inner conflict between drives and fears beyond individual's awareness which, having been repressed, now fight their way back into consciousness via neurotic symptoms
B. Character or personality disorder—manifestation of pathology exaggerated to a point that behavior, destructive to the individual or to others, becomes distorted or restricted and is a source of distress to himself or others
C. Psychophysiologic disorder—manifestation of emotions (or their symbolic representation) that cannot be discharged effectively through behavior or speech and that find expression in a somatic fashion in the structured or functional alteration of an organ or organ system

2. **Etiology and symptomatology characteristic of psychoneurotic, character or personality, and psychophysiologic disorders**
A. Etiology
1. Maternal deprivation in first few years of ego-integrative development

2. Lack of individual's capacity to give equitable expression to drives, especially to aggressive ones, can lead to emotional and social self-destructive attitudes

3. Inconsistency, excessive harshness, or undue permissiveness on the part of the parents may result in a disordered functioning of the superego (primary disorder—feelings of worthlessness)

4. Severe conflict that cannot be dealt with through symptom formation (i.e., conversion) may lead to severe restrictions in ego function and impaired capacity to learn and develop new skills

B. Classification and symptomatology of psychoneurotic, character or personality, and psychophysiologic disorders

1. Psychoneurotic disorders
   a. Hysterical neurosis, conversion type—a defense against intensive psychic threat, by means of a transformation or conversion of psychic stimuli into physical manifestation; special senses or voluntary nervous system elements are attacked, causing such symptoms as blindness, deafness, and/or paralyses; individual often exhibits an inappropriate lack of concern about symptoms
   b. Hysterical neurosis, dissociative type—characterized by alterations in state of individual's consciousness or in identity, producing symptoms of amnesia, fugue somnambulism, and multiple personality
   c. Anxiety neurosis—characterized by anxious overconcern, extending to panic; frequently associated with somatic symptoms; not to be confused with normal apprehension or fear that occurs in realistically dangerous situation
   d. Phobic neurosis—characterized by intensive fear of an object or situation that the individual consciously recognizes as having no real danger; phobias are generally attributed to fears displaced to the phobic object from some other object of which the patient is unaware
   e. Obsessive-compulsive neurosis—characterized by persistent intrusion of unwanted thoughts, urges, or actions that the individual is unable to stop; the thoughts may consist of single words, ideas, or trains of thought often perceived by individual as nonsensical; the actions vary from simple movements to complex rituals such as repeated handwashing
   f. Depressive neurosis—characterized by excessive reaction of depression due to internal conflict or to identifiable event such as loss of love object

2. Character or personality disorders

3. Psychophysiologic disorders
   a. Gastric ulcer—lesion may be result of excessive production of gastric juice and chronic repression of primitive and explosive methods of expressing aggression
   b. Neurodermatitis—skin responds to repressed tension in same manner as true visceral organ
   c. Ulcerative colitis—patient suffering from ulcerative colitis may give anal or intestinal values as compensation for oral receptivity and aggressiveness
   d. Asthma—may be physical expression of anxiety related to unmet anxiety needs
   e. Essential hypertension—may be manifestation of psychoneurotic condition based upon excessive and inhibited hostile impulses
   f. Rheumatoid arthritis—general psychodynamic background of many patients may be that of inhibited, hostile, aggressive state and excessive masochistic need to do for others
   g. Migraine headache—evidence suggests that conflict situations such as hostile destructive aims toward beloved person set off migrainous attacks

3. **Character and personality disorders**

A. Inadequate personality—characterized by ineffectual responses to emotional, social, intellectual, and physical demands; individual seems neither physically nor mentally deficient but manifests lack of adaptability, as well as ineptness, poor judgment, social instability, and lack of physical and emotional stamina

B. Schizoid personality—characterized by

shyness, oversensitivity, seclusiveness, avoidance of close or competitive relationships, and eccentricity; often succumb to daydreaming with an inability to express hostility and ordinary aggressive feelings; individuals react to disturbing experiences and conflicts with apparent detachment

C. Cyclothymic personality (affective personality)—characterized by recurring and alternating periods of depression and elation; periods of elation are marked by ambition, warmth, enthusiasm, optimism, and high energy; periods of depression are marked by worry, pessimism, low energy, and a sense of futility; these mood variations are not readily attributable to external circumstances

D. Paranoid personality—characterized by hypersensitivity, rigidity, unwarranted suspicions, jealousy, envy, excessive self-importance, and a tendency to blame others and ascribe evil motives to them; these symptoms interfere with the ability to maintain satisfactory interpersonal relations

4. **Sociopathic personality disorders**
A. Antisocial personality—characterized by an inability to conform to social or legal standards; marked by great irresponsibility, egocentricity, poor judgment, inability to profit from experience, and inability to develop lasting and meaningful relationships with others
    1. Addiction
        a. Alcoholism—episodic, habitual or addictive types characterized by emotional immaturity, dependency and instability, extremely low frustration tolerance, feelings of isolation, tendency to act impulsively with hostility and rebellion, little ability to persevere
        b. Drug addiction—characterized by addiction to or dependency on drugs other than alcohol, tobacco, and ordinary caffeine-containing beverages; personality profile similar to that seen in alcoholism; drugs commonly used include morphine, cocaine, bromides, barbituric acid, heroin, and Demerol
        c. Drug abuse—a process characterized by nonaddictive usage of drugs to produce mood changes and sensory stimulation
            (1) Marijuana (*Cannabis sativa*)—

mild intoxicant and/or hallucinogen, depending on amount used and personality predisposition of user
            (2) LSD (lysergic acid diethylamide), psilocybin (found in certain mushrooms), mescaline (peyote buttons), jimsonweed (*Datura stramonium*), and mandrake (*Mandragora*)—hallucinogenic properties evoking profound mental changes and exceptional sensory stimulation
            (3) Glue sniffing, gasoline or solvent inhalation (volatile intoxicants)—usage may lead to brain damage

5. **Nurse's role in understanding, identifying, and meeting needs of individual with impaired functional-adaptational development**
A. Individual's inability to establish and maintain meaningful relationships must be understood as being the result of unresolved psychic conflict
B. Therapeutic nurse-patient relationship must be based upon the concept that positive behavior will receive approval; negative behavior will be accepted but will not receive approval
    1. Frustration and anxiety should be identified and allowed to be expressed
    2. Realistic and appropriate praise and encouragement should be given
C. Hostility and aggression expressed by the patient should be accepted and channeled into appropriate outlets
D. Nurse must accept that she, too, may experience anxiety, frustration, hostility, aggression in the process of developing a meaningful relationship with the patient

6. **Methods of treatment used for individuals with impaired functional-adaptational development**
A. Psychoanalysis—method of treatment that utilizes free association to bring repressed conflictual material back into consciousness so that the individual, on the basis of a greater understanding of needs and motives, may find a real solution to the conflict; goal is to uproot the neurosis rather than to focus on the symptoms alone; therapist assumes nonjudgmental role (passive-objective); relaxed listening allows relationship to develop into transference, therapist wait-

ing for patient to acquire motivation and work through resistance to reach unconscious and the repressed material
1. Psychoanalytic methods and concepts
   a. Free association—verbalization of whatever thoughts come into mind, freely associating events from whole life-span of experiences, feelings, fantasies, and dreams without concern for logic or continuity
   b. Transference phenomenon—emotional reaction of patient to therapist, in which patient relives conflicts and emotions emerging from the past and the unconscious; emotions and feelings toward significant others in childhood and past are transferred to therapist
B. Psychotherapy—method of uncovering unconscious material in order to strengthen the ego's ability to handle repressed emotional conflicts
1. General types
   a. Supportive—aimed at helping patient deal with problems
   b. Uncovering—uncovers and gives meaning to repressed conflicts
2. More participation and interpretative intervention by therapist (active-objective)
C. Brief psychotherapy—developed as result of increased demand for mental health services and lack of personnel; roots in psychoanalytic theory; limited to removing or alleviating specific symptoms; intervention may lead to some reconstruction of personality; main purpose—to improve or maintain the individual's ability to function; secondary purpose—to prevent development of deeper neurotic or psychotic symptoms after critical life situations
1. Basic methods
   a. Focus is on current reality
   b. Concentration on target symptoms
   c. Face-to-face dialogue intense and of short duration
   d. Regressive dependency and ambivalent transference are avoided
   e. Therapist is active
   f. Termination of treatment is preset
D. Group psychotherapy—method of treating emotional problems of individual in a group setting; individuals are encouraged to be honest and direct, as well as supportive and comforting; in the immediate experience new relationships are formed, multiple transferences are established, repressed and suppressed material may be uncovered
1. Types of group therapy—psychodrama, sensitivity, "T" groups, encounter, confrontation, marathon
E. Crisis intervention—seeks to resolve immediate crisis when individual's important life goals are for a time obstructed and usual problem-solving methods fail; periods of disorganization and upset result while many abortive attempts at solution are made
1. General approach—focus is on particular kind of crisis, with direct encouragement of adaptive behavior, general support, environmental manipulation, anticipatory guidance
2. Individual approach—interpersonal and intrapsychic processes of individual are assessed; treatment deals with the "now"; little or no concern for developmental past; emphasis upon immediate causes of disequilibrium, with aim to regain a precrisis or higher level of functioning
3. Steps in crisis intervention
   a. Assessment of individual and problem
      (1) Determine onset of crisis
      (2) Determine precipitating factor
      (3) Determine degree of disruption to individual and to others in his life circle
      (4) Determine individual's strengths, past methods used in coping, who are significant others in his life who may help
   b. Planning therapeutic intervention
      (1) With information gained through assessment, begin to search for alternative coping methods that for some reason are not being used
   c. Intervention—dependent upon preexisting skills, creativity, and flexibility of therapist and upon rapidity of response of individual
      (1) Establish intellectual understanding of crisis; show relationship between precipitating factor (event in life) and crisis
      (2) Reduce immobility caused by anxiety, by helping to bring out those immediately accessible repressed feelings of grief, rage, anger, etc.

(3) Explore coping mechanisms; search reservoir of experiences for successful coping devices used in past or devise new methods

(4) Reopen social world; attempt to establish new supportive and meaningful relationships and experiences

d. Resolution and anticipatory planning—reenforcement of successful coping devices by therapist; summary to allow for confirmation and reenforcement; assistance given as needed to make realistic future plans; indication as to how present experience may help in coping with future crises

e. Crisis intervention techniques include the following

(1) Crisis intervention should be directed toward a one-to-one relationship directed at identification and resolution of a problem

(2) The individual's reservoir of past experiences and coping methods is tapped, in seeking alternative methods of dealing with problem

7. Role of occupational therapy in mental health

A. Encourages individual to become involved in activities that reestablish old skills and knowledge or initiate new abilities, which may serve as a hobby or basis for establishing other challenging interests

B. Self-esteem and self-confidence are developed in an effort to establish ability to cope with life outside hospital

8. Role of recreational therapy in mental health

A. Encourages individual to become involved in familiar recreational activities and to learn to participate in new activities

B. Activities are planned to allow individuals to relate to one another in a structured social or recreational setting (resocialization)

C. Allows for the outlet and expression of physical energy in competitive games

D. Allows for the satisfaction of participating in sedentary activities for elderly patients

9. Contributions of social work in mental health

A. Interpreting the significance of patient's social environment to all members of the interdisciplinary treatment team

B. Helping the patient and his family to effectively use the health and social resources available to them

C. Helping the patient and his family to understand and accept the need for hospitalization

D. Helping the patient and his family by explaining the admission procedure

E. Working with the interdisciplinary treatment team, the patient, and his family to plan for discharge

F. Helping discharged patients find community interests and jobs

G. Psychiatric social workers with specialty training are therapists and cotherapists along with psychiatrists, psychologists, and nurses

10. Responsibilities of community in mental health

A. Priorities must be established for the expenditure of public funds for the restoration, maintenance, and establishment of diagnostic, treatment, and institutional facilities

B. Programs designed to educate and enlighten the public about the developments and needs in the field of mental health need to be sponsored

C. Programs in sex education need to be established in grade schools and high schools in an effort to

1. Provide intelligent social, emotional, and physiologic sex education for children

2. Prepare young people for the responsibilities of marriage and parenthood

D. Recreational facilities must be established for all age groups

E. Day and night care facilities, sheltered workshops, "foster homes" for all age groups, aftercare, halfway houses must be considered in community planning

F. Multiple community efforts in the areas of alcohol and drug abuse must be coordinated for maximum efficiency and community benefit

UNDERSTANDING THE INDIVIDUAL WITH DISINTEGRATIVE EMOTIONAL PROCESSES

1. Differentiation between psychoneurotic reactions and psychotic disorders

A. Psychoneurosis—process of substitution used to maintain anxiety at a tolerable level; the individual uses other techniques, as well, as a way of making unacceptable impulses acceptable; the neurotic symptom is an adaptive reaction; the major function is to prevent disintegration of personality and promote repair

B. Psychosis—results when the repressed aspects of personality emerge into conscious awareness; these aspects are alien to the ego and disruptive to the usual, conventional, acceptable social processes; the individual withdraws from reality, becomes wholly preoccupied with fantasy, and engages in a psychic struggle that consists of intense rage, stuporous immobility, or a combination of both

2. **Affective reactions—manic-depressive; involutional depression**

A. Causes, types, and symptomatology characteristic of affective reactions
   1. Causes
      a. Biogenetic factor thought to contribute but has yet to be proved; incidence twenty-five times as high among the siblings of manic-depressive patients as in average population
      b. Definite, disturbing life situations exist in 80% of the attacks; changes in environment or threats to social, economic, or physical security may precipitate the mood swings
      c. Cyclothymic personalities having wide spectrum of mood swings suggest predisposition
   2. Symptoms of manic phase of manic-depressive reaction
      a. Pronounced and sustained elated mood and affect
      b. Overtalkativeness
      c. Flight of ideas
      d. Excessive psychomotor activity
      e. Narcissism, little tolerance of criticism, loss of insight
   3. Symptoms of depressed phase of manic-depressive reaction
      a. Pronounced morbid depression of mood and affect
      b. Extreme psychomotor retardation and inhibition
      c. Verbal responses monosyllabic
      d. Vacillation and perplexity in decision-making
      e. Feelings of unworthiness, to the

extremes of self-destruction or mutilation

4. Interpretation of manic-depressive reactions
   a. Manic phase is essentially a massive denial of the underlying depression
   b. Depressive phase represents a penance for repressed hatred, aggressiveness, and impulses that have given rise to guilt; rigid superego forces redirection of hostile, aggressive tendencies against self

5. Symptoms and factors of involutional depression
   a. Symptoms
      (1) Progressive hypochondriasis
      (2) Progressive insomnia
      (3) Self-depreciation
      (4) Self-doubt and indecision
      (5) Profound depression
      (6) Delusions of disease and impending death
      (7) Extreme anxiety and agitation
      (8) Suicidal impulses
   b. Factors
      (1) Age—periods of psychophysiologic stress (males, late fifties; females, late forties); threat to personality through loss of prized biologic functions and imminence in aging process along with extensive changes in metabolic and vegetative activities of the body
      (2) Prepsychotic personality—superego-dominated; history of anxious, insecure childhood; personality inventory reveals person to be compulsive, inhibited, quiet, serious, chronically worrisome, intolerant, sensitive, scrupulously honest, frugal, apprehensive, with narrowed interests
      (3) Predisposing elements—realization that early dreams and desires cannot be fulfilled, zenith of life has passed, with opportunities for success diminished, plus loneliness, loss of physical attractiveness, children growing up and leaving home, friends dying, loss of feeling that he is needed, ebbing potency in male

B. Nursing care in affective reactions

1. Nursing care of hyperactive patient (manic phase)
   a. Reduce environmental stimuli
   b. Provide safe and appropriate outlet for excessive energy, remembering that fatigue produces excitement—not tranquility
   c. Anticipate and prevent combative, destructive behavior
   d. Maintain nutritional and fluid intake
   e. Provide safe environment and opportunities for rest
   f. Maintain accepting, nonjudgmental attitude
2. Nursing care of underactive patient (depressed phase)
   a. Prevent suicide
   b. Maintain patient's physical appearance
   c. Provide undemanding tasks to allow for simple accomplishment avoiding frustration
   d. Stimulate reasonable and appropriate activity
   e. Reactivate old, familiar recreational and occupational skills and initiate undemanding, satisfying new ones
   f. Make decisions for patient
   g. Maintain nutritional and fluid intake
   h. Observe patient for signs of dehydration and acidosis
   i. Check bowel movements to avoid constipation
   j. Maintain accepting, nonjudgmental attitude
C. Types of therapy used in treating affective reactions
   1. Electroshock—highly effective (90%) treatment for depressive reaction
      a. Nurse's pretreatment responsibility to patient receiving electroshock treatment
         (1) Make certain patient has not eaten within 8 hours
         (2) Make certain patient has not received sedatives within 8 hours
         (3) Remove dentures
         (4) Toilet patient
         (5) Stay with patient prior to treatment, providing calm and reassurance
         (6) Avoid using the terms "electric shock" or "convulsion"; refer to procedure as "the treatment"
         (7) Assure patient that there will be no pain
         (8) Explain to patient that he will remember nothing but will desire to sleep
         (9) Reassure the patient that he will not be left alone
         (10) Take temperature, pulse, respiration, and blood pressure; report any unusual findings to appropriate person
         (11) Nurse must be aware of her own potential anxiety over this treatment and not project onto patient
      b. Nurse's posttreatment responsibility to patient receiving electroshock treatment
         (1) Stay until respiration and pulse are within normal limits and patient is asleep
         (2) Posttreatment confusion and excitement are common; do not leave patient unattended; use side rails on bed
         (3) Orient patient when awake in calm, reassuring manner
         (4) Return patient with assistance when ambulatory
         (5) Help patient to occupy time during the remainder of day and evening with meaningful, interesting activities designed to allow for the development of a positive relationship with others
         (6) Reassure patient and family that some disorientation and/or amnesia is a common response to the treatment and that it will resolve itself shortly after completion of the designated number of treatments
   2. Psychotherapy—elastic, nondemanding, active interpretive approach in treating depressed phase; avoid responding to rejection provocation in manic phase
   3. Pharmacologic therapy
      a. Phenothiazines — tranquilizing agents used in manic phase
         (1) Side effects and untoward reactions
            (a) Side effects of tranquilizing agents
               (1) Complications reasonably uncommon and

no absolute contrain-
dications
(2) Increase in all toxic
effects with increase
in dosage and length
of time drug given
(3) Marked potentiation
of effects of barbitu-
rates and alcohol
(4) Drowsiness
(5) Dryness of mouth,
nasal congestion, con-
stipation
(6) Mild fever
(7) Increased appetite and
weight gain
(8) Vomiting and diarrhea
(b) Untoward reactions
(1) Jaundice
(2) Postural hypotension
(3) Symptoms closely re-
sembling parkinsonian
reaction
(4) Skin rash, especially
after undue exposure
to sun
(5) Delirium
(6) Agranulocytosis, al-
though infrequent,
may be serious
(7) Lower convulsive
threshold
(8) Lactation in female
patients
b. Lithium carbonate—highly effective in chronic and recurrent mania:
effective in damping depressive
phase of cyclic reaction
(1) Side effects and untoward
reactions
(a) Side effects
(1) Diarrhea
(2) Vomiting
(3) Drowsiness
(4) Ataxia
(5) Dizziness
(6) Excessive thirst
(7) Large output of urine
(b) Untoward reactions—because of high toxicity for
kidney function, drug is
contraindicated when his-
tory of kidney disease is
present or in heart dis-
ease, epilepsy, and the
elderly

c. Antidepressants—effective in elevating mood during depressive phase
(1) Side effects similar to those of
tranquilizing agents
d. Responsibility of nurse to patient
receiving drug therapy
(1) Make certain patient is taking
medication
(2) Persuade reluctant patient to
take medications regularly
(3) Know all possible side effects
and untoward reactions, observe patient carefully, report
symptoms to appropriate person
(4) Since drug therapy will make
the patient more accessible to
therapeutic interpersonal intervention, the nurse should make
effort to establish an accepting,
nonjudgmental relationship
(5) Plan creative, appropriate so-
cializing activities that will
neither overstimulate the manic
patient nor overly extend the
depressed
(6) Participate actively in observing, evaluating, and reporting
the quality and the quantity
of the patient's interaction to
the therapeutic interdisciplinary team which plans a treatment program for patient
D. Prognosis of affective reactions
1. Manic-depressive reactions
a. Prepsychotic personality traits influence prognosis as to both duration and outcome; being flexible,
tolerant, conciliatory, reasonably secure, without defensive of compensatory traits and having varied and
wholesome interests, promise more
favorable prognosis
b. Average untreated attacks of mania
last 6 months; average depressive
episodes last 9 months
c. Depressions increase in length with
advancing age
d. Depression more likely to become
chronic than mania
e. The more frequent the attacks the
poorer the prognosis
f. Prognosis worse when precipitation
is related directly to an actual loss
(exogenous cause) than when it is
due to covert experiences or factors
(endogenous)

g. Even after repeated episodes the mind is unchanged in its intellectual, affective and cognitive aspects; a disorganization of the personality does not follow

3. **Psychoses characterized by deterioration of personality—schizophrenic reactions**

A. Causes, onset, types, and symptomatology characteristic of schizophrenic reactions
 1. Causes
  a. Genetic—consistent evidence shows risk of schizophrenia increases to 50% if family member is affected, 85.5% in twins
  b. Prepsychotic personality—shy, insecure, limited sociability, narrow acquisition of emotional relations with extrafamily members during adolescence and adulthood; limited development of personal skills; perceptual discrimination and sense of personal autonomy necessary for effective social and heterosexual adaptation in adult life are lacking
  c. Emotional conflict—disturbed parental investment in child, limitation of mothering process, impaired sense of identity within family structure
 2. Onset—throughout entire life-span; highest incidence in adolescence; perplexed by new problems (sex, religion, vocation, and social relations), the individual may be in conflict over a desire for independence and the crippling effects of too long a dependence
 3. Types and symptoms
  a. Simple type
   (1) Progressive social maladaptation
   (2) Progressive eccentricity
   (3) Limited interests
   (4) Progressive indifference
   (5) Progressive dulling of affect
   (6) Hallucinations, rare and fleeting
  b. Catatonic type
   (1) Stupor or excitement
   (2) Negativism
   (3) Automation
   (4) Characteristic posturing
   (5) Hallucinations
  c. Hebephrenic type
   (1) Gross personality disintegration

   (2) Extreme autism
   (3) Bizarre and grossly inappropriate speech and behavior
   (4) Regressive behavior (bed-wetting, soiling)
   (5) Hallucinations
  d. Paranoid type
   (1) Ideas of reference
   (2) Delusions of persecution
   (3) Aggressive hostility
   (4) Auditory hallucinations
   (5) Suspiciousness and grandiosity

B. Nursing care of schizophrenic patient
 1. Provide a nonthreatening, safe environment in which a therapeutic interpersonal relationship may be established
 2. Develop and encourage opportunities and stimulate social activities through which the patient may develop a sense of self and a feeling of trust
 3. Encourage and help patient to maintain good personal hygiene and physical well-being to develop the continuing sense of self
 4. Maintain a constant effort to keep alive and reestablish an affective contact with reality

C. Types of therapy used in treatment of patients with schizophrenic reactions
 1. Psychotherapy—goals are to develop a more stable and adaptive personality, relieve anxiety, develop ego identity and function
 2. Group psychotherapy—can be used alone or in conjunction with individual psychotherapy; valuable for those who are inhibited in individual psychotherapy and those with major defects in group living
 3. Milieu therapy—emphasis on social rehabilitation stresses active social participation in group and an opportunity to gain satisfaction through learned adaptive behavior
 4. Pharmacologic treatment—provides relief of anxiety and symptoms of tension, impulsiveness, psychomotor overactivity, agitation, aggressive outbursts, destructiveness, and antagonistic paranoid reactions
  a. Phenothiazines
   (1) Chlorpromazine (Thorazine) —indicated for all types of schizophrenia
   (2) Trifluoperazine (Stellazine)— effective in treatment of with-

drawn, apathetic, and depressed schizophrenic
  (3) Thioridazin (Mellaril)—effective for all types of schizophrenia; fewer side effects
  (4) Perphenazine (Trilafon)—effective for all types of schizophrenia; does not cause photosensitivity
  5. Electroshock treatment—largely discontinued since advent of tranquilizing agents
  6. Insulin therapy—largely discontinued since advent of tranquilizing agents
  7. Prefrontal lobotomy—historically significant; discontinued since advent of tranquilizing agents
D. Prognosis for patients with schizophrenic reactions
  1. Incidence of recovery influenced by effectiveness of prepsychotic personality adjustment
  2. Sudden, acute onset indicates more favorable prognosis than slow, insidious onset
  3. Early diagnosis and treatment directly related to favorable prognosis
  4. Catatonic reactions thought to have more favorable prognosis than hebephrenic or paranoid reactions
E. Prevention of schizophrenic reactions
  1. Promotion of healthful patterns of living, thinking, and feeling to prevent the establishment of subterfuges and substitutions that result in imbalance of personality
  2. Stable home life with loving, understanding, and accepting parents
  3. More child guidance clinics and programs in schools
  4. Early detection and attention for shy, withdrawn, retiring, seclusive unsociable child and for those exhibiting antisocial behavior
  5. Continued mental health education for teachers to enable them to assist in early detection and in social and emotional development of children
  6. More and better-trained mental health professionals
  7. Continued and expanded mental health research
4. **Contributions of occupational and recreational therapy**
A. Encourages individual to become involved in activities that reestablish all skills and knowledge or initiate new abilities which may serve as a hobby or basis for establishing other challenging interests
B. Self-esteem and self-confidence are developed in an effort to establish ability to cope with life outside hospital
C. Encourages individual to become involved in familiar recreational activities and to learn and participate in new activities
D. Activities are planned to allow individuals to relate to one another in a structured social or recreational setting (rehabilitation)
E. Allows for the outlet and expression of physical energy in competitive games
F. Allows for the satisfaction of participating in sedentary activity for elderly patients
5. **Community responsibilities in mental health; losses due to high incidence of personality deterioration**
A. Community responsibilities in mental health
  1. Priorities must be established for the expenditure of public funds for the restoration, maintenance, and establishment of diagnostic treatment and institutional facilities
  2. Programs designed to educate and enlighten the public about the developments and needs in the field of mental health need to be sponsored
  3. Programs in sex education need to be established in grade schools and high schools in an effort to
    a. Provide intelligent social, emotional, and physiologic sex education for children
    b. Prepare young people for the responsibilities of marriage and parenthood
  4. Recreational facilities must be established for all age groups
  5. Day and night care facilities, sheltered workshops, foster homes for all age groups, aftercare, halfway houses must be considered in community planning
B. Community losses due to high incidence of schizophrenia
  1. More patients ill in United States each year with schizophrenia than with all other illnesses combined
  2. Schizophrenia strikes youth (17 to 25) more frequently than any other illness
  3. Schizophrenic reactions often become

chronic, thus costing community millions of dollars

4. In addition to cost of care of chronically ill patients, nation loses value of the talents, abilities, and manpower these people could provide

5. Homes from which patients come suffer in many ways from loss of these members; not least of this suffering is a feeling of shame and guilt—common attitudes in our society about mentally ill relatives

UNDERSTANDING THE PERSONALITY DISORGANIZATION IN BEHAVIOR PATTERNS RESULTING FROM TOXIC AND/OR ORGANIC BRAIN DISORDERS

1. **Symptomatology**
A. Clouded consciousness, accompanied by bewilderment, restlessness, confusion, disorientation, and impairment in thinking
B. Progressive deterioration and loss of memory
C. Progressive deterioration and impairment of judgment
D. Progressive disorientation as to time and place
E. Progressive language difficulties; defect in coherent train of expression
F. Lability of mood
G. Limited attention span
H. Frequent delusions and hallucinations

2. **Types of brain disorders**
A. Personality disorganization resulting from acute brain disorder
   1. Brain disorders with intracranial or systemic infection
      a. Etiology—infection and inflammation of brain tissue, or disturbance of blood supply to brain
      b. Symptomatology
         (1) Delirium
      c. Treatment
         (1) Medical and/or surgical treatment of infection
         (2) Bed rest
         (3) Sedation (tranquilizer or hypnotic)
         (4) Reduction of environmental stimuli
         (5) Adequate food and fluid intake
         (6) Vitamin replacement
         (7) Maintenance of normal acid-base equilibrium
   2. Brain disorders with drug or poison intoxication

a. Delirium with drugs or exogenous poisons
   (1) Etiology
      (a) Drug intoxication due to complications of drug therapy or occurring as secondary effect of suicidal attempt, self-medication, or accidental ingestion
      (b) Intoxication due to poisoning in suicidal or homicidal attempt, industrial accident, or accidental ingestion
   (2) Symptomatology
      (a) Mild intoxication—confusion, drowsiness, defective judgment, transient nystagmus, unsteady gait, slurred speech
      (b) Moderate intoxication—gross confusion, heavy drowsiness and sleep with arousal only on vigorous stimulation, constant nystagmus, dysarthria, slow respirations, depression of tendon reflexes
      (c) Severe intoxication—unarousable coma, absence of all reflexes, periodic respirations, signs of shock
   (3) Treatment
      (a) Identification and withdrawal of intoxicant (drug or poison)
      (b) Bed rest
      (c) Monitoring of vital signs
      (d) Adequate fluid intake
      (e) Maintenance of acid-base equilibrium
      (f) High-caloric diet
      (g) Safety precautions for delirious patient
b. Acute brain syndrome associated with alcohol intoxication
   (1) Types
      (a) Delirium tremens
      (b) Acute hallucinosis
      (c) Korsakoff's psychosis
   (2) Etiology
      (a) Delirium tremens—prolonged nutritional and vitamin deficiency and deprivation, especially of vitamin B

(b) Acute hallucinosis—clinical characteristics determined by personality factors; possible identification of schizophrenic reaction released by alcohol

(c) Korsakoff's psychosis—vitamin B deficiency due to chronic alcoholism, impaired gastrointestinal absorption, dietary deficiency consisting of high-caloric alcohol and little or no vitamin intake

(3) Symptomatology
   (a) Delirium tremens—clouding of consciousness, misidentification of people, auditory and tactile hallucinations, extreme fear (especially in relation to hallucinations), fumbling and picking at bedclothes, excessive profuse perspiration, tremors, rapid weak pulse, temperature elevation

   (b) Acute hallucinosis—accusatory and threatening auditory, olfactory, and visual hallucinations with marked fear and panic; rapid and elaborative delusional system develops

   (c) Korsakoff's psychosis—superficial clarity of consciousness; memory loss, amnesia, with confabulation in an attempt to relate fictitious memories to conceal actual amnesia; jovial disorientation; polyneuropathy (especially in lower extremities)

(4) Treatment
   (a) Discontinue use of alcohol
   (b) Bed rest, adequate fluid intake, high-caloric diet with addition of vitamin B
   (c) Control of hyperactivity through use of sedative medication, cold wet sheet packs, and sedative tub baths
   (d) Psychotherapy following

recovery from acute episode

(5) Nursing care of patient having personality disorder, with infection or intoxication
   (a) Provide constant nursing supervision
   (b) Provide sedative environment conducive to relaxation and sleep
   (c) Reduce fear by simplifying environmental stimuli
   (d) Maintain good oral hygiene
   (e) Maintain nutritional and fluid intake
   (f) Calmly accept hallucinations, illusions, and disorientation as part of the illness
   (g) Provide sympathy, reassurance, and understanding
   (h) Avoid use of mechanical restraints

B. Personality disorganization resulting from chronic brain disorder
   1. Disorders associated with trauma
      a. Psychopathology following brain lesion or trauma is an expression of the result of the cerebral lesion *and* the efforts of a damaged personality to adapt to these changes and to demands that can no longer be met because of defects
      b. Symptomatology
         (1) Mental deterioration
         (2) Convulsions
         (3) Personality changes
            (a) Easy distractibility
            (b) Emotional instability
            (c) Outbursts of rage and violence
            (d) Defects in memory and judgment
            (e) Extreme irritability
            (f) Progressive loss of interests
            (g) Confusion
      c. Treatment for personality change following brain injury will depend upon severity of the lesion, pretraumatic personality of the patient, and rapidity of the initiation of rehabilitation; no final assessment of the degree of damage should be

made in less than 12 to 18 months after the injury

2. Disorders associated with new growth
   a. Symptoms depend upon location, size, and type of growth
   b. Symptomatology
      (1) Physical symptoms
         (a) Headache
         (b) Unsteady gait
         (c) Projectile vomiting
         (d) Seizures
      (2) Mental symptoms
         (a) Sluggishness
         (b) Poor attention
         (c) Lethargy
         (d) Irritability
         (e) Stupor
         (f) Marked personality change noted when frontal lobe is site of growth
   c. Treatment
      (1) Surgical removal only treatment of permanent value; successful surgical intervention depends upon site, size, and type of tumor
      (2) Growth of tumor may be stopped temporarily or inhibited by x-ray therapy
3. Disorders associated with degenerative and arteriosclerotic changes
   a. Types
      (1) Senile reaction patterns
      (2) Disorders associated with circulatory disturbances
      (3) Disorders associated with changes of the nervous system that are of uncertain cause
         (a) Huntington's chorea
         (b) Multiple sclerosis
   b. Etiology
      (1) Causes of senile reaction patterns attributed to
         (a) Atrophy of brain
         (b) Formation of senile plaques
         (c) Arteriosclerotic changes
         (d) Failure to maintain interests in life
         (e) Inability to meet personal problems brought on by aging
      (2) Cerebral arteriosclerosis caused by the closing or narrowing of lumen of blood vessel, as large patches or plaques of fatty and calcified material deposited
      (3) Huntington's chorea a familial disease transmitted directly from parent to child as simple mendelian dominant
      (4) Cause of multiple sclerosis unknown; patches of sclerotic degeneration appear at widely scattered spots in brain and spinal cord and cause wide variety of symptoms, depending upon position of sclerotic foci
   c. Symptomatology
      (1) Simple senile deterioration
         (a) Loss of memory for recent events
         (b) Tendency to reminisce
         (c) Intolerance of change
         (d) Disorientation
         (e) Restlessness
         (f) Insomnia
         (g) Failure of judgment
      (2) Delirious and confused senile reaction
         (a) Extreme restlessness
         (b) Misidentification of people
         (c) Combative and resistive behavior
         (d) Incoherence
         (e) Complete disorientation
      (3) Cerebral arteriosclerosis
         (a) Painful anxiety
         (b) Crying spells
         (c) Outbursts of irritability
         (d) Excessive preoccupation with symptoms
         (e) As condition becomes chronic, patient loses initiative, endurance diminishes, and concentration becomes difficult and trying
      (4) Huntington's chorea develops in middle life, with twitching of face and with purposeless movements of trunk and limbs; slow intellectual deterioration and personality changes expressed by irritability and outbursts of temper
      (5) Multiple sclerosis usually begins in early adult life and progresses slowly

(a) Symptoms are of numerous types and varying degrees of severity

(b) Mental changes occur in advanced and chronic forms and consist largely of emotional instability, tendency to euphoria, gradual blunting of mental activity, and progressive tendency to sluggishness and indifference

d. Treatment for patients suffering from disorders associated with degenerative and arteriosclerotic changes

(1) No specific treatment for these diseases

(a) Patients should be maintained with dignity in safe, happy, and comfortable environment

(b) Avoid irritating situations, changes in habits of eating, resting, working, or living

(c) Utilize simple occupational and recreational therapy

(d) Institutional care is frequently necessary

4. Disorders associated with defective organic conditions

a. Types

(1) Disorders associated with mental deficiency

(2) Disorders associated with epilepsy or convulsive disorders

b. Causes

(1) Mental deficiency—lack of intellectual capacity, derived from an innately imposed limitation in cerebral development, a result of disease or injury to the brain suffered before, during, or in the period immediately after birth; a result of genetic defects; or the consequence of impaired maturation due to sensory and environmental deprivation from familial and cultural sources

(2) Epilepsy—disturbance in the electrophysicochemical activity of the discharging cells of the brain; may be produced by brain trauma, brain tumor, brain infection, alcoholism; or may exist in the absence of demonstrable brain defects

c. Treatment

(1) Mentally defective

(a) Training in special schools that assist such an individual to attain his maximum level of intellectual and social functioning

(b) Institutionalization indicated for many mentally defectives, for their safety and because of inability of families and society to cope with and accept their problems

(2) Epilepsy

(a) Phenobarbital, Dilantin, and Mesantoin are principal drugs used to control grand mal epilepsy

(b) Tridione and Paradione are used specifically to control petit mal seizures

(c) Institutionalization is indicated for small number of epileptics who suffer personality disorganization

5. Nurse's role in care of patients suffering from chronic brain disorders

a. Provide dignified, safe, simple, carefully regulated daily routine

b. Recognize emotional and intellectual limitations

c. Protect against judgmental defects

d. Avoid emotional upsets

e. Provide simple occupational diversion

f. Supervise personal hygiene carefully

g. Provide simple, well-balanced, easily digested diet

h. Keep patients as happy and comfortable as possible

i. Provide security and reassurance

j. Use kind, sympathetic approach

k. Help patients to utilize intellectual capacity to the fullest

6. Significance to society of personality disorganization occurring with disorders associated with impairment of brain tissue function

a. Society's responsibilities

(1) Alcoholism is on increase

throughout country; recognized as major United States health problem with the attendant emotional, social, and economic pressures it causes for individuals, families, communities, and the nation; casual attitudes toward abuse of alcohol must be be corrected by intensified programs of education

(2) Auto manufacturers, consumer groups, state and federal agencies, and the public must recognize that, as highway traffic accidents increase, incidence of posttraumatic encephalopathy increases

(3) Society has not yet elected to establish high priorities for the care, treatment, rehabilitation, and education of its mentally retarded children and adults

(4) Sheltered workshops, rehabilitation programs, and colonies for severely handicapped epileptics are needed in every state, along with programs designed to correct public misconceptions and misinformation regarding epileptics

(5) The increasing number of aged persons in our society need to be guaranteed the right to live in dignity, with opportunity to have meaningful occupation and continued use of the skills they have developed over decades; they also need opportunity for socialization and the feeling that they are a part of, not apart from, mainstream of society

b. Prevention
(1) Individual, familial, social attitudes toward casual abuse of alcohol and taboos associated with alcoholism must be changed; more clinics and programs for alcoholics and the members of their families need to be established; mental health professionals need to appreciate and better utilize the unique and effective role played by Alcoholics Anonymous

(2) More extensive medical and

social research is needed to prevent, interrupt, and retard senile reaction patterns; community must accept responsibility to incorporate the aged in all programs

REVIEW QUESTIONS FOR PSYCHIATRIC NURSING
Multiple choice

Read each question carefully and consider all possible answers. When you have decided which answer is best, blacken in the corresponding space on the answer sheet. There is only one best answer for each question (or implied question).

1. Donald R (questions 1 to 4), a 19-year-old college sophomore, has been admitted through the university health service. He had become increasingly withdrawn, unkempt, isolated, and depressed. The referring psychiatrist has detected strong suicidal tendencies. A contributing factor appears to be a very recent broken romance with a 22-year-old senior. His grades have fallen to the extent that he is in danger of failing all his courses. He had been a B to B+ student throughout high school and his freshman year. Donald's prognosis for reasonably rapid recovery is
   1. Poor, since he has suicidal tendencies
   2. Bad, since he is failing in all sectors of his life
   3. Fair, since he is intelligent enough to pull himself together
   4. Good, since the onset is fairly sudden and no previous emotional problems existed

2. Donald's parents have just concluded a visit with him. They have been telling him how pleased they are that he broke up with that "older woman" and how distressed they are that he will fail his courses. They have clearly indicated to him that they are ashamed that he is in a psychiatric hospital, but have told him that they would be afraid to take him home because he might kill himself. A positive and healthy response by Donald would be
   1. "I'm sorry I caused you all this trouble. I know how terrible you must feel."
   2. "I was pretty confused, but I think I can sort things out now."
   3. "It's always how you feel, how ashamed you are, what you want, isn't it?"
   4. "I don't give a damn how you feel. It's my life."

3. On the second day after his admission Donald asks the nurse why he is being observed around-the-clock and restricted as to his freedom of movement. The nurse's most appropriate reply would be
   1. "Your doctor has ordered it. He's the one you should ask."

2. "Why do you think we are observing you?"
3. "We are concerned that you might try to harm yourself."
4. "What makes you think that, Donald?"

4. On the fourth day Donald tells the nurse, "Hey look! I was feeling pretty depressed for a while, but I'm certainly not going to kill myself." Which comment by the nurse best responds to the patient's communication?
   1. "Kill yourself? I don't understand."
   2. "We have to observe you until your doctor tells us to stop."
   3. "Suppose we talk some more about this?"
   4. "You do seem to be feeling better."

Situation: Mr. J is a handsome and smooth-talking bright young man who has been forced to marry 3 different girls because each named him as the father of her child. Each of his wives divorced him within a few months because of his irresponsible and unfaithful behavior. He says that he has never loved any of these girls, that he does not intend to support his children, and that he has no reason to be sorry for anything he has ever done. His parents brought him to the hospital for psychiatric help, since they can no longer tolerate the disgrace that he brings upon them. He has told the psychiatrist that there is nothing wrong with him and that he does not need treatment. Questions 5 through 14 apply to this patient.

5. Mr. J's behavior would fall into which of the following psychiatric classifications?
   1. Obsessive-compulsive reaction
   2. Psychoneurotic reaction
   3. Anxiety reaction
   4. Sociopathic personality disturbance
6. Mr. J's behavior may be due to defective personality development in which area?
   1. Id development
   2. Ego development
   3. Superego development
   4. Sexual development
7. In working with Mr. J the nurse should adopt the following kind of attitude:
   1. Sincere, cautious, and consistent
   2. Strict, punishing, and restrictive
   3. Accepting, supportive, and friendly
   4. Sympathetic, motherly, and encouraging
8. Ms. Moody, student nurse, is taking a new patient on an admission-orientation tour of the service when another patient, Mr. J, rushes down the hallway and asks her to sit and talk to him. Which would be the most appropriate action by the nursing student?
   1. Excuse herself from the new patient and speak with Mr. J
   2. Suggest to Mr. J that he talk with another staff member
   3. Introduce Mr. J and suggest that he might join them on the tour
   4. Tell Mr. J that she will speak with him later
9. Mr. J responds to her suggestion by smiling broadly and saying "Ms. Moody, you sure do look messy today." Which would be the most appropriate response by the student nurse?
   1. "That's not a nice thing to say, Mr. J."
   2. "Don't you feel well today, Mr. J?"
   3. "I didn't get a chance to set my hair last night."
   4. "You're angry with me Mr. J."
10. Mr. J takes Ms. Moody by the shoulder, suddenly kisses her, and shouts "I like you." Which would be the most appropriate response for the student nurse to make?
    1. "I like you too, but please don't do that again."
    2. "I wish you wouldn't do that."
    3. "Don't ever touch me like that again."
    4. "Thank you, I liked that very much."
11. In the previous situation Ms. Moody should consider which rule of appropriate behavior?
    1. The professional role must not be confused with the social one
    2. Never become personally involved with a patient
    3. Always be prepared to meet the patient's needs
    4. Limits must be realistically and objectively set.
12. The new patient waits until Mr. J has left and whispers to Ms. Moody, "He's one of the ones who were trying to poison me." Ms. Moody's most appropriate response to the patient's comment is
    1. "I don't understand. Mr. J has been trying to poison you?"
    2. "Don't worry. Let me introduce you to some of the other patients."
    3. "That's crazy talk. You'll never get well thinking like that."
    4. "It couldn't have been him. He's been locked up here for months."
13. Mr. J has just been given the first day pass from the hospital. He is due to return at 6:00 P.M. At 5:00 P.M., Mr. J telephones the nurse in charge of the ward and says "Six o'clock is too early. I feel like coming back at 7:30 P.M." Which approach by the nurse would be most therapeutic at this time?
    1. Tell him to return immediately
    2. Tell him to return on time or he will be restricted
    3. Tell him to come back some time between 6:00 and 7:30 P.M. No one is likely to notice
    4. Tell him to come back whenever he feels like it; he is to set his own limits
14. Ms. Moody's psychiatric experience will be over in 2 weeks. She tells Mr. J that she is leaving. Which response would indicate that he is progressing in his ability to maintain more mature relationships?
    1. He tells her that he too must get well enough, by then, so that he may also leave
    2. He wishes her good luck and thanks her for helping him
    3. He tells her that her leaving is just another loss he must adjust to
    4. He informs her that, since she is leaving, this should be their last meeting

Situation: Ms. Black was brought to the hospital for psychiatric treatment because her behavior has interfered with her daily functioning. Her symptoms included an uncontrollable and constant desire to scrub herself and the walls and furniture of her home with strong disinfectants because she felt that everything was contaminated with virulent disease germs. Although she realized that it was not sensible, Ms. Black was unable to mingle in crowds because of fear of being contaminated. Questions 15 through 19 apply to this patient.

15. Such symptoms are usually thought of as belonging to which of the following categories?
    1. Manic-depressive reaction
    2. Anxiety reaction
    3. Obsessive-compulsive reaction
    4. Dissociative reaction
16. Ms. Black's preoccupation with thoughts of the contaminating germs in her home is called
    1. Compulsion   3. Delusion
    2. Obsession   4. Anxiety
17. When Ms. Black carries on a regimen of continuous scrubbing, she is exhibiting the mechanism of adaptive behavior that is called
    1. Sublimation   3. Projection
    2. Suppression   4. Displacement
18. When Ms. Black is unable to control repetitive behavior that she considers illogical, she is exhibiting a symptom called
    1. Delusion   3. Phobia
    2. Compulsion   4. Hysteria
19. Ms. Black's symptom of morbid fear of disease germs is called
    1. Delusion   3. Phobia
    2. Hallucination   4. Illusion

Situation: Mr. T, a successful corporation lawyer, came to the hospital for psychiatric treatment because of symptoms of persistent gastric distress that accompanied all food intake. Although he had received a great deal of medical help from specialists in the field of internal medicine, it was suggested that he needed psychiatric care. His history included 5 years of emotional stress after his marriage to a successful actress who refused to accept the role of homemaker and mother and who was admired by many other men. Recently he had lost 2 important legal cases. The only time his wife gave him much attention was during his hospitalizations, which had become increasingly numerous. Questions 20 through 26 apply to this patient.

20. Mr. T's illness can be classified as
    1. An affective reaction
    2. A chronic brain disorder
    3. A psychophysiologic disorder
    4. A psychotic disorder
21. Mr. T is employing the mechanism of adjustive behavior which is called
    1. Repression
    2. Projection
    3. Suppression
    4. Sublimation
22. In encouraging Mr. T to become involved in activities the nurse should
    1. Heap praise on all his efforts
    2. Insist that he is expected to participate
    3. Show interest in his efforts on and off the ward

4. Show him the fine work done in O.T., by other patients
23. The goal of the therapeutic environment is to
    1. Help the patient become popular
    2. Improve the patient's ability to relate to others
    3. Help the staff with their daily work
    4. Make the hospital atmosphere more home-like
24. Mr. T moves uncomfortably from one foot to the other, hangs his head low, does not look up when he says "Ms. Moody, you're so nice to take the time to talk to me. It must be boring for you to have to listen to me. I'm so sick and I say such things." Ms. Moody's most appropriate reply would be
    1. "I have to learn how to talk to sick people, Mr. T."
    2. "The sicker you are the more you need to talk."
    3. "I don't understand what you're trying to tell me, Mr. T."
    4. "It's easy to talk with you, Mr. T, you're such a nice person."
25. Mr. T has been attending the group sessions for the past 3 weeks. He seems uncomfortable, polite, reserved, and uninvolved in the verbal exchanges. He reveals to Ms. Moody that he is ashamed to have to attend these sessions and that listening to the exchange among the group members only further serves to heighten his anticipation of rejection by the others. Ms. Moody can best help Mr. T cope with these feelings by
    (a) Encouraging group sessions in which members point out each other's positive qualities
    (b) Telling Mr. T that the longer he resists involvement the weaker and more frightened he will become
    (c) Telling him that there are others who are sicker than he; he has nothing to lose by participating
    (d) Carefully observing and pointing out to Mr. T his strengths and accomplishments
    1. a and b   3. a and d
    2. c and d   4. b and c
26. During a later group meeting Mr. T tells everyone of his fear of his impending discharge from the hospital. Which response by the group leader would be most appropriate?
    1. "Maybe you're not ready to be discharged."
    2. "Maybe others in the group have similar feelings."
    3. "You ought to be happy that you're leaving."
    4. "How many in the group feel that Mr. T is ready to be discharged?"

Situation: Ms. R, an attractive unmarried 24-year-old teacher, has been referred for psychiatric evaluation following the sudden onset of the following symptoms: panic, apprehension, palpitations, vague overwhelming fears, general weakness, excessive perspiration in the palms of her hands, and a feeling of constricting tightness in her chest. Her father is a 68-year-old cardiac patient with a history of frequent admissions to hospitals for "heart attacks" that are precipitated by family quarrels. Her symptoms began about 2 months ago when her fiance insisted that she resign her position and marry. A series of examinations by medical specialists reveal no organic illness. For the past month she has remained in bed most of the day and night. Questions 27 through 34 apply to this patient.

27. Ms. R's symptoms fall into the following classification
    1. Obsessive-compulsive reaction
    2. Phobic reaction
    3. Depressive reaction
    4. Anxiety reaction
28. Why is the information that her father is a cardiac patient with a history of frequent hospitalizations for "heart attacks," which are precipitated by family quarrels, important?
    1. Ms. R's anxiety is due to her fear that if she quarrels she will have a heart attack
    2. Her symptoms have become a learned type of response to emotional stress.
    3. Ms. R blames her father for her own illness
    4. Ms. R's family blames her for her father's heart attacks
29. Which of the following mechanisms of adjustment is Ms. R using?
    1. Projection   3. Displacement
    2. Sublimation   4. Introjection
30. Ms. Moody and the patient walk to a quiet corner of the ward. Ms. R's anxiety mounts. She becomes increasingly restless, moving rapidly from one foot to the other, and wringing her hands. Her face is contorted as though in pain. Ms. Moody suddenly feels uncomfortable and wishes she could leave the scene. The probable reason for her feeling is
    1. Her inability to tolerate any more crazy behavior
    2. Her desire to go off duty
    3. The empathic communication of anxiety
    4. Her fear of the patient
31. Just before she is to go off duty for the day Ms. Moody is confronted by Ms. R, who says "that feeling, it's coming back. I'm so afraid that the evening staff won't like me like this. They'll seclude me." Ms. Moody can best assist the patient by saying
    1. "Don't worry. I told you that you'd be all right."
    2. "I have to go now. Can we talk about this in the morning?"
    3. "Tell me more about what you're feeling now."
    4. "I'll ask the staff not to lock you up."
32. The next afternoon Ms. R meets Ms. Moody in the hallway. She says, "That was a terrible feeling I had yesterday. I'm so afraid to talk about it." Ms. Moody's most useful response would be
    1. "Okay, let's not talk about it."
    2. "It's best that you tell me all about it."
    3. "What were you doing yesterday when you first noticed the feeling?"

4. "Don't worry; tnat feeling won't come back."
33. Later Ms. R tells Ms. Moody that she is still uncomfortable and says that she feels helpless to control her discomfort. To intervene effectively, the student nurse will need to know
    1. What kind of medication she takes when she feels like this
    2. How Ms. R responds to seclusion
    3. How long she has been feeling like this
    4. What she has done in the past to help relieve anxiety
34. While Ms. Moody, the student nurse, stands quietly beside her, Ms. R moves from one foot to the other, wringing her hands, and suddenly says "I don't know what to do with myself. I can't stop this. I can't sit still." Ms. Moody's most therapeutic response would be
    1. "What makes you so restless?"
    2. "Why don't we play some Ping-Pong?"
    3. "Would you like me to stay with you?"
    4. "I don't mind it at all."

Situation: Mr. F, 21, is an only child who has never earned his own living and has always been pampered and coddled by his domineering mother and ignored by his quiet, retiring father. When he started dating, his mother chose the girls he took out. Recently Mr. F married a girl several years older than he, even though his mother seriously disapproved of her. Despite this, he brought his wife to his home to live. Both the mother and the wife were unhappy with this arrangement. Mr. F had many guilt feelings about his marriage and soon began to complain of pain in his right arm, which progressed to the point of paralysis. After seeking help from competent orthopedic specialists he was referred for psychiatric evaluation. Questions 35 through 39 apply to this patient.

35. Mr. F's symptoms may be an unconscious attempt to solve a conflict concerning
    1. Hostile feelings toward his home
    2. Ambivalent feelings toward his wife
    3. Needs to be a dependent child and an independent adult
    4. Inadequate feelings in regard to assuming the role of husband
36. In dealing with Mr. F the nurse should realize that
    1. This symptom is necessary in order for Mr. F to cope with his present situation
    2. This symptom is an unconscious method of attention getting
    3. Mr. F can get well if he is helped to focus on other things
    4. His problems will be solved when he leaves his wife
37. Mr. F's symptoms seem to indicate that he is suffering from
    1. Depressive reaction
    2. Anxiety reaction
    3. Phobic reaction
    4. Conversion reaction
38. What could be said about Mr. F's prognosis after appropriate treatment?
    1. His symptoms of paralysis will spread to other parts of his body

2. Continuous psychiatric treatment will be required to maintain him as a functioning individual
3. Recovery of the use of the arm can be expected, but under stress he may utilize similar symptoms
4. It is not possible to predict what the future for this patient holds

39. In relating with Mr. F the nurse should understand that interpersonal relationships will be affected by
   1. The situation
   2. The personalities of both the nurse and the patient
   3. Careful listening
   4. All of these

Situation: Ms. L, a 23-year-old bride, has been married 3 months. She was admitted to a psychiatric hospital after a month of unusual behavior that included eating and sleeping very little, talking or singing constantly, charging hundreds of dollars' worth of furniture to her father-in-law, and picking up dates on the street. In the hospital, Ms. L monopolized conversation, insisted upon unusual privileges, and frequently became demanding, bossy, and sarcastic. She had periods of great overactivity and sometimes became destructive. She frequently used vulgar and profane language. Ms. L had formerly been witty, gay, and the "life of the party." Her many friends say she was always ladylike in spite of her fun-loving ways and was a kind, sympathetic person. Questions 40 through 50 apply to this patient.

40. The symptoms that Ms. L exhibited are suggestive of which of the following diagnostic entities?
   1. Manic reaction
   2. Schizophrenic reaction
   3. Depressive reaction
   4. Involutional reaction
41. Ms. L's prepsychotic personality can be described by which of the following statements?
   1. Hostile, suspicious, unsociable
   2. Warm, friendly, outgoing
   3. Rigid, meticulous, compulsive
   4. Immature, shy, sensitive
42. The treatment of choice for Ms. L would be
   1. Psychoanalysis
   2. Recreational therapy
   3. Psychotherapy
   4. Group therapy
43. The prognosis for a patient with Ms. L's symptoms can be described by which of the following?
   1. Guarded, because the present attack will probably continue indefinitely
   2. Good, for the immediate attack; but recurrences can be expected
   3. Poor, because the future will bring alternating attacks
   4. Guarded, because the symptoms of overactivity will continue to increase
44. When Ms. L's language becomes vulgar and profane, the nurse should
   1. Comment: "We don't like that kind of talk around here."
   2. Comment: "When you can talk in an acceptable way, we will talk to you."

3. Recognize it as part of her illness but set limits on it

45. During Ms. L's phase of extreme elation and hyperactivity the nursing staff should consider her nutritional needs by
   1. Following her around the dining room with her tray
   2. Providing her with frequent high-caloric feedings that can be held in the hand
   3. Adopting the attitude that she will eat when she is hungry
   4. Allowing her to prepare her own meals and eat when she pleases
46. When coming on duty the staff nurse is met by an attendant who states, "What a time you're going to have with Ms. L; she's been acting crazy all day." The best reply would be
   1. "Thanks, I'm glad you warned me."
   2. "Haven't they given her enough sedation?"
   3. "What's she been doing?"
   4. "Have you reported this to her doctor?"
47. Ms. L's hyperactivity might be redirected therapeutically in which of the following ways?
   1. Give her cleaning equipment and suggest that she assist with the ward work
   2. Ask her to guide other patients as they clean their cubicles
   3. Suggest that she initiate social activities on the ward for the patient group
   4. Give her a pencil and paper and encourage her to write
48. In supervising Ms. L's personal hygiene the nurse would
   1. Keep makeup away from her because she will apply it too freely
   2. Suggest that she wear hospital clothing
   3. Encourage her to dress attractively and in her own clothing
   4. Allow her to apply makeup in whatever manner she chooses
49. The attendant has just reported that Ms. L is in the washroom, shampooing her hair in the toilet. The nurse should
   1. Call Ms. L's doctor to report the incident
   2. Tell the attendant to get help and remove Ms. L from the washroom
   3. Go to the washroom with the attendant (to evaluate the situation)
   4. Send the attendant back with instructions to be sure to flush all the soap out
50. Ms. Moody and 3 of her classmates are newly assigned to the floor on which Ms. L is a patient. During their orientation tour, Ms. L greets them by saying, "Welcome to the Funny Farm. I'm Jo-Jo the Head Yo-Yo." This comment might mean that the patient is
   1. Looking for attention
   2. Unable to distinguish fantasy from reality
   3. Anxious over the arrival of the new students
   4. Trying to frighten the students

Situation: Ms. S, a 45-year-old housewife, was recently admitted to the psychiatric hospital because of a history of hopelessness, anxiety, and suicidal attempts. In the hospital she paces the halls, cries, and says that the terrible condition of the world is her fault. She believes that her insides are decayed, that her husband and children are dead, and that the food she eats is of no nutritional value to her. Ms. S has 3 daughters, all of whom are away at college. Her life has always centered about her family and her meticulously kept home. She has never had any hobbies or outside interests, and her moral standards have been strict and unbending. Questions 51 through 63 apply to this patient.

51. Ms. S's prepsychotic personality can best be described by which of the following statements?
    1. Withdrawn and seclusive, with an active fantasy life
    2. Rigid, narrow, overly conscientious
    3. Suspicious, sensitive, aloof
    4. Dependent, immature, insecure
52. Such a symptom picture as Ms. S presents is typical of which reaction type?
    1. Paranoid reaction
    2. Anxiety reaction
    3. Manic-depressive reaction
    4. Involutional reaction
53. Probably one of the most effective treatments that psychiatry can offer a patient with Ms. S's problems would be
    1. One of the tranquilizing agents
    2. Electroshock therapy
    3. Psychotherapeutic interviews
    4. Narcosis therapy
54. Ms. S's symptom picture includes
    1. Somatic delusions
    2. Autistic thinking
    3. Paranoid ideas
    4. Ideas of depersonalization
55. Ms. S's symptoms also include
    1. Disorientation
    2. Self-accusatory ideas
    3. Euphoria
    4. Ideas of reference
56. This illness is usually precipitated by
    1. Severe headaches, backaches, nervous tension, insomnia
    2. Loss of a love object, change in status, fear of loss of personal attractiveness
    3. Compulsive house cleaning, rigid daily routine, meticulous personal grooming
    4. "Hot flashes," physical weakness, lethargy, anorexia
57. Ms. S has been hospitalized because
    1. She is a problem to her family
    2. She is a difficult person to live with
    3. Her physical symptoms require medical attention
    4. She is a danger to herself
58. One of the nurse's primary responsibilities in giving care to Ms. S is
    1. Helping her realize that her children are not dead
    2. Protecting her against her suicidal impulses
    3. Reassuring her that she is a good woman
    4. Keeping up her interest in the outside world
59. One of the nursing responsibilities is to help Ms. S pace the halls less frequently, since this wears her out physically. This can best be accomplished by
    1. Supplying her with simple monotonous tasks

    2. Restraining her in a chair
    3. Requesting a sedative order for her
    4. Placing her in a single room
60. In reassuring Ms. S concerning the many fears that are upsetting to her, it would be helpful to say
    1. "Your daughters and your husband love you very much."
    2. "You know that you are not a bad woman."
    3. "Ms. S, those ideas of yours are just in your imagination."
    4. "Those ideas are part of your illness and will change as you improve."
61. Ms. Moody continues to sit with Ms. S, although there is little verbal communication. One day, Ms. S asks her, "Do you think they'll ever let me out of here?" Ms. Moody's best response is
    1. "Why are you asking me?"
    2. "You have the feeling that you might not leave?"
    3. "Everyone says you're doing just fine."
    4. "Why don't you ask your doctor?"
62. Ms. S confides to Ms. Moody that she has been thinking about suicide. Which statement best explains her action?
    1. She feels safe with Ms. Moody and can share her feelings with her
    2. She wishes to frighten Ms. Moody
    3. She is fearful of her own impulses and is seeking protection from them
    4. She wants attention
63. Ms. S is on Suicide Observation. She has managed to elude the staff member assigned to observe her. Ms. Moody accidentally discovers her in the bathroom with a piece of broken glass in her hand. What should be the student nurse's *first* action?
    1. Report this finding to the head nurse
    2. Call the patient's doctor immediately
    3. Ask Ms. S if she will give her the piece of glass
    4. Scream for help

Situation: The staff and patients have just learned that, while on a weekend pass from the hospital, Sally F has suicided. A meeting is called to attempt to deal with the feelings which this incident has aroused among staff and patients alike. The collective mood of the group is tense and restless. Questions 64 through 66 apply to this situation.

64. Ms. Moody, sitting beside Ms. S, observes that she is sobbing and rocking back and forth in a sitting position while she hugs her arms around herself. Ms. Moody hears her moaning softly, "I'm next. Oh, my God, I'm next. They couldn't stop Sally and they can't protect me." Ms. Moody's response should be
    1. "Sally was a lot sicker than you are, Ms. S."
    2. "It's different, Ms. S, Sally was home; you're here."
    3. "You are afraid you will hurt yourself, Ms. S?"
    4. "Don't worry. All passes will be cancelled for awhile."

65. Jim M, a friend of Sally's, stands up and shouts, "Oh! I know what you're all thinking, you think that I should have known that she was going to kill herself. You think that I helped her plan this." The group leader's response should be
    1. "Oh no, Jim, we all know you liked Sally."
    2. "You feel we're blaming you for Sally's death, Jim?"
    3. "It'll ease your conscience if you tell us the truth, Jim."
    4. "Helping her plan her suicide and not telling anyone would be like murder."

66. During the group discussion it is learned that Sally had not shared her strong suicidal feelings and had successfully masked her depression. The group leader should be prepared primarily to deal with
    1. The guilt that the group feels because it could not prevent Sally's suicide
    2. The fear and anxiety which some members of the group may have that their own suicidal urges may go unnoticed and unprotected
    3. The guilt, fear, and anger of the staff, that they have failed to anticipate and prevent Sally's suicide
    4. The lack of concern over Sally's suicide expressed by some of the group

Situation: Ms. H, 19 years of age, came to the psychiatric hospital from a girl's dormitory on a nearby college campus where she was a freshman. Throughout high school she had always been an excellent student who was interested in modern art, ballet, dancing, symphony concerts, and good literature. She played the violin very well. She had no close friends and was considered a lone wolf. Her family states that she always has been sensitive, and different from other girls. She was admitted to the psychiatric hospital when she refused to get out of bed and go to classes. Her personal appearance deteriorated steadily during the past month and recently she did not bother to comb her hair or put on makeup. In the hospital she talks to unseen people, voids on the floor, sometimes masturbates openly, occasionally eats with her hands, and refuses to shower or wear her own clothes. Questions 67 through 75 apply to this patient

67. The best description of Ms. H's prepsychotic personality would include the words
    1. Suspicious, haughty, paranoid
    2. Shy, cool, aloof, schizoid
    3. Warm, outgoing, cyclothymic
    4. Immature, dependent, oral

68. The symptoms that Ms. H exhibits would place her problem in what diagnostic category?
    1. Psychopathic personality
    2. Obsessive-compulsive reaction
    3. Psychoneurotic reaction
    4. Schizophrenic reaction

69. The nurse's efforts should be directed especially toward which aspect of Ms. H's care?
    1. Frequent rest periods to avoid exhaustion
    2. Appropriate attempts to establish a meaningful relationship with her

3. Reduction of environmental stimuli and maintenance of dietary intake
    4. Improving social relations with her peer group.

70. The most appropriate way to begin to help Ms. H accept the realities of daily living would be to
    1. Encourage her to join the other patients in group singing
    2. Assist her to care for her own personal hygiene
    3. Encourage her to take up the playing of the violin again
    4. Leave her alone when she is disinterested in the activity at hand

71. When Ms. H openly masturbates, the nurse should most appropriately
    1. Restrain her hands
    2. Not react to the behavior
    3. Put her in seclusion
    4. Remind her that such behavior is not acceptable

72. The nurse could best handle the problem of voiding on the floor by
    1. Making the patient mop the floor
    2. Restricting the patient's fluids throughout the day
    3. More frequent toileting with supervision
    4. Withholding privileges each time the patient voids on the floor

73. When Ms. H eats with her hands, the nurse can handle this problem by
    1. Commenting, "I thought college girls had better manners than that."
    2. Placing the spoon in her hand and suggesting that she use it
    3. Removing the food and saying, "You can't have any more until you can use your spoon."
    4. Saying in a joking way, "Well, fingers were made before forks."

74. While watching TV in the day room Ms. H suddenly screams, bursts into tears, and runs out of the room to the far end of the hallway. What would be the most therapeutic action for Ms. Moody to take?
    1. Write up the incident on the patient's chart while it is still fresh in her memory
    2. Ask another patient what made Ms. H act as she did
    3. Walk to the end of the hallway where Ms. H has run off to
    4. Accept the action as just being the impulsive behavior of a sick person

75. Ms. H has been observed watching Ms. Moody, student nurse, for a few days. She suddenly walks up to her and shouts, "You think you're so damned perfect and pure and good. I think you stink." What would be the most appropriate response for Ms. Moody?
    1. "I can't be all that bad can I?"
    2. "You seem angry with me."
    3. "Stink? I don't understand."
    4. "You don't smell so good yourself."

Situation: Ms. X, 22, a tall thin college student, came into the psychiatric hospital last week because she refused to leave her room at home. For weeks she had done nothing but sit and stare into space.

For several days she had not eaten and would not bathe or change clothing. Her mother told the social worker that until recently she had done well in school but had been shy and backward, had few friends, and had taken part in no extracurricular activities. Her major interests are mathematics and modern art. Although she had been extremely attached to her father, she had never been interested in boys. Two months ago her father died. She refused to return to school after the funeral. In the hospital she speaks to no one, does not appear to recognize what is going on about her, resists all nursing procedures, and assumes and holds unusual body positions. Recently she became very loud, profane, and noisy for a 24-hour period. During this time she called out to her father, became combative, and tore her clothing into small pieces. Since then she has returned to her motionless state. Questions 76 through 82 apply to this patient.

76. The doctor would probably place Ms. X in what diagnostic classification?
    1. Manic-depressive reaction
    2. Schizophrenic reaction, catatonic type
    3. Schizophrenic reaction, simple type
    4. Schizophrenic reaction, paranoid type
77. Among the symptoms that Ms. X has shown during hospitalization is (are)
    1. Somatic delusions
    2. Suicidal ideas
    3. Flight of ideas
    4. Withdrawal from reality
78. Another symptom that Ms. X has shown during hospitalization is
    1. Agitation
    2. Paranoid ideas
    3. Depersonalization
    4. Autism
79. Ms. X's prepsychotic personality would best be described as
    1. Warm, outgoing, friendly, well-socialized
    2. Hostile, suspicious, aggressive
    3. Aloof, poorly socialized, reserved
    4. Rigid, meticulous, unbending
80. Prognosis for a patient showing the symptoms that Ms. X exhibits is
    1. Poor, because the illness developed so early in life
    2. Only fair, because she is likely to become mentally ill again when her mother dies
    3. Favorable, because she is getting treatment early in her illness
    4. Unpredictable, since it depends upon her prepsychotic adjustment and the effectiveness of the treatment
81. The precipitating factor in Ms. X's illness could be
    1. Low grades in school
    2. Shyness
    3. Too much studying
    4. Loss of a loved one
82. The nursing care for Ms. X should be directed toward
    1. Helping her substitute new interests for old ones
    2. Helping her dress more attractively
    3. Helping her establish a relationship with another person
    4. Helping her forget the past and become interested in the present

Situation: Ms. A, 29, was a capable librarian before her marriage. However, she was always very sensitive, aloof, withdrawn, and lacking in the ability to feel warmly toward others; she rarely joined any organizations and distrusted people in general. Shortly after the birth of her last child she was admitted to a psychiatric hospital for care. At this time she was convinced that the neighbors were accusing her of indiscretions and that they had her home "bugged" so that they might overhear any conversations taking place there. After hospital admission she remained aloof from the other patients, paced the floor, believed that the hospital was a house of torture, that the doctors were trying to kill her, and that the food was poisoned. She thought that the other patients were spying on her and said, "This whole thing is a plot to keep me from my children." Questions 83 through 94 apply to this patient.

83. One of the symptoms presented by Ms. A is called
    1. Flight of ideas
    2. Auditory hallucinations
    3. Depersonalization
    4. Paranoid delusion
84. Such a symptom picture as Ms. A exhibits would probably carry the diagnosis of
    1. Anxiety reaction
    2. Schizophrenic reaction, paranoid type
    3. Schizophrenic reaction, catatonic type
    4. Manic-depressive reaction, depressive type
85. Ms. A's prepsychotic personality might be described as
    1. Suspicious, socially inadequate
    2. Rigid, meticulous
    3. Dependent, immature
    4. Controlling, grasping
86. Nursing interventions should appropriately be directed toward
    1. Convincing her logically that the hospital is trying to help her
    2. Helping her enter into group recreational activities
    3. Arranging the hospital environment so that she can avoid association with others
    4. Helping her learn to trust the hospital staff, through selected experiences
87. An evaluation of this patient's prognosis would probably indicate
    1. Good, for the immediate attack, but recurrences to be expected
    2. Good, if she can return to her position as a librarian
    3. Guarded, because use of these delusions makes adjustment to life's pressures possible for her
    4. Complete recovery can be expected after a series of electroshock treatments
88. Ms. A frequently refuses to eat because she believes that the food is poisoned. One of the most appropriate ways in which the nurse might initially handle this situation is to
    1. Tell her simply that it is not poisoned
    2. Suggest that food be brought to her from home
    3. Taste the food in her presence
    4. Tell her that she will have to be tube fed if she will not eat

89. After the appropriate initial intervention the nurse should pursue the matter of Ms. A's belief that the food is poisoned, by saying
    1. "You're not the only one who thinks the food is so bad that it's poisoned."
    2. "You feel someone wants to poison you?"
    3. "That's crazy talk. No one poisons food around here."
    4. "You'll be safe with me. I won't let anyone poison you."

90. Ms. A has refused to eat for 36 hours. She states that the voice of her dead father has commanded her to atone for her sins by fasting for 40 days. What initial intervention on the part of the nurse might contribute to the interruption of the delusional system?
    1. Get the doctor to write an order for tube feeding
    2. Ask Ms. A exactly what she has heard
    3. Tell Ms. A that her father wants her to eat
    4. Suggest other means of atonement

91. Ms. A remains aloof from all other patients. What might the nurse, with whom Ms. A has developed a friendly relationship, do to help her participate in some ward activity?
    1. Invite another patient to take part in an activity that the nurse and Ms. A are sharing
    2. Ask the doctor to speak to Ms. A about entering into ward activities
    3. Find solitary pursuits that Ms. A can enjoy on the ward
    4. Speak to her about the importance of entering into activities

92. Ms. A has been given a bed in the large dormitory of the ward to which she has been assigned. The night nurse reports that she has been awake for several nights. What is the probable cause of her prolonged wakefulness?
    1. She is fearful of the other patients
    2. She is worrying about her family
    3. She is a light sleeper and hospital noises keep her awake
    4. She is watching for an opportunity to escape

93. The nurse could most appropriately begin to help Ms. A with her sleep problem by saying
    1. "You'll sleep when you're tired."
    2. "I'll report your problem to your doctor."
    3. "I'll get you the sedative your doctor ordered."
    4. "You seem unable to sleep at night?"

94. While talking with Ms. Moody, student nurse, about her problem of not being able to make friends with any of the other patients, Ms. A begins to cry. What action on the part of Ms. Moody would be most therapeutic at this time?
    1. Suggest that they play a game of Scrabble
    2. Tell her that her crying isn't going to help her
    3. Sit quietly with her
    4. Leave her to cry privately

Situation: Mr. G, 36, was admitted to the general hospital for the repair of an inguinal hernia. His history indicates that he is a chronic alcoholic and once had delirium tremens. When he was admitted, he had not had a drink for 3 weeks; but following the operation he became sullen, irritable, and confused. Although his physical condition is good, he calls his nurse by his wife's name and calls his doctor "Joe." Mr. G believes that he is in prison and that the drapes at the windows are ropes put there to help him to escape. He hears voices telling him to run away. The designs on the upholstered chair in his hospital room suggest whiskey bottles to him, and he keeps trying to reach them. His hands tremble as he plucks at the sheets. Questions 95 through 100 apply to this patient.

95. Which one of the following symptoms was *not* exhibited by Mr. G following the operation?
    1. Disorientation
    2. Auditory hallucinations
    3. Somatic delusions
    4. Visual illusions

96. A nursing care plan for Mr. G might appropriately include which of the following suggestions?
    1. Reassure him by telling him that he is going to be all right
    2. Remind him repeatedly that you are his nurse and not his wife
    3. Prolong his bath, back rub, and other nursing procedures
    4. Remove the drapes and upholstered chair from his room

97. Which of the following suggestions ought to be omitted in giving nursing care to Mr. G?
    1. Allow only one or two visitors for very short periods of time
    2. Give him frequent and large doses of a sedative drug
    3. Keep a soft light burning in the room at night
    4. Explain procedures simply and in a low, firm voice

98. The type of personality that resorts to excessive use of alcohol as a method of adjustment is best described as
    1. Emotionally immature
    2. Morally inadequate
    3. Lacking in will power
    4. Pathologically selfish

99. Most individuals who resort to excessive use of alcohol do so for which of the following reasons?
    1. Alcohol is a sedative and quiets the nerves
    2. Alcohol is a stimulant and speeds up brain action
    3. Alcohol aids the socially inadequate in making friends
    4. Alcohol furnishes a temporary release from emotional tension

100. What appropriate help could be offered to Mr. G to assist him in overcoming his problem of chronic alcoholism after the acute symptoms have subsided and he is physically well again?
    1. Mr. G's minister might help him by suggesting that he use his will power and act like a man
    2. His family might help him by giving him more financial aid

3. His employer might help him by giving him a promotion and more responsibility
4. Alcoholics Anonymous might provide a social milieu in which he can feel accepted and talk to others with problems like his own

101. Dr. K, a 45-year-old physician, is admitted to the psychiatric unit of the general hospital. He is restless, loud, aggressive, and resistive during the admission procedure. He shouts at the nurse who is trying to take his admission blood pressure, "I'm a physician. Do you think you're more qualified than I? I'll do it myself, nurse." The most therapeutic response by the nurse would be
    1. "Right now, doctor, you're just another patient."
    2. "If you'd rather, doctor, I'm sure you'll do it OK."
    3. "I'm sorry but I can't allow that. I must take it."
    4. "If you won't cooperate, I'll get the attendants in to hold you down."

102. After the admission examination Ms. Moody is assigned to introduce the new patient to the other patients. He tells her that he wishes to be introduced as Dr. K. Ms. Moody's response should be
    1. "I can't do that. It's better they don't know."
    2. "That's fine, Dr. K."
    3. "All the patients here call one another by their first names."
    4. "Why do you insist on being called doctor?"

103. Mr. Y, a 58-year-old depressed schoolteacher, has come to Ms. Moody to tell her that one patient, Dr. K, has advised him that the only thing which will save him from "lifelong insanity" is a lobotomy. Mr. Y asks, "That's when they operate on your brains, isn't it, Ms. Moody? Will they need to do that to me?" Ms. Moody's reply should be
    1. "No Mr. Y, Dr. K is a patient and is giving out wrong information."
    2. "Actually, Mr. Y, a lobotomy is not as complicated as most brain surgery."
    3. "They ought to operate on his brains, not yours."
    4. "Yes, Mr. Y, that is the operation on the frontal lobe of the brain."

104. By the time Dr. K has been a patient on the service for 3 days he has questioned everyone's authority, has advised other patients that their treatments were all wrong, and has talked 4 other patients into forming a "counter-encounter." The staff's most appropriate response to this would be to
    1. Ignore him, and he'll stop trying to disrupt the ward
    2. Understand that his acting out is getting more bizarre and that he is unable to control it
    3. Tell the other patients that he is just another crazy patient and not to worry
    4. Seclude him until he stops bothering everyone

Situation: Ms. O is a 46-year-old woman who came into the psychiatric hospital because she drank poison and slashed her wrists. She cries a great deal, refuses food, and says that she is not fit to live. The doctor has ordered electroshock treatment (EST or ECT) for her. Questions 105 through 108 apply to this patient.

105. What condition is relieved most effectively by electroshock therapy?
    1. Schizophrenic withdrawal
    2. Obsessive-compulsive behavior
    3. Depressed mood
    4. Paranoid idea

106. Which of the following physical problems occurs when anectine is administered before electroconvulsive therapy?
    1. Dislocation of jaw
    2. Compression fracture of vertebrae
    3. Respiratory arrest
    4. Electrocution

107. Ms. O has just awakened from her first electroconvulsive therapy treatment. The most appropriate nursing intervention would be to
    1. Get Ms. O up and out of bed as soon as possible and back into her normal routine
    2. Orient Ms. O to time and place and tell her that she has just had a treatment
    3. Arrange for the attendant to bring her a lunch tray
    4. Take her BP and TPR every 15 minutes until she is fully awake

108. In a staff discussion, a new nurse admits that she feels ECT is frightening. Which of the following statements would demonstrate a mature response on her part?
    1. "It's a horrible thing, but I'll never let the patients know I feel that way about it."
    2. "I just won't let anyone know how I feel about it. I'm a professional nurse and I can handle it."
    3. "I have to deal with my own anxiety over ECT."
    4. "You'll never get me to assist with ECT; I'll faint."

109. Two 20-year-old female patients have become very much attached to one another and were recently found in bed together. They became angry and sarcastic when the nurse asked one of them to return to her own bed. How can this situation best be handled by the nurse?
    1. Ask the doctor to transfer one patient from the ward
    2. Supervise the girls carefully and separate them when possible throughout the day and night
    3. Restrict both girls' privileges for several days because their behavior is undesirable and immature
    4. Adopt a matter-of-fact, noncondemning attitude toward these patients, while escorting one back to her own bed

110. Which one of the following factors is characteristically found in the life histories of individuals who need psychiatric help?
    1. Unsatisfactory family relationships
    2. Brain injury
    3. Lack of educational opportunity
    4. Inadequate discipline

111. The unconscious mechanism by which a person excludes from awareness those thoughts and feelings which are painful and unacceptable to his self-esteem is called
    1. Rationalization
    2. Repression
    3. Substitution
    4. Projection
112. The area of the mind in which awareness of reality situations is found is called the
    1. Preconscious
    2. Subconscious
    3. Conscious
    4. Unconscious
113. The term "affect" is a synonym for
    1. Stimulus
    2. Feeling tone
    3. Behavior
    4. Response
114. The sum of traits and characteristics that to a large degree determine behavior in an individual is known as
    1. Reaction pattern
    2. Character
    3. Total response
    4. Personality
115. The human personality develops as a result of
    1. Heredity
    2. Environmental and cultural influences
    3. Influence of the group
    4. All of the above
116. The part of the mind that distinguishes right from wrong and acts as the censor of behavior is called the
    1. Libido
    2. Id
    3. Ego
    4. Superego
117. An individual's simultaneous experiencing of two opposing emotions about the same situation is referred to as
    1. Tension
    2. Feeling
    3. Aggression
    4. Ambivalence
118. Temper tantrums are frequently a result of
    1. Poor inheritance
    2. Physical handicaps
    3. Lack of love
    4. Frustration
119. All behavior can be said to be
    1. A response to a stimulus
    2. A conditioned response
    3. An intellectual reaction
    4. An emotional reaction
120. When an individual is given an intelligence test, the psychologist may assign him an intelligence quotient as a result of the test findings. This intelligence quotient tells us about
    1. Intellectual maturity
    2. Mental age in relation to chronologic age
    3. Academic achievement
    4. Mental growth
121. Which of these suggestions would be particularly helpful in organizing a work situation for a patient who has an intelligence quotient of 70?
    1. Offer challenging, competitive situations
    2. Offer simple, repetitive tasks
    3. Concentrate upon teaching detailed tasks
    4. Offer complete directions at the beginning of the work period
122. Which one of the following symptoms is *not* characteristic of a patient whose behavior is classified as a personality disturbance?
    1. Pronounced selfishness
    2. Failure to profit by experience
    3. Satisfactory emotional adjustment
    4. Inability to withstand frustration
123. Which of the following factors is one of the most frequent causes of adult homosexuality?

1. Inadequate physical development of the sexual organs
2. Deficiency of gonadal and pituitary hormones
3. Failure to progress normally through the stages of psychosexual development
4. Poor adjustment, due to association with homosexual companions

124. The main psychological tasks ascribed to adulthood are adjustments in
    1. Trust vs. mistrust
    2. Intimacy vs. isolation
    3. Generativity vs. stagnation
    4. Self-indulgence vs. selflessness
125. The head nurse has noticed that one of the staff nurses on the ward constantly avoids having contact with one particular patient. Which statement seems most correct?
    1. The patient is a very hostile, irritable, and demanding person and is better left alone
    2. The nurse may be avoiding the patient because some of the patient's behavior makes her uncomfortable
    3. The nurse is waiting for the patient to initiate the contact
    4. There are so many other things to do each day, and she hasn't had time to relate to this particular patient
126. When a patient refuses to talk with a particular nurse, avoiding her whenever possible, we should be aware that
    (a) The patient needs to learn useful, satisfying, and appropriate interpersonal skills
    (b) The nurse needs to examinne her own behavior and its effect on the patient
    (c) The patient is communicating something by this behavior
    (d) The patient may be reverting to an earlier method used to relate to significant people
      1. a and d
      2. a, c, and d
      3. c and b
      4. All of the above
127. A young male patient greeted Ms. Moody and the other student nurses by screaming obscenities, pointing, and shouting "You! You know who I mean! I hate you." Ms. Moody is upset and reports the incidents to the head nurse. Which statement indicates Ms. Moody's best attempt to understand the situation?
    1. "He's crazy. He can't help it. I should not be upset."
    2. "I don't know why this particular situation upset me."
    3. "That patient should be put in seclusion the next time he verbally assaults anyone."
    4. "I don't understand why he attacked me."
128. For most nurses the most difficult part of the nurse-patient relationship is
    1. Developing an awareness of self and her role in the relationship
    2. Being able to understand and accept the patient's behavior
    3. Accepting responsibility in evaluating the real needs of the patient
    4. Remaining therapeutic and professional at all times
129. The purpose of realistically preparing a patient for termination reasonably early in the nurse-patient relationship is to

(a) Deal with possible resultant feelings of rejection
(b) Allay anxiety
(c) Deal with the reality of the situation and the relationship
(d) Define the relationship as a therapeutic one
    1. a and d   3. a and b
    2. b, c, and d   4. All of the above

130. An irresistible impulse to carry out some act is called
    1. Delusion   3. Obsession
    2. Phobia   4. Compulsion

131. Which of the following aspects of nursing care is not helpful for psychoneurotic patients?
    1. Recognize that his symptoms are necessary ego-protective devices
    2. Appropriately praise him for his accomplishments
    3. Approach him with a tolerant and accepting attitude
    4. Sympathize openly with him about his problems

132. A young female patient believes that doorknobs are contaminated and refuses to touch them, except with the aid of a paper tissue. What attitude should the nurse adopt toward this behavior?
    1. Force her to touch doorknobs by removing all available paper tissue until her anxiety becomes intolerable
    2. Explain to her that her idea about doorknobs is foolish
    3. Encourage her to scrub the doorknobs with a strong antiseptic
    4. Supply her with paper tissues to help her function until her anxiety is reduced

133. Symptoms such as those exhibited by the patient who uses tissues to touch doorknobs develop because she is
    1. Unconsciously using this method of punishing herself
    2. Unconsciously controlling unacceptable impulses or feelings
    3. Listening to voices that tell her the doorknobs are unclean
    4. Fulfilling a need to punish others by carrying out a procedure that annoys everyone

134. Therapeutic treatment for the patient who touches doorknobs with paper tissue would be directed toward helping her to
    1. Forget her fears, by treating her with deep narcosis therapy
    2. Understand her behavior as caused by unconscious impulses that she fears
    3. Redirect her energy, by encouraging her to help others
    4. Learn that her behavior is inconveniencing others

135. Ms. E complains constantly that her "heart is failing and the pulse is gone." She asks the nurse to take her pulse and to listen to her heart several times each hour. How should the nurse handle this problem?
    1. Tell her that there is nothing wrong with her heart and to stop worrying

    2. Count her pulse and explain in a kind voice that is is beating at a normal rate
    3. Tell her that she is annoying all of the other patients with her imaginary complaints
    4. Listen to her complaints and attempt to involve her in activities

136. A patient suffering from a psychoneurotic reaction cried bitterly after a conference with her psychiatrist. She pounded the bed and threatened to kill herself. What should the nurse do about this situation?
    1. Pat her reassuringly on the back and say, "I know it is hard to bear."
    2. Sit beside her and listen attentively if she wishes to talk about the situation
    3. Ask her to talk about her troubles and tell her that other people have problems

137. A characteristic symptom exhibited by patients suffering from the manic type of manic-depressive reaction is
    1. Withdrawal from reality
    2. Retardation of activity
    3. Inappropriate laughter
    4. Overactivity in all spheres of behavior

138. Also characteristic of the manic patients is (are)
    1. Memory loss
    2. Flight of ideas
    3. Marked suicidal tendencies
    4. Ideas of depersonalization

139. The manic patient may fail to eat because
    1. He feels that he does not deserve the food
    2. He believes that he does not need the food
    3. He wishes to avoid the crowd in the dining room
    4. He is so busy that he does not take time to eat

140. In approaching a patient who is showing great overactivity it is essential to keep which of the following aspects of care in mind?
    1. Anticipate and physically control his hyperactivity
    2. Use a firm warm consistent approach
    3. Allow the patient to choose the activities in which he will participate
    4. Isolate the patient and ignore him

141. Mr. B, a hyperactive elated patient who exhibits flight of ideas, is assigned to you. Your nursing care plan should appropriately include
    1. Encouragement to talk as much as he seems to need to
    2. Arousal and focus of his interest in reality
    3. Encouragement to complete any task that he has started
    4. Provision for constructive channels for redirecting his excess energy

142. Which of the following statements is true of patients who are suffering from either the manic or the depressed phase of the manic-depressive reaction?
    1. The major disturbance is in the area of the mood
    2. There is intellectual deterioration
    3. Distractibility is a prominent symptom
    4. Suicide is the major nursing problem

143. A symptom that is characteristic of schizophrenic patients is

1. Memory loss   3. Autistic thinking
2. Flight of ideas   4. Disassociation

144. Bizarre behavior by the schizophrenic patient is
    1. The patient's response to his environment
    2. The result of psychophysiologic turmoil
    3. Meaningful to the patient
    4. Unrelated to his feelings

145. To a large degree the prognosis for a patient suffering from any type of affective reaction is dependent upon
    1. Age
    2. Intellectual ability
    3. Prepsychotic adjustment
    4. Treatment provided

146. The nursing care plan for the patient with senile brain deterioration should include which of the following?
    1. Reeducate the patient extensively
    2. Give protective and supportive care
    3. Introduce new interests
    4. Help the patient gain insight into his problems

147. In planning care for the patient with senile brain deterioration the nurse should appropriately
    1. Maintain the daily routine of living with which the patient is familiar
    2. Discuss current events with the patient
    3. Teach the patient new social skills to help him participate in ward activity
    4. Encourage the patient to talk of his youth

Situation: Ms. Smith has been admitted to a psychiatric hospital because of emotional problems that have been diagnosed as a senile psychotic reaction. Questions 148 through 150 apply to this patient.

148. Which of the following symptoms would Ms. Smith be least likely to demonstrate?
    1. Resistance to change
    2. Preoccupation with personal appearance
    3. Tendency to dwell on the past and ignore the present
    4. Inability to concentrate on new activities or interests

149. Which of the following approaches would *not* be helpful in meeting Ms. Smith's needs?
    1. Simplifying the environment as much as possible, eliminating choices
    2. Providing a simple, highly nutritious diet of familiar foods
    3. Developing a consistent nursing plan to provide for emotional and physical needs
    4. Providing an opportunity for many alternative choices in the daily schedule, to stimulate interest

150. How would the nurse expect a patient like Ms. Smith to use defense mechanisms in her relations with others?
    1. Seek new defense mechanisms to meet new life situations
    2. Cease utilizing defense mechanisms altogether
    3. Make exaggerated use of old familiar mechanisms
    4. Choose one method of defense and utilize it in all instances

BE SURE YOUR MARKS ARE HEAVY AND BLACK.
ERASE COMPLETELY ANY ANSWER YOU WISH TO CHANGE.

13

REHABILITATION NURSING

Bergstrom, D.: Care of patients with bowel and bladder problems: a nursing guide, Minneapolis, 1968, American Rehabilitation Foundation.

Bergstrom, D., and others: Rehabilitative nursing techniques, Minneapolis, 1964, American Rehabilitation Foundation.

Brower, P., and Hicks, D.: Maintaining muscle function in patients on bed rest, American Journal of Nursing 72:1250, July, 1972.

Burgess, E. M., Traub, J. E., and Wilson, A. B.: Immediate postsurgical prosthetics in the management of lower extremity amputees, Washington, D. C., 1967, Veterans Administration, Prosthetics and Sensory Aids Service, Department of Medicine and Surgery.

Carnevali, D.: Immobilization: reassessment of a concept, American Journal of Nursing 70:1502, July, 1970.

Coles, C. H.: A procedure for passive range of motion and self-assistive exercises, Minneapolis, 1964, Kenny Rehabilitation Institute.

Coles, C. H., and Bergstrom, D. A.: Basic positioning procedures, Minneapolis, 1971, Kenny Rehabilitation Institute.

David, J. H., Hanser, J. E., and Madden, B. W.: Guidelines for discharge planning, Downey, Calif., 1968, Attending Staff Association of Rancho Los Amigos Hospital, Inc.

Delehanty, L., and Stavino, V. D.: Achieving bladder control, American Journal of Nursing 70:312, Feb., 1970.

Do it yourself again: self-help devices for the stroke patient, New York, 1965, American Heart Association.

Elementary rehabilitative nursing care, U. S. Public Health Service, Pub. no. 1436, Washington, D. C., 1966, U. S. Government Printing Office.

Fahland, B. B.: Wheelchair selection—more than choosing a chair with wheels, Minneapolis, 1967, American Rehabilitation Foundation.

Fordyce, W. E.: Some implications of learning in problems of chronic pain, Journal of Chronic Diseases 21:179, 1968.

Haynes, U.: The role of nursing in programs for patients with cerebral palsy and related disorders, New York, 1962, United Cerebral Palsy Association Inc.

Homemaking aids for the disabled, Minneapolis, 1963, American Rehabilitation Foundation.

Kelly, M. M.: Exercises for bedfast patients, American Journal of Nursing 66:2209, Oct., 1966.

Klinger, J., Frieden, F., and Sullivan, R.: Mealtime manual for the aged and handicapped, New York, 1970, Simon & Schuster, Inc.

Kottke, F. J.: The effects of limitation of activity upon the human body, J.A.M.A. 196:825, 1966.

Krusen, F. H., and others: Handbook of physical medicine and rehabilitation, ed. 2, Philadelphia, 1971, W. B. Saunders Co.

Lawton, E. B.: Activities of daily living for physical rehabilitation, New York, 1963, McGraw-Hill Book Co.

Lowman, E., and Klinger, J.: Aids to independent living, New York, 1969, McGraw-Hill Book Co.

Madden, B., and Affeldt, J. E.: To prevent helplessness and deformities, American Journal of Nursing 62:59, Dec., 1962.

McCarthy, J. A.: Immobility—effects on gastrointestinal function, American Journal of Nursing 67:785, April, 1967.

Merlino, A. F.: Decubitus ulcers: cause, prevention, and treatment, Geriatrics 24:119, 1969.

Montero, J., Wasserman, K., and Feldman, D. J.: Respiratory problems of the chronically ill, Archives of Physical Medicine 46:386, 1965.

Montgomery, J., and Inaba, M.: Physical therapy techniques in stroke rehabilitation, Clinical Orthopedics and Related Research 63:57, 1969.

Olsen, E., and Wade, M.: The hazards of immobility—effects on metabolic equilibrium, American Journal of Nursing 67:793, April, 1967.

Pigott, R., and Brickett, F.: Visual neglect, American Journal of Nursing 66:101, Jan., 1966.

Peabody, S. R.: Assessment and planning for continuity of care, Nursing Clinics of North America 4:303, June, 1969.

Rehabilitation nursing techniques, 1964. Available at American Rehabilitation Foundation, 1600 Chicago Ave., Minneapolis, Minn. 55404.

Rehabilitative aspects of nursing, programmed instruction: Unit I, Concepts and goals; Unit II, Physical therapeutic measures, New York, 1967, National League for Nursing.

Rosenberg, C.: Simple self-help devices to make for the handicapped, Atlanta, 1965, Damon & Kay Printing Co.

Rothberg, J. S.: Why nursing diagnosis? American Journal of Nursing 67:1040, May, 1967.

Rothberg, J. S.: The challenges for rehabilitative nursing, Nursing Outlook 17:37, Nov., 1969.

Rusk, H. A.: Rehabilitation medicine, ed. 3, St. Louis, 1971, The C. V. Mosby Co.

Sarno, J., and Sarno, M.: Stroke, New York, 1969, McGraw-Hill Book Co.

Sister Regina Elizabeth: Sensory stimulation techniques, American Journal of Nursing 66:281, Feb., 1966.

Sorenson, L., and Ulrich, P.: Ambulation—a manual for nurses, Minneapolis, 1966, American Rehabilitation Foundation.

Stryker, R. P.: Rehabilitative aspects of acute and chronic nursing care, Philadelphia, 1972, W. B. Saunders Co.

Taylor, M.: Understanding aphasia: a guide for family and friends, New York, 1958, The Institute of Rehabilitation Medicine.

Toohey, P., and others: Range of motion exercise: key to joint mobility, Minneapolis, 1968, American Rehabilitation Foundation.

Ujhely, G.: Determinants of the nurse-patient relationship, New York, 1968, Springer Publishing Co., Inc.

Up and about, New York, 1966, American Heart Association.

Verhonick, P. J.: Decubitus ulcer care, American Journal of Nursing 61:68, Aug., 1961.

Whitehouse, F.: Stroke—some psychosocial problems it causes, American Journal of Nursing 63:81, Oct., 1963.

Wright, B.: Physical disability: a psychological approach, New York, 1960, Harper & Row Publishers, Inc.

---

1. Concepts of rehabilitation

A. Principal aims
  1. To recognize
     a. The individual, intrinsic worth of persons
     b. The right of persons to receive necessary help
     c. The community's responsibility in providing help
     d. That the individual must be treated as a whole person
     e. That abilities—not disabilities—must be stressed
     f. That activity strengthens and inactivity weakens
     g. That treatment must be started early (at the time of onset) and continued without interruption for as long as necessary
  2. To strengthen the person's self-worth despite overwhelming difficulties
     a. To protect his personal integrity
     b. To enhance his sense of self-respect
     c. To provide the person with opportunities for success
     d. To help him acquire a sense of independence and control
  3. To help disabled persons attain their full potential of function (physical, psychological, social) as members of society
     a. To establish function where none existed—habilitation, as for a child born without limbs
     b. To restore function that has been lost—rehabilitation, as for an adult who has lost a limb
     c. To expand or enhance limited functional abilities

B. Who requires rehabilitation?
  Infants, children, adolescents, adults, aged persons

C. What conditions require rehabilitation?
  All chronic diseases and any acute problems that incapacitate or immobilize the individual for more than a short period of time; examples are listed
  1. Congenital problems—retardation, cerebral palsy, congenital malformations (cleft lip and/or palate, spina bifida, amelia, etc.)
  2. Vascular problems—especially heart attacks and strokes
  3. Cancer—all forms, particularly after mutilating surgery such as amputation of breast or limb, maxillofacial resection, and the "ostomies"
  4. Degenerative diseases—multiple sclerosis, parkinsonism, arthritis, etc.
  5. Neuromuscular disorders—muscular dystrophy and atrophies, myasthenia gravis, etc.
  6. Traumatic injury—paraplegia, quadriplegia, brain injury, limb amputation, fractures and other orthopedic conditions
  7. Sensory deficits—blindness, hearing loss
  8. Epilepsy
  9. Psychological and psychiatric problems

D. Factors influencing rehabilitation outcome
  1. Age
  2. Age at onset
  3. Type of onset
  4. General physical condition
  5. Type of disability and resultant physical dependence

6. Previous medical, psychological, and social history
7. Psychological status, intelligence level, attitude
8. Approach and attitude of family and of professional staff
9. Availability of professional health workers and necessary facilities
10. Availability of community resources

E. Symptoms commonly occurring in persons requiring rehabilitation
1. Diminished or disturbed sensory reception—hemiplegia, blindness, spinal cord injury, pernicious anemia
2. Increased, decreased, or disturbed sensation or motion
   a. Pain—arthritis, hemiplegia
   b. Spasm—spinal cord injury
   c. Tremor—multiple sclerosis, parkinsonism
   d. Seizures—epilepsy
   e. Rigidity—parkinsonism
3. Disturbances of integration, coordination, or balance—hemiplegia, parkinsonism, cerebellar ataxia
4. Diminished or absent motion or mobility (paresis, paralysis)—hemiplegia, spinal cord injury, arthritis, myasthenia gravis, muscular dystrophy
5. Disturbances in communication—stroke, cerebral palsy
6. Bladder and bowel problems—spinal cord injury, multiple sclerosis, hemiplegia, spina bifida

F. Common results of any prolonged immobilization
1. Decreased circulatory efficiency
   a. Edema of extremities
   b. Orthostatic hypotension upon being placed in upright position (sitting or standing)
2. Decreased respiratory efficiency—inability to aerate lungs, to cough and produce secretions
3. Generalized muscle weakness—disuse atrophy, loss of bone density and strength
4. Contracture deformities—shortening of connective tissue of joints, with resultant decrease in functional range of motion, especially hip and knee flexion contractures and foot drop
5. Loss of skin integrity—decubitus ulcers over bony prominences
6. Urinary stasis—infections, development of calculi

7. Disturbances in food absorption and metabolism—constipation, fecal impaction
8. Disturbances in psychological status—anxiety, depression, withdrawal, sensory distortions, etc.

2. **Rehabilitation nursing—overview**
A. Is basic component of all nursing care of persons with acute and chronic illnesses
B. Is practiced in the generalized hospital, in specialized hospitals and centers, in the extended care facility, in the nursing home, in the outpatient health center, and in the patient's home
C. Its immediate goals are to help
1. Restore function
2. Maintain existing function
3. Prevent further dysfunction
D. Its long-range goals are to help the patient
1. Learn new skills
2. Develop new patterns of activity
3. Develop new concepts about himself
E. Its focus is on
1. Patient and his family (as opposed to organ or to disease orientation)
2. Multiple facets—psychological and social factors in addition to physical problems
3. Teaching of patient and family
4. Eventual outcomes for patient
   a. Where will he go?
   b. How will he fare?
   c. How independent will he be in functional living?
   d. What type of continuing assistance will he need?
F. The rehabilitation nurse needs to understand
1. The physiology of the basic pathologic process causing the person's disability
2. The rationale for his therapeutic regimen
3. That all individuals going through a recovery process experience a variety of emotional responses (denial, fear, anxiety, anger, hostility, mourning, withdrawal, frustration, depression, etc.)
4. That the patient needs help in accepting that his personality and his being continue despite his changed physical status
5. That disabilities affect the person's whole life, not just a part of it
6. That previous life style and status will

exert powerful influences on the restorative process

7. That every individual has capabilities and strengths (examples: physical strength, emotional maturity, a supportive family) that can be utilized to offset his disabilities
8. That the patient and family need to set and maintain realistic goals of independent living
9. That some persons may be able to make only modest gains toward functional independence
10. That energy and endurance levels will affect the patient's ability to perform and learn
11. That time and space are powerful tools, which may be helpful in the process of restoration, equally, they can cause serious adverse effects
12. That patients need many opportunities to experience successful performances
13. That professionals only *help* a person rehabilitate himself, and therefore he must have a voice in decisions made regarding his care
14. That the nurse must often become the patient's advocate on the rehabilitation team
15. That rehabilitative care is rewarding and full of hope

G. Responsibilities of rehabilitation nurse
1. Assess the patient's needs for nursing care in physical, psychological, and social areas
2. Define, in cooperation with the patient and family, goals for nursing care
3. Establish a plan to carry out goals
4. Select appropriate methods, resources, and personnel to meet identified needs and determined goals
5. Institute nursing intervention
6. Evaluate, with patient and other team members, response to intervention
7. Be knowledgeable about and skilled in
   a. Proper body mechanics—her own and her patient's
   b. Turning, positioning, transfer, and ambulation techniques
   c. Range of motion exercises
   d. Use of specialized assistive devices
   e. Individualized methods of training for activities of daily living (ADL) such as personal hygiene, bathing, bladder and bowel care, dressing, feeding, and mobility

f. Preventing sensory overload or its opposite (lack of stimulation), through environmental control and sensory stimulation techniques

8. Help the patient cope with psychological relations to disability by
   a. Encouraging the patient and family to verbalize their feelings
   b. Learning what the disability means to the patient and family
   c. Accepting the patient's feelings without minimizing them
   d. Reassuring the patient that his reactions are not unusual
   e. Offering encouragement toward improvement and some degree of independence
   f. Offering opportunities for successful performance of activities of daily living
   g. Involving the patient in the planning of activities and care
   h. Providing information to the patient and family

3. **Rehabilitation nursing methods—general**
A. Maintenance of intact skin
1. Assess need for skin care
2. Establish a turning schedule of every 1 to 2 hours for changing patient's position and inspecting skin for signs of pressure
3. Check especially (on each side)
   a. Sacrum, vertebrae, scapula
   b. Heel, ankle, toes, dorsum of foot, and tibia
   c. Back of head, chin, and jaw
   d. Iliac crest, patella, groin
   e. Elbow, humerus, wrist
4. Turn and move patient carefully, using turning sheet or frame
5. Secure even distribution of body weight and/or change of pressure points by use of
   a. Alternating-pressure mattress—air mattress
   b. Flotation mattress—water bed
   c. Gel pads—in bed and wheelchair
   d. Foam rubber, polyurethane, sheepskin pads; air cushions
   e. Stryker frame, Foster frame, CircOlectric bed
   f. Trapeze to enable patient to shift weight
6. Teach patient to relieve body pressure as soon as possible by turning himself in bed and doing wheelchair push-ups;

protect pressure points in wheelchair, as well as in bed; keep patient, clothing, bed linen clean and dry; linens should be wrinkle free
7. Lightly massage areas of body that are subjected to pressure; use external heat with caution; especial care is necessary for patients with diminished or lack of sensation
8. Check circulation and skin condition frequently when appliances such as casts, braces, splints, elastic hose, or elastic wraps are used
9. Teach patient technique of regular self-inspection of skin using long-handled mirror
10. Teach skin care to the family
B. Maintenance of normal posture
1. In bed
   a. Immobility and inactivity lead to contraetural shortening deformities of joints (especially of flexor surfaces), pain, subluxation, edema, peripheral vascular stasis, hypoxia, and pneumonia; avoid these by establishing a turning and positioning schedule of at least every 2 hours, to be followed by all staff
   b. Utilize all positions unless contraindicated (e.g., right side, supine, left side, prone—in sequence)
   c. Position extremities in a variety of ways to maintain or increase range of motion and to prevent edema; stress extension of joints and correct alignment of extremities in positioning
   d. Prevent foot drop, hip or knee contracture, external rotation of leg
   e. Maintain correct body alignment, utilizing pillows, sandbags, footboards, handrolls, chest restraints, slings, etc.
   f. For patients with contractures, spasticity, or edema, special positioning techniques as well as supports to maintain desired position are necessary
      (1) Contractures: slowly move the joint through its range of motion to the extent possible without producing pain before positioning
      (2) Spasticity: move part slowly and allow time for muscle relaxation before positioning at

completion of range of movement
      (3) Edema: when positioning an edematous extremity in raised position, take care not to encourage flexion contractures of proximal joints
   g. Use turning sheet under the patient from shoulder to below buttock to facilitate change of position
   h. Distribute body weight evenly so that pressure is off bony prominences of the ear, shoulder, hip
2. In wheelchair
   a. Check sitting posture; correct a hunched sitting position, especially in wheelchair (or in bed); secure and support flaccid extremities in proper position; do not allow foot or arm to dangle over side of wheelchair
   b. Determine that wheelchair is proper size to permit good posture
3. On a frame
   a. Purposes of frames
      (1) Hyperextension
      (2) Immobilization
      (3) Correction of deformities
      (4) Facilitation of turning
      (5) Relief of pressure
   b. Types of frame
      (1) Bradford
      (2) Whitman (curved Bradford)
      (3) Balkan (overhead bars used with traction)
      (4) Stryker or Foster (reversible paired Bradford frames with specially constructed turning device) allows for horizontal turning of patient
      (5) CircOlectric bed
         (a) Allows for vertical turning of patient
         (b) Patient may be placed in various positions—Trendelenburg, standing, supine, prone
         (c) One nurse can turn patient
         (d) Electric motor provides power
         (e) Attachments permit application of traction
   c. General principles
      (1) Size—width should equal distance between tips of shoul-

ders; length, length of patient's body plus 6 inches

(2) Frame cover made of heavy canvas; tighten canvas daily

(3) Provide foot support; foot exercises beneficial for frame patients

(4) Side-lying and sitting on frame not permitted; for change of position, patient should lie prone; twin frames such as Stryker frame or Foster bed useful for this purpose; patient strapped (sandwichlike) between frames and turned

(5) Turning done all in one piece; patient rolled without twisting spine, in loglike fashion

(6) Patient should not reach out to side for tray while eating; provide table that can cross over bed, or feed patient

(7) Patient's clothes should open down back; avoid disturbance of spinal rest, caused by lifting patient to put garments over head or under buttocks; provide support to prevent foot drop and external rotation of the legs

C. Maintenance of functional range of joint motion (ROM)

1. Plan an exercise regimen for joints and muscles to meet needs and problems of individual patient

2. Purpose is to achieve or maintain that degree of motion in joints necessary to perform daily activities; patient should be taught early to actively exercise uninvolved extremities and to carry out as many activities as possible, as a preventive measure

3. Types of ROM exercises
   a. Passive: nurse or therapist does exercise for patient
   b. Assistive: patient voluntarily assists in carrying out exercise
   c. Active: patient carries out exercise independently after being instructed in proper method

4. Combinations of exercise types are usual in the same patient; for example, patient may do active upper extremity exercise but require passive range of motion type for legs
   a. Move all joints through full range twice daily

   b. Incorporate ROM exercises with other activities such as bathing, dressing, etc.
   c. Maintain firm support under joints while handling extremities
   d. Exercise slowly and smoothly and do not go beyond the point of pain without guidance from physician

5. Teach patient active muscle setting (isometric contraction and relaxation of muscles without joint movement), especially in quadriceps, gluteal, and abdominal muscles

6. Provide opportunities and encourage the patient to perform activities that are within his functional capabilities

7. Request assistance from physical therapist and/or occupational therapist in planning and implementing exercise program

8. Encourage family members to participate so they can help in the hospital as well as in the home

D. Maintenance of bowel function

1. Determine patient's bowel habits prior to illness

2. Determine whether patient is aware of need or act of defecation

3. Eliminate impaction if present

4. Offer bedpan or commode at time of day consistent with previous normal habit

5. It is preferable, if at all possible, for patient to use commode or toilet

6. Supply diet adequate in bulk, roughage, and bowel-stimulating properties

7. Encourage sufficient fluid intake (1,500 to 2,000 ml.)

8. Utilize suppositories, stool softeners, digital stimulation as needed

9. Use enemas only as a last resort

10. Teach family the bowel-training program

11. Provide for adaptation of equipment as necessary (e.g., raised toilet seat, padded backrest, grab bars, flat bedpan)

E. Maintenance of bladder function

1. Determine patient's bladder habits prior to illness

2. Determine whether patient is aware of need or act of voiding

3. Respond promptly to signs of need

4. If patient is on catheter, keep it clean, patent, and properly taped

5. In females, when recumbent, tape to

inner aspect of thigh; in males, to suprapubic area

6. Give perineal care daily
7. Plan with physician for early removal of catheter and bladder-retraining program
8. In patients with spinal cord injury, be alert for early signs of autonomic hyperreflexia due to distended bladder
9. Utilize physical and psychological techniques to stimulate voiding reflex
10. Manual expression of urine via Credé method may be of use
11. Encourage an adequate amount of fluids (2,500 ml.); maintain an intake-output record
12. Offer fluids during the waking hours; restrict fluids somewhat in the evening to control incontinence during sleep
13. Establish a voiding schedule to provide opportunity to void before incontinence occurs
    a. Start with an hourly schedule and gradually extend time interval
    b. Most patients can be maintained on a scheduled voiding pattern without the use of an indwelling catheter
14. Assist the patient to assume, as early as possible, a normal position for voiding; if the patient must use a urinal or bedpan, help him to use it
15. Provide privacy in toileting activities
16. Keep the patient clean and dry; use an external urinary collecting device, if necessary
17. Provide clothing that allows the patient to function independently in toilet activities
18. Communicate the patient's bladder control program to all staff
19. Teach the family the techniques of the patient's bladder program

F. Maintenance of independence in activities of daily living (ADL); nurse participates with physician and therapists in
1. Assessing present ability to perform skills
2. Evaluating factors that might interfere with self-care functions
3. Planning realistic ADL objectives, a training program, and necessary assistive devices to enable the patient to function at his maximum level
   a. Initiate program early, before discouragement is overwhelming
   b. Allow extensive time and do not rush patient
   c. Begin with familiar, easily accomplished tasks in order to motivate the patient; reinforce successes in those tasks; ignore or minimize failures
   d. Teach appropriate techniques and provide any necessary adaptive equipment to enable the patient to perform self-care tasks; see following examples
      (1) One-handed techniques for dressing
      (2) Selection of suitable clothing and assistive devices (e.g., shirt or dress large enough to slip on easily over the head, shoes that do not require lacing, Velcro fastenings, large buttons, buttonhooks, long-handled shoehorn)
      (3) Simplified methods and adaptive equipment for hygiene, bathing, and toileting (e.g., suction brush for dentures, movable shower head, soap mitt, shower chair)
      (4) Feeding devices (e.g., plateguard, knife, fork, long-handled straw, spillproof cup)
   e. Encourage the patient to repeat activities until they become habitual; teach patient to incorporate affected extremities in as many functional tasks as possible
   f. Utilize opportunities in the hospital for having patient practice housekeeping activities (bed making, dusting, etc.)
   g. Take special precautions with patient in whom sensation is diminished or absent
      (1) Test temperature of bath water to avoid burns; teach patient always to test temperature of water in any water-related activity
      (2) Avoid bumps, pressure, bruises, etc. when ambulating or getting into or out of wheelchair; examine skin for signs of pressure from bed and chair positioning, braces, splints, shoes
      (3) Teach patient to compensate for loss of sensation

(a) Use a footboard to stimulate pressure sensations and proprioception

(b) Provide opportunity for patient to touch, grasp, and manipulate objects of different sizes, weights, and textures, to stimulate tactile sensations

(c) Make patient aware of ignored body segments by reminding him to look at both extremities, to shave both sides of the face, to comb both sides of his hair, etc.

(d) Protect ignored limbs by using sling during functional activities and by providing proper positioning of extremities during transfer activities

(e) Teach patient to use his unaffected extremities to manipulate and move his affected ones and to use involved extremity as stabilizer

G. Transfer and ambulation activities; nurse participates with physician and physical and occupational therapists in
1. Evaluating
    a. Sitting tolerance, balance, skin condition, fatigue level, strength, and endurance
    b. Comprehension and motivation
2. Assessing need for and selection of assistive devices (wheelchair, crutches, canes, walker, hydraulic lift, trapeze, sliding board, etc.)
3. Planning mobility program
    a. Select most appropriate transfer method (either standing transfer or sitting transfer) to move to and from bed, chair, toilet, tub, etc.
    b. After the patient learns transfer technique, select appropriate method of ambulation with proper assistive device (e.g., wheelchair, cane, walker, crutches)
4. Transfer and ambulation instruction
    a. Use sliding board, two-man lift, mechanical lift, side rails and rope, grab bars, etc. in transfers
    b. Patient should wear shoes for standing transfers
    c. Use transfer belt and, in wheelchair, a safety strap if necessary
    d. Teach patient and family the transfer techniques and gait training—stressing safety factors, especially locking of wheelchair brakes during transfer
    e. Instruct in manner the patient can comprehend and at a pace he can maintain
    f. Teach patient to transfer while bed is set at the same level as his bed at home
    g. Maintain correct proximity and visual relationship of wheelchair to bed
    h. Ensure that patient has adequate assistance during transfers
    i. Teach patient and his family the proper use, handling, and care of wheelchair or other aids
    j. Instruct family about the installation of necessary grab bars, elevated toilet seat, ramps and the removal of hazardous conditions—scatter rugs, doorsills, slippery floors, etc.
5. Crutch walking instruction
    a. Selection of crutches
        (1) Proper length—with patient lying supine, measure from anterior fold of axilla to point 6 inches out from heel
        (2) Rubber crutch tips—intact, of good quality
        (3) Axillary bar not padded unless requested by physician; bar top should be about 2 inches below axilla
        (4) Handbar should allow almost complete extension of arm with elbow flexed about 30 degrees when patient places weight on palms
    b. Preparation for using crutches
        (1) Patient should have period of dangling before standing is attempted; also should do push-up exercises and other types of bed exercise to strengthen wrist extensors, elbow extensors, and shoulder depressors
        (2) Shoes should be firm and well fitting; avoid bedroom slippers
        (3) Guard patient so that he is not afraid; see that obstruc-

tions are eliminated (throw rugs, light cords, etc.)

(4) Patient should wear safety (transfer) belt if necessary to enable nurse to support and steady him

(5) Patient must learn to balance on crutches before attempting to walk; see that posture is good—chest high and body in full extension, particularly hips and knees

(6) Patient must learn to bear body weight largely on hands and should not lean on crutches with axillae; tendency causes crutch paralysis

c. Type of crutch walking will depend on disability

(1) Four-point gait—right crutch, left foot, left crutch, right foot —for patients who can manipulate both extremities, as in poliomyelitis, arthritis

(2) Two-point gait—more rapid version of above—right crutch and left foot advanced together

(3) Three-point gait—when one leg is unable to bear full weight of body (amputation, fractured hip, etc.); patient stands on good leg and places both crutches equal distance in advance; then swings himself forward slightly ahead of crutches, placing weight again on sound leg; regains balance before advancing crutches for another step

(4) Swinging-to or swinging-through gait—with crutches placed ahead, patient raises body off floor and up to or through crutches; for paraplegia, and other severe involvement of lower limbs

(5) Tripod—for patients who cannot lift body off floor; tripod position assumed, patient drags body up to crutches

d. Common mistakes in crutch walking

(1) Tendency to use body in poor mechanical fashion

(2) Hiking of hip with abduction gait (common in amputees)

(3) Trying to lift crutches while still bearing down on them

(4) Tendency to bear body weight on underarms (axillae)

(5) Hunching of shoulders (crutches usually too long) or stooping with shoulders (crutches usually too short)

(6) Walking on ball of foot with foot turned outward, flexion at hip or knee level

6. Use and care of braces and splints

a. Purposes

(1) Prevent and correct deformity

(2) Support body weight, assist weak muscles, and provide joint stability

(3) Relieve pain

(4) Prevent further injury

(5) Control involuntary movement

(6) Provide immobilization and rest

(7) Provide for improvement of function

b. General principles of care

(1) Brace can be kept in good condition with saddle soap or naphtha; joints should be oiled each week; excess oil should be wiped off and lint eliminated; straps, laces, and elastic should be replaced when frayed or worn

(2) Patient should be taught purpose and care of brace, and parent instructed as to when brace may be removed

(3) Skin should be examined daily for abrasions, evidence of pressure; metal of brace should not rub the skin

(4) Keep shoes in good repair

(a) Low-heeled walking shoe desirable

(b) Shoe that opens over the toes, if spasticity present

(c) High-top shoe to hold heel down in shoe

(5) Check alignment of brace— knee joint at level of the femoral condyles; hip joint opposite the greater trochanter

(6) Desirable to have an extra brace

(7) Recognize signs that patient is outgrowing brace

(8) If there are loose pieces at-

tached to brace, such as knee pads, secure when brace is removed so that they do not become lost

(9) Know purpose of each pad and apply correctly

(10) Leg braces

(a) Attachment to shoe—caliper (prongs fit into shoe heel), stirrup (brace fastened to the shoe), or foot plate (fits inside shoe)

(b) Ankle joint "stops" control ankle motion

(c) T straps at ankle control pronation and supination

(d) Knee lock allows for flexion of knee

(e) Leg cuffs and knee pads used to prevent "buckling of knee" (weak quadriceps), genu recurvatum (weak hamstrings), and genu varum or valgum

(f) Long leg brace with pelvic band designed to control hip joint movements

(11) Back braces should grasp pelvis and trochanters firmly

(a) See that upright bars are in center of back

(b) Begin lacing from below

(c) Do not save time by lacing in alternate holes, as this does not give proper support

(d) Allow patient to sit up in back brace before leaving him, to see that no metal pieces are pressing into groin or axilla

NURSING THE PATIENT WITH ARTHRITIS

1. **Common types of arthritis (inflammation of the joint)**

A. Osteoarthritis (degenerative, nonankylosing)—common progressive degenerative disorder, particularly of middle and old age

1. Cause unknown

a. Women more frequently affected; more common in the elderly, but may occur at any age as a result of trauma

2. Symptoms

a. Associated with aging process and the "wearing out" of articular cartilage and overgrowth of juxta-articular bone

b. Roughened cartilage causes trauma to synovium and joint capsule

c. Muscle spasm and inflammation result in swelling and pain, which result in limitation of joint motion

d. Heberden's nodes, deforming bony protuberances, develop at distal interphalangeal joints of fingers

e. Weight-bearing joints more frequently involved; degenerative joint disease of hips is most disabling form

f. Obesity increases joint stress

3. Methods of treatment—no specific measures

a. Main objectives of therapy

(1) Relief of pain

(2) Prevention of avoidable disability

(3) Reassurance that disease is not likely to spread and that serious disability is unusual

(4) Stress on need to maintain general health via proper diet, rest, exercise

b. Measures for relief of pain

(1) Drugs—salicylates usually adequate

(2) Rest of affected joint

(3) Phenylbutazone used occasionally

c. Physical therapy

(1) Maintain muscle strength, prevent contractures, maintain range of motion by use of exercise

(2) Correct poor body mechanics (faulty weight bearing)

(3) Protect joints against unnecessary deformity

(4) Encourage activity (alternate with short rest periods)

d. Local heat—hot soaks, packs, or heating pads to painful joints

e. Use of cane or crutches—can relieve pain and protect joint against added trauma

f. Diet—limit in calories, if patient overweight; otherwise, adequate diet fortified with vitamins

g. Maintain shoe corrections

h. Provide reassurance; eliminate worry and other emotional disturbances

i. Surgical procedures (usually arthroplasty) may be necessary when severe joint destruction, pain, or limitation of motion is present

B. Rheumatoid arthritis (Still's disease, infectional form, polyarthritis, ankylosing, and Marie-Strümpell disease)—systemic disease of connective tissue primarily, with widespread joint inflammation and destruction; involvement of back, sacroiliac joints, and shoulders occurs in addition to disease of extremities

1. Cause unknown
   a. Theories pertaining to cause include autoimmune mechanisms as most likely; also virus or other infections
   b. Occurs in all age groups; most frequent in fourth decade, although not infrequent in children below 14 years
   c. Occurs three times more frequently in women than in men
2. Symptoms
   a. Characterized by exacerbations and remissions
   b. Onset is insidious with ill-defined aching and stiffness, followed by swelling, warmth, redness, and tenderness of joints
   c. Symmetric involvement of both sides; small joints of hands and feet almost always affected
   d. Silent loss of range of motion (at extremes of range); muscle weakness and atrophy common
   e. Early morning stiffness
   f. General weakness, fatigue, loss of appetite and weight, anemia; systemic effects are very pronounced during acute stage
   g. Deformity and loss of joint motion caused by the inflammatory process, synovial membrane changes, pain, and muscle spasm
3. Diagnostic procedures (not specific for arthritis)
   a. Latex agglutination
   b. Erythrocyte sedimentation rate
   c. X-ray films
4. Treatment—based on recognition that rheumatoid arthritis is a systemic disease
   a. Adequate diet; avoid overweight condition
   b. Rest—both systemic and local, using very well fitted supports

c. Improvement in posture, and prevention of deformity; muscle spasm holds joint in position of greatest comfort (flexion and adduction); joints may ankylose in these positions if provision for relieving muscle spasm is not made; provide for functional positions, maintaining good body alignment, with regular change of position

d. Heat—used to relax muscles and to relieve pain and stiffness; given by means of electric pad, baths, hot packs, paraffin wax

e. Exercise—may include active, passive, resistance
   (1) Build and maintain muscle strength and range of joint motion (should be carefully prescribed)
   (2) Especial attention to lower extremities as a crucial area to prevent permanent disability due to contractures of hips
   (3) Avoid fatigue and pain

f. Drug therapy
   (1) Salicylates (aspirin most commonly used)—relieve pain, tend to lessen joint inflammation; very large dosage over long periods may cause gastric problems and ototoxicity
   (2) Phenylbutazone—relieves pain, stiffness; may have undesirable side effects
   (3) Indomethacin — anti-inflammatory drug; may cause side effects
   (4) Hydroxychloroquine — antimalarial drug; periodic eye examination necessary
   (5) Corticosteroids—decrease inflammation, pain, stiffness; patient may experience recurrence of pain as drug is decreased or discontinued
   (6) Hydrocortisone—injected directly into joint; used with varying degrees of success in controlling pain in specific joint, thus enabling patient to continue joint motion and prevent ankylosis

g. Helping patient understand condition; lessen worry and anxiety; prevent self-pity and apathy

h. Use of assistive devices for ADL to

encourage independence and decrease pain during activities such as dressing, bathing, etc.
  i. Use of braces and splints
    (1) Give support, protect joint
    (2) Prevent contractures
    (3) Give rest to acute joint
  j. Use of cane or crutches—protect weight-bearing joints
  k. Properly fitted shoes essential
  l. Encourage therapeutic and diversional crafts, particularly those that promote functional use of hands, arms, and legs
  m. Surgical procedures (not necessary to wait until disease "burned out")
    (1) Prophylactic surgery—to prevent destruction of joint
    (2) Reconstructive surgery—to restore joint motion and correct deformities
    (3) Surgical procedures include synovectomy, arthroplasty, osteotomy, arthrodesis, and soft tissue procedures
  n. Rehabilitation plans need to be developed jointly with patient at an early stage of illness
C. Gouty arthritis
  1. Cause—disturbance in purine metabolism
  2. Occurs more frequently in men than in women
  3. Metatarsophalangeal joint of great toe usually affected first
  4. Urates deposited in periarticular structures
  5. Treatment

NURSING THE PATIENT WITH CEREBRAL PALSY

1. **Common types**
A. Spastic
B. Athetoid
C. Ataxic
2. **Causes varied**
A. Prenatal or postnatal trauma or infection
B. Natal trauma, anoxia
C. Nutritional status of mother during pregnancy and Rh factor possible causes of malformation and brain injury
3. **Complexity of condition demands many professionals working as a coordinated team**
A. Physicians of various specialties
  1. Pediatrician   3. Physiatrist
  2. Neurologist   4. Orthopedist, etc.
B. Nurse
C. Physical therapist
D. Occupational therapist
E. Speech clinician
F. Teacher
G. Social worker
4. **Rehabilitation is difficult, perhaps because of**
A. Combination of problems and sites involved
  1. Type of neuromuscular involvement
  2. Parts of body involved
  3. Degree of involvement
  4. Degree of brain damage and retardation, resulting in deficits in vision, hearing, speech perception, or intelligence
B. Age of patient and his social environment
5. **Methods of treatment**
A. Physical therapy highly complex
  1. Specially trained workers needed
  2. Treatment aimed at teaching child to relax and to perform movements from relaxed positions
  3. Performance of functional, everyday activities stressed at as early a stage as possible
B. A number of neuromuscular reeducation, reflex, sensory stimulation and/or sensory inhibition techniques are being tried by various therapists
  1. None has shown itself to be completely effective to date
  2. Purpose of each method is to help the child develop the patterns of movements necessary to perform activities of daily living
C. Experts feel that efforts should first be directed to get child to speak and use hands and arms; walking not primary requisite
6. **Priorities in rehabilitation—to be performed in as nearly normal a manner as is possible**
A. Bed and wheelchair activities
  1. Bed and wheelchair activities are taught by nurse
    a. Personal hygiene
    b. Feeding
    c. Toileting
    d. Dressing
    e. Handling a wheelchair
B. Maximum use of hands
  1. Occupational therapist teaches fine-hand skills
C. Walking activities
  1. Walking instruction and advanced

therapy exercise routines are directed by physical therapist

7. **General rehabilitation considerations**

A. Child must learn to be as independent as possible; home furnishing should be constructed to assist him toward greater independence, and safety precautions should be instituted

B. Deformities often present—particularly flexion and adduction deformities and stooped shoulders

C. Parent education and psychological support (and/or treatment) are highly essential; coddling, overprotection, or rejection of child may hamper progress

D. Hospital or special school should provide classwork and treatment for child who cannot attend regular school

E. Patients do not belong in general hospital, but many need to be admitted for surgery such as tenotomies, neurotomies, and for correction of established deformities; or may require admission to the Rehabilitation Center for training in ADL, for application of braces, or for intensive speech and hearing evaluation and therapy

F. Evaluation of home, family, and community resources is an important part of whole process

NURSING THE PATIENT WITH AN AMPUTATION

1. **Prevention of flexion contracture in lower extremity amputation**

A. See that bed does not sag under hips

B. Eliminate pillow under stump as soon as danger of hemorrhage passes

C. Encourage patient to lie prone and to extend hip several times during day, to stretch out any developing flexion contractures of hip and knee

D. Instruct patient to maintain hip and knee in extension and adduction at all times possible

E. When patient begins to walk, note particularly that he does not keep the hip in slight flexion; teach him to avoid hiking of shoulder and abduction of artificial leg

2. **Care of stump**

A. Stump shrinkage is an important early stage; two elements in shrinkage are
1. Reduction of subcutaneous fat by pressure of constrictive bandage and socket of prosthesis

2. Atrophy of disuse occurring in involved muscles; use of prosthesis prevents excessive atrophy

B. Compression bandage
1. Several cotton elastic bandages will be necessary
2. Two sets needed so that they can be washed between applications

C. Apply bandages snugly, compressing the end of the stump into smooth, rather conical shape, working from distal end to proximal

D. When patient begins to wear prosthesis, he will need several all-wool stump socks
1. Must be kept in good condition by frequent washing
   a. Warm soft water
   b. Mild soap
   c. Thorough rinsing

E. Instruct patient to report to physician any skin irritation or other abnormality that occurs in stump

3. **General health and physical condition must not be overlooked during preoperative or postoperative period**

A. Exercise activities must be planned to maintain strength, balance, posture, and overall muscle tone

B. Immediate postsurgical prosthetic fitting for lower extremity amputee
1. Done in United States since 1964, principally in military and Veterans Administration Hospitals
2. Found to be very effective with both young and aged adults
3. Patients are fitted with prostheses immediately after surgery, and ambulation training is begun on the first postoperative day

C. Lower extremity amputee must be taught
1. Arm and shoulder girdle exercises (e.g., wheelchair push-ups or pull-ups in overhead rings)—to develop muscle strength for crutch walking
2. Crutch walking techniques
3. Balance training—at bedside, against a wall, or in parallel bars
4. Exercises for remaining extremity, to prevent disuse atrophy and hamstring contractures and to maintain quadriceps tone
5. Purpose of prosthesis is weight bearing and ambulation

D. Upper extremity amputee must be taught
1. Correct posture and asymmetric balance to avoid poor posture and gait habits

2. Bilateral shoulder exercises to prepare for fitting of prosthesis
3. Purpose of prosthesis is prehension (picking up and transporting objects) Amount of function is very dependent on level of amputation
   Mastery of upper extremity prosthesis more complex than that of lower extremity
4. Prosthesis components
   Terminal device replacing hand (cosmetic *or* functional), wrist device, forearm segment, elbow mechanism, upper arm segment, and harness

4. **Psychological adjustments**
A. Are often difficult
B. Patient has to adjust to a new body image and at the same time he has to develop skill in utilizing his prosthesis
C. Patient requires support, encouragement, and understanding

NURSING THE PATIENT WITH SPINAL CORD INJURY

1. **Transportation of patient with back injury**
A. Avoid flexion, hyperextension, or rotation of the vertebrae
2. **Immediate care**
A. Observe for
   1. Respiratory difficulty (if injury in cervical area); maintain patent airway; keep equipment available for tracheotomy, suctioning, and administration of oxygen
   2. Level of consciousness and signs of confusion—intracranial involvement
   3. Hyperthermia; cause may be of central origin
   4. Bladder distention
      a. Catheterize (if ordered)
      b. Save specimen
B. Give I.M. drugs, parenteral fluids, and/ or blood as ordered
C. Equipment for doing spinal puncture should be available
3. **Type of bed (as prescribed)**
A. Firm mattress
   1. Sponge rubber
   2. Alternating-pressure pad
   3. CircOlectric bed—facilitates turning of the paralyzed patient
   4. Stryker or Foster frame
B. Equipment for head traction if required
C. Protective bed covering to facilitate changes of linen

4. **On-going care**
   (See review of rehabilitation nursing methods, p. 627.)
A. Maintain cervical vertebrae in position of extension or hyperextension as prescribed
B. Observe for loss of motion or muscle strength and for change in skin sensation
C. Encourage deep breathing
D. Observe for autonomic hyperreflexia
E. Check on patency of bladder catheter
F. Observe for distention (paralytic ileus); relief provided with drugs or suctioning with stomach tube
G. Prevent fecal impaction
H. Prevent deformity
   1. Correct body alignment with frequent and regular changes of position
   2. Maintain functional positions
   3. Maintain normal range of joint motion (actively or passively)
5. **After stabilization of acute condition**
   (See review of rehabilitation nursing methods, p. 627.)
A. Encourage and teach self-help and self-care (activities of daily living)
B. Exercises to strengthen shoulder, arm, and back muscles—aid in performing ADL and in crutch walking
C. Tilt table
D. Bracing—to facilitate ambulation
E. Ambulation in parallel bars—progress to crutches
F. Provide high-protein diet; high fluid intake
G. Elimination
   1. Bowel
      a. Prevent fecal impactions
      b. Bowel-training program
   2. Bladder
      a. Program for development of independent bladder function (if prescribed)
      b. Catheter care, sterile technique, closed catheter drainage
      c. Prevention of urinary tract infection and calculi
      d. Use of antibiotics as ordered
H. Active life—wheelchair or braces and crutches—goal for all patients
I. Teach patient and family all aspects of care—prepare home for return
J. Help patient and family to accept situation and to plan for realistic goals
K. Vocational planning and training should be instituted early

NURSING THE PATIENT WITH A STROKE

1. **Main types**
A. Completed stroke—stroke that has produced its full neurologic damage
   1. Cerebral thrombosis: occlusion of intracranial vessel, resulting in ischemia of area of brain; usually due to arteriosclerosis
   2. Cerebral hemorrhage: bleeding within the brain, usually due to ruptured intracranial vessel
   3. Cerebral embolism: obstruction of intracranial vessel by clot or other substance arriving from elsewhere in the body
B. Transient ischemic attacks (TIA)
   1. Short episodes of localized neurologic dysfunction caused by cerebrovascular disease
   2. Often are first signs of pending strokes (above)
2. **Etiology**
A. May occur at any age including childhood
B. Peak incidence from 40 to 70 years
C. Recent increase among women of childbearing age who are using various forms of the "Pill" for contraception
3. **Symptoms and tests**
A. Symptoms differ with type of vascular incident
   1. Rapid sudden onset, with hemorrhage and embolism
   2. Prodromal symptoms (dizziness, weakness, headache, etc.), with thrombosis
B. Most frequently observed symptoms
   1. Headache
   2. Mental confusion with varying levels of consciousness
   3. Coma
   4. Focal neurologic signs
   5. Arterial hypertension
C. Diagnostic tests
   1. Neurologic examination
   2. Spinal tap
   3. Skull x-ray film
   4. Cerebral angiography
   5. Electroencephalography
   6. Blood chemistry and gas analysis
4. **Treatment**
A. For transient ischemic attack
   1. Identification of patients at risk
   2. Identification of cause
   3. Prevention of progression of disease and harmful sequelae, via
      a. Thorough physical examination
      b. Appropriate use of medication (e.g., anticoagulants)
      c. Diet therapy
      d. Regimen of rest, exercise, avoidance of stress
      e. Instruction of patient and family in their responsibility for promotion of health
      f. Surgical procedures
B. For completed stroke
   1. Emergency lifesaving measures
   2. Complete rest with head slightly elevated
   3. Thrombolytic medication to dissolve thrombosis
   4. Anticoagulant medication to prevent clotting
   5. Surgery—to repair ruptured vessel; to remove expanding clot in brain or from occluded vessel (e.g., carotid artery)
   6. Prevention of further dysfunction
5. **Nursing care**
A. In acute situation, institute lifesaving measures for maintenance of vital body functions
   1. Careful observation of vital signs and level of consciousness
   2. Maintain adequate airway; prevent aspiration
   3. Maintain circulation
   4. Institute eye and mouth care
   5. Give catheter care as necessary
   6. Be prepared to deal with seizures
B. Concurrently, institute measures to prevent further dysfunction
   1. Maintenance of intact skin
   2. Proper positioning
   3. Passive range of motion
      (See review of rehabilitation nursing methods, p. 627, for details.)
   4. Maintain appropriate fluid and nutritional intake
   5. Maintain adequate bladder and bowel function—p. 627
C. Institute measures to
   1. Prevent self-harm due to perceptual loss, especially with visual loss of half of visual field (hemianopia) and with psychological ignoring of body parts, by placing bedside table on unaffected side, protecting ignored parts, etc.
   2. Compensate for diminished or lost sensation
   3. Relieve patient and family's anxiety through reassurance and explanation

4. Cope with the many psychological re-actions to stroke that patient and family have
5. Motivate patient to participate in re-habilitation process

D. For all patients with stroke, anticipate communication problems
1. Evaluate extent of patient's ability to understand and express himself at a simple level
2. Confirm to the patient that he has a problem in communicating
3. Speak slowly, clearly, in short sentences and phrases that patient can understand
4. Use gestures, picture board, writing, etc. as alternative means of communication
5. Attempt to stimulate patient's communication without pushing him to point of frustration
6. Seek help from speech therapist in establishing a functional level of communication with patient so as to be able to meet at least his minimal needs in daily activities (e.g., requesting a drink)

E. As soon as medically feasible, encourage patient to
1. Undertake activities of daily living in personal hygiene, feeding, etc.
2. Start transfer and ambulation training —p. 632

F. Long-range rehabilitation will include, as appropriate
1. Vocational training (or retraining)
2. Homemaking activity training

REVIEW QUESTIONS FOR REHABILITATION NURSING
Multiple choice

Read each question carefully and consider all possible answers. When you have decided which answer is best, blacken in the corresponding space on the answer sheet. There is only one best answer for each question (or implied question).

Situation: Following a car accident, Ed, an 18-year-old high school senior, is taken to the local hospital with a back injury. He did not lose consciousness and remembers that he was unable to move his legs following the accident. Questions 1 through 17 relate to this patient.

1. Following an accident when there is a questionable back injury, the individual involved
(a) May be transported in sitting position, if necessary, to secure immediate medical care
(b) May be transported in any position because position is not important, since damage to the cord has already occurred
(c) May be transported in the supine position unless there is bleeding from the nose and mouth; then he should be placed in prone position
(d) Should be protected from flexion and hyperextension of the spine
(e) May be transported best when placed in the side-lying position
1. a   3. c and d
2. c and e   4. a and b

2. Following examination, the doctor indicated that Ed was paraplegic. This means
1. Both lower and upper extremities are paralyzed
2. Upper extremities are paralyzed
3. One side of the body is paralyzed
4. Lower extremities are paralyzed

3. When caring for a paraplegic patient, the nurse should recognize that various deformities may develop in a relatively short time if nursing measures are not instituted. Which of the following deformities are most likely to develop?
(a) Hip contracture   (c) Foot drop
(b) Knee contracture   (d) Wrist drop
1. All of these   3. b and d
2. a and c   4. a, b, and c

4. When caring for a paraplegic, the nurse will remember that a high intake of fluid is necessary to help
1. Prevent elevation of temperature
2. Maintain electrolyte balance
3. Prevent dehydration
4. Prevent urinary tract infection

5. Good nursing care of the paraplegic will provide that he be turned every 2 hours. This is necessary mainly to
(a) Keep the patient comfortable
(b) Prevent pressure sores
(c) Improve circulation in the lower extremities
(d) Prevent flexion contractures of the extremities
1. a and b   3. c and d
2. b and d   4. All of these

6. The development of contractures of the joints of the lower extremities in a paraplegic can be prevented by
(a) Changing bed position every 2 hours
(b) Maintaining proper bed positions
(c) Passively moving the extremities through a full range of motion several times daily
(d) Providing the patient with active exercise instructions
1. a, b, and c   3. All of these
2. b and d   4. c and d

7. The paraplegic patient frequently loses calcium from the skeletal system. Which of the following factors contributes to this condition?
1. Inactivity
2. Decreased calcium intake
3. Inadequate kidney function
4. Inadequate fluid intake

8. Formation of urinary calculi is a complication that may be encountered by the paraplegic patient. Factors that contribute to this condition are

(a) Inadequate fluid intake
(b) Increased intake of calcium
(c) Inadequate kidney function
(d) Increased loss of calcium from the skeletal system
   1. a, b, and c   3. a and d
   2. b and d   4. c and d

9. The tilt table is used to help
(a) Overcome orthostatic hypotension
(b) Prevent pressure sores
(c) Prevent loss of calcium from long bones
(d) Encourage increased activity
   1. a, b, and c   3. a and c
   2. b and c   4. a, b, and d

10. Rehabilitation plans for the paraplegic
   1. Should be considered and planned for, early in his care
   2. Are not necessary, since he will return to his usual activities following hospitalization
   3. Should be left up to the patient and his family
   4. Are not necessary, since he will not be able to work again

11. Teaching Ed to care for himself while in the hospital
   1. Is not necessary, since he will be back to normal when he leaves the hospital
   2. Is too complicated to be undertaken by a lay person
   3. Is not necessary, since his family will not be able to care for him in the home situation
   4. Is an essential part of his nursing care

12. Since Ed has paraplegia, the nurse recognizes that one major early problem will be
   1. Use of mechanical aids for ambulation
   2. Patient education
   3. Quadriceps setting
   4. Bladder control

13. The nursing care of Ed should be directed toward
(a) Preventing decubiti
(b) Maintaining nutrition
(c) Providing emotional support
(d) Proper positioning
(e) Conditioning exercises
   1. All of these   3. a, c, and d
   2. All but e   4. a, b, and d

14. It may be expected that Ed will have some spasticity of the lower extremities. To prevent the development of contractures, careful consideration must be given to
   1. Proper positioning   3. Active exercise
   2. Use of tiltboard   4. Deep massage

15. The rehabilitation of Ed will include very close cooperation of the following team members:
(a) Professional nurse
(b) Physiatrist
(c) Physical therapist
(d) Social worker
(e) Vocational counselor
   1. All but b   3. All but e
   2. All of these   4. a, c, and d

16. During the convalescent phase of Ed's illness, emphasis should be placed on
(a) Job placement
(b) Activities of daily living
(c) Muscle-strengthening exercises

(d) High-protein, high-caloric diet
   1. b, c, and d   3. b and d
   2. All of these   4. a and d

17. When Ed is transferred to a rehabilitation center, therapy will be directed toward
(a) Ambulation
(b) Job training
(c) Maintaining independence
(d) Preparation for braces
   1. a and d   3. All of these
   2. a and c   4. a, b, and d

Situation: Mrs. B, 35 years of age, has had a mid-thigh amputation following injury in an automobile accident. Questions 18 through 26 apply to Mrs. B.

18. To promote early and efficient ambulation the nurse would
   1. Place pillows under the stump
   2. Encourage the patient to lie supine
   3. Turn patient to the prone position frequently to prevent flexion contracture of the hip
   4. Keep backrest elevated

19. When the patient is allowed to be up, she should
   1. Keep hip in extension and adduction
   2. Keep hip in extension and abduction
   3. Lift shoulder and hip of affected side when taking a step
   4. Walk with crutches until permanent prosthesis is secured; this will prevent the development of faulty walking habits

20. Before ambulation is started, the following activity will make walking with crutches easier:
   1. Frequent use of the trapeze to strengthen the biceps muscles
   2. Push-up exercises with sawed-off crutches to strengthen the triceps, finger flexors, wrist extensors, and elbow extensors
   3. Sitting in a chair until strength is regained
   4. Keeping limb in extension and abduction

21. Crutch gait adaptable to the patient with a single leg amputation wearing a prosthesis is
   1. Tripod crutch gait
   2. Four-point gait
   3. Three-point gait
   4. Swinging-through type of crutch gait

22. Preparing Mrs. B for ambulation with crutches will include teaching her
(a) To stand and maintain balance
(b) To ambulate several hours a day for practice
(c) To do active exercises for muscle strengthening
(d) To use a gait suited for her
(e) To sit down and stand up
   1. a and d   3. a, b, and c
   2. a, c, and d   4. All but b

23. Rehabilitation of the amputee begins
   1. Before the surgery
   2. During the convalescent phase
   3. Upon discharge from the hospital
   4. When he is ready for a prosthesis

24. If Mrs. B had an immediate postsurgical prosthetic application, this would have meant that
(a) She would be out of bed and weight bearing about 24 hours after surgery
(b) Her stump would have been wrapped in

an external plaster bandage in the operating room

(c) A temporary prosthetic unit would be attached to the rigid dressing during or before the first postoperative day

(d) No drains would be necessary, since hemorrhage does not usually occur
   1. All but d   3. b and c
   2. All but a   4. b and d

25. There are several "don'ts" for the patient with a mid-thigh amputation. These include: Don't
   (a) Hang the stump over the bed
   (b) Sit in a wheelchair with stump flexed
   (c) Rest stump on crutch handle
   (d) Abduct stump
   (e) Place pillow between thighs
      1. b, c, and d   3. a, b, and d
      2. All of these   4. All but e

26. Stump shrinkage is an important factor in the healing stage. There are two elements in such shrinkage. They are
   (a) Reduction of subcutaneous fat
   (b) Development of skin tension
   (c) Atrophy of disuse
   (d) Postoperative edema
      1. b and c   3. c and d
      2. a and d   4. a and c

Situation: Mr. D, a 52-year-old accountant, has been admitted to the hospital in an unconscious state due to a cerebrovascular accident. Questions 27 through 34 relate to this patient.

27. The nurse's immediate responsibilities include
   (a) Maintaining a patent airway
   (b) Maintaining adequate circulation
   (c) Maintaining proper positioning
   (d) Maintaining an intact skin
      1. a and b   3. c and d
      2. All of these 4. a, b, and c

28. When Mr. D regains consciousness, evaluation indicates that he has a left hemiplegia. The nurse contributes to his rehabilitation by
   (a) Referral to the physical therapist
   (b) Not moving the affected arm and leg unless necessary
   (c) Beginning passive exercises
   (d) Positioning to prevent deformity and decubiti
      1. c and d   3. a, b, and d
      2. a and b   4. b and d

29. Mr. D has expressive aphasia. The nurse
   1. Places him away from other patients so he will not become frustrated in not being able to speak
   2. Raises her voice to help him understand her
   3. Uses alternate means (such as gestures) to stimulate his ability to communicate
   4. Does not expect him to be able to perform ADL, since he can't speak

30. In aiding Mr. D to develop independence, the nurse
   (a) Demonstrates ways he can regain independence in activities
   (b) Reinforces success in tasks accomplished
   (c) Establishes long-range goals for the patient
   (d) Points out his errors in performance
      1. c and d   3. a and b
      2. All of these 4. a, b, and c

31. Mr. D has been incontinent of feces. The nurse establishes a bowel-training program. The program includes the following steps:
   (a) Determine the patient's previous bowel habit
   (b) Eliminate impaction
   (c) Offer bedpan at accustomed time
   (d) Provide sufficient fluid and roughage in diet
   (e) Use enemas as part of training program
      1. All but b   3. All but e
      2. a, c, and d   4. b, c, and d

32. The rehabilitation of Mr. D should include
   (a) ADL training
   (b) Psychosocial understanding
   (c) Therapeutic exercise
   (d) Providing encouragement and praise for accomplishment
   (e) Evaluation of the total patient
      1. b, c, and d   3. All of these
      2. c, d, and e   4. a, b, and d

33. Some important aspects of rehabilitation of the stroke patient are
   (a) His return to a satisfactory level of social functioning
   (b) Help in adjusting to the acute situation
   (c) Involving the family in the rehabilitation program
   (d) Retraining for employment
      1. All of these   3. a, b, and c
      2. b and d   4. a and d

34. Some problems that may be encountered in the rehabilitation of the stroke patient are
   (a) Age and chronic disease
   (b) Lack of desire for independence
   (c) Unwillingness to cooperate
   (d) Lack of community resources
   (e) The subculture of the aged
      1. a and d   3. Only c
      2. d and e   4. All of these

Situation: Mrs. C, a 32-year-old woman who has intermittently been having painful swollen knee and wrist joints during the past 3 months, is being admitted to the hospital for treatment of rheumatoid arthritis. Questions 35 through 50 apply to Mrs. C.

35. One would expect the doctor to order the following diet for Mrs. C:
   1. High-protein
   2. Salt-free
   3. General diet, supplemented with vitamins and iron
   4. Bland diet

36. To relieve Mrs. C's painful knees, the doctor will probably prescribe
   1. Codeine 30 mg. every 4 hours
   2. Aspirin 0.6 Gm. every 4 hours
   3. Codeine 30 mg. every 4 hours p.r.n.
   4. Nembutal 90 mg. every h.s.

37. As to bed position, the nurse will encourage Mrs. C to
   1. Assume position in which she is most comfortable
   2. Place pillows beneath her knees
   3. Assume Fowler position
   4. Maintain limbs in extension

38. To prevent deformity of the knee joint, the doctor will

1. Immobilize joint in cylinder cast for a period of several weeks
2. Discourage use of the knee joint
3. Encourage motion of joint within limits of pain
4. Put patient on bed rest
39. The most common deformity of the knee joint in arthritis is
1. Flexion contracture
2. Ankylosis in an extended position
3. Ankylosis with genu varum deformity
4. Ankylosis with genu valgum deformity
40. The doctor may inject hydrocortisone into the knee joint. The *most* important reason for doing this is to
1. Prevent ankylosis of the joint
2. Reduce inflammation
3. Provide psychotherapy
4. Relieve pain
41. Which of the following laboratory tests or procedures would be helpful in making the diagnosis of arthritis?
1. Latex agglutination
2. Lipase
3. Bence Jones protein
4. Phosphatase alkaline
42. Heberden's nodes are associated with
1. Osteomyelitis
2. Rheumatoid arthritis
3. Hypertrophic arthritis
4. Syndactylism
43. Which of the following terms would refer to hypertrophic arthritis?
(a) Degenerative
(b) Nonankylosing
(c) Herberden's nodes
(d) Marie-Strümpell
    1. a and b   3. c and d
    2. b, c, and d   4. a, b, and c
44. Mrs. C's condition would indicate that a primary consideration in her care should be directed toward
1. Motivation   3. Control of pain
2. Education   4. Surgery
45. Since Mrs. C does not have marked crippling, preventive efforts are important. This will require a team approach and should include the following team members:
(a) Physician
(b) Professional nurse
(c) Physical therapist
(d) Occupational therapist
    1. All but d   3. c and d
    2. All of these   4. a, b, and c
46. After medical evaluation, therapy for Mrs. C may include
(a) Range of motion exercises
(b) Braces
(c) Massage
(d) Conductive heat
(e) Well-balanced diet
    1. a, b, and c   3. All but a
    2. c, d, and e   4. All but b
47. In helping Mrs. C toward self-reliance and independence the team should approach the problem with
1. A positive attitude toward the eventual outcome
2. The understanding that little can be accomplished

3. A feeling that efforts should be made to place the patient in an extended care facility
4. Limited objectives
48. The patient with rheumatoid arthritis must be protected against injury to the joints. Therefore, therapeutic exercise should be
1. Only passive
2. Avoided
3. Preceded by heat
4. Active assistive
49. Through motivation and teaching, Mrs. C may
1. Learn to perform most ADL
2. Become vocationally employed
3. Ambulate with crutches
4. Be transferred to a halfway house
50. Destructive changes in joints as a result of arthritis
(a) Are more incapacitating in joints of the lower extremities because of weight-bearing requirements
(b) Require establishment of self-care goals for upper extremities
(c) Are due to bone and cartilage erosion
(d) Cause loss of joint motion in the intermediate range before loss in the extremes of the range
    1. b and c   3. d
    2. a and b   4. a, b, and c

Situation: Mrs. S, a small 78-year-old woman, fell in her backyard. Because of pain, she was unable to get to her feet when assisted by a neighbor; she was transported to the local hospital by ambulance. X-ray films were taken and the attending surgeon told Mrs. S that she had fractured her hip (fractured neck of the femur). She was admitted to the hospital and Buck's extension was applied to her limb. The following day, she was given a general anesthetic, the fracture was reduced, and a Smith-Petersen nail inserted. Questions 51 through 62 apply to Mrs. S.

51. On examination of Mrs. S, the nurse would expect to find
1. Shortening of the affected extremity with internal rotation
2. Shortening of the affected extremity with external rotation
3. Abduction with external rotation
4. Adduction with internal rotation
52. Following fracture of the neck of the femur, the desirable position for the limb is
1. External rotation with flexion of the knee and hip
2. External rotation with extension of the knee and hip
3. Internal rotation with extension of the knee
4. Internal rotation with flexion of the hip and knee
53. Side rails are placed on the bed of the elderly patient primarily
1. To be used as hand holds and to facilitate patient's moving
2. As a precautionary measure, since many patients in this age group become disoriented
3. Because of hospital regulations

4. Because the patient will rest better with the rails in place
54. Buck's extension was applied to Mrs. S's limb. The chief reason for applying traction is to
   1. Help reduce the fracture and to relieve muscle spasm and pain
   2. Keep patient from turning and moving in bed
   3. Facilitate nursing care
   4. Maintain the limb in a position of external rotation
55. Following application of traction to the lower extremity, it is important to know that the patient can dorsiflex the foot. Inability to do this may indicate
   1. Atrophy of the tibialis anticus muscle
   2. Poor circulation in the extremity
   3. A painful ankle joint
   4. Peroneal nerve damage
56. When Mrs. S is helped from the bed to a chair after nailing of her hip, it is desirable that she stand on her good leg before sitting in a chair (no weight bearing on the involved limb). This is true because
   1. There is usually insufficient help to lift her from bed to chair
   2. This will help maintain strength in her good limb
   3. This is the quickest method of getting her to and from the bed
   4. There is less danger of injuring her hip
57. When in the side-lying position, it is necessary that Mrs. S have a firm pillow placed between her thighs and that the entire length of her uppermost limb be supported. The most important reason for this is to
   1. Prevent adduction contracture of the involved hip and strain on the fracture site
   2. Make the patient more comfortable
   3. Prevent flexion contractures of the hip joint
   4. Prevent skin surfaces from rubbing together
58. Contractures that develop most frequently following fracture of the hip are
   1. Hyperextension of the knee joint with drop foot deformity
   2. Internal rotation with abduction
   3. Flexion and adduction of the hip, with flexion of the knee
   4. External rotation with abduction
59. When Mrs. S is ready to walk with crutches, she will be taught
   1. Four-point crutch walking
   2. Two-point crutch walking
   3. Swing-through gait
   4. Three-point crutch walking
60. When teaching crutch walking, one instructs the patient to place her weight on
   1. The axillary region
   2. Palms of the hands and axillary region
   3. Palms of the hands
   4. Both extremities, with partial weight bearing
61. Aseptic necrosis of the head of the femur is a complication of fracture of the neck of the femur. It is caused by
   1. Wound infection
   2. Immobilization following reduction of the fracture
   3. Loss of blood supply to head of the femur
   4. Weight bearing before fracture is healed
62. Intramedullary nailing is used in the treatment of
   1. Fracture of the shaft of the femur
   2. Fracture of the neck of the femur
   3. Slipped epiphysis
   4. Intertrochanteric fracture of the femur

QUESTIONS FOR STUDY AND DISCUSSION

1. Differentiate between the various types of cerebral palsy.
2. Discuss the responsibility of the nurse pertaining to the care of a child with cerebral palsy from the standpoint of
   a. Speech therapy
   b. Nutritional and feeding problems
   c. Toilet training and self-help activities
   d. Play activities and selection of toys
   e. Education and vocational guidance
   f. Preoperative and postoperative nursing care
   g. Care of the child in braces
   h. Guidance of parents
3. Discuss the nursing care responsibilities for the child with spina bifida.
   a. Nutritional and feeding problems
   b. Toilet training and self-help activities
   c. Play activities and selection of toys
   d. Education and vocational guidance
   e. Preoperative and postoperative nursing care
   f. Care of the child in braces
   g. Guidance of parents
4. List danger signals that would indicate that a cast is interfering with the circulation of the involved extremity.
5. Discuss instructions to be given a mother pertaining to the care of a 9-month-old baby in a hip spica cast.
6. Discuss and demonstrate finishing of cast edges and methods of protecting a cast from urine.
7. Describe the nursing care you would provide for the elderly patient with fracture of the neck of the femur. Include possible complications and the nursing care necessary to prevent them.
8. Differentiate between atrophic, hypertrophic, and traumatic forms of arthritis.
9. Discuss the following as they relate to arthritis:
   a. Exercise, including range of motion
   b. Drug therapy
   c. Nursing measures to prevent deformity
   d. Surgical procedures for the arthritic patient
   e. Rehabilitation of the arthritic patient
10. Differentiate between skin and skeletal traction.
11. When caring for a patient in traction, list factors to be observed pertaining to
    a. Effectiveness of the traction
    b. Comfort and safety of the patient
    c. Prevention of secondary deformities
    d. Exercises
12. Describe the psychological mechanisms to be expected in a young adult with a sudden disabling injury. Compare these with the mechanisms operating in a middle-aged person with a slowly progressive disabling disease.
13. Persons with brain injury may have disturbances of perception. Perceptual disturbances may cause disruption in normal activities of

·daily living. Why? What can the nurse do to aid such patients?

14. Compare two male patients, 20 years of age, who have fresh spinal cord injuries—one with injury below C7, the other below T12. What functions can you expect each will be able to accomplish at the end of a year? What critical factors influence the eventual functional level attained? What differences can be expected in their nursing care requirements?

1	5
2	6
3	7
4	8

NAME _____ LAST _____ FIRST _____ MIDDLE _____ DATE _____

SCHOOL _____ CITY _____

DATE OF BIRTH _____

GRADE OR CLASS _____ INSTRUCTOR _____

NAME OF TEST _____

AGE _____ SEX _____ M OR F

PART _____

DIRECTIONS: Read each question and its numbered answers. When you have decided which answer is correct, blacken the corresponding space on this sheet with the special pencil. Make your mark as long as the pair of lines, and move the pencil point up and down firmly to make a heavy black line. If you change your mind, erase your first mark completely. Make no stray marks; they may count against you.

SAMPLE:

1—1 a country
1—2 a mountain
1—3 an island
1—4 a city
1—5 a state

1. Chicago is

BE SURE YOUR MARKS ARE HEAVY AND BLACK.
ERASE COMPLETELY ANY ANSWER YOU WISH TO CHANGE.

Questions 1–150 arranged in answer grid columns with choices 1 2 3 4 5.

1 2 3 4 5 · 31 · 61 · 91 · 121

Printed by the International Business Machines Corporation, Endicott, N. Y., U. S. A.

IBM FORM I. T. S. 1000 B 108